Section 1 Gene

Section 2 Perioperative Care and Anesthesia

Section 3 Otology and Neurotology

Section 4 Rhinology

Section 5 Laryngology and the Upper Aerodigestive Tract

Section 6 Head and Neck Surgery

Section 7 Endocrine Surgery in Otolaryngology

Section 8 Pediatric Otolaryngology

Section 9 Facial Plastic and Reconstructive Surgery

Appendices

Index

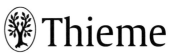

Handbook of Otolaryngology
Head and Neck Surgery
Second Edition

David Goldenberg, MD, FACS
The Steven and Sharon Baron Professor of Surgery
Professor of Surgery and Medicine
Chief, Division of Otolaryngology–Head and Neck Surgery
Milton S. Hershey Medical Center
The Pennsylvania State University College of Medicine
Hershey, Pennsylvania

Bradley J. Goldstein, MD, PhD, FACS
Associate Professor
Department of Otolaryngology, Graduate Program in Neuroscience, and
Interdisciplinary Stem Cell Institute
University of Miami Miller School of Medicine
Miami, Florida

164 illustrations

Thieme
New York • Stuttgart • Delhi • Rio de Janeiro

Executive Editor: Timothy Hiscock
Managing Editor: J. Owen Zurhellen IV
Director, Editorial Services: Mary Jo Casey
Developmental Editor: Judith Tomat
Production Editor: Kenny Chumbley
International Production Director: Andreas Schabert
Editorial Director: Sue Hodgson
International Marketing Director: Fiona Henderson
International Sales Director: Louisa Turrell
Director of Institutional Sales: Adam Bernacki
Senior Vice President and Chief Operating Officer: Sarah Vanderbilt
President: Brian D. Scanlan

Library of Congress Cataloging-in-Publication Data

Names: Goldenberg, David, 1962- editor. | Goldstein, Bradley J., editor.
Title: Handbook of otolaryngology : head and neck surgery / [edited by] David Goldenberg, Bradley J. Goldstein.
Other titles: Head and neck surgery
Description: Second edition. | New York : Thieme, [2018] | Includes bibliographical references and index.
Identifiers: LCCN 2017028786| ISBN 9781626234079 (pbk. : alk. paper) | ISBN 9781626234086 (e-book)
Subjects: | MESH: Head--surgery | Neck--surgery | Handbooks
Classification: LCC RF51 | NLM WE 39 | DDC 617.5/1059--dc23
LC record available at https://lccn.loc.gov/2017028786

© 2018 Thieme Medical Publishers, Inc.
Thieme Publishers New York
333 Seventh Avenue, New York, NY 10001 USA
+1 800 782 3488, customerservice@thieme.com

Thieme Publishers Stuttgart
Rüdigerstrasse 14, 70469 Stuttgart, Germany
+49 [0]711 8931 421, customerservice@thieme.de

Thieme Publishers Delhi
A-12, Second Floor, Sector-2, Noida-201301
Uttar Pradesh, India
+91 120 45 566 00, customerservice@thieme.in

Thieme Publishers Rio de Janeiro, Thieme Publicações Ltda.
Edifício Rodolpho de Paoli, 25º andar
Av. Nilo Peçanha, 50 – Sala 2508
Rio de Janeiro 20020-906, Brasil
+55 21 3172 2297

Cover design: Thieme Publishing Group
Typesetting by Prairie Papers

Printed in India by Replika Press Pvt. Ltd.   5 4 3 2 1

ISBN 978-1-62623-407-9

Also available as an eBook:
eISBN 978-1-62623-408-6

Important note: Medicine is an ever-changing science undergoing continual development. Research and clinical experience are continually expanding our knowledge, in particular our knowledge of proper treatment and drug therapy. Insofar as this book mentions any dosage or application, readers may rest assured that the authors, editors, and publishers have made every effort to ensure that such references are in accordance with **the state of knowledge at the time of production of the book.**

Nevertheless, this does not involve, imply, or express any guarantee or responsibility on the part of the publishers in respect to any dosage instructions and forms of applications stated in the book. **Every user is requested to examine carefully** the manufacturers' leaflets accompanying each drug and to check, if necessary in consultation with a physician or specialist, whether the dosage schedules mentioned therein or the contraindications stated by the manufacturers differ from the statements made in the present book. Such examination is particularly important with drugs that are either rarely used or have been newly released on the market. Every dosage schedule or every form of application used is entirely at the user's own risk and responsibility. The authors and publishers request every user to report to the publishers any discrepancies or inaccuracies noticed. If errors in this work are found after publication, errata will be posted at www.thieme.com on the product description page.

Some of the product names, patents, and registered designs referred to in this book are in fact registered trademarks or proprietary names even though specific reference to this fact is not always made in the text. Therefore, the appearance of a name without designation as proprietary is not to be construed as a representation by the publisher that it is in the public domain.

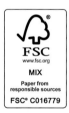

This book is dedicated in loving memory of our dear, sweet daughter Ellie
Goldenberg (ז״ל) 1994–2017

From the last song Ellie sang for us:

I am there in music
I am there in sky
I don't know why this thing did happen
But this much is clear
Anytime or anywhere
I am there

William Finn

—David Goldenberg, MD, FACS

To my wife, Liz, and to my children, Ben and Eva.

—Bradley J. Goldstein, MD, PhD, FACS

Contents

Foreword *by David W. Eisele*. xv
Preface xvii
Acknowledgments xix
Contributors xxi

Section 1	General Otolaryngology. 1
1.0	Approach to the Otolaryngology–Head and Neck Surgery Patient 3
1.1	Diagnostic Imaging of the Head and Neck. 6
1.2	Hematology for the Otolaryngologist. 13
1.3	Obstructive Sleep Apnea 20
1.4	Benign Oral and Odontogenic Disorders 25
1.5	Temporomandibular Joint Disorders .34
1.6	Geriatric Otolaryngology. 38
1.7	Lasers in Otolaryngology. 43
1.8	Complementary and Alternative Otolaryngologic Medicine 47

Section 2	Perioperative Care and Anesthesia for the Otolaryngology–Head and Neck Surgery Patient. . . .51
2.0	Preoperative Assessment. 53
2.1	Airway Assessment and Management 54
2.2	Anesthesia 70
2.2.1	Principles of Anesthesia 70
2.2.2	Regional Anesthesia Techniques 73
2.2.3	Anesthesia Drugs 76
2.2.4	Anesthetic Emergencies. 86
2.3	Fluids and Electrolytes 89
2.4	Common Postoperative Problems 91

Section 3	Otology and Neurotology 99
3.0	Embryology and Anatomy of the Ear 101
3.1	Otologic Emergencies 108
3.1.1	Sudden Hearing Loss. 108

3.1.2	Ear and Temporal Bone Trauma	110
3.1.3	Acute Facial Paresis and Paralysis	115
3.1.4	Ear Foreign Bodies	120
3.2	Otitis Media	122
3.2.1	Acute Otitis Media	122
3.2.2	Chronic Otitis Media	126
3.2.3	Complications of Acute and Chronic Otitis Media	132
3.2.4	Cholesteatoma	140
3.3	Otitis Externa	145
3.3.1	Uncomplicated Otitis Externa	145
3.3.2	Malignant Otitis Externa	149
3.4	Audiology	154
3.4.1	Basic Audiologic Assessments	154
3.4.2	Pediatric Audiologic Assessments	159
3.4.3	Objective/Electrophysiologic Audiologic Assessments	163
3.5	Hearing Loss	165
3.5.1	Conductive Hearing Loss	165
3.5.2	Sensorineural Hearing Loss	169
3.5.3	Hearing Aids	174
3.5.4	Cochlear Implants	177
3.5.5	Other Implantable Hearing Devices	180
3.6	Vertigo	182
3.6.1	Balance Assessment	182
3.6.2	Benign Paroxysmal Positional Vertigo	186
3.6.3	Ménière's Disease	190
3.6.4	Vestibular Neuritis	193
3.6.5	Migraine-Associated Vertigo	196
3.7	Tinnitus	200
3.8	Cerebellopontine Angle Tumors	203
3.9	Superior Semicircular Canal Dehiscence Syndrome	210
3.10	Otologic Manifestations of Systemic Diseases	213
Section 4	**Rhinology**	**219**
4.0	Anatomy and Physiology of the Nose and Paranasal Sinuses	221
4.1	Rhinologic Emergencies	224
4.1.1	Acute Invasive Fungal Rhinosinusitis	224
4.1.2	Orbital Complications of Sinusitis	228
4.1.3	Intracranial Complications of Sinusitis	230
4.1.4	Cerebrospinal Fluid Rhinorrhea	233
4.1.5	Epistaxis	237
4.2	Rhinosinusitis	241
4.2.1	Acute Rhinosinusitis	241
4.2.2	Chronic Rhinosinusitis	244
4.3	Rhinitis	250
4.3.1	Nonallergic Rhinitis	250
4.3.2	Allergy	253
4.4	Inverted Papillomas	256
4.5	Anosmia and Other Olfactory Disorders	260

| 4.6 | Taste Disorders | 262 |
| 4.7 | Rhinologic Manifestations of Systemic Diseases | 264 |

Section 5	**Laryngology and the Upper Aerodigestive Tract**	**269**
5.0	Anatomy and Physiology of the Upper Aerodigestive Tract	271
5.1	Laryngeal and Esophageal Emergencies	277
5.1.1	Stridor	277
5.1.2	Laryngeal Fractures	280
5.1.3	Caustic Ingestion	282
5.1.4	Laryngeal Infections	285
5.2	Neurolaryngology	289
5.3	Voice Disorders	295
5.3.1	Papillomatosis	295
5.3.2	Vocal Fold Cysts, Nodules, and Polyps	298
5.3.3	Vocal Fold Motion Impairment	300
5.3.4	Voice Rehabilitation	303
5.4	Swallowing Disorders	307
5.4.1	Zenker's Diverticulum	307
5.4.2	Dysphagia	310
5.4.3	Aspiration	313
5.5	Acid Reflux Disorders	318
5.6	Laryngeal Manifestations of Systemic Diseases	321

Section 6	**Head and Neck Surgery**	**325**
6.0	Anatomy of the Neck	327
6.1	Neck Emergencies	330
6.1.1	Necrotizing Soft Tissue Infections of the Head and Neck	330
6.1.2	Ludwig's Angina	332
6.1.3	Deep Neck Infections	334
6.1.4	Neck Trauma	337
6.2	Approach to Neck Masses	342
6.3	Head and Neck Cancer	346
6.3.1	Chemotherapy for Head and Neck Cancer	352
6.3.2	Radiotherapy for Head and Neck Cancer	356
6.3.3	Sinonasal Cancer	360
6.3.4	Nasopharyngeal Cancer	365
6.3.5	Oral Cavity Cancer	370
6.3.6	Oropharyngeal Cancer	378
6.3.7	Human Papillomavirus and Head and Neck Cancer	382
6.3.8	Cancer of Unknown Primary	385
6.3.9	Hypopharyngeal Cancer	388
6.3.10	Laryngeal Cancer	392
6.3.11	Speech Options after Laryngectomy	401
6.3.12	Referred Otalgia in Head and Neck Disease	403
6.3.13	Neck Dissection	406
6.3.14	Robotic-Assisted Head and Neck Surgery	409
6.3.15	Skin Cancer of the Head, Face, and Neck	412
6.3.15.1	Basal Cell Carcinoma	412

6.3.15.2	Cutaneous Squamous Cell Carcinoma	417
6.3.15.3	Melanomas of the Head, Face, and Neck	423
6.3.16	Malignant Neoplasms of the Ear and Temporal Bone	430
6.3.17	Lymphomas of the Head and Neck	434
6.3.18	Idiopathic Midline Destructive Disease	440
6.3.19	Paragangliomas of the Head and Neck	442
6.3.20	Peripheral Nerve Sheath Tumors	445
6.4	The Salivary Glands	447
6.4.0	Embryology and Anatomy of the Salivary Glands	447
6.4.1	Salivary Gland Disease	452
6.4.2	Benign Salivary Gland Tumors	456
6.4.3	Malignant Salivary Gland Tumors	460
6.4.4	Sialendoscopy	466

Section 7	**Endocrine Surgery in Otolaryngology**	**469**
7.0	Embryology and Anatomy of the Thyroid Gland	471
7.1	Physiology of the Thyroid Gland	473
7.2	Thyroid Evaluation	475
7.3	Thyroid Nodules and Cysts	479
7.4	Hyperthyroidism	483
7.5	Hypothyroidism	487
7.6	Thyroid Storm	491
7.7	Thyroiditis	492
7.8	Thyroid Cancer	496
7.9	Embryology, Anatomy, and Physiology of the Parathyroid Glands	509
7.10	Hyperparathyroidism	512
7.11	Hypoparathyroidism	517
7.12	Calcium Disorders	518

Section 8	**Pediatric Otolaryngology**	**523**
8.1	Pediatric Airway Evaluation and Management	525
8.2	Laryngomalacia	529
8.3	Bilateral Vocal Fold Paralysis	531
8.4	Laryngeal Clefts	534
8.5	Tracheoesophageal Fistula and Esophageal Atresia	537
8.6	Vascular Rings	541
8.7	Subglottic Stenosis	545
8.8	Pierre Robin's Sequence	549
8.9	Genetics and Syndromes	552
8.10	Diseases of the Adenoids and Palatine Tonsils	560
8.10.1	Adenotonsillitis	560
8.10.2	Adenotonsillar Hypertrophy	563
8.11	Congenital Nasal Obstruction	567
8.12	Pediatric Hearing Loss	571
8.13	Infectious Neck Masses in Children	582
8.14	Hemangiomas, Vascular Malformations, and Lymphatic Malformations of the Head and Neck	586
8.15	Branchial Cleft Cysts	589
8.16	Congenital Midline Neck Masses	593

8.17	Congenital Midline Nasal Masses	596
8.18	Choanal Atresia	599
8.19	Cleft Lip and Palate	601

Section 9	**Facial Plastic and Reconstructive Surgery**	**609**
9.1	Craniomaxillofacial Trauma	611
9.1.1	Nasal Fractures	611
9.1.2	Naso-Orbito-Ethmoid Fractures	614
9.1.3	Zygomaticomaxillary and Orbital Fractures	618
9.1.4	Frontal Sinus Fractures	621
9.1.5	Midface Fractures	624
9.1.6	Mandible Fractures	628
9.1.7	Burns of the Head, Face, and Neck	634
9.2	Facial Paralysis, Facial Reanimation, and Eye Care	639
9.3	Facial Reconstruction	648
9.3.1	Skin Grafts	648
9.3.2	Local Cutaneous Flaps for Facial Reconstruction	651
9.3.3	Microvascular Free Tissue Transfer	657
9.3.4	Bone and Cartilage Grafts	661
9.3.5	Incision Planning and Scar Revision	665
9.4	Cosmetic Surgery	669
9.4.1	Neurotoxins, Fillers, and Implants	669
9.4.2	Rhytidectomy	674
9.4.3	Brow and Forehead Lifting	677
9.4.4	Chemical Peels and Laser Skin Resurfacing	682
9.4.5	Blepharoplasty	687
9.4.6	Otoplasty	692
9.4.7	Rhinoplasty	695
9.4.8	Deviated Septum and Septoplasty	700
9.4.9	Liposuction of the Head, Face, and Neck	703
9.4.10	Hair Restoration	705

Appendix A	**Basic Procedures and Methods of Investigation**	**711**
A1	Bronchoscopy	711
A2	Esophagoscopy	712
A3	Rigid Direct Microscopic Laryngoscopy with or without Biopsy	713
A4	Tonsillectomy	715
A5	Adenoidectomy	716
A6	Open Surgical Tracheotomy	717
A7	Cricothyroidotomy	718

Appendix B	**The Cranial Nerves**	**721**

Appendix C	**ENT Emergencies Requiring Immediate Diagnostic and/or Therapeutic Intervention**	**733**

Index		**735**

Foreword

With this second edition of this popular clinical reference textbook, edited by Dr. David Goldenberg and Dr. Bradley Goldstein, two outstanding clinicians and educators, the reader has available, in one succinct text, a wealth of information spanning the breadth of the specialty of otolaryngology–head and neck surgery. This makes this text a valuable resource not only for medical students, residents, and fellows, but also active practitioners.

The book's content has been updated with the second edition, ensuring up-to-date clinical information. Each section has an editor and multiple expert content contributors. Chapters are organized within subspecialty sections around specific clinical scenarios using a uniform-content format. In each chapter, key features of the specific disorder are highlighted, followed by epidemiology, clinical presentation, evaluation, therapeutic options, and follow-up.

Dr. Goldenberg and Dr. Goldstein continue their success with the second edition of this popular text, which is a beneficial trove of clinical information for students, specialty trainees, and established practitioners alike.

David W. Eisele, MD, FACS
Andelot Professor and Director
Department of Otolaryngology–
Head and Neck Surgery
Johns Hopkins University School of Medicine
Baltimore, Maryland

Preface

The vision for *Handbook of Otolaryngology–Head and Neck Surgery* arose when, several years ago, the editors felt that a truly practical clinical guide of sufficient quality was lacking. In an effort to fill this void, the first edition was designed to present key information in a highly organized format, covering the broad spectrum of otolaryngology subjects. From the start, this product was intended to be most useful as a clinical handbook, especially for students, residents, or other clinicians seeking rapid and reliable guidance relating to clinical care.

In the six years since the first edition was published, our specialty has witnessed continual expansion and innovation. Accordingly, the second edition builds upon the original 160 chapters to incorporate necessary changes. Without increasing the overall size of the book, we have sought to update existing chapters, combine redundant subjects, reorganize certain topics more logically, and include entirely new subjects where necessary. Whenever available, we have incorporated accepted evidence-based guidelines or recommendations.

We are grateful to all of our original contributors who helped develop the first edition content. The second edition acknowledges the new section editors who have worked to update and revise our original material. Readers will notice that references were removed, as their value in a clinical handbook is limited, while precious page space is consumed. Similarly, diagnosis-code information was eliminated, since we now have a vastly expanded ICD10 system, which is difficult to list efficiently.

We are thankful to all of those who have used our handbook, and we hope that this second edition will serve its readers well. As always, we are especially grateful to students who continue to challenge and teach us and who are our future.

"It goes without saying that no man can teach successfully who is not at the same time a student." —Sir William Osler

David Goldenberg, MD, FACS
Bradley J. Goldstein, MD, PhD, FACS

Acknowledgments

The contributing authors are true experts in the topics at hand and have put forth great effort into preparing exceptional sections and chapters that are informative, readable, and concise. We would like to thank them for their willingness to participate. Also, we thank the people who provided us with our training—faculty, fellow residents, and patients.

The thirteen chapters of this book that include cancer staging information have been thoroughly updated with data from Amin MB, Edge S, Greene F, et al, eds. *AJCC Cancer Staging Manual 8th Edition* (Springer, 2017), with the kind permission of the American Joint Committee on Cancer and of Springer.

Contributors

Eelam A. Adil, MD, MBA, FAAP
Assistant Professor of Otology and
    Laryngology
Harvard Medical School
Boston, Massachusetts
**6.3.3–6.3.10, 6.3.12, 6.3.13,
    6.3.15–6.3.20, 8.13**

Benjamin F. Asher, MD, FACS
Asher Integrative Otolaryngology
New York, New York
1.8

Daniel G. Becker, MD, FACS
Clinical Professor
Department of Otolaryngology
University of Pennsylvania
Philadelphia, Pennsylvania
9.4.7

Paul J. Carniol, MD
Clinical Professor and Director of
    Facial Plastic Surgery
Rutgers New Jersey Medical
    School–UMDNJ
Summit, New Jersey
1.7

**Michele M. Carr, MD, DDS, PhD,
FRCSC**
Professor
Division of Otolaryngology–Head
    and Neck Surgery
West Virginia University
Morgantown, West Virginia
Section Editor: Pediatric, 6.4.4

Ara A. Chalian, MD
Professor of Otorhinoaryngology–
    Head and Neck Surgery
The University of Pennsylvania
    Hospital
Philadelphia, Pennsylvania
9.3.3

Donn R. Chatham, MD
Clinical Instructor
Department of Otolaryngology
University of Louisville Medical
    College
Chatham Facial Plastic Surgery
Louisville, Kentucky
9.4.9

Gregory L. Craft, MD
Oregon Anesthesiology Group
Salem Hospital
Salem, Oregon
2.2

David Culang, MD
Otolaryngologist
Department of Otolaryngology
Beth Israel Medical Center
New York, New York
8.14

Sharon L. Cushing, MD, MSc, FRCSC
Assistant Professor
Department of Otolaryngology–
  Head and Neck Surgery
University of Toronto
Hospital for Sick Children
Toronto, Ontario, Canada
8.9, 8.10, 8.12, 8.19

Christine T. Dinh, MD
Assistant Professor of
  Otolaryngology
Otology, Neurotology, and Skull
  Base Surgery
University of Miami Miller School
  of Medicine
Miami, Florida
**Section Editor: Otology and
  Neurotology**

Carole Fakhry, MD, MPH
Associate Professor
Department of Otolaryngology–
  Head and Neck Surgery
The Johns Hopkins University
Baltimore, Maryland
8.2, 8.4

Renee Flax-Goldenberg, MD
Assistant Professor
Department of Radiology
The Pennsylvania State University
  College of Medicine
Hershey, Pennsylvania
1.1

John L. Frodel Jr., MD
Director, Facial Plastic Surgery
Department of Otolaryngology–
  Head and Neck Surgery
Geisinger Medical Center
Danville, Pennsylvania
Atlanta Medical Day Spa and
  Surgicenter
Atlanta and Marietta, Georgia
9.3.4

David Goldenberg, MD, FACS
The Steven and Sharon Baron
  Professor of Surgery
Professor of Surgery and Medicine
Chief, Division of Otolaryngology–
  Head and Neck Surgery
Milton S. Hershey Medical Center
The Pennsylvania State University
  College of Medicine
Hershey, Pennsylvania
Chief Editor

Bradley J. Goldstein, MD, PhD, FACS
Associate Professor
Department of Otolaryngology,
  Graduate Program in Neuroscience,
  and Interdisciplinary Stem Cell
  Institute
University of Miami Miller School
  of Medicine
Miami, Florida
Chief Editor

**Jerome C. Goldstein, MD, FACS,
FRCSEd**
Past Chair, Otolaryngology
Albany Medical College
Albany, New York
Past Executive Vice President
American Academy of
  Otolaryngology–Head and Neck
  Surgery
Wellington, Florida
1.8.5

Neerav Goyal, MD, MPH
Director of Head and Neck Surgery
Assistant Professor of Surgery
Division of Otolaryngology–Head
  and Neck Surgery
Milton S. Hershey Medical Center
The Pennsylvania State University
  College of Medicine
Hershey, Pennsylvania
**Section Editor: Head and
  Neck, Endocrine Surgery in
  Otolaryngology**

Colin Huntley, MD
Assistant Professor of
  Otolaryngology–Head and Neck
  Surgery
Thomas Jefferson University
Philadelphia, Pennsylvania
8.15, 8.16

Jon E. Isaacson, MD
Associated Otolaryngology of
  Pennsylvania
Camp Hill, Pennsylvania
**3.0, 3.1.1, 3.1.4, 3.2.1, 3.2.2, 3.3.1,
  3.3.2, 3.5.5**

Robert M. Kellman, MD, FACS
Professor and Chair
Department of Otolaryngology and
  Communication Sciences
SUNY Upstate Medical University
Syracuse, New York
9.1.6

Ayesha N. Khalid, MD, MBA
Clinical Instructor
Harvard Medical School
Adjunct Lecturer
Harvard–MIT HST Program
Boston, Massachusetts
9.4.5

Christopher K. Kolstad, MD
Kolstad Facial Plastic Surgery
La Jolla, California
8.19, 9.4.3

Theda C. Kontis, MD, FACS
Assistant Professor
Department of Otolaryngology–
  Head and Neck Surgery
The Johns Hopkins University
Facial Plastic Surgicenter Ltd
Baltimore, Maryland
9.4.1

Melissa M. Krempasky, MS, CCC-ALP
Scottsdale, Arizona
5.3.4, 6.3.11

J. David Kriet, MD, FACS
Professor
The W. S. and E. C. Jones Chair in
  Craniofacial Reconstruction
Department of Otolaryngology–
  Head and Neck Surgery
University of Kansas School of
  Medicine
Kansas City, Kansas
9.1.5

Devyani Lal, MD, FARS
Associate Professor and Consultant
Endoscopic Sinus and Skull Base
  Surgery
Otolaryngology–Head and Neck
  Surgery
Mayo Clinic
Phoenix, Arizona
4.3.1

Phillip R. Langsdon, MD, FACS
Professor
University of Tennessee
Memphis, Tennessee
Chief of Facial Plastic Surgery and
  Director
The Langsdon Clinic
Germantown, Tennessee
9.4.4

Gregory T. Lesnik, MD
Otolaryngologist
William W. Backus Hospital
Norwich, Connecticut
3.6.4

Adam J. Levy, MD
Head and Neck Cosmetic Surgeon
    Associates LLC
The Advanced Center for Specialty
    Care
Chicago, Illinois
3.6.5, 3.10

Jessyka G. Lighthall, MD
Assistant Professor
Division of Otolaryngology–Head
    and Neck Surgery
Milton S. Hershey Medical Center
The Pennsylvania State University
    College of Medicine
Hershey, Pennsylvania
Section Editor: Facial Plastic

Heath B. Mackley, MD, FACRO
Professor of Radiology, Medicine,
    and Pediatrics
Penn State Hershey Cancer Institute
Milton S. Hershey Medical Center
The Pennsylvania State University
    College of Medicine
Hershey, Pennsylvania
6.3.1, 6.3.2

E. Gaylon McCollough, MD, FACS
Clinical Professor of Facial Plastic
    Surgery
University of South Alabama
    Medical School
Mobile, Alabama
President and CEO, McCollough
    Plastic Surgery Clinic
Founder, McCollough Institute for
    Appearance and Health
Gulf Shores, Alabama
9.4.2

Johnathan D. McGinn, MD, FACS
Associate Professor
Division of Otolaryngology–Head
    and Neck Surgery
Milton S. Hershey Medical Center
The Pennsylvania State University
    College of Medicine
Hershey, Pennsylvania
**Section Editor: General
    Otolaryngology; Laryngology and
    the Upper Aerodigestive Tract**

Elias M. Michaelides, MD
Director, Yale Hearing and Balance
    Center
Associate Professor of
    Surgery–Otolaryngology
Yale School of Medicine
New Haven, Connecticut
**3.5.1, 3.5.2, 3.5.4, 3.6.2–3.6.5,
    3.7–3.10**

Ron Mitzner, MD
ENT and Allergy Associates LLP
Lake Success, New York
2.4

Kari Morgenstein, AuD, FAAA
Assistant Professor
Director, Children's Hearing
    Program
Department of Otolaryngology
University of Miami Miller School
    of Medicine
Miami, Florida
3.4

Michael P. Ondik, MD
Montgomery County ENT Institute
Elkins Park, Pennsylvania
8.18, 9.1.1

Stuart A. Ort, MD
ENT and Allergy Associates
Old Bridge, New Jersey
3.1.2, 3.1.3, 3.2.3

Stephen S. Park, MD
Professor and Vice Chair
Department of Otolaryngology–
Head and Neck Surgery
Director, Division of Facial Plastic
Surgery
University of Virginia
Charlottesville, Virginia
9.3.2

Vijay Patel, MD
Division of Otolaryngology–Head
and Neck Surgery
Milton S. Hershey Medical Center
The Pennsylvania State University
College of Medicine
Hershey, Pennsylvania
8.11

**Wayne Pearce, BTh, MBBCh,
MMed(Anes), FCA(CMSA)**
Assistant Professor
Department of Anesthesiology and
Perioperative Medicine
The Pennsylvania State University
College of Medicine
Hershey, Pennsylvania
**Section Editor: Perioperative Care
and Anesthesia**

Sarah E. Pesek, MD
St. Peters Health Partners Medical
Associates
Albany, New York
8.5, 8.6

Daniel I. Plosky, MD, FACS
Ear, Nose, and Throat Surgeons of
Western New England LLC
Springfield, Massachusetts
3.7

Rafael Antonio Portela, MD
Portela ENT
Nicklaus Children's Hospital
Miami, Florida
2.4

Julie A. Rhoades, AuD, CNIM
Audiologist/Neurophysiologist
NuVasive Clinical Services
Hershey, Pennsylvania
3.4.1, 3.4.3, 3.5.3, 3.6.1

Christopher A. Roberts, MD
Department of Otolaryngology–
Head and Neck Surgery
West Virginia University
Morgantown, West Virginia
8.14

Francis P. Ruggiero, MD
ENT Head and Neck Surgery of
Lancaster
Lancaster, Pennsylvania
6.3.19, 6.3.20, 9.3.1

John M. Schweinfurth, MD
Professor of Otolaryngology
University of Mississippi Medical
Center
Jackson, Mississippi
9.3.5

Dhave Setabutr, MD
Assistant Professor
Hofstra University/Northwell Health
Cohen's Children's Hospital
New Hyde Park, New York
9.1.4

Sohrab Sohrabi, MD
VA Central California Health Care
System
Fresno, California
6.3.15.1, 6.3.15.2, 6.3.15.3, 8.1

Scott J. Stephan, MD
Assistant Professor
Facial Plastic and Reconstructive
Surgery
Otolaryngology–Head and Neck
Surgery
Vanderbilt University Medical Center
Nashville, Tennessee
9.3.2

Jonathan M. Sykes, MD, FACS
Director of Facial Plastic and
    Reconstructive Surgery
Professor
Department of Otolaryngology–
    Head and Neck Surgery
University of California Davis
    Medical Center
Sacramento, California
8.19, 9.4.3

Travis T. Tollefson, MD, MPH, FACS
Professor and Director
Facial Plastic and Reconstructive
    Surgery
Department of Otolaryngology–
    Head and Neck Surgery
University of California Davis
    School of Medicine
Sacramento, California
9.1.3

Robin Unger, MD
Assistant Professor
Department of Dermatology
Icahn School of Medicine at Mount
    Sinai
New York, New York
9.4.10

Jeremy Watkins, MD
Fort Worth ENT
Fort Worth, Texas
9.4.4

1 General Otolaryngology

Section Editor

Johnathan D. McGinn

Contributors

Benjamin F. Asher

Paul J. Carniol

Renee Flax-Goldenberg

David Goldenberg

Bradley J. Goldstein

Jerome C. Goldstein

Johnathan D. McGinn

1.0 Approach to the Otolaryngology–Head and Neck Surgery Patient

This book is organized into brief chapters addressing specific clinical entities. To enable readers to focus readily on their information needs, the chapters are arranged in a similar manner:

- Key Features
- Epidemiology
- Clinical
  - Signs and symptoms
  - Differential diagnosis
- Evaluation, including history, exam, imaging, and other testing
- Treatment options, including medical and surgical treatments
- Follow-up care

This first chapter is an exception because it deals entirely with the evaluation step. Specifically, we review in detail the approach to an efficient and effective otolaryngology patient history and physical examination, which should be especially useful to those new to the care of such patients.

◆ History

The generally accepted organization of the history and physical examination for a new patient is outlined in **Table 1.1**.

The History of Present Illness is the subjective narrative regarding the current problem. It should include a focused summary of the complaint, including location, time of onset, course, quality, severity, duration, associated problems, and previous testing or treatment.

◆ Physical Exam

The physical examination in otolaryngology is typically a complete head and neck exam. This should include an evaluation of the following:

General

- The general appearance of the patient (i.e., well- or ill-appearing, acute distress)
- Vital signs (temperature, heart rate, blood pressure, respiratory rate, weight, possibly BMI)
- Stridor, abnormal respiratory effort/increased work of breathing

Head

- Normocephalic, evidence of trauma
- Description of any cutaneous lesions of the head and neck

Ear

- Pinnae, ear canals, tympanic membranes, including mobility
- 512-Hz tuning fork testing (Weber, Rinne)

Nose

- External nasal deformities
- Anterior rhinoscopy noting edema, masses, mucus, purulence, septal deviation, perforation

Oral Cavity/Oropharynx

- Noting any masses, mucosal lesions, asymmetries, condition of dentition, presence/absence of tonsils and appearance
- Consider palpation of floor of mouth and base of tongue
- Hypopharynx and larynx
- Presence of hoarseness or phonatory abnormality
- Direct fiber optic or indirect mirror exam of the nasopharynx, hypopharynx, and larynx
- Laryngeal exam should note vocal fold mobility, mucosal lesions, and masses as well as assess the base of the tongue, valleculae, epiglottis, vocal folds, and piriform sinuses

Neck

- Inspection and palpation of the parotid and submandibular glands
- Inspection and palpation of the neck for adenopathy or masses
- Inspection and palpation of the thyroid gland for enlargement or masses
- Cranial nerve function

Other, more specialized aspects of an examination are discussed in the various sections that follow, such as vertigo assessment and nasal endoscopy.

◆ Endoscopic Exam

If the mirror examination does not provide an adequate assessment of the nasopharynx, hypopharynx, or larynx, a flexible fiberoptic nasolaryngoscopy is performed. Usually, the nose is decongested with oxymetazoline (Afrin, Schering-Plough Healthcare Products Inc., Memphis, TN) or phenylephrine (Neo-Synephrine, Bayer Consumer Health, Morristown, NJ) spray. Topical Pontocaine or lidocaine spray may be added for anesthetic. Surgilube jelly (E. Fougera & Co., Melville, NY) is helpful to reduce irritation. Antifog is applied to the tip of the flexible laryngoscope. The patient is best examined sitting upright. The tip of the scope is inserted into the nostril and under direct vision is advanced inferiorly along the floor of the nose into the nasopharynx. If septal spurring or other intranasal deformities prevent advancement of the scope, the other nostril may be used. The nasopharynx is assessed for masses or asymmetry, adenoid hypertrophy, and infection. In the sleep apnea patient, the presence of anteroposterior (AP) or lateral collapse of the retropalatal region is remarked. The scope is then guided inferiorly to examine the base of the tongue, valleculae, epiglottis, piriform sinuses (piriform fossae), arytenoids, and vocal folds. Again, mucosal lesions, masses, asymmetries, and vocal fold mobility are noted. Asking the patient to cough, sniff, and phonate will reveal vocal fold motion abnormalities. The piriform sinuses may be better visualized if the patient puffs out the cheeks (exhalation with closed lips and palate).

◆ Other Tests

Often, laboratory studies, audiograms, or imaging studies are reviewed. These are summarized in the note after the physical exam section. Whenever possible, radiology images (CT, MRI) should be personally reviewed to confirm that one agrees with the reports.

◆ Impression and Plan

In the documentation of the patient's visit, the note concludes with an impression and plan. Generally, a concise differential diagnosis is given, listing the entities that are considered most relevant. A plan is then discussed, including further tests to confirm or exclude possible diagnoses as well as medical or surgical treatments that will be instituted or considered. Timing of a return or follow-up visit, if needed, is noted.

A copy of one's note, or a separate letter, should always be sent to referring physicians.

Table 1.1   Organization of the history and physical exam for a new patient

Chief complaint
History of present illness
Past medical history
Past surgical history
Current medications
Medication allergies
Social history
Family history
Review of systems
Physical examination
Laboratory testing/imaging
Impression
Plan

1.1 Diagnostic Imaging of the Head and Neck

Many of the structures of the head and neck are deep and inaccessible to direct visualization, palpation, or inspection. Therefore, valuable information may be obtained by the use of various radiographic techniques. Advances in technology have supplemented simple X-ray procedures with computed tomography (CT), magnetic resonance imaging (MRI), ultrasound, and positron emission tomography (PET). Other imaging modalities are used for specific conditions, such as angiography for vascular lesions or barium swallow cinefluoroscopy for swallowing evaluations.

◆ Computed Tomography

A contrast-enhanced CT scan is typically the first imaging technique used to evaluate many ear, nose, throat, and head and neck pathologies. The CT scan is an excellent method for the staging of tumors and identifying lymphadenopathy. A high-resolution CT scan may be used in cases of trauma to the head, neck, laryngeal structures, facial bones, and temporal bone. Temporal bone CT is used to assess middle ear and mastoid disease; paranasal sinus CT is the gold standard test for assessing for the presence and extent of rhinosinusitis and many of its complications. A CT scan is superior to MRI in evaluating bony cortex erosion from tumor. A CT scan is also widely used for posttreatment surveillance of head and neck cancer patients.

Working Principle of CT

In CT, the X-ray tube revolves around the craniocaudal axis of the patient. A beam of X-rays passes through the body and hits a ring of detectors. The incoming radiation is continuously registered, and the signal is digitized and fed into a data matrix, taking into account the varying beam angulations. The data matrix can then be transformed into an output image (**Fig. 1.1**). The result is usually displayed in "slices" cross-sectionally. Different tissues attenuate radiation to varying degrees, allowing for the differentiation of tissue subtypes (**Table 1.2**). This absorption is measured in Hounsfield units. When one views an image, two values are displayed with the image: Window and Level. The Window refers to the range of Hounsfield units displayed across the spectrum from black (low) through the grayscale to white (high). Level refers to the Hounsfield unit on which middle gray is centered. By adjusting the window and level, certain features of the image can be better assessed or emphasized.

Recent advances have improved the quality of CT imaging. Multidetector scanners have several rows of photoreceptors, enabling the simultaneous acquisition of several slices. Helical techniques allow the patient table to move continuously through the scanner instead of stopping for each slice. These advances have significantly decreased scan times and radiation exposure while improving spatial resolution. Improved resolution and computing power enable cross-sectional images to be reformatted into any plane (axial, coronal, sagittal), as well as three-dimensional anatomy or subtraction images to be displayed when necessary or helpful (e.g., three-dimensional reconstruction of airways). Newer in-office flat-plate cone-beam scanners

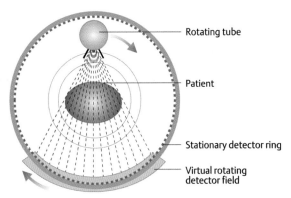

Rotating tube

Patient

Stationary detector ring

Virtual rotating detector field

Fig. 1.1 Working principle of computed tomography. The X-ray tube revolves continuously around the longitudinal axis of the patient. A rotating curved detector field opposite to the tube registers the attenuated fan beam after it has passed through the patient. Taking into account the tube position at each time point of measurement, the resulting attenuation values are fed into a data matrix and further computed to create an image. (Used with permission from Eastman GW, Wald C, Crossin J. *Getting Started in Clinical Radiology: From Image to Diagnosis*. New York: Thieme; 2006:9.)

Table 1.2   Attenuation of different body components

Body Component	Hounsfield Units (HU)
Bone	1000–2000
Thrombus	60–100
Liver	50–70
Spleen	40–50
Kidney	25–45
White brain matter	20–35
Gray brain matter	35–45
Water	–5 to 5
Fat	–100 to –25
Lung	–1000 to –400

Data from Eastman GW, Wald C, Crossin J. *Getting Started in Clinical Radiology: From Image to Diagnosis*. Stuttgart/New York: Thieme; 2006.

can rapidly acquire 1-mm slice thickness images of the sinuses and temporal bone with very low radiation exposure.

Contrast Media

Intravenous contrast media are used in CT to visualize vessels and the vascularization of different organ systems. This allows better differentiation of vessels versus other structures. Some tissues also take up greater amounts of contrast natively, as well as in certain disease states (e.g., infection, neoplasm, edema). Luminal contrast material containing iodine or barium can also be used in some structures (e.g., gastrointestinal tract) to clarify anatomy.

Computer-Assisted Surgical Navigation

CT scanning data can be utilized for computer-assisted surgical navigation. There are several systems in use. The axial CT image data, acquired at 1-mm slice thickness or less, are loaded onto the image guidance system in the operating room. The system utilizes the CT data and compares them to the patient's facial features or landmarks via an infrared camera or electromagnetic field disturbance to determine point location in three-dimensional space. Various surgical instruments can be registered and detected. The location of an instrument tip is then displayed on the previous CT images in three planes. This is most often used in sinus and skull base surgery.

◆ Magnetic Resonance Imaging

MRI provides the physician with high-definition imaging of soft tissue without exposing the patient to ionizing radiation. MRI is useful for detecting mucosal tumors, neoplastic invasion of bone marrow, and, at times, perineural invasion of large nerves. MRI is valuable in assessing intracranial extension of tumors of the head and neck. Gadolinium-enhanced MRI of the brain with attention to the internal auditory canal is the gold standard test for diagnosis of vestibular schwannoma or meningioma, easily identifiable on postcontrast T1-weighted images. The disadvantages of MRI include limited definition of bony detail and cost. Magnetic resonance angiography (MRA) is a useful modality for imaging vascular anatomy or vascular pathology without the intravascular infusion of iodine contrast medium, which is used in traditional angiography with X-ray fluoroscopy.

Working Principle of MRI

MRI is a technique that produces cross-sectional images in any plane without the use of ionizing radiation. MR images are obtained by the interaction of hydrogen nuclei (protons), high magnetic fields, and radiofrequency pulses. This is done by placing the patient in a strong magnetic field, which initially aligns the hydrogen nuclei in similar directions. The intensity of the MRI signal that is converted to imaging data depends on the density of the hydrogen nuclei in the examined tissue (i.e., mucosa, fat, bone) and on two magnetic relaxation times (**Table 1.3**). MRI imaging is more time-intensive to perform and thus more vulnerable to motion

Table 1.3   Definitions of terms used in magnetic resonance imaging

TR	Time to repetition
TE	Time to echo
Ti	Time to inversion
T1	Time to magnetize (regrowth); also known as spin lattice relaxation time
T2	Time to demagnetize (DK); also known as spin relaxation time

artifact, as the patient must remain still for minutes (versus seconds in CT imaging).

Contraindications to MRI

- Implanted neural stimulators, cochlear implants, and cardiac pacemakers (MRI may cause temporary or permanent malfunction)
- Ferromagnetic aneurysm clips or other foreign bodies with a large component of iron or cobalt, which may move within the body or heat up in the MRI scanner
- Metallic fragments within the eye (e.g., may be seen in patients who weld or grind metals)
- Placement of a vascular stent, coil, or filter in the past 6 weeks
- Ferromagnetic shrapnel
- Relative contraindications include claustrophobic patients, critically ill patients, morbidly obese patients who cannot physically fit in the MRI scanner, and those having metal implants in the region of interest and possibly tattoos with ferromagnetic ink.

◆ Ultrasound

Ultrasound or ultrasonography is an inexpensive and safe method of gaining real-time images of structures of the head and neck. Neck masses can be assessed for size, morphologic character (i.e., solid, cystic, or combined solid and cystic, also known as complex), and association with adjacent structures. Vascularity may also be assessed. High-resolution ultrasound is used for head and neck anomalies such as thyroglossal duct cysts, branchial cleft cyst, cystic hygromas, salivary gland masses, abscesses, carotid body and vascular tumors, and thyroid masses. There is growing emphasis on using ultrasound, when possible, in pediatric patients to reduce the use of ionizing radiation from CT imaging.

Ultrasound, combined with fine-needle aspiration biopsy (FNAB) and cytology, is helpful both in providing a visual description and as an aid for specific localization sampling of a mass for cytologic evaluation. Until recently, ultrasounds were performed mainly by radiologists. However, many otolaryngologists are now performing their own in-office ultrasounds and ultrasound-guided FNABs.

Working Principle of Ultrasound

An alternating electric current is sent through a piezoelectric crystal; the crystal vibrates with the frequency of the current, producing sound waves of that frequency. In medical ultrasound, typical frequencies vary between 1 and 15 MHz. Ultrasound gel acoustically couples the ultrasound transducer to the body, where the ultrasound waves can then spread. Inside the body the sound is absorbed, scattered, or reflected. Fluid-filled (cystic) structures appear dark and show acoustic enhancement behind them. Bone and air appear bright because they absorb and reflect the sound, showing an "acoustic shadow" behind them (**Fig. 1.2**). Linear transducers with a width

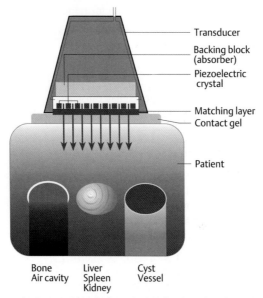

Fig. 1.2 Working principle of ultrasonography. (Used with permission from Eastman GW, Wald C, Crossin J. *Getting Started in Clinical Radiology: From Image to Diagnosis*. New York: Thieme; 2006:11.)

of 7.5 to 9 cm and frequencies of 10 to 13 MHz are typically used for evaluating the neck and thyroid.

◆ Barium Esophagram

An esophagram (also known as a barium swallow) is designed to evaluate the pharyngeal and esophageal mucosa; it is distinct from a modified barium swallow (MBS), which evaluates functional aspects of the upper swallow process and is usually performed in conjunction with a speech pathologist. These techniques are performed utilizing fluoroscopy. Fluoroscopy with intraluminal contrast is invaluable for studying the functional dynamics of the pharynx and esophagus.

An MBS evaluates the coordination of the swallow reflex. It is most often used to determine the etiology and severity of food bolus processing issues as well as the risk and/or presence of airway aspiration. A speech pathologist is usually in attendance and administers barium suspensions of varying thickness (thin liquid, thick liquid, nectar, paste, and solid) while the radiologist observes fluoroscopically, primarily in the lateral but also in the anteroposterior projections. One can also assess for esophageal motility/dysmotility, Zenker diverticulum, stricture, mass, hiatal hernia, or obvious free reflux.

Contrast Media

Barium suspension is the most commonly used fluoroscopic contrast agent. If a perforation of the hypopharynx or esophagus is suspected, there is a risk for barium extravasation into the soft tissues of the neck or chest. Therefore, in these cases, water-soluble contrast agents are often used (such as Gastrografin, Bracco Diagnostics, Inc., Princeton, NJ). However, it is important to note that these agents may cause a chemical pneumonitis or severe pulmonary edema if aspirated into the airway, so they must be cautiously used if concern for aspiration exists.

◆ Nuclear Medicine Imaging

Positron Emission Tomography with Computed Tomography

PET-CT is essentially a positron emission tomography scan performed and superimposed upon a simultaneous computed tomography scan to allow precise correlation between increased function (enhanced cellular activity) and anatomic evaluation provided by the CT. The PET scanning portion is a functional imaging technique that measures metabolic activity through the use of molecules tagged with positron-emitting isotopes such as the glucose precursor ^{18}F-fluoro-deoxyglucose (FDG), the most commonly used radiotracer, which has a half-life of ~ 110 minutes. ^{18}F is produced in a cyclotron and immediately extracted from solution, incorporated into the carbohydrate molecule, and administered.

Working Principle of PET-CT

After being emitted from the atom, the positron travels in the tissue for a short distance until it encounters an electron and forms a positronium, which immediately annihilates (converts its mass to energy), forming two photons. These annihilation photons travel in opposite directions from each other and are picked up by the detectors placed around the patient. Simultaneous detection of these photons relates them to the same annihilation event, allowing the event to be localized in space. Detection of annihilation by the dedicated PET scanner yields spatial resolution and sensitivity. The spatial resolution of the final reconstructed images is limited by the number of collected events.

FDG is taken up by glucose transporters. Normally, glucose enters into a cell, is phosphorylated by hexokinase, and then enters directly into either the glycolytic or glycogenic pathway. FDG, a glucose analogue, is subsequently unable to continue into the usual glucose metabolic pathways (because of the substitution of fluorine for a hydroxyl group) and is essentially trapped in the cell as FDG-phosphate. Because neoplastic cells have higher rates of glycolysis and glucose uptake, localized areas of intracellular activity on a PET scan may represent neoplastic disease. Tumor concentration of FDG generally peaks at 30 minutes, remains constant for 60 minutes, and then declines.

Note that FDG can also accumulate nonspecifically in other cells that have active glycolysis, such as organs with high glucose metabolism (e.g., brain and kidneys) as well as areas of active inflammation and infection. This may lead to a false positive PET-CT scan. Other activities that may cause false positive findings include muscular activity, foreign bodies, and granulomas. False negatives in PET-CT scans may occur when the tumor threshold is too small (< 0.5 cm in diameter). In PET scanning, quantification of FDG uptake intensity is generally expressed on an arbitrary scale as standard uptake values (SUVs).

Thyroid Scintigraphy

Thyroid scintigraphy renders, at one point in time, information about the global and regional functional status of the thyroid. It is observer-independent and reproducible with low inherent radiation exposure. Scintigraphic imaging of the thyroid helps determine whether solitary or multiple nodules are functional when compared with the surrounding thyroid tissue. Findings for a nodule may be normal functional (warm), hyperfunctional (hot), or hypofunctional (cold). Scintigraphy can also help determine whether cervical masses contain thyroid tissue, and it can demonstrate whether metastases from well-differentiated thyroid cancer concentrate iodine for the purpose of radioiodine therapy. For thyroid scintigraphy the following radionuclides are in use: technetium-99m (^{99m}Tc), iodine-123 (^{123}I), and iodine-131 (^{131}I).

Working Principle of Thyroid Scintigraphy

The technique of thyroid scintigraphy is based on the principle that functional, active thyroid cells incorporate iodine and a gamma camera can then be used to detect the accumulated radionuclide.

Parathyroid Scintigraphy

Several radiotracers are available for parathyroid scintigraphy. At present, the radiotracer of choice is ^{99m}Tc-sestamibi (also called sestamibi, methoxy-isobutylisonitrile, or MIBI). ^{99m}Tc-sestamibi is a lipophilic cation that is taken up in the mitochondria of the cells. Of note, this radiotracer can be used with a wide variety of imaging techniques, including planar multiplex ion-beam imaging (MIBI), single-photon emission computed tomography (SPECT), and fused SPECT-CT.

Working Principle of Parathyroid Scintigraphy

Sestamibi accumulates in the thyroid and parathyroid tissues within minutes after IV administration, but it has a different washout rate from these two tissues. It is released faster from the thyroid than from the parathyroid. The presence of large numbers of mitochondria-rich cells in parathyroid adenomas is thought to be responsible for their slower release of ^{99m}Tc-sestamibi from hyperfunctioning parathyroid tissue than from the adjacent thyroid tissue. Thus, on 2- to 3-hour washout images, after thyroid uptake has dissipated, the presence of a retained area of activity allows one to identify and localize a parathyroid adenoma. Overall, ^{99m}Tc-sestamibi parathyroid scintigraphy has good sensitivity for the detection and localization of a single adenoma in patients with primary hyperparathyroidism. Correlation with ultrasound findings can also be helpful.

Single-Photon Emission Computed Tomography

SPECT scanning for parathyroid disease allows increased accuracy of routine sestamibi scanning by ~ 2 to 3%. SPECT scanning can be performed within the first several hours after a patient is injected with the sestamibi. During the scan, multiple images are taken of the patient's head and neck. These images are assembled to provide a three-dimensional picture. SPECT scanning is typically used when ordinary planar sestamibi scans are inconclusive.

Four-Dimensional Parathyroid CT (4D-CT)

4D-CT is a specialized imaging study that was first introduced in 2006 for the purpose of identifying abnormal parathyroid glands in the planning of parathyroid surgery. 4D-CT includes image sets in three planes (axial, coronal, sagittal) from the angle of the mandible to the mediastinum. The "fourth" dimension of 4D-CT is the perfusion information derived from multiple contrast phases. It is most commonly performed with three phases: noncontrast, arterial, and delayed-phase imaging. 4D-CT has a higher radiation dose than scintigraphy.

1.2 Hematology for the Otolaryngologist

◆ Key Features

> • Head and neck surgery patients may require screening for, and correction of, hematologic disorders.

An overview of blood components, disorders, and transfusion complications is provided in this chapter.

◆ Blood Loss Management

Estimated Blood Volume (EBV)

- 95–100 mL/kg for premature infant
- 85–90 mL/kg for full-term infant
- 80 mL/kg for infants up to 12 months
- 70–75 mL/kg for adult males
- 65–70 mL/kg for adult females

    Allowable blood loss = [EBV × (Hct – target Hct)]/Hct
    Replace every 1 mL blood loss with 3 mL crystalloid, 1 mL colloid, or 1 mL packed red blood cells (PRBCs).

PBRC Transfusion Guidelines

- One unit PRBCs increases Hct ~ 3% and hemoglobin (Hb) ~ 1 g/dL in adults.
- 10 mL/kg PRBCs increases Hct ~ 10%

Compatibility Testing

- **Type specific:** ABO-Rh typing only; 99.80% compatible.
- **Type and screen:** ABO-Rh and screen; 99.94% compatible.
- **Type and crossmatch:** ABO-Rh screen, and crossmatch; 99.95% compatible. Crossmatching confirms ABO-Rh typing, detects antibodies to the other blood group systems, and detects antibodies in low blood titers.
- **Screening donor blood:** Hematocrit is determined; if normal, the blood is typed, screened for antibodies, and tested for hepatitis B, hepatitis C, syphilis, human immunodeficiency virus-1 (HIV-1), HIV-2, and human T cell lymphotropic viruses 1 and 2.

Blood Component Therapy

The archaic perioperative axiom of transfusing patients to maintain Hb of 10 and a hematocrit of 30 has fallen by the wayside. Although these are indeed safe guidelines for patients with coronary artery disease, transfusions are currently guided by hemodynamics, intraoperative blood loss, and laboratory values such as the arterial blood gas. Blood replacement in a complex surgical patient is part of goal-directed fluid therapy guided by the clinical response seen in continuously monitored flow parameters (see **Chapter 2.3**).

- **Whole blood:** 40% hematocrit; used primarily in hemorrhagic shock.
- **PRBCs:** Each unit has a volume of 250 to 300 mL with a hematocrit of 70 to 85%.
- **Platelets:** A normal platelet count is 150,000 to 400,000/mm^3. Thrombocytopenia is defined as <150,000/mm^3. Intraoperative bleeding increases with counts between 40,000 and 70,000/mm^3, and spontaneous bleeding can occur with counts <20,000/mm^3. During most surgeries, platelet transfusions are probably not needed unless the count is less than 50,000/mm^3. One unit of platelets will increase platelet count 5000 to 10,000/mm^3. The usual dose is 1 unit of platelets per 10 kg body weight. Platelets are stored at room temperature; ABO compatibility is not necessary.
- **Fresh frozen plasma (FFP):** Acute reversal of warfarin requires 5 to 8 mL/kg of FFP. ABO compatibility is mandatory. A 250 mL bag contains all coagulation factors except platelets. 10 to 15 mL/kg will increase plasma coagulation factors to 30% of normal. Fibrinogen levels will increase by 1 mg/mL of plasma transfused.
- **Cryoprecipitate:** Indications include hypofibrinogenemia, von Willebrand's disease, and hemophilia A. ABO compatibility is not necessary. Each 10 to 20 mL/bag contains 100 units of factor VIII-C, 100 units of von Willebrand factor (vWF), 60 units of factor XIII, and 250 mg of fibrinogen.

◆ Massive Transfusions

A massive transfusion is defined as the replacement of a patient's total blood volume in less than 24 hours. It also applies to the acute administration of more than half the patient's estimated blood volume per hour.

◆ Universal Donor Blood

Group O, Rh-negative blood should be reserved for patients close to exsanguination. If time permits, crossmatched or uncrossmatched type-specific blood should be administered. Group O, Rh negative blood should not be given as whole blood. The serum contains high anti-A and anti-B titers, which may cause hemolysis of recipient blood.

If more than 4 units of group O, Rh-negative whole blood is administered, type-specific blood should not be given subsequently because the potentially high anti-A and anti-B titers could cause hemolysis of the donor blood.

Patients administered up to 10 units of group O, Rh-negative PRBCs may be switched to type-specific blood, since there is an insignificant risk of hemolysis from the small volume of plasma administration with PRBCs.

◆ Complications of Transfusions

Immune Reactions (Hemolytic versus Nonhemolytic)

Hemolytic Reactions

● *Acute Hemolytic Reaction.* An acute hemolytic reaction occurs when ABO-incompatible blood is transfused, resulting in acute intravascular hemolysis; the severity of a reaction often depends on how much incompatible blood has been given. Symptoms include fever, chills, chest pain, anxiety, back pain, and dyspnea; in anesthetized patients, the reaction may present with fever, tachycardia, hypotension, hemoglobinuria, and diffuse oozing in the surgical field. Free Hb in plasma or urine is evidence of a hemolytic reaction. Risk of a fatal hemolytic transfusion reaction: 1:600,000 units.

● *Delayed Hemolytic Reaction.* Typically, this reaction is delayed 2 to 21 days after the transfusion. The symptoms are generally mild and may include malaise, jaundice, and fever; treatment is supportive. A delayed hemolytic reaction is caused by incompatibility of minor antigens (i.e., Kidd, Duffy, Kelly, etc.), causing hemolysis.

Nonhemolytic Reactions

● *Febrile Reaction.* A febrile reaction is the most common nonhemolytic reaction (0.5–1.0% of RBC transfusions and up to 30% of platelet transfusions). The reaction is the result of the action of recipient antibodies against donor antigens present on leukocytes and platelets; treatment includes stopping or slowing the infusion and antipyretics.

● *Urticarial Reaction.* An urticarial reaction occurs in 1% of transfusions; it is thought to be due to sensitization of the patient to transfused plasma proteins. It is characterized by erythema, hives, and itching without fever. Treat with antihistamine drugs.

● *Anaphylactic Reaction.* Anaphylactic reactions are rare (1:500,000). Patients with IgA deficiency may be at an increased risk because of the transfused IgA reaction with anti-IgA antibodies.

Transfusion-Related Lung Injury

Transfusion-related lung injury (TRALI) is due to a transfusion of anti–histocompatibility leukocyte antigen (HLA) antibodies that interact with and cause the patient's white cells to aggregate in the pulmonary circulation. Risk: 1:6000. Treatment is supportive, using a similar therapy as for managing acute respiratory distress syndrome (ARDS).

Graft-versus-Host Disease

Graft-versus-host disease is most commonly seen in immunocompromised patients. Cellular blood products contain lymphocytes capable of mounting an immune response against the compromised host.

Posttransfusion Purpura

Due to the development of platelet alloantibodies; the platelet count typically drops dramatically one week after the transfusion.

Immune Suppression

Transfusion of leukocyte-containing blood products appears to be immunosuppressive. Blood transfusions may increase the incidence of serious infections following surgery or trauma. Blood transfusions may worsen tumor recurrence and mortality rate following resections of many cancers.

Infectious Complications

Viral Infections

- **Hepatitis:** Risk of hepatitis B virus (HBV) is 1:137,000; risk of hepatitis C virus (HCV) is 1:1,000,000
- **HIV/acquired immunodeficiency syndrome (AIDS):** Risk of HIV is 1:1,900,000
- **Cytomegalovirus (CMV) and Epstein-Barr virus:** Common and usually cause asymptomatic or mild systemic illness

Bacterial Infections

Gram-positive and gram-negative bacteria contamination of blood is rare. Specific bacterial reactions transmitted by blood include syphilis, brucellosis, salmonellosis, yersiniosis, and various rickettsioses.

Parasitic Infections

Malaria, toxoplasmosis, and Chagas's disease are very rare.

◆ Other Complications Related to Blood Transfusion

Metabolic Abnormalities

- Decreased pH secondary to increased hydrogen ion production
- Increased potassium: Due to cell lysis (increases with length of storage)
- Decreased 2,3-diphosphoglycerate (2,3-DPG): Consumed by RBCs; P50 decreases to 18 mm Hg after 1 week and to 15 mm Hg after 3 weeks.

- Citrate toxicity: Citrate metabolism to bicarbonate may contribute to metabolic alkalosis; binding of calcium by citrate could result in hypocalcemia and the ability of the liver to metabolize citrate to bicarbonate.

Microaggregates

Microaggregates consisting of platelets and leukocytes form during the storage of whole blood. Micropore filters may help remove these particles.

Hypothermia

The use of blood warmers (except for platelets) greatly decreases the likelihood of transfusion-related hypothermia.

Coagulopathies

Coagulopathies occur after massive transfusions (>10 units).

Dilutional Thrombocytopenia

Dilutional thrombocytopenia is a common cause of abnormal bleeding in the setting of massive transfusion. It typically responds quickly to platelet transfusion.

Factor Depletion

Factors V and VIII are very labile in stored blood and may decrease to levels as low as 15 to 20% of normal (this is usually enough for hemostasis).

Disseminated Intravascular Coagulation

Disseminated intravascular coagulation (DIC) is a hypercoagulable state caused by activation of the clotting system leading to deposition of fibrin in microvasculature, causing secondary fibrinolysis, leading to consumption of platelets and factors.

◆ Treatment of Hemolytic Transfusion Reactions

1. Stop the transfusion.
2. Check for error in patient or donor identification.
3. Send donor unit and newly obtained blood sample to blood bank for re-crossmatch.
4. Treat hypotension with fluids and pressors as needed.
5. If transfusion is required, use type O-negative PRBCs and type AB FFP.
6. Maintain the urine output at a minimum of 75 to 100 mL/h by generously administering IV fluids; consider mannitol, 12.5 to 50 g, or furosemide, 20 to 40 mg.
7. Monitor for signs of DIC clinically or with laboratory tests.
8. Send patient blood sample for direct antiglobulin (Coombs) test, free Hb, haptoglobin; send urine for Hb.

◆ Coagulation Studies

Partial Thromboplastin Time (PTT)

- By adding particulate material to a blood sample, which activates the intrinsic coagulation system, the PTT can be determined.
- PTT measures the clotting ability of all factors in the intrinsic and common pathways except factor XIII.
- PTT is abnormal (prolonged) if there are decreased amounts of coagulation factors, if the patient is on heparin, or if there is a circulating anticoagulant present.
- Normal values are between 25 and 37 seconds.

Prothrombin Time (PT)

- Performed by measuring the time needed to form a clot when calcium and a tissue extract are added to plasma.
- PT evaluates the activity of fibrinogen, prothrombin, and factors V, VII, and X; evaluates the intrinsic coagulation system and vitamin K–dependent factors.
- Normal PT is 10 to 12 seconds (depending on control).

International Normalization Ratio (INR)

INR is a means of standardizing PT values: it is the ratio of the patient's PT to the control PT value. INR values are commonly used as a guide for warfarin therapy.

Activated Clotting Time (ACT)

The ACT is a simple test that provides a global measurement of hemostatic function and is measured after the whole blood is exposed to a specific activator of coagulation. The time for clot formation after whole blood is exposed to Celite (diatomaceous earth) is defined as the ACT.

There is a linear relationship between ACT and heparin dose, which provides a convenient method to measure response to heparin anticoagulation. Normal values are 90 to 120 seconds. The ACT lacks sensitivity to clotting abnormalities.

Platelet Function

Detailed evaluation of possible platelet aggregation disorders requires complex hematology testing. However, a screening platelet function test (via the use of the PFA analyzer) is available and can rapidly screen for platelet function abnormality without identifying a specific cause (e.g., recent aspirin use, von Willebrand's disease). Thus, abnormal PFA-100 test should prompt detailed work-up, whereas a normal test is reassuring in the setting of planned elective surgery, such as tonsillectomy.

✦ Hematologic Disorders

Sickle Cell Anemia

Sickle cell anemia is a hereditary hemolytic anemia resulting from the formation of an abnormal Hb (HbS); sickle Hb has less affinity for oxygen and decreased solubility. Patients are typically asymptomatic. Vigorous physical activity, high altitude, air travel in unpressurized planes, and anesthesia are potentially hazardous.

Clinical features include signs and symptoms of anemia (Hb levels 6.5–10 gm/dL), obstructive or hemolytic jaundice, lymphadenopathy, hematuria, epistaxis, priapism, finger clubbing, and skeletal deformities.

The disease manifests as periodic exaggeration of symptoms or sickle crises. There are four types of crises:

- Vaso-occlusive crisis: caused by sickled cells blocking the microvasculature; characterized by sudden pain frequently without a precipitating event.

- Hemolytic crisis: seen in patients with sickle cell disease and glucose-6-phosphate dehydrogenase (G6PD) deficiency; manifests as sudden hemolysis.

- Sequestration crisis: red blood cells are sequestered in the liver and spleen, leading to splenohepatomegaly and acute fall in hematocrit. This can progress to circulatory collapse.

- Aplastic crisis: characterized by transient episodes of bone marrow depression; often occurs after viral illness.

Management of Sickle Cell Anemia

The practice of transfusion to an end point of 70% HbA and less than 30% HbS preoperatively is controversial. Patients should be well oxygenated and hydrated intraoperatively to lessen the chance of sickling. Acidosis and hypothermia can also trigger a crisis and should also be avoided.

Factor Deficiencies

Factor VIII Deficiency (Hemophilia A)

The half-life of factor VIII is 8 to 12 hours. Treatment includes lyophilized factor VIII, cryoprecipitate, or desmopressin. Infusion of 1 unit of factor VIII per kg will increase the factor VIII activity by 2%. Levels of 20 to 40% are desirable prior to surgery.

Factor IX Deficiency (Hemophilia B; Christmas's disease)

The half-life of factor IX is 24 hours. Therapy consists of factor IX concentrates of FFP. To ensure surgical hemostasis, activity levels of 50 to 80% are needed. Infusion of 1 unit per kg of factor IX will increase the factor IX level by 1%.

von Willebrand's Disease (VWD)

VWD is the most common of all the inherited bleeding disorders. It occurs in ~1 of every 100 to 1000 people. VWD affects both males and females, with three forms. von Willebrand factor (VWF) is involved in platelet adhesion and in carrying factor VIII.

- Type 1 VWD: Most common, usually mild; low VWF, possibly low factor VIII.
- Type 2 VWD: Abnormal function of VWF; various forms.
- Type 3 VWD: Rare, severe. Usually no VWF and low factor VIII.

Testing for VWD includes platelet function assay, VWF levels, ristocetin cofactor assay to assess VWF function, factor VIII levels, and VWF multimers.

Management of von Willebrand's Disease

The goal of therapy is to correct the defect in platelet adhesiveness (by raising the level of effective VWF) and the defect in blood coagulation (by raising the factor VIII level). Desmopressin (1-diamine-8-D-arginine vasopressin, DDAVP) is used to increase VWF/factor VIII release. Most experience in treating individuals with VWD is with intravenous infusion, with which the response is rapid (peak VWF levels within ~45–90 minutes of infusion). Doses may be repeated at intervals of 12 to 24 hours for continued bleeding or for postoperative use. Pediatric dosage is 0.3 µg/kg IV.

VWF/factor III infusion can be given for more severe cases. Plasma-derived factor VIII concentrates that contain VWF in high molecular weight can be used, and cryoprecipitate contains multimeric VWF. Humate-P (Centeon, L.L.C., King of Prussia, PA) and Alphanate (Grifols, S.A., Barcelona, Spain) are other forms of factor VIII/VWF. Aminocaproic acid (Amicar, Pfizer Pharmaceuticals, New York, NY) inhibits fibrinolysis via inhibition of plasminogen activator substances and, to a lesser degree, through antiplasmin activity. Amicar (pediatric dosing 100 mg/kg/dose orally every 4–6 hours) can be useful in cases of mucosal bleeding.

1.3 Obstructive Sleep Apnea

◆ Key Features

- Sleep apnea is a cessation of breathing during sleep.
- Sleep apnea may be central, obstructive, or mixed.
- Obstructive sleep apnea is caused by upper airway collapse and narrowing.
- Cardinal symptoms are disruptive snoring, witnessed apneas, and daytime sleepiness.

Obstructive sleep apnea (OSA) is characterized by repetitive episodes of complete (apnea) or partial (hypopnea) upper airway obstruction occurring during sleep. Apnea is a cessation of breathing for at least 10 seconds. Hypopnea is a transient reduction of breathing for less than 10 seconds. Hypopneas must be associated with oxygen desaturation of at least 4%, whereas apneic events are not required to be associated with a decrease in oxygen saturation.

◆ Epidemiology

Estimates of the prevalence of sleep-disordered breathing vary widely in the literature, with most quoting at least 2 to 4% of the general population. Men have a higher prevalence than women (3–8 times), except that risk equalizes in postmenopausal females. The prevalence increases with age and body mass index (BMI) above 25, but it may remain undiagnosed in the majority of patients. Other risk factors include family history, obesity, left ventricular heart failure, advanced age, and allergy.

◆ Clinical

Signs and Symptoms

The signs and symptoms of sleep apnea include witnessed nocturnal apnea events, snoring, daytime sleepiness, headaches, depression, restless sleep, trouble concentrating, irritability, nighttime awakenings or gasping for air, and decreased libido.

Differential Diagnosis

Sleep disturbance and respiratory events can be caused by nonobstructive alveolar hypoventilation, asthma, chronic obstructive pulmonary disease, congestive heart failure, narcolepsy, periodic limb movement disorder, sleep deprivation, and medication, drug, and alcohol use. The differential diagnosis may also include laryngospasm related to gastroesophageal reflux disorder (GERD).

◆ Evaluation

History

The history taken from the patient and his or her bed partner will include reports of snoring, witnessed apneas or gasping events at night, daytime sleepiness, decreased libido or sexual dysfunction, and motor vehicle or work accidents. Bed partner reporting is helpful to evaluate a pretest risk of OSA but is not a good predictor of the severity of sleep-disordered breathing. The Epworth Sleepiness Scale (8 questions scored 0–3) is often used to assess daytime sleepiness; score >11 may correlate with OSA.

Physical Exam

- Body habitus (weight, BMI)
- Congenital craniofacial abnormalities

- Oral exam: large tongue base, elongated soft palate, enlarged uvula, narrow oropharyngeal inlet, modified Mallampati and tonsil staging (**Table 1.4**)
- Nasal exam: deviated septum, hypertrophic conchae, polyposis nasi
- Facial skeleton abnormalities: e.g., retrognathia, midface hypoplasia, craniofacial anomalies
- Neck circumference: men ≥ 17 inches (≥ 43 cm), women ≥ 15.5 inches (≥ 39 cm) is predictive of OSA

Imaging

Consider a chest X-ray to rule out right-sided heart failure.

Labs

Laboratory testing is not necessary.

Other Tests

Flexible fiberoptic nasopharyngoscopy can be useful to assess the retropalatal and retrolingual spaces for narrowing or dynamic collapse. Some surgeons utilize a Müller maneuver (patient inspires with closed mouth and nose) to assess for possible collapse that may indicate regions of anatomic concern during OSA events. Drug-induced sleep endoscopy (DISE) is a better predictor of possible anatomic sites of obstruction. This procedure involves flexible endoscopy with the patient under sedated anesthesia in an attempt to reproduce conditions similar to natural sleep.

Nocturnal *polysomnography* (PSG), or sleep study, is the gold standard for diagnosing and quantifying obstructive sleep apnea; multiple physiologic parameters are measured while the patient sleeps in a laboratory. Data are collected in the presence of a qualified technician. Typical parameters in a sleep study include eye movement observations (to detect rapid-eye-movement [REM] sleep), electroencephalography (EEG; to determine arousals from sleep), chest wall and abdominal monitors, nasal and oral airflow

Table 1.4   Mallampati and tonsil staging

Mallampati scoring		Tonsil grading	
Class I	Soft palate, uvula, faucial arches, pillars visible	0	Tonsils absent
Class II	Soft palate, portion of the uvula and faucial arch visible	1	Tonsils occupy ≤ 25% of interpillar space
Class III	Soft palate and base of uvula visible	2	Tonsils occupy 26–50% of interpillar space
Class IV	Only hard palate visible	3	Tonsils occupy 51–75% of the interpillar space
		4	Tonsils occupy ≥ 75% of the interpillar space

measurements, an electrocardiogram (ECG), an electromyogram (to look for limb movements that cause arousals), and oximetry.

Obstructive apnea is defined as an apneic event associated with increased respiratory effort throughout. *Central apnea* is an apneic event without associated respiratory effort. *Mixed apnea* begins as central, but then respiratory effort resumes.

The *apnea-hypopnea index (AHI)* is the most common summary measure used to describe respiratory disturbances during sleep. AHI is the total number of episodes of apnea and hypopnea during sleep, divided by the hours of sleep time. AHI values can be summarized for the sleep period or computed for different sleep stages and body position. An AHI >5 is required for the diagnosis of OSA; mild OSA is defined as AHI values of 5 to 15, moderate OSA for values of 16 to 30, and severe OSA for values ≥ 30.

The *respiratory disturbance index (RDI)* is a similar measure to AHI and includes apneas, hypopneas, and respiratory-related arousal events (arousal with some respiratory perturbations that does not meet criteria for apnea or hypopnea).

The *arousal index (AI)* is the number of arousals per hour of sleep, which can be computed from an EEG. The AI may be correlated with AHI or RDI, but ~20% of apneas and desaturation episodes are not accompanied by arousals, or other causes of arousals are present. Some sleep centers utilize portable home monitors that measure only heart rate, pulse oximetry, and nasal airflow to diagnose OSA.

In *pediatric sleep studies*, EEG traces have different categories of activities. Apneic events are counted if duration is at least 2 baseline breaths. Hypopneas are associated with at least 3% O_2 desaturation or arousal.

◆ Treatment Options

Medical

Mild OSA may be managed conservatively by weight loss or avoidance of alcohol and certain medications. *Weight loss* is the simplest treatment for OSA in obese patients. Even a modest (10%) weight loss may eliminate apneic episodes by reducing the mass of the posterior airway. Positional mild OSA may be improved as well by sleep positioning maneuvers (e.g., avoidance of supine position by those with supine-predominant OSA).

Continuous positive airway pressure (CPAP) or *bilevel positive airway pressure (BiPAP)* treatment is the primary medical management for patients who have symptomatic mild or any moderate or severe obstructive sleep apnea. CPAP improves upper airway patency by the application of positive pressure to the collapsible upper airway. CPAP use can improve multiple cardiac and respiratory parameters as well as GERD, ED, and depression. Effective pressures typically range from 3 to 15 cm H_2O. The most common problem with CPAP is noncompliance. BiPAP independently provides inspiratory and expiratory pressures. CPAP failure may be caused by perceived discomfort, claustrophobia, nasal congestion, inadvertent dislodgement of mask during sleep, and panic attacks. *Contraindications* include cerebrospinal fluid (CSF) leak, pneumocephalus, pneumothorax or bullae, aspiration risk, and hypotension.

Oral appliances may be useful. *Mandibular advancement devices* are designed to advance the mandible forward and increase the retrolingual space or, at the very least, reduce mandible and tongue retrusion with sleep.

Surgical

A variety of procedures may improve OSA in properly selected patients. The challenge is identifying the likely anatomic site of obstruction to be corrected. Many surgeons advocate a potentially staged approach to treat additional sites if improvement is not achieved with the initial procedure. Sites of obstruction may include the nasal airway (septum, conchae, nasal valve), the palatine tonsils and soft palate/uvula, the base of tongue/lingual tonsils, and the mandible. Common procedures include:

- Septoplasty with or without inferior concha reduction may improve nasal breathing and reduce mouthbreathing. It may enable CPAP to be used at a lower pressure with a nasal-only device, but it is unable to generate any significant change in AHI.
- Adenoidectomy or adenotonsillectomy may be performed, especially in children with OSA.
- Uvulopalatopharyngoplasty (UPPP) involves the removal of part of the soft palate, some or all of the uvula and redundant oropharyngeal tissues, including the tonsils, and then subsequent resuspension of pharyngopalatal tissues, with various described techniques (palatal advancement or uvulopalatal flaps).
- Tongue base reduction procedures include a midline glossectomy, lingual tonsillectomy (with or without transoral robotic technique), radiofrequency/Coblation (Smith & Nephew, London, UK) treatment of base of tongue. Risks: bleeding, hematoma, lingual artery or nerve injuries, dysgeusia.
- Orthognathic surgery may consist of genioglossal, mandibular, or maxillomandibular advancement. Risks include nonunion, deformity, temporomandibular joint (TMJ) disorder, and nerve injury.
- Base of tongue or hyoid suspension may be attempted.
- Hypoglossal nerve stimulation implant involves a sensing lead from the intercostal muscles, a battery-powered implantable pulse generator, and a stimulation lead secured to a hypoglossal nerve. Excellent outcomes have been reported.
- Tracheotomy is the most effective therapeutic maneuver for obstructive apnea, as it bypasses the obstructed region, but it is a procedure of last resort. It is indicated for patients who are most severely affected by OSA or obstructive sleep hypopnea and who cannot utilize CPAP effectively.

◆ Outcome and Follow-Up

Prognosis for improvement is excellent with proper treatment. Polysomnography is often repeated ~3 months following surgical treatment or following weight loss achievement. Surgical success is often defined as at least a 50% reduction in AHI or reduction of AHI to below 5. A 50% reduction may not be a cure, and either retitration of CPAP or additional staged treatment may be required.

OSA is frequently undiagnosed and untreated and can have long-term sequelae, including poorly controlled hypertension, arrhythmias, cerebral vascular accidents, pulmonary vascular disease, heart failure, and further weight gain with its associated morbidities. The adverse effects of hypersomnolence may include loss of employment, motor vehicle accidents, and sexual dysfunction.

1.4 Benign Oral and Odontogenic Disorders

◆ Key Features

- Pathology may arise from any of the tissue types within the oral cavity—mucosal, glandular, nervous, vascular, immunologic, osseous, and dental.
- Lesions may present symptomatically or be noted on routine screening.
- Squamous papilloma is the most common oral mucosal papillary lesion (2.5% of all oral lesions).
- Benign lesions should be differentiated from malignancy, which when indicated requires biopsy.

Benign oral lesions are common and may be manifestations of local or systemic disorders. The appearance of the lesion, associated symptoms, temporal relationship to other illnesses, and, when necessary, biopsy will enable the appropriate therapy to be determined. Differentiation of benign and malignant lesions is important for proper and expedient care.

◆ Etiology

Lesions may be infectious, inflammatory, neoplastic, traumatic, vascular, or congenital/developmental. They may be isolated phenomena or be related to underlying medical disease or systemic disorder. The pathophysiology varies widely and is mentioned in connection to specific lesions in the Clinical section, below.

◆ Clinical

Signs and Symptoms

Lesions of the oral cavity may present asymptomatically or may be noted by the patient or dental provider. Associated symptoms may include pain, bleeding, recurrent trauma, dental pain, malocclusion, or loose dentition. Benign lesions of varied etiology may share morphologic features. Many lesions appear as white plaques (i.e., leukoplakia) or ulcerations. Epithelial changes involving alteration in maturation (e.g., hyperplasia, dysplasia, carcinoma) often appear white in the moist environment of the oral cavity. Time course of the lesion and associated symptoms may guide the clinician as to the nature of the pathology.

Differential Diagnosis

For patients with oral cavity lesions or periodontal findings, several considerations must be taken into account in generating the differential diagnosis: color of the lesion (e.g., white, red, normal), thickness (e.g., exophytic, plaque, erosive), presence of pain, subsite within the oral cavity/oropharynx (e.g., hard palate, soft palate, gingiva, buccal mucosa, lips), type of apparent tissue involved (e.g., mucosa alone, bony, salivary), and underlying induration or fluctuance. Lesions may involve local factors or may be related to systemic illnesses. Systemic lupus erythematosus, sarcoidosis, Sjögren's disease, Kawasaki's disease, drug reaction, amyloidosis, viral infections, immune deficiencies, Crohn's disease, HIV, and nutritional and metabolic deficiencies are among the possibilities.

Exophytic Mucosal Lesions

Squamous Papilloma

Squamous papilloma is a common benign epithelial growth caused by human papillomavirus (HPV). The lesion is usually pink to red with typical verrucous appearance. These may be singular or multiple (more often in immunocompromised patients). Excision to include the base of the lesion is typically curative, but lesions can recur from incomplete resection or other cells infected with HPV.

Fibromas

Fibromas are nodular swellings with fibrotic submucosal reaction related to trauma or chronic irritation. These may occur anywhere but are more common on the buccal, labial, and lingual mucosa. Excision may be carried out for diagnosis or if repeated trauma is occurring because of the lesion size.

Congenital Epulis

Congenital epulis is a benign lesion occurring along the alveolar region in infants, with a female predominance. Simple excision may be done for comfort or diagnosis.

Lobular Capillary Hemangioma (Pyogenic Granuloma)

Lobular capillary hemangioma (pyogenic granuloma) was long thought to be an inflammatory lesion but has been reclassified as a benign vascular neoplasm. It may be found on any mucosal surface in all demographics, but there is some association with pregnancy. Although vascular in nature, it may become increasingly fibrotic with time. Simple excision is the treatment of choice, but recurrence is not unusual.

Granular Cell Tumor

Granular cell tumor is a benign neoplasm originating with Schwann cells. They most often form on the lingual dorsum and may have some mild surrounding induration. Simple excision is typically curative.

Oral Hairy Leukoplakia

Oral hairy leukoplakia occurs on the tongue, often along the lateral border, and appears as rough white plaques. It is caused by Epstein-Barr virus (EBV) and occurs most often in immunocompromised patients, such as HIV-positive individuals. The appearance can fluctuate. Typically this is asymptomatic, but occasionally some mild discomfort or taste aberration may be present. No specific treatment is required.

Hairy Tongue

In contrast to the preceding, hairy tongue occurs along the tongue dorsum and may be darkly pigmented, pink, or even colored by other agents, such as coffee or mouthwash. It is associated with smoking, poor oral hygiene, local radiation, and antibiotic use. The filiform papillae of the tongue fail to desquamate normally and hence become elongated (or "hairy"). The condition is usually asymptomatic, but some patients relate a tickling sensation or find it unsightly. Treatment involves limiting the potential offending agents, along with tongue brushing or use of a commercially available tongue scraper.

Mucoceles

Mucoceles are cystic, ballottable swellings related to salivary gland trauma, often occurring on the lips or buccal mucosa. They may be clear, pink or even bluish in color. They may spontaneously resolve or may be excised to avoid repeated trauma or for diagnosis.

Gingival Hyperplasia

Gingival hyperplasia involves excessive growth of the gingival (gum) tissue. This may occur in response to inflammatory conditions, but when more pronounced, it is more often related to side effects of medications, including phenytoin, cyclosporin, and some calcium channel blockers.

Mesenchymal Tumors

Mesenchymal tumors may arise in the oral cavity. These include hemangioma, leiomyoma, rhabdomyoma, schwannoma, and neurofibroma. Local excision is usually adequate in these lesions, except hemangioma which, in pediatric patients will often regress.

Salivary Gland Adenomas

Salivary gland adenomas may occur in the mucosa of the oral cavity. Pleomorphic and monomorphic lesions may occur. These should be distinguished from minor salivary gland malignant lesions, which are more common.

Surface Mucosal Lesions

Leukoplakia

"Leukoplakia" is a term that may be used to describe any white plaque in the oral mucosa. It typically is related to some epithelial maturation issue, ranging from hyperkeratosis to dysplasia to carcinoma. Leukoplakias may occur as a result of chronic irritation, such as trauma (e.g., dentures, chewing on edentulous alveolus) or tobacco use (e.g., chew/"dip," smoking). Excisional or incisional biopsy may be indicated for diagnostic purposes to rule out early carcinoma.

Nicotine Stomatitis

Nicotine stomatitis is a leukoplakic lesion, located along the hard and soft palate and caused by the heat from cigar, pipe, or, less commonly, cigarette smoking. Often it is diffuse in nature with white irregular patches mixed with red spots. If consistent historically, it does not require biopsy unless clinical concerns are present.

Fordyce Granules

Fordyce granules are flat to slightly raised yellow clustered lesions occurring on the buccal mucosa and lip. They represent sebaceous glands within the mucosa and require no treatment beyond patient reassurance.

Lichen Planus

Lichen planus is a dermatologic condition that may also involve the oral mucosa. Classically it appears as pink to purple patches with surrounding white "lacy" lines. Often this is asymptomatic, but it may be painful in the erosive subtype. Biopsy is necessary for definitive diagnosis. Treatment is not often necessary for the asymptomatic lesions, but topical or systemic steroids may be necessary in the painful erosive circumstances. A slightly elevated risk of oral squamous cell carcinoma is associated with lichen planus, particularly the erosive subtype. Lichen planus should be monitored during regular semiannual dental visits.

Kawasaki's Disease

Kawasaki's disease is a febrile vasculitis disorder affecting young children. Symptoms include prolonged fever, nonexudative conjunctivitis, uveitis, perianal erythema, "strawberry tongue" with fissures, lymphadenopathy, erythema and edema of the palms and soles, and possible coronary arteritis with possible aneurysm formation. This last issue should be evaluated with echocardiogram, as it can lead to death. The etiology remains unknown, but some suspect an infectious trigger. Treatment includes supportive care, monitoring for cardiac issues, and intravenous immunoglobulins.

Tattoo

Tattoo may be present on the mucosa from embedded pigmented materials or dental amalgam. These may be located away from the point of introduction secondary to uptake of the material and migration by macrophages. No treatment is necessary.

Racial Pigmentation

Racial pigmentation of the oral mucosa involves diffuse and symmetric melanotic coloration, most commonly on the gingival and labial regions. This should be contrasted to melanosis, as follows.

Melanosis

Melanosis is increased melanin production from irritants (e.g., smoker's melanosis), genetic disorders (e.g., Peutz-Jeghers's syndrome), endocrine disorders (e.g., Addison's disease), or true neoplasm (e.g., melanotic nevus, melanoma).

Ecchymosis, Hematoma, and Petechiae

Ecchymosis, hematoma, and petechiae are different types of collections of extravascular blood. Ecchymoses are bruises and may be purple, red, or blue. Hematoma is a collection of blood in the soft tissues, with swelling and a purple to dark blue color. Petechiae are round and small red lesions. Each of these will typically resolve without treatment. However, unless a specific etiology is known (e.g., local trauma), concern for coagulopathy should be investigated. An expanding hematoma of the floor of the mouth or pharynx can potentially cause airway compromise. Therefore, these patients should be monitored for worsening or be prophylactically intubated to prevent airway compromise.

Candidiasis

Candidiasis is a local fungal infection and may be asymptomatic or painful. The lesions typically appear as multiple white plaques on an erythematous base, with the white material able to be scraped off. Predisposing factors include prior radiation to the head and neck, xerostomia, antibiotic therapy, dentures, steroid inhaler use, and immunosuppression (e.g., diabetes, AIDS). Treatment often involves topical antifungals, although systemic therapy may be useful in particular cases.

Erosive Mucosal Lesions

Mucositis

Mucositis is a general term for inflammation of the oral epithelium. This may be caused by medications, radiation, chemotherapy, and local irritants. The mucositis may be generalized or patchy. Mucosal erythema or erosion may be present, but it is typically superficial. Deeper ulcerations are concerning for alternative diagnoses.

Viral Stomatitis

Viral stomatitis represents multiple possible infectious agents. Herpes simplex virus may cause vesicular and ulcerative lesions, typically associated with pain. The virus typically lies latent and may cause localized eruptions periodically. Primary herpetic gingivostomatitis occurs in children, and less often in adults. It is associated with tender cervical adenopathy, fever, and malaise. Antiviral agents may be helpful in symptomatic treatment. Varicella primarily affects the skin, but reactivation of varicella (herpes zoster) may involve sensor nerve distributions of the skin and oral mucosa. Herpangina caused by coxsackievirus

A involves fever, malaise, pharyngitis, nausea, and diarrhea, with vesicular or ulcerative lesions along the soft palate and tonsillar pillars. Hand, foot, and mouth disease is also caused by coxsackievirus and involves similar symptoms along with rash of the hands and feet. Rubeola is associated with Koplik spots, which appear as red macules with white centers along the buccal mucosa. Rubeola causes more severe systemic illness but is rare, given vaccinations.

Recurrent Aphthous Ulcers (Canker Sore)

Recurrent aphthous ulcers (canker sores) are common ulcerative lesions with a quick onset and typical 7 to 14 day course. They occur on nonkeratinized mucosa, such as the lip, buccal mucosa, unattached gingiva, soft palate, and floor of the mouth. The etiology is unclear, although some family history is not uncommon. Occurrences may be sporadic or related to psychosocial stressors, illness, and menstrual cycle. The lesions are typically painful at first, and the pain may abate before the ulcer is fully healed. They are shallow ulcers covered with a yellow to gray membrane. Treatment may be supportive, although topical steroids speed resolution. Most lesions are singular or few but may occur in a "herpetiform" fashion. "Major" aphthous ulcers are large and can be debilitating. This form may be associated with longer duration and healing with scarring.

Pemphigus Vulgaris

Pemphigus vulgaris is an autoimmune disorder in which the patient develops antibodies to the epithelial desmosomes, creating a loss of cellular adhesion and subsequent sloughing. Bullae form but are often quickly ruptured within the oral cavity. Nikolsky sign may be present on intact bullae. Incisional biopsy with immunofluorescent staining is required for diagnosis. Treatment includes immunosuppressive agents, including corticosteroids.

Pemphigoid

Pemphigoid is similar to pemphigus, but with the antibodies directed at the basement membrane. A Nikolsky sign is less common but may be present. Scarring may occur in this condition.

Benign Migratory Glossitis

Benign migratory glossitis may also be known as geographic tongue. The disorder manifests as lingual erythema, papillary atrophy, fissures, and serpiginous white hyperkeratotic regions. These findings wax and wane over time. The etiology is unknown, but the condition has been associated with psoriasis, granulomatous disease, and certain HLA types. Diagnosis is made through classic features on examination. Many cases are asymptomatic, but some patients have sensitivity to spicy or hot foods. If the condition is severe, possible topical retinoids or corticosteroids have been tried.

Necrotizing Sialometaplasia

Necrotizing sialometaplasia is a process involving salivary acini that undergo ischemia and necrosis. The lesions may involve swelling with some central necrosis and ulceration, and because of this appearance, they can be mistaken for squamous cell carcinoma. Incisional biopsy should be done for diagnosis, but the lesion typically spontaneously resolves.

Vitamin Deficiencies

Certain vitamin deficiencies may have oral manifestations. Deficiencies of vitamin B_2 (riboflavin) and vitamin B_3 (niacin) may be associated with angular cheilitis and with magenta or red-colored tongue with filiform papilla atrophy. Vitamin B_{12} (cobalamin) deficiency may produce angular cheilitis as well but also aphthous ulcerations, general mucositis, glossitis, and taste aberration.

Odontogenic Lesions

Odontogenic infections may occur in any tooth-bearing region and may extend into the neck.

Periodontal Abscess

Periodontal abscess occurs when infection accumulates in the periodontal space. This may present as swelling and pain around a tooth or tooth remnant. Bony erosion may be present. Spontaneous drainage may occur. Incision and drainage with dental follow-up is recommended.

Periapical Abscess

Periapical abscess is an infection within the periapical region of the tooth, which can be seen on radiography. These may be asymptomatic or may preset with surrounding cellulitis, pain, or drainage. If a fistula tract leads to the oral mucosa, a soft tissue swelling may occur, called a parulis or gumboil. An associated soft tissue abscess should be drained, but otherwise therapy includes possible dental extraction or root canal by a dental professional.

Torus Mandibularis and Torus Palatini

Torus mandibularis and torus palatini are common bony protrusions from the mandibular bone and hard palate, respectively. Torus palatini occurs along the midline and may be broad and smooth or may have a nodular appearance, sometimes with a narrower base. Torus mandibularis occurs along the medial mandible from the region above the mylohyoid muscle attachment. No treatment is needed, although they can complicate the fitting of dentures.

Exostoses

Exostoses are benign bony protuberances located on the buccal aspect of the upper (more common) or lower alveolus. The etiology is not clear, although it may involve bruxism and genetic contributors. As with torus mandibularis and torus palatini, no treatment is required, although, again, they may interfere with denture fitting. If larger, they may also contribute to periodontal disease.

Odontogenic Tumors and Cysts

Some odontogenic tumors and cysts may present with oral swelling or distortion of the alveolus, while others may be noted only on imaging studies. On oral examination they are not classically distinguished.

Odontogenic Keratocyst (OKC)

An odontogenic keratocyst (OKC) is a developmental cyst from the dental lamina that occurs in either the upper or lower jaw. It appears as a well-defined radiolucency in the bone. The cyst is lined with a parakeratinizing epithelium. The OKC can cause local aggressive destruction of bone and has a moderate recurrence risk. Resection can be conservative (e.g., enucleation curettage) or aggressive (e.g., complete resection). Recurrence rates are higher for conservative therapy, although a balance of recurrence versus surgical morbidity must be determined. This lesion may be associated with nevoid–basal cell syndrome (Gorlin's syndrome).

Dentigerous Cyst

A dentigerous cyst is a cystic lesion associated with the crown of an unerupted tooth. The cyst is lined with enamel epithelium. The cyst may become large enough to jeopardize mandible stability. Treatment may include excision of the cyst and origin tooth.

Calcifying Epithelial Odontogenic Tumor (Pindborg's Tumor)

A calcifying epithelial odontogenic tumor (Pindborg's tumor) is a rare odontogenic tumor of unclear tissue origin. It is slow growing and favors the posterior mandible. The radiography shows a heterogeneous mixed osseous pattern. Complete excision is recommended.

Fibrous Dysplasia

Fibrous dysplasia is a dysplastic process of bone growth, with a mixed pattern of osseous and fibrous tissue. Generally, it is self-limited and slow growing. The lesion may cause cosmetic deformity or impingement on other structures, depending on location. Resection is reserved for functional or severe cosmetic concerns.

Ossifying Fibroma

An ossifying fibroma is a slow-growing, well-circumscribed tumor consisting of lamellated bone with fibrous stroma, which can act aggressively locally. It may appear similar to fibrous dysplasia on imaging. Treatment favors resection, given the concern of more aggressive growth.

Ameloblastoma

Ameloblastoma is a benign tumor of ameloblasts (enamel-forming cells) more common in the mandible. It is more common in men in their 30 to 40s. The lesion tends to grow in an expansile fashion. Radiographically it has a "soap bubble" appearance, with multiloculated features. Resorption of tooth roots may be seen. Though histologically benign, these tumors can be aggressive and therefore complete surgical resection is the treatment of choice, as the tumor is poorly sensitive to radiation and chemotherapy.

Systemic Disorders

Amyloidosis

Amyloidosis may occur locally in the oral cavity or as part of a systemic illness. Classically, amyloid (immunoglobulin light chains) deposits in the tongue, buccal, and gingival tissue. This may cause expansion and induration. With severe tongue involvement, this may prevent the tongue fitting in the oral cavity or being retrodisplaced with airway restriction. Diagnosis is via biopsy, with "apple-green" birefringence on Congo red staining with polarized light microscopy. Treatment may involve systemic therapy, but local resection may assist if airway obstruction is an issue.

Sarcoidosis

Sarcoidosis is a systemic granulomatous disease affecting many organ systems, with predilection for the respiratory system. Salivary glands and oral mucosa may be involved. Sarcoid lesions may appear as red or violaceous nodular swellings of the lips, palate, and gingiva. Xerostomia may also be present secondary to salivary gland involvement and dysfunction. Biopsy is diagnostic and should show noncaseating granulomatous vasculitis. Serum angiotensin-converting enzyme (ACE) levels may be elevated in active disease. Treatment is with corticosteroids and cytotoxic drugs.

Systemic Lupus Erythematosus

Systemic lupus erythematosus is a systemic autoimmune disorder that can involve multiple organs, including ulcerative mucosal lesions.

Sjögren's Syndrome

Sjögren's syndrome is an autoimmune disease affecting the exocrine glands, primarily salivary and lacrimal. This results in keratoconjunctivitis sicca. Primary Sjögren's syndrome occurs in isolation, whereas secondary Sjögren's syndrome is associated with another connective tissue disorder. Diagnosis may be made by minor salivary gland biopsy, usually from the lip, looking for lymphocytic infiltrate. Serology may demonstrate SS-A/Ro and SS-B/La antibodies. Treatment is symptomatic, with an emphasis on good dental care. Five percent of Sjögren's syndrome patients will develop a lymphoid malignancy, most commonly non-Hodgkin's lymphoma.

◆ Evaluation

A detailed history of the lesion and any associated symptoms should be elicited. Past medical history should be taken, focused on possible inflammatory disorders, malignancy, autoimmune or connective tissue disorders, immunodeficiencies, and nutritional or metabolic conditions. The use of tobacco in any form should be noted. Dental and denture history may be helpful in odontogenic disorders and in some traumatic concerns (e.g., poorly fitting dentures, edentulous mastication, fractured teeth causing trauma to buccal mucosa or tongue).

Oral cavity examination should include all mucosal surfaces, keeping in mind that some regions require manipulation to evaluate (e.g., gingivolabial sulcus, posterior floor of mouth). In addition to inspection of the mucosal surfaces, the dentition should be evaluated. Palpation of the floor of mouth; the tongue, including the base; and, when appropriate, the buccal and labial structures should be performed to identify depth of involvement of a lesion. Lesions can be initially characterized by their color (e.g., leukoplakia, erythroplakia), depth (e.g., ulcerative/erosive, plaque, exophytic, expansile), and location (e.g., gingival, palatal). These features allow refining a differential diagnosis and evaluation plan.

If any question exists as to the nature of the lesion, biopsy is an appropriate evaluation tool. Most biopsies can be sent for routine histopathologic evaluation, but some diagnoses require special techniques and staining. Examples include pemphigus versus pemphigoid, where immunoglobulin staining is done and tissue should be sent fresh.

CT and MRI imaging may be indicated if there is concern for the depth of the lesion, involvement of deeper structures, or proximity to vital structures or if the concern is for submucosal disease presenting luminally. CT provides good soft tissue resolution and the relationship to underlying osseous structures, including abutment to the bone, erosion/invasion of the bone, or even development from the bone itself. While some use of ultrasound intraorally has been described for evaluation of peritonsillar abscess identification and fluid collection, this requires clinician training in the technique. Rarely other imaging such as angiography and sialography may be indicated.

◆ Treatment Options

Individual disease treatments are outlined in the preceding section with the corresponding diseases. The concern of oral cavity squamous cell or minor salivary gland carcinoma must also be considered, and if questions remain after a detail exam and history, biopsy is advised.

1.5   Temporomandibular Joint Disorders

◆ Key Features

- After toothache, temporomandibular joint (TMJ) disorders are the most common cause of facial pain.
- Most patients respond to conservative management.
- Surgical treatments can repair or replace severe damage.

Disease of the temporomandibular joint (TMJ) is often classified as myogenous or arthrogenous, involving a primary problem of muscle tension versus joint anatomy. Patients present with pain, headache, discomfort with chewing, and popping of the TMJ.

◆ Anatomy and Physiology

The TMJ connects the jaw and skull at the condyle of the mandible and the squamous portion of the temporal bone. The articular surface of the temporal bone is formed by the articular eminence anteriorly and the glenoid fossa posteriorly. The articular surface of the mandible consists of the top of the condyle. The surfaces are separated by an articular disk, the meniscus. The joint meniscus is made of fibrocartilage and is important for smooth joint function. The meniscus has a thick anterior band, a thin intermediate zone, and a thick posterior band; pathologic changes can contribute to TMJ disorders. A dense fibrous capsule surrounds the joint. Joint motion involves both a rotational component and a sliding translational component.

◆ Epidemiology

TMJ disease is more common in women, with a female-to-male ratio of 4:1. The highest incidence is among young adults, aged 20 to 40 years. The disorder is seen more frequently in persons of European descent than in persons of African descent.

◆ Clinical

Signs and Symptoms

Signs and symptoms include TMJ pain, earache, joint popping, joint locking, crepitus, tenderness, and spasm of the mastication muscles. Headache, neck ache, and tooth sensitivity are common. A history of poor sleep or other sleep disorders is common.

Differential Diagnosis

For patients presenting with complaints in the TMJ region, important considerations, in addition to TMJ disorders, include disease involving the ear, such as otitis externa or otitis media, and sources of referred otalgia such as malignancy of the larynx or pharynx. TMJ disorders may be related to rheumatoid arthritis, degenerative joint disease, ankylosis, dislocations, infections, congenital anomalies, and neoplasm. Dental malocclusion, jaw clenching, bruxism, increased pain sensitivity, and stress and anxiety should be considered. TMJ disorders may be mistaken for migraine, or these may be concurrent disorders.

◆ Evaluation

History

As in other areas, a careful history is important to guide the clinical assessment. Particular attention to prior dental problems, dental procedures, and head and neck injuries is important. Prior diagnosis of psychologic disorders, chronic pain, migraine, or other headache disorders should be noted. A detailed, accurate medication list is required, with attention to chronic analgesic or anxiety medication use.

Physical Exam

A full head and neck examination is performed. It is necessary to assess for evidence of active otologic disease, which could be a source of pain. Also, it is important to visualize the pharynx and larynx to exclude an obvious lesion that could be a source of referred pain. Assess for dental malocclusion, abnormal dental wear, absent teeth, and visible clenching or spasm of the ipsilateral neck muscles. Evaluate jaw motion, which may be reduced in TMJ disease. Normal range of motion for opening is 5 cm. The joint should be palpated, inferior to the zygomatic arch 1 to 2 cm anterior to the tragus, in both open and closed positions. The examiner should feel for muscle spasm, muscle or joint tenderness, crepitance, and limitation of joint motion or asymmetry of motion between sides.

Imaging

CT can provide information on degenerative changes, bony irregularity of the joint, erosions, and fractures. MRI can provide detailed evidence of soft tissue derangements, particularly of the articular cartilage. Imaging is recommended prior to consideration of surgery.

Pathology

Two categories of TMJ disease exist:

1. *Myogenous temporomandibular disease:* Muscular hyperactivity and dysfunction due to dental malocclusion. Psychological factors may be contributory, such as anxiety leading to habitual clenching of the jaw. Factors contributing to muscle spasm include malocclusion, jaw clenching, bruxism, increased pain sensitivity, personality disorders, stress and anxiety, and a history of trauma.
2. *Articular temporomandibular disease:* Joint dysfunction related either to (a) displacement of the meniscus disk or (b) diseases causing degenerative changes to the joint anatomy. Meniscus displacement is the most common cause. Abnormal anterior displacement of the posterior band between the condyle and the eminence leads to signs and symptoms. Muscular hyperactivity/spasm in this situation is secondary. Conditions causing degenerative changes to the joint anatomy include rheumatoid arthritis, degenerative joint disease, ankylosis, dislocations, infections, trauma, congenital anomalies, and neoplasm.

◆ Treatment Options

Medical

Most patients can be managed with conservative treatment, involving joint rest, anti-inflammatories, muscle relaxants, dental occlusal splints/nightguards. Joint rest is achieved with the use of a soft diet and the avoidance of chewing gum. Nightguard splints can be fashioned using dental impressions and will likely reduce nighttime bruxism and masticator muscle clenching.

The main goal of physical therapy is to stabilize the joint and restore mobility, strength, endurance, and function. Modalities include relaxation training, friction massage, and ultrasonic treatment.

Relevant Pharmacology

- Antiinflammatory medication for 4 weeks, then taper:
  - Ibuprofen 200 to 400 mg orally every 4 to 6 hours; not to exceed 3.2 g/d
  - Naproxen 500 mg orally, followed by 250 mg every 6 to 8 hours; not to exceed 1.25 g/d
- Muscle relaxants:
  - Cyclobenzaprine (Flexeril, Ortho-McNeil-Jansson Pharmaceuticals, Titusville, NJ) 20 to 40 mg/d orally divided into two or four doses; not to exceed 60 mg/d
  - Diazepam (Valium, Roche Pharmaceuticals, Nutley, NJ) for mild spasms: 5 to 10 mg PO every 4 to 6 hours as needed
  - Adverse effects include sedation, depression, and addiction.
- Other:
  - OnabotulinumtoxinA (Botox, Allergan, Dublin, Ireland) has been injected to reduce muscle spasm.

Surgical

- Absolute indications: tumor, severe ankylosis
- Relative indications: failed conservative management

Arthrocentesis

Arthrocentesis is a minimally invasive procedure, usually performed under either IV sedation or general anesthesia. A 22-gauge needle is inserted in the superior joint space, and a small amount of saline is injected to distend the joint space, after which the fluid is withdrawn and evaluated. With reinjection, the joint is then lavaged; steroids and/or local anesthetics can be injected into the joint space.

Arthroscopic Surgery

Indications include internal derangements, adhesions, fibrosis, and degenerative disk changes. Arthroscopic lysis and lavage can be a minimally invasive alternative to open procedures.

Arthroplasty

Arthroplasty is open TMJ surgery, including disk repositioning, discectomy, and joint replacement. Disk repositioning is used when the meniscus has become displaced. Under general anesthesia, an incision is made to access the joint, and the displaced disk is repositioned with or without plication. Repair of surrounding ligaments may be required.

Discectomy is indicated for TMJ internal derangement involving disk position and integrity; it is typically done as an open procedure under general anesthesia.

In cases of articular eminence anatomic derangement, articular eminence contouring, a procedure to reduce and smooth the articular eminence, may be indicated.

If TMJ damage cannot be repaired, the patient may be a candidate for removal and replacement of part or all of the TMJ components. Conditions requiring surgery may include severe degenerative disease, congenitally deformed TMJs, and advanced rheumatoid arthritis. Options for a partial joint replacement are (a) articular fossa replacement and (b) mandibular condyle replacement using either autologous bone, such as a rib, or a metal prosthesis. In a total joint procedure, the condyle and fossa are both replaced using prosthetic components.

Complications

A mandible dislocation may occur iatrogenically, typically during intubation, the use of a mouth prop during oral cavity and oropharyngeal surgery, or endoscopy. Typically the condylar head is dislocated anteriorly and sits anterior to the articular eminence. Typically, the jaw can be relocated manually. Support the head. If the patient is awake, give diazepam and consider morphine to provide relaxation and analgesia of muscle spasm so as to permit reduction. Place thumbs behind the last molar on either side of the mandible and grasp the inferior surface of the mandible with fingers on each side. Exert downward pressure on the lower molars to free the condyle from its entrapped position anterior to the articular eminence. Ease the mandible posteriorly to return it to its anatomic position. The teeth should close rapidly.

◆ Outcome and Follow-Up

In most cases the prognosis is good, and patients respond to conservative management. Surgical outcomes tend to be favorable in properly selected cases.

1.6 Geriatric Otolaryngology

◆ Key Features

- The elderly population is expanding rapidly worldwide.
- The elderly often present with multiple comorbidities.
- Disease presentation in the elderly may be atypical.
- For safe performance of surgery in the elderly, thorough preoperative management is important.

◆ Epidemiology

The proportion of the U.S. population aged 65 and older is predicted to expand from 12.4% in 2000 to 19.6% (or 71 million persons) in 2030. Moreover, the over-80 age group is expected to expand from 9.3 million

Table 1.5 General approach to the elderly patient

History of present illness: Patient may be a poor historian; obtain primary care records if possible.
Medications: Obtain accurate current medication list; consider polypharmacy issues.
Social: DNR status; end-of-life care wishes, advance directives; tobacco and alcohol use; functional status; elder neglect and abuse.
Preoperative: Careful consideration of risk factors. Testing including CBC, PT, PTT, BMP, chest X-ray, 12-lead ECG. Consider cardiac echo or stress test if risk factors.
Anesthesia: Consider local, local with IV sedation, versus general.
Examination: Ancillary testing to consider: audiology, VNG study, videostroboscopy, modified barium swallow.

Abbreviations : DNR, do not resuscitate; CBC, complete blood count; PT, prothrombin time; PTT, partial thromboplastin time; BMP, basic metabolic panel; ECG, electrocardiogram; IV, intravenous; VNG, videonystagmographic.

persons to 19.5 million by 2030. Many diseases affecting the elderly involve otorhinolaryngologic care. Comorbidities such as cardiovascular disease, renal disease, and polypharmacy may increase the complexity of safe and effective medical and surgical care for these patients.

◆ Clinical

The clinical approach to the geriatric otolaryngology patient should follow the same general organization as is used for other patients. However, certain areas of the evaluation require specific attention (**Table 1.5**), as discussed in the Evaluation section.

Diseases

Several aspects of otolaryngology—head and neck surgery are directly impacted by aging. Age-related changes may affect hearing, balance, voice, swallowing, nutrition, olfaction, sleep quality, and cosmetic concerns. Many head and neck neoplasms also have an increased incidence with advanced age. A consideration of some common conditions, by area, follows.

Otology
- Ceruminosis
- Serous otitis
- Presbycusis
- Tinnitus
- Balance dysfunction
  - Benign paroxysmal positional vertigo (BPPV)
  - Ménière's disease

o Medication side effects
o Nonvestibular dizziness (related to loss of sensation, proprioception, neuromuscular coordination)

Rhinology
- Presbyosmia
- Rhinitis
- Epistaxis
- Sinusitis
- Nasal obstruction from structural collapse (e.g., ptosis, valve collapse)

Laryngology and Oropharyngeal
- Presbylarynx
- Neurolaryngeal disorders
- Xerostomia
- Dysphagia
- Aspiration
- Reflux

Endocrine
- Hyperparathyroidism with osteopenia
- Thyroid disorders or malignancy

Head and Neck
- Upper aerodigestive tract malignancy
- Parotid neoplasm
- Cutaneous malignancies of the head and neck

◆ Evaluation

History

Obtaining a good history from a debilitated, chronically ill elderly patient or a patient suffering from dementia may be difficult. If possible, input from a close relative or friend may be helpful. In addition, the primary care provider (PCP) and/or facility (e.g., nursing home) records should be obtained. For instance, the patient may be unable to state how long a lump has been present, but knowledge of the duration or growth rate of a mass will have a direct impact upon how the mass will or will not be evaluated. Previous medical or surgical treatments for the current problem might be unknown to the patient but are of great relevance. The same is true of previous testing or evaluation, such as laboratories or imaging. The general past medical and surgical history should be thorough; again, PCP records should be sought. It is not uncommon for the elderly patient to forget to mention important facts, such as the presence of a pacemaker, that are crucial to consider when planning procedures such as surgery or an MRI scan.

Medication History

The importance of obtaining an accurate, current medication list cannot be overstated. Medication reconciliation, or ensuring that pretreatment, current treatment, and posttreatment medication lists are accurate, has become an issue of great importance to regulation bodies such as the Joint Commission because of emerging data regarding the consequences and frequency of medication errors. Fortunately, the growing use of electronic medical records is making legible and detailed medication lists more rapidly available. In the elderly, polypharmacy is a widespread problem. Complaints such as dysequilibrium, xerostomia, dysphagia, dyspepsia, and parosmias can be a consequence of medication side effects. This should be considered during the assessment of the elderly. Also, when surgical therapy is being considered, the accurate medication list is critical. The use of cardiac medications such as β-blockers must be considered perioperatively in accordance with current (rapidly evolving) guidelines. Medications such as warfarin, aspirin, rivaroxaban, or clopidogrel must be considered regarding potential risks associated with holding medications preoperatively. Herbs, nutritional supplements, and any complementary and alternative medicine treatments should not be overlooked.

Social History

A key factor to consider when treating elderly patients involves a consideration of end-of-life care wishes. Often the otolaryngologist is not directly involved in these time-consuming and emotional conversations, which may involve multiple family members, close friends, and clergy. Ideally, the PCP can and should address these issues with clearly written documentation. When considering surgical intervention in the elderly, one should be sure that advanced directives have been discussed and properly documented.

Physical Exam

The head and neck exam in the elderly patient does not, in general, differ from that in the general population. There are some generalizations to consider. The incidence of presbycusis or other forms of hearing loss is such that most geriatric patients should be considered for screening audiologic assessment. The incidence of hyposmia in the geriatric group, especially the over-80 group, is exceedingly high. The use of videostroboscopy in the geriatric patient with voice complaints can be of great value in elucidating stiffness and atrophic or other subtle vocal fold changes, thus facilitating appropriate voice rehabilitation choices. Although the otolaryngologist does not generally focus on the physical exam outside of the head and neck, the ability to examine briefly for obvious signs of congestive heart failure, such as peripheral edema or jugular venous distention (JVD), may prompt appropriate preoperative testing.

Review of Systems

Review of systems is especially important in stratifying preoperative risk. Angina, dyspnea on exertion, chronic renal disease, liver failure, and

Table 1.6   Conditions used to identify patients at risk for increased perioperative morbidity and mortality

Cardiovascular: Coronary artery disease, congestive heart failure, presence of arrhythmias, peripheral vascular disease, severe hypertension, recent MI **Respiratory:** Smoking history >20 pack-years, morbid obesity, preexisting pulmonary disease, PO_2 <60 or PCO_2 >50 **Renal:** Renal insufficiency (BUN >50, creatinine >3.0) **Hepatic:** Cirrhosis, hepatitis **Endocrine:** Diabetes mellitus, hyperthyroidism or hypothyroidism, chronic steroid therapy **Hematologic:** Coagulopathy, anemia, thrombocytopenia **General:** Age >70, bedridden/debilitated, malnutrition, emergency surgery

Abbreviations: MI, myocardial infarction; BUN, blood urea nitrogen.

severe chronic obstructive pulmonary disease (COPD) all must be factored in when considering surgery. General surgeons traditionally have used classifications such as the Goldman criteria to consider major surgical risk factors (**Table 1.6**). An important factor to assess in the elderly is the frailty factor. Frailty is the decline in the cognitive and physical state with reduced physiologic reserve over multiple organ systems. It is not a disease or syndrome but rather a variable state of illness and functional status. Frailty can be a strong predicator of adverse postoperative morbidity and mortality, as well as a predictor for the need of long-term institutionalization. Multiple frailty indexes have been proposed, with most focusing on factors such as fatigue, weight loss, comorbid illnesses, and restrictions on normal ambulation.

It has been stated that "there is nothing like an operation or an injury to bring a patient up to chronological age." The elderly patient with potentially limited reserve, impaired organ function, and/or polypharmacy requires particular attention, especially when considering surgical intervention. The reader is directed to resources from the recently formed American Society of Geriatric Otolaryngology (ASGO); for mission, meeting, membership, and other information about ASGO, go to www.geriatricotolaryngology.com. Also, consult the online e-book from the American Academy of Otolaryngology–Head and Neck Surgery Foundation, *Geriatric Care Otolaryngology,* at www.entnet.org. As the aging population expands, and economic and physician workforce issues evolve, there is likely to be increasing need for practicing otolaryngologists to provide appropriate and efficient geriatric care.

1.7 Lasers in Otolaryngology

◆ Key Features

- The carbon dioxide (CO_2) laser is the most commonly used laser in otolaryngology–head and neck surgery and facial plastic surgery.
- Complications of laser surgery include eye damage, airway fire, and infection via smoke plume.

Surgical management of the head and neck has some distinctive features. Access to specific areas may be restricted by limiting anatomy. Many types of disorders involve highly vascular tissues or pathology. Lasers are tools that are adaptable to certain of the necessary surgical procedures in these regions. Use of lasers has some advantages regarding hemostasis. The energy in the laser beam exists as focused light and may be used for diagnostic and therapeutic interventions.

◆ Laser Biophysics

The word "laser" was originally an acronym for Light Amplification by Stimulated Emission of Radiation. A laser contains a substance called the *lasing medium*, which a power source *excites* by pumping energy into it. The medium releases this energy in the form of light at a uniform wavelength (frequency) that is *coherent*, meaning that all the waves are in phase. As such, the laser provides a source of relatively uniform, concentrated power with predictable effects. The effects of laser light, applied to tissues, depend on several variables, including the specific targeted chromophore, competing chromophores, pulse duration, pulse frequency, pulse pattern, beam diameter, and depth of penetration. Furthermore, associated tissue cooling techniques can also alter the effects of the laser.

A *chromophore* is a substance that absorbs a specific wavelength of light. Some of the chromophores directly targeted by current laser technology include water, melanin, oxyhemoglobin, deoxyhemoglobin, and ink pigments. Lasers can also affect a competing chromophore; that is, something other than the targeted substance that also absorbs that particular wavelength. Depending on the goals of treatment, this may provide added benefit or may be undesirable. Laser wavelength selection is therefore key in order to generate the desired tissue effect.

When using lasers, it is important to consider how far the laser energy travels inside the treated tissues. This depth effect is important to consider because the laser beam might fail to reach its target or might reach well beyond its target. The actual depth of laser penetration depends on multiple factors including, but not limited to, the laser wavelength, the beam diameter, tissue characteristics (e.g., presence or absence of chromophore), and the amount of scatter. Relative scatter can also vary depending on the diameter of the laser beam.

In addition to the depth of penetration, the extent of associated tissue interactions is also related to *adjacent thermal effects*. Adjacent thermal effects can alter the effects of the laser treatment, beneficially (e.g., such as by stimulating neocollagen production in the heated tissues) or not. These effects can extend laterally within the horizontal plane of the treated tissues as well as deeper to these tissues. Adjacent thermal effects can vary depending on pulse duration, number of pulses, rate of energy absorption, sequencing, beam diameter, any associated cooling techniques, and whether the beam is passing through previously laser-treated tissues with secondarily altered characteristics, such as residual "char." For some lasers, residual char can act as a heat sink, increasing adjacent changes.

Fluence is the measure of the laser's energy per unit of area (usually reported in joules per square centimeter). This is an important measure for use in medicine. Typically, a certain amount of fluence is necessary to achieve a given effect. For some procedures, subthreshold fluence may provide no benefit. However, on other occasions "low-energy" lasers may be beneficial. Alternatively, excessive fluence can result in undesirable excessive thermal effects.

◆ Laser Applications

Specific laser applications in otolaryngology—head and neck surgery include:

- **General otolaryngology:** treatment of benign oral lesions, sleep medicine
- **Otology:** middle ear surgery, stapedotomy
- **Rhinology:** treatment of nasal polyposis, reduction of conchal hypertrophy, management of bleeding from the Kiesselbach area in chronic recurrent nasal bleeding, control of epistaxis in patients with hereditary hemorrhagic telangiectasia
- **Laryngology:** treatment of exudative lesions of the Reinke space, intracordal mucosal or epidermal cysts, sulcus vocalis, webs, recurrent respiratory papilloma, vocal fold vascular lesions/ectasias, laryngeal and tracheal stenosis, some laryngeal cancers
- **Facial plastic surgery:** treatment of vascular anomalies of the skin, facial skin rejuvenation, hair removal, pigment removal

Laser selection for a specific application will vary depending upon the desired effects and the laser characteristics. Optimal device selection for any application can be challenging because lasers are an evolving technology. As with all procedures in medicine, risk/benefit ratios should be considered. Only well-constructed studies can determine whether there is an optimal device for a given procedure.

◆ Types of Laser

The types of lasers commonly used in otolaryngology–head and neck surgery and facial plastic surgery are described in the following paragraphs and summarized in **Table 1.7**.

Carbon Dioxide Laser

The CO_2 laser is the most commonly used laser; it emits at 10.6 μm, in the (invisible) midinfrared region, with water being the primary tissue chromophore. A visible red helium-neon (HeNe) laser is accurately aligned with the

Table 1.7 Lasers commonly used in otolaryngology—head and neck surgery and facial plastic surgery

Laser type	Wavelength	Uses
Carbon dioxide	10,600 nm	Incision, vaporization, skin resurfacing
Holmium:YAG	2100 nm	Osseous and soft tissue ablation
Neodymium:YAG	1064 nm	Hair removal, vascular lesion ablation
KTP	532 nm	Vascular lesion ablation
Er:YAG	2940 nm	Skin resurfacing
Diode	635–2200 nm	Tissue ablation, photocoagulation
Argon	488 nm	Vascular lesion ablation
Dye	580–600 nm	Vascular lesion ablation, photodynamic therapy

CO_2 beam to act as an aiming beam. The CO_2 laser has excellent tissue-cutting properties with very little lateral tissue damage. The CO_2 laser integrates well with operating microscopes; however, its light cannot be propagated through a traditional fiber optic cable. There are some new hollow-core fibers that can be used to deliver a CO_2 laser beam in a flexible modality.

Holmium:Yttrium-Aluminum-Garnet (Ho:YAG) Laser

The Ho:YAG laser is a pulsed infrared laser with output at 2.1 μm (2100 nm). Its lasing medium is an yttrium-aluminum-garnet crystal doped with holmium. The laser is excited by a xenon arc flash lamp. It is used in nasal surgery and tonsillectomy. The Ho:YAG laser light can be propagated through a fiber optic cable.

Neodymium:Yttrium-Aluminum-Garnet (Nd:YAG) Laser

The Nd:YAG laser emits in the near infrared at 1064 nm; it is capable of vaporizing large volumes of tissue and is well suited for hemostasis by coagulation. The Nd:YAG laser light can be propagated through a fiber optic cable.

Potassium Titanyl Phosphate (KTP) Laser

A potassium titanyl phosphate (KTP) laser is a Nd:YAG laser that is frequency-doubled by passing the beam through a potassium titanyl phosphate (KTP) crystal. Doubling the frequency halves the wavelength (from 1064 nm to 532 nm), converting the infrared light to visible green light. The beam appears to be continuous but is in fact rapidly pulsed. A KTP laser integrates well with an operating microscope. A KTP laser beam can be propagated through a fiber optic cable.

Erbium:Yttrium-Aluminum-Garnet (Er:YAG) Laser

The Er:YAG laser's lasing medium is an yttrium-aluminum-garnet crystal doped with erbium; it emits at 2940 nm (an infrared wavelength that is strongly absorbed by water), which, like the CO_2 laser, requires hollow-core optical fibers. It is used for facial skin rejuvenation.

Diode Laser

The diode laser is an electronic device that consists of an array of semiconductor diode junctions as its lasing medium, excited by the electric current flowing through them. An emission in the far infrared at 810 μm is most suited for otolaryngologic applications. It can be used in both near-contact and contact mode (thermal effect).

Argon Laser

The argon laser produces a blue-green beam of light (several frequencies in the range 455–529 nm, especially 488 nm), which is selectively absorbed by red pigment. This characteristic of argon laser light has been successfully applied in the treatment of vascular anomalies of the skin, particularly portwine stains. Argon lasers spare epithelial tissue and photocoagulate subepithelial vascular tissue with little or no scarring.

Dye Laser

A dye laser is one that uses an organic dye as the lasing medium, usually in liquid form (compared with the gases or solids used as media in the lasers previously discussed), so that it may emit a wide range of appropriate wavelengths. It may be used for photodynamic therapy (PDT) of small cancers and premalignant conditions; it activates a hematoporphyrin derivative that is selectively retained by malignant tissues, causing destruction of the malignant cells with no damage to surrounding normal tissues.

◆ Laser Safety Considerations

Special complications of laser surgery include direct or indirect ocular exposure to laser irradiation, fire, explosion, or electric shock and transmission of infection via smoke plume or tissue spatter. Other complications include scarring or synechia (adhesion) surrounding tissue damage.

Whenever using a laser, it is important to follow the proper safety precautions. According to the U.S. Food and Drug Administration (FDA), the most common safety-related incidents associated with lasers are eye injuries. In general, laser light between the wavelengths of 380 and 1400 nm (visible to near infrared) can pass through the cornea and cause retinal injuries. Laser light of wavelengths longer than 1400 nm usually can cause injury to the cornea. To avoid eye injuries, it is important to wear protective eyewear designed for the wavelength that is being used. Eyewear that protects for one wavelength may not provide protection for another wavelength. All laser eyewear should be clearly labeled as to the laser wavelengths for which it provides protection. It is important that everyone in the laser room, including the patient, the physician, and any observers, wear proper protective eyewear. Both direct and reflected laser beams can be hazardous. Many lasers, such as the CO_2 laser, do not emit in the visible light spectrum yet still may cause ocular injury.

Lasers also present fire and skin hazards, which require specific precautions. Depending upon the laser being used and the area being treated, these may include but are not limited to limiting potentially flammable materials or substances near the laser, wetting surgical drapes, using laser-approved endotracheal tubes, and having water on the surgical table and an appropriate fire extinguisher available. In terms of potential flammability of surgical scrubs, prep solutions, and topical ointments, it is best to review the products' informational inserts and, if necessary, check with the manufacturer as to laser safety. Volatile agents such as alcohol and acetone should not be used to clean the skin for injections or skin prep prior to using a laser. Oxygen-rich environments can be created in body spaces, cavity lumen, and beneath drapes, increasing the risk of surgical fire. Surgical fires require fuel (e.g., drapes, hair, endotracheal tube, char), an oxidizer (e.g., oxygen, nitrous oxide, room air), and an ignition source (e.g., laser, electrosurgical unit, light sources). Taking care to control as many of these factors as possible is key to reducing fire risk.

If a laser produces a significant plume, then it is important to protect against potential biocontaminants. Currently, protection against airborne biocontaminants includes the use of both a smoke evacuator and appropriate surgical masks. It is important to keep the smoke evacuator within 2 cm of the source of the laser plume. The masks should have antiviral 0.3-μm (0.3-micron) filters.

1.8 Complementary and Alternative Otolaryngologic Medicine

◆ Key Features

- Patients often use complementary and alternative medicine (CAM); it is important to inquire about use.
- There is evidence that some CAM treatments may be effective for allergies, sinusitis, and bronchitis in certain cases.
- Nutritional supplements and herbal remedies should be avoided 2 weeks prior to elective surgery.
- The two editors of this book do not endorse the use of CAM but provide this information as a resource because many patients and physicians do use these treatments.

The use of complementary and alternative medicine (CAM) therapeutic modalities by patients is common in the United States and elsewhere. These may include traditional Chinese medicine including acupuncture, herbal medications, massage, chiropractic and osteopathic manipulations, Ayurvedic medicine, mind-body medicine, naturopathy, and homeopathy. As their use becomes more and more prevalent, more research on them is being performed. Otolaryngologic conditions for which patients may seek out CAM products include seasonal and perennial allergic rhinitis, acute and chronic rhinosinusitis, upper respiratory infections, head and neck cancer, tinnitus, and vertigo. Patients may be drawn to complements and alternatives to conventional medical therapies for various reasons, including (1) failure of the conventional medical therapy to treat a chronic medical condition, (2) perceived lack of potential side effects from a CAM modality, and (3) patient appreciation of the philosophy of the alternative practitioner regarding their treatment paradigm. Possible uses of CAM therapies are discussed here, organized by the otolaryngologic condition for which they have been advocated. As more high-quality research is done, there may be further evidence-based recommendations for novel therapies based on CAM practices.

◆ CAM for Allergic Rhinitis, Acute Sinusitis, and Asthma

The herb butterbur (*Petasites* spp.) contains the active ingredient petasin. This appears to act upon leukotrienes. The supplement Petadolex, standardized to 7.5 mg petasin, has been shown to be as effective as cetirizine hydrochloride for allergic rhinitis.

The use of probiotics (bacteria that are ingested in the form of a nutritional supplement to restore the normal gastrointestinal tract flora) has shown effectiveness in the prevention of seasonal allergic rhinitis symptoms.

A combination of herbs from traditional Chinese medicine (Reishi, shrubby Sophora, and Chinese licorice) has been advocated for asthma therapy in an effort to avoid systemic steroids. It is reported that both the herbal combination and prednisone improve FEV1 and decrease Th2 inflammatory cytokines; the herbal combination increases cortisol and interferon gamma levels, whereas prednisone has the opposite effect.

The African herb *Pelargonium sidoides* has been positively reviewed by the Cochrane Database for use in acute sinusitis and acute bacterial bronchitis. The report comments on "eight randomized clinical trials with acceptable methodologies. Two trials showed that *P. sidoides* was effective in relieving all symptoms, and in particular cough and sputum production in adults with acute bronchitis. . . . Similarly, *P. sidoides* was effective in resolving symptoms of acute bronchitis in two out of three pediatric studies. In acute sinusitis and the common cold *P. sidoides* was effective in resolving all symptoms including headaches and nasal discharge in adults when taken for an extended time period."

◆ CAM for Upper Respiratory Infections

In several double-blind placebo controlled trials, North American ginseng (*Panax quinquefolius*) has been found to be efficacious for influenza and common cold prevention.

Imu-Max (Ortho Molecular Products, Woodstock, IL), a proprietary blend of propolis, echinacea (*E. angustifolia* and *E. purpurea*), and vitamin C, is reported to be effective for cold prevention in children. Also, the use of milk fortified with probiotics was found to reduce the incidence of upper respiratory infections in children.

However, the Cochrane Database reviewed the use of echinacea and vitamin C for both cold prevention and treatment and found them both to be ineffective.

Oscillococcinum is used for influenza and meta-analysis indicates some reduction in duration of symptoms.

◆ CAM for Head and Neck Cancer

The prognoses for many head and neck cancers remain poor, and hence alternatives to the traditional therapies may be sought by the patient. While many chemotherapeutic agents have been derived from plants, no specific herbal medications have been shown to provide benefit in management of head and neck cancer.

Two areas of CAM which may have beneficial effect in this patient population are nutritional therapies and mind-body. Given the frequent limitations for proper nutrition in head and neck cancer patients (e.g. reduced ability to eat, coincident alcoholism) as well as cancer related cachexia, nutritional deficiencies are not uncommon. Dietary balance may be of benefit in restoring immune function and healing potentials. Depression is common in head and neck cancer, and mind-body techniques may serve as behavioral and psychological interventions which reduce psychological stress and improve immune function (natural killer cells).

◆ CAM for Tinnitus and Vertigo

Coenzyme Q_{10} supplementation in individuals with coenzyme Q_{10} deficiency and tinnitus has been reported to result in an improvement in tinnitus. Ginkgo biloba and acupuncture are ineffective in all studies for tinnitus treatment. Biofeedback is helpful in some patients.

A homeopathic remedy, Vertigoheel (Heel, Inc., Albuquerque, NM), is suggested to be as effective as betahistine hydrochloride for moderate vertigo. Cocculus indicus is an herb with some antivertigo benefits, likely through a GABA-ergic mechanism.

The Clinical Practice Guideline: Tinnitus, published by the American Academy of Otolaryngology–Head & Neck Surgery in 2014, recommended against the use of ginkgo biloba, melatonin, zinc, or other dietary supplements in the management of tinnitus, with either a concern over study methodology or a lack of preponderance of benefit over harm.

◆ Acupuncture

As with the rest of traditional Chinese medicine, acupuncture has been practiced for thousands of years. Its efficacy has been established for multiple medical conditions. The National Institutes of Health position paper on acupuncture supports its efficacy and use for seasonal allergic rhinitis and asthma.

◆ Herbal and Nutritional Supplements and Surgery

Many herbal and nutritional supplements interact with general anesthetics and with the coagulation system; therefore, all supplements and herbs should be avoided 2 weeks preoperatively (**Table 1.8**).

Homeopathic *Arnica montana* has not been found to be effective for hematoma prevention postoperatively.

◆ Dangerous CAM Practices

Ear candling is ineffective for cerumen removal and can result in severe burns. Ephedra (from the plant *Ephedra sinica*, known in traditional Chinese medicine as "ma huang") may cause arrhythmias and hypertension and was removed from the market by the FDA in 2004. High doses of licorice may elevate blood pressure and cause potassium depletion (deglycyrrhizinated licorice, or DGL, does not cause these side effects).

Herbal agents do not have strict federal standards for dosing and purity as in allopathic medications. Therefore quality and consistency cannot be assured in some cases.

CAM options are being used by many patients, and physicians should solicit that information from them. This allows for a frank discussion of options and improve the safe use of CAM in combination with proven therapeutic interventions. Patients need to be aware of the risk of some CAM techniques and that "natural" does not denote inherent safety. Engaging patients in their own care, both traditional and CAM, may improve outcomes and patient satisfaction.

Table 1.8   Herbal and nutritional supplements and surgery

Herbal supplements and vitamins known or suspected to increase bleeding risk
Ginkgo biloba Garlic Ginseng Fish oil Dong quai Black cohosh Glucosamine/chondroitin Feverfew Vitamin E
Supplements with sedating effects that may prolong effects of anesthesia
Kava St. John's wort Valerian root
Supplements with cardiovascular effects
Ephedra Hoodia Garlic
Supplements with drug interactions
Licorice St. John's wort Kava Valerian Echinacea Goldenseal

2 Perioperative Care and Anesthesia for the Otolaryngology–Head and Neck Surgery Patient

Section Editor

Wayne Pearce

Contributors

David Goldenberg

Bradley J. Goldstein

Gregory L. Craft

Ron Mitzner

Wayne Pearce

Rafael Antonio Portela

2 0 Preoperative Assessment

The aims of the Preoperative Assessment are risk stratification and identifi-cation of medical conditions and their severity (**Table 2.1**). An additional goal is to ensure that medical management is optimized preoperatively. A review of medications, allergies, NPO (nothing by mouth) status (guidelines are summarized in **Table 2.2**), and previous experiences with anesthesia should be obtained. Laboratory and physiologic tests and screens can be ordered and reviewed prior to surgery. The American Society of Anesthesiologists (ASA) physical status classification (**Table 2.3**) stratifies patient risk associ-ated with general anesthesia based on physical status and existing diagnoses (it is not differentiated by type of operation or patient age).

Table 2.1 Preoperative assessment

System	Assessment
Cardiac	Does the patient have hypertension, congestive heart failure, or coronary artery disease? What medications are currently prescribed? Does the cardiac status prohibit the patient from achieving 5 METS (up flight of stairs) without shortness of breath? Review of recent (past-month) ECG for patients older than 45 or those with symptoms Review of cardiac notes and tests
Respiratory	Does the patient have asthma, COPD, OSA, or reactive airway disease? Is the patient on medications, home oxygen, or a CPAP device? Is the patient a smoker? Does the patient have shortness of breath related to pulmonary conditions? Review of PFTs, sleep studies, and pulmonary notes
Metabolic	Does the patient have diabetes mellitus or thyroid disease? Are these conditions optimized? What medications is the patient currently taking?
NPO status	Has the patient followed the ASA NPO guidelines? (see also **Table 1.3**)
Alcohol/substance abuse/chronic pain	Does the patient have substance abuse issues that will interact with the pharmacology of an anesthetic? Will postoperative pain management be complicated by existing opioid dependence? Has alcohol or drug abuse contributed to organ dysfunction?

Abbreviations: ASA, American Society of Anesthesiologists; CPAP, continuous positive airway pressure; COPD, chronic obstructive pulmonary disease; ECG, electrocardiogram; METS, metabolic equivalents (of oxygen consumption); NPO, nothing by mouth; OSA, obstructive sleep apnea; PFT, pulmonary function test.

Table 2.2   American Society of Anesthesiologists NPO guidelines

Ingested material (unlimited quantity)	Fasting period before anesthesia/ procedure begins (minimum time)
Water and clear liquids	2 hours
Infant formula/Nonhuman milk	6 hours
All other liquids and/or a light meal[1]	6 hours
Breast milk	4 hours
Postpyloric feedings (J-tube)	Do not stop
Gastric (G-tube) feedings	6 hours
Full meal[2]	8 hours

1. *Similar to toast and a clear liquid.*
2. *Includes meats, fried and/or fatty foods.*
Abbreviations: NPO, nothing by mouth.

Table 2.3   American Society of Anesthesiologists (ASA) Physical Status Classification System

ASA Class	Definition
1	Patient has no organic, physiologic, biochemical, or psychiatric disturbance. The pathologic process for which the procedure is to be performed is localized and does not entail systemic disturbance.
2	Patient has mild to moderate systemic disturbance caused either by the condition to be treated surgically or by other pathophysiologic processes.
3	Patient has severe systemic disturbance or disease; variable degree of disability.
4	Patient has severe systemic disorders that may be life-threatening, not always correctable by operation.
5	Seriously ill patient has little chance of survival but has submitted to the operation in desperation.
6	Patient has met brain death criteria and is undergoing organ procurement.

2.1   Airway Assessment and Management

All forms of surgery in the head and neck region require consideration of airway management, maintenance of ventilation with an adequate form of anesthesia, and prevention of concentration of oxygen in the operative field in the presence of cautery or laser. Various forms of airway management are discussed in the following paragraphs, considering anatomy, innervation, indications, instrumentation and equipment, and clinical context. The specific situation of the difficult airway is then discussed.

◆ Airway Anatomy

There are two physiologic entry points to the airway: the nose and the mouth. The epiglottis, located at the base of the tongue, separates the oro-pharynx from the hypopharynx. The larynx is made up of a cartilaginous structure supported by muscles and ligaments.

Innervation

The sensory innervation above the epiglottis is provided by the trigeminal nerve (cranial nerve V, abbreviated CN V) and the glossopharyngeal nerve (CN IX); below the epiglottis, by the superior laryngeal and recurrent laryngeal branches of the vagus nerve (CN X). For more information on the cranial nerves, see **Appendix B**.

- Nasal mucosa: by the pterygopalatine ganglion branch of the middle (maxillary) division of the trigeminal nerve (CN V$_2$)
- Posterior pharynx (including uvula and tonsils): by the continued branches from the pterygopalatine ganglion
- Oropharynx and supraglottic area: by the glossopharyngeal nerve; branches of this nerve include the lingual, pharyngeal, and tonsillar branches
- Trachea: by the recurrent laryngeal nerve
- Larynx: sensory and motor innervation from the vagus nerve
  - Sensory: above the vocal folds, innervation is supplied by the internal branch of the superior laryngeal nerve; below the vocal folds, by the recurrent laryngeal nerve.
  - Motor: all muscles are supplied by the recurrent laryngeal nerve except for the cricothyroid muscle, which is supplied by the external branch of the superior laryngeal nerve.

◆ Airway Equipment

Oral and Nasal Airways

In anesthetized patients, loss of airway tone allows the tongue and epiglottis to contact the posterior pharyngeal tissue, leading to obstruction. Artificial airway devices can be placed in the nose or mouth to provide an air passage. Nasal airways carry a risk of epistaxis and should be avoided in anticoagulated patients. These devices should also be avoided in patients with basilar skull fractures to avoid intracranial penetration of the airway device. If an airway device is indicated in a lightly anesthetized patient, the nasal route is generally tolerated better.

Facemasks

The facemask is designed to contour and conform to a variety of facial features, with the intention of creating an airtight seal capable of delivering gases from the anesthesia equipment.

Laryngoscopes

The intubating laryngoscopes most commonly used by the anesthesiology team have curved (Macintosh) or straight (Miller) blades and an open-blade design. Newer fiberoptic video rigid laryngoscopes are useful, such as the GlideScope (Diagnostic Ultrasound Corporation, Bothell, WA). There are a variety of operative laryngoscopes that may be useful for intubation, such as the Holinger or Dedo laryngoscope.

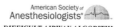

DIFFICULT AIRWAY ALGORITHM

1. **Assess the likelihood and clinical impact of basic management problems:**
   - **Difficulty with patient cooperation or consent**
   - **Difficult mask ventilation**
   - **Difficult supraglottic airway placement**
   - **Difficult laryngoscopy**
   - **Difficult intubation**
   - **Difficult surgical airway access**

2. **Actively pursue opportunities to deliver supplemental oxygen throughout the process of difficult airway management.**

3. **Consider the relative merits and feasibility of basic management choices:**
   - **Awake intubation vs. intubation after induction of general anesthesia**
   - **Non-invasive technique vs. invasive techniques for the initial approach to intubation**
   - **Video-assisted laryngoscopy as an initial approach to intubation**
   - **Preservation vs. ablation of spontaneous ventilation**

4. **Develop primary and alternative strategies:**

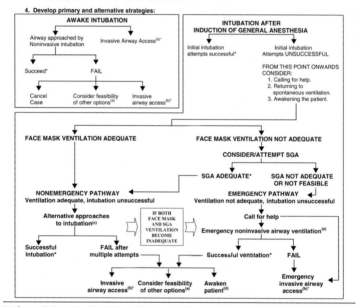

*Confirm ventilation, tracheal intubation, or LMA placement with exhaled CO2.

a Other options include (but are not limited to): surgery utilizing face mask or LMA anesthesia, local anesthesia infiltration, and regional nerve blockade. Pursuit of these options usually implies that mask ventilation will not be problematic. Therefore, these options may be of limited value if this step in the algorithm has been reached via the Emergency Pathway.

b Invasive airway access includes surgical or percutaneous tracheotomy or cricothyrotomy.

c Alternative noninvasive approaches to difficult intubation include (but are not limited to): use of different laryngoscope blades, LMA as an intubation conduit (with or without fiberoptic guidance), fiberoptic intubation, intubating stylet or tube changer, light wand, retrograde intubation, and blind oral or nasal intubation.

d Consider repreparation of the patient for awake intubation or canceling surgery.

e Options for emergency noninvasive airway ventilation include (but are not limited to): rigid bronchoscope, esophageal-tracheal Combitube ventilation, and transtracheal jet ventilation.

Fig. 2.1 The American Society of Anesthesiologists (ASA) Difficult Airway Algorithm (DAA). (Used with permission from Apfelbaum JL, Hagberg, CA, Caplan RA, et al. Practice guidelines for management of the difficult airway: an updated report by the American Society of Anesthesiologists Difficult Airway Algorithm (ASA DAA). Anesthesiology 2013;118:251-270.)

◆ Airway Assessment

A complete airway examination looks at several aspects of the airway. It would be important to take note of difficulty with patient cooperation or consent or of the appropriateness of, or difficulty with, supraglottic airway placement, as well as difficult surgical airway access (see revised ASA Difficult Airway Algorithm [DAA], **Fig. 2.1**). There is a population of patients where the clinical examination belies the extent of their disease. However, the first priority is to identify patients who may be difficult to mask-ventilate or intubate. This is critically important: induction of general anesthesia without subsequently being able to ventilate the patient adequately is an acute, life-threatening emergency. Thus, identification of a patient with a potentially difficult airway before induction will enable the operative and anesthetic team to institute an appropriate plan and backup plans and to assemble and test airway equipment ahead of time.

- **Mallampati classification:** Used to predict the ease of intubation by looking at the anatomy of the oral cavity while the patient is sitting upright in the neutral position (**Fig. 2.2**).
- **Thyromental distance:** Measured from the upper edge of the thyroid cartilage to the chin with head in full extension. A short thyromental distance (< 6 cm) equates with an anterior (superior) laryngeal position that is at a more acute angle, which makes the larynx difficult to visualize via direct laryngoscopy. It is a relatively unreliable test unless combined with other tests.
- **Mouth opening:** Less than two finger-widths of mouth opening (trismus) suggests difficulty with intubation.
- **Cervical spine movements:** Mobility of the atlantooccipital and atlantoaxial joints may be assessed by asking the patient to extend the head while the neck is in flexion. Extension of the head with atlantoaxial joint immobility results in greater cervical spine convexity, which pushes the larynx anteriorly and impairs laryngoscopic view.

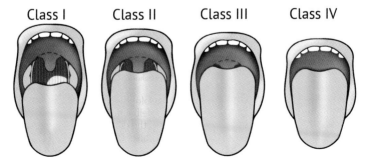

Fig. 2.2 The Mallampati classification of oral opening. Class 1: visualization of soft palate, hard palate, uvula, and tonsillar pillars. Class 2: visualization of soft palate, hard palate, and portion of uvula. Class 3: visualization of soft palate, hard palate, and base of uvula. Class 4: visualization of hard palate only.

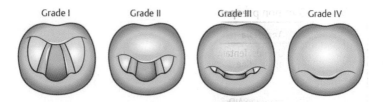

Fig. 2.3 Cormack and Lehane grades. Grade I: visualization of entire laryngeal aperture. Grade II: visualization of posterior part of the laryngeal aperture. Grade III: visualization of epiglottis only. Grade IV: not even the epiglottis is visible. (Used with permission from Bernal-Sprekelsen M, Vilaseca I, eds. *Transoral Laser Microsurgery of Benign and Malignant Lesions*. Stuttgart: Thieme, 2016:27.)

- **Temporomandibular joint (TMJ) mobility:** Assessed by asking the patient to protrude the jaw while sitting up in the neutral position. Decreased mobility suggests greater difficulty with intubation.
  - ○ Grade A: Lower incisors in front of upper incisors (good mobility)
  - ○ Grade B: Lower incisors up to upper incisors
  - ○ Grade C: Lower incisors cannot be protruded to touch upper incisors (poor mobility).
- **Cormack and Lehane grade:** Used to classify the view on direct laryngoscopy. Previous documentation of laryngoscopy should include the grade of glottic view (**Fig. 2.3**).
- **Preoperative Endoscopic Airway Evaluation:** An airway evaluation technique that is readily available, is minimally invasive, and may provide enough information to reduce the use of awake intubation. The information sought by the anesthesiologist from this examination differs from that sought by the surgeon. The surgeon is interested in the extent and location of disease, the degree of preservation of function, and whether immediate intervention is required. The anesthesiologist wants to know whether there is sagittal plane access to the larynx, whether there are lesions that might interfere with supraglottic airway placement (such as an LMA), and whether there are lesions in the anterior part of the glottic opening that may be damaged by traditional laryngoscopy.

◆ Preoperative Medication

Medications are often administered preoperatively to alleviate anxiety, to provide analgesia, or as aspiration prophylaxis (**Table 2.4**).

◆ Airway Management

Endotracheal Intubation

Indications for Endotracheal Intubation

- Need for protection from aspiration
- Altered level of consciousness (Glasgow Coma Score [GCS] score <8)

Table 2.4 Common preoperative medications

Anxiolysis	Analgesia	Aspiration prophylaxis
Diazepam	Opioids: fentanyl, morphine, meperidine	Bicitra
Midazolam		Metoclopramide
Lorazepam	Nonsteroidal antiinflammatory drugs (NSAIDs)	Famotidine
	COX2 inhibitors	
	Acetaminophen	
	Gabapentin	

- Respiratory distress
- Severe pulmonary or multiorgan failure
- Facilitation of positive pressure ventilation
- Operative position other than supine
- Operative site involving the upper airway
- Disease involving the upper airway
- One-lung ventilation

Confirmation of Endotracheal Intubation

- Direct visualization of endotracheal tube passing between the vocal folds
- Carbon dioxide present in exhaled gases in at least four consecutive breaths (positive end-tidal CO_2)
- Bilateral breath sounds
- Absence of air entry during epigastric auscultation
- Condensation of water vapor in endotracheal tube (ETT) during exhalation
- Maintenance of arterial oxygenation
- Chest X-ray with tip of ETT between the carina and thoracic inlet

Endotracheal Tube Size Recommendations

- ETT size (mm): Age/4 + 4 for patients >2 years old.
- Length of insertion: 12 + Age/2. Add 2 to 3 cm for nasal intubation.
- Pediatrics: Uncuffed ETTs are generally used in patients <8 years old.

Types of Endotracheal Tube

● *Ring-Adair-Elwyn endotracheal tubes.* Ring-Adair-Elwyn (RAE) endotracheal tubes are preformed to fit in the nose or mouth and are commonly used in oral or pharyngeal surgery, particularly adenoidectomy or tonsillectomy. The shape prevents obstruction of the surgical field and fits surgical retractors such as the Crow-Davis retractor.

● *Armored endotracheal tubes.* These tubes are commonly used in head and neck surgery. They prevent kinking of the tube when the head is manipulated. This tube works well through a tracheotomy, as it can be curved inferiorly out of the surgical field without kinking and sutured in place temporarily.

● *Laser-resistant endotracheal tubes.* Laser-resistant ETTs are used in laser surgery, particularly treatment of laryngeal lesions. By preventing an interaction of inhaled oxygen with the laser, these tubes help prevent airway fires. The portion of the tube beyond the cuff(s) without laser-resistant metal wrap is flammable, and conflagration can still ensue if the laser breaches the barrier constituted by the cuff(s) and saline-soaked blocking pledgets and enters an oxygen-enriched tracheal environment.

● *Nerve-monitoring endotracheal tubes.* For thyroid and parathyroid surgery, a tube with contact electromyographic electrodes positioned at the level of the vocal folds permits intraoperative monitoring of recurrent laryngeal nerve integrity.

◆ Endotracheal Intubation Procedure

● Preoperative evaluation will help determine the route (oral vs. nasal) and method (awake vs. anesthetized) for tracheal intubation.
● Equipment: laryngoscope with working light, appropriate-sized ETTs, oxygen supply, functioning suction catheter, functioning intravenous (IV) line, and anesthetic medications.
● Cricoid pressure: an assistant's thumb and forefinger depress the cricoid cartilage downward, compressing the esophagus against the underlying vertebral body. This prevents spillage of gastric contents into the pharynx during the period of time from induction of unconsciousness to placement of the ETT in the trachea.
● Induction of anesthesia can be achieved by using IV or inhaled agents.

◆ Endotracheal Intubation Complications

During intubation, possible complications include aspiration, dental damage, laceration of lips/gingiva/palate, laryngeal injury, esophageal intubation, endobronchial intubation, bronchospasm, and activation of sympathetic nervous system (elevated heart rate [HR] and blood pressure [BP]).

After intubation, possible complications include aspiration, laryngospasm, transient vocal fold incompetence, pharyngitis, and tracheitis.

Orotracheal Intubation

If there is no history of cervical spine instability, the patient's head is extended into a "sniffing" position. This position aligns the oral, pharyngeal, and laryngeal axes such that the passage from the lips to the glottic opening is a straight line. The height of the operating room (OR) table should be manipulated so that the patient's head is at the level of the clinician's xiphoid cartilage (**Fig. 2.4**).

The laryngoscope is introduced into the right side of the mouth. Advancing the blade posteriorly and toward the midline, the tongue is displaced to the left. Check that the lower lip is not pinched between the blade and the incisors. Placement of blade depends on which style has been selected:

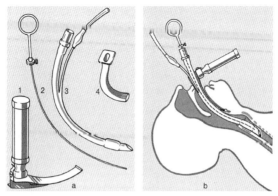

Fig. 2.4 Intubation. **(a)** Necessary instruments. 1, Macintosh laryngoscope; 2, stylette; 3, tube with cuff; 4, Guedel tube. **(b)** Introduction of the tube. (Used with permission from Becker W, Naumann HH, Pfaltz CR. *Ear, Nose, and Throat Diseases: A Pocket Reference*. 2nd ed. Stuttgart/New York: Thieme; 1994:450.)

- Macintosh (curved) blade: The tip of the blade is advanced until the tip enters the vallecula (the space between the epiglottis and the base of the tongue).
- Miller (straight) blade: The tip of the blade is passed below the laryngeal surface of the epiglottis, which is then lifted to expose the vocal folds.

Regardless of the blade selected, the laryngoscope is lifted upward and forward in the direction of the long axis of the handle. The upper incisors should *not* be used as a fulcrum for leverage, as this may damage teeth.

The vocal folds should be visualized prior to advancement of the ETT. Passing the ETT from the right, little resistance should be encountered. The balloon cuff of the ETT should pass 1 to 2 cm past the vocal folds. Once the proper position of the ETT is confirmed, it should be secured in place.

Nasotracheal Intubation

Prior to instrumentation, a vasoconstrictor (e.g., oxymetazoline) should be applied to nasal mucosa. After induction of anesthesia and mask ventilation is established, the ETT can be placed.

The naris and ETT should be generously lubricated. The tube can be softened by placing it in warm water prior to induction. The tube is placed in the nose parallel to the palate, aiming inferiorly to avoid skull base injury, until a loss of resistance is encountered, consistent with entrance into the pharynx.

Placement under direct visualization can be performed using a laryngoscope and McGill forceps to direct the ETT past the glottic opening. Alternately, a fiberoptic bronchoscope can be placed through the tube and directed past the vocal folds.

Rapid-Sequence Intubation

Indications include aspiration risk (full stomach, history of gastroesophageal reflux disease [GERD], pregnancy, trauma) in a patient who does not appear to be a difficult intubation on physical examination.

Nonparticulate antacids, H2 blockers, and metoclopramide can be administered to decrease the acidity and volume of gastric contents. As with a standard intubation already described, instrumentation should be prepared and available. Preoxygenation with 100% O_2 by mask for 3 to 5 minutes or 4 maximal breaths over 30 seconds is sufficient. Once the paralytic and induction agents are administered, no further ventilation is given.

Induction is accomplished with any induction agent, and the procedure is followed immediately with the administration of a paralytic agent. As the medications are being delivered, cricoid pressure should be applied. Succinylcholine (1–1.5 mg/kg), because of its speed of onset, is the drug of choice for rapid-sequence induction. As soon as jaw relaxation is present, intubation should be performed. Cricoid pressure should continue until tracheal placement of the ETT is verified.

Conscious Intubation

Indications include history of difficult intubation, acute infectious/inflammatory process that may involve the airway, mandibular fractures or other facial deformities, morbid obesity, and certain neoplasms involving the upper aerodigestive tract.

The indications and plan should be discussed with the patient. As with a standard intubation, all necessary equipment should be available and checked prior to induction. A backup plan should be formulated should intubation be difficult, such as the creation of a surgical airway.

Preparing the airway by decreasing secretions with an antisialagogue (glycopyrrolate 0.2 mg 30 minutes before intubation) will help with visualization. If the nasal route is desired, administer 4 drops of 0.25% phenylephrine to each naris to reduce bleeding. After standard monitors are placed, sedation with fentanyl, midazolam, low-dose ketamine, or dexmedetomidine should be considered.

Topical anesthesia can be achieved using topical agents or nerve blocks. Topical agents include lidocaine jelly, nebulized lidocaine, nasal cocaine, or Cetacaine (Cetylite Industries, Pennshauken, NJ) spray. Regional anesthesia, either alone or in combination with topical agents, is useful in conscious intubations. Each major nerve (as described previously under "Airway Anatomy") should be approached.

Fiberoptic-Assisted Tracheal Intubation

Indications for a fiberoptic-assisted tracheal intubation include upper airway obstruction, mediastinal mass, subglottic edema, congenital upper airway abnormalities, immobile cervical vertebrae, and confirmation of proper double lumen ETT placement.

Nasal Technique

After vasoconstriction and anesthetizing of the airway (see above), the ETT is advanced through the naris into the nasopharynx. The bronchoscope is then inserted into the ETT until the epiglottis and glottic opening are visualized. The scope is then passed through the opening until the carina is in view. As the carina is maintained in sight, the ETT is passed over the scope.

Oral Technique

A bite block should be inserted to protect the fiberoptic scope after anesthetizing of the airway (see above). The tracheal tube is inserted into the oropharynx (8–10 cm), and the bronchoscope is inserted through the ETT. The epiglottis and glottic opening should be in view. The ETT is advanced over the scope as the carina is kept in view.

Transtracheal Ventilation

Transtracheal ventilation serves as a temporizing measure if mask ventilation and oxygenation become inadequate or impossible. A catheter (12- or 14-gauge) is inserted into the trachea through the cricothyroid membrane and connected to a jet-type ventilator capable of delivering gas at a pressure of 50 psi. The gas is then delivered using the handheld jet ventilator. Ventilation is best assessed by observing chest rise and fall. It is advised that an inspiration:expiration (I:E) ratio of 1:4 be utilized.

Complications include catheter displacement (caused by high pressure), pneumothorax, and pneumomediastinum.

Laryngeal Mask Airway (LMA)

Indications for the LMA

- Can be used in place of a face mask or ETT
- Can be used in place of an ETT for controlled ventilation as long as the peak pressure does not exceed 30 cm H_2O
- Can aid in the management of difficult airways by providing ventilation or as a guide for fiberoptic intubation

Contraindications for the LMA

- Does not protect against gastric regurgitation and aspiration because it does not provide an airtight seal of the airway
- If periglottic pathology (periglottic masses, large abscesses, large hematomas, hemorrhage of the airway, radiation-induced changes, epiglottitis, and laryngeal stenosis) causes a "Cannot Intubate, Cannot Ventilate" emergency, a supraglottic airway such as an LMA is not a good choice as a rescue device.

Insertion of the LMA

- The backside of the LMA should be lubricated with a water-soluble lubricant.
- Unconsciousness is rendered with an induction agent of choice. Typically, propofol at doses of 2 to 3 mg/kg produces reliable jaw and pharyngeal muscle relaxation.
- With the LMA held like a pencil, it is placed into the midline of the mouth and advanced with pressure against the hard palate as it slides into the hypopharynx. When the upper esophageal sphincter is encountered, resistance is felt. The LMA is then inflated.

- When placed properly, the black vertical line on the back of the LMA faces backward toward the head of the patient.
- The LMA is then removed upon emergence when the patient can follow commands.

Table 2.5   Conditions associated with difficult airway and intubation

Condition	Examples
Tumors	Cystic hygroma
	Hemangiomas
	Hematoma
Infections	Submandibular abscess
	Peritonsillar abscess
	Epiglottitis
Congenital anomalies	Pierre Robin's syndrome
	Treacher Collins's syndrome
	Laryngeal atresia
	Goldenhar's syndrome
	Craniofacial dystocias
Trauma	Laryngeal fracture
	Mandibular/maxillary fracture
	Inhalational burn
	Cervical spine injury
Inadequate neck extension	Rheumatoid arthritis
	Ankylosing spondylitis
	Halo traction
Anatomic variations	Micrognathia
	Prognathism
	Large tongue
	Arched palate
	Short neck
	Prominent upper incisors
Obesity	
Airway foreign body	

Complications of the LMA

- Possible regurgitation/aspiration.
- Negative pressure pulmonary edema can result when an LMA is placed improperly in a spontaneously breathing patient.
- LMA malfunction in patients with pharyngeal or esophageal disease.
- Placement requires neck extension, which is often contraindicated with cervical spine disease.

The GlideScope

The GlideScope is a video laryngoscope that can be a useful alternative to the fiberoptic scope for placement of an endotracheal tube if a difficult airway is expected. The blade is curved like the Macintosh blade with a 60° curvature to match the anatomic alignment. The GlideScope has a digital camera incorporated in the blade, displaying a view of the vocal folds on a monitor. Under visualization on the monitor, an ETT is passed between the vocal folds.

Surgical Laryngoscopes

Closed cylinder style rigid laryngoscopes with bright fiberoptic light guides, such as the Dedo or Holinger, are used by the otolaryngologist and have advantages that permit visualization of the glottis and intubation.

◆ The Difficult Airway

Among otolaryngology–head and neck surgery patients, a high percentage presents with a difficult airway (**Table 2.5**). By definition, a patient with a difficult airway potentially poses difficulty with ventilation or ETT placement. The goal of history, physical exam, and chart review is to identify patients with difficult airway before they arrive in the OR. Evaluation by the otolaryngologist and review of diagnostic studies can provide invaluable information to the anesthesiologist when a difficult airway is suspected. Conditions associated with difficult airway are discussed in the following paragraphs.

The induction of anesthesia in otolaryngology patients should not be initiated until a plan is formulated between the surgical and anesthesia teams. As outlined in the 2013 ASA DAA (**Fig. 2.1**), the plan should address the likelihood and clinical impact of basic (1) management problems, (2) management choices, and (3) the development of primary and alternative strategies (see preamble to the algorithm). A "skeletonized" version of the algorithm reveals the overall strategy and the two main root induction points (**Fig. 2.5**). The degree of laryngeal inlet visualization with preoperative endoscopic examination can be combined with respiratory symptoms

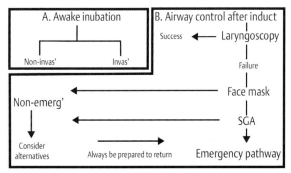

Fig. 2.5 "Skeletonized" version of the ASA DAA. (Adapted with permission from Abdelmalak B, Doyle DJ, eds. *Anesthesia for Otolaryngologic Surgery*. New York, NY: Cambridge University Press; 2013:51.)

Table 2.6   Airway grades based on respiratory symptoms and degree of laryngeal inlet visualization

Grade	Symptoms	Airway mass	Laryngeal view	Root point of ASA-DAA[a]
0	None	No lesion	Complete view	B
1	Hx smoking, no hoarseness	Small lesion	Complete view	B
2a	Hoarse voice, no difficulty in breathing	Laryngeal or supraglottic lesion	Clear view of vocal folds partial or fully	B
2b	Hoarse voice, no difficulty in breathing	Large laryngeal or supraglottic lesion	Partial view of parts of vocal folds	A
3	Hoarse voice, some difficulty in breathing	Large laryngeal or supraglottic lesion	Difficult to view vocal folds. May be seen only on inspiration	A
4		Large mass	Vocal folds cannot be visualized	A[b]

[a]*Root points of the ASA Difficult Airway Algorithm are Box A: awake intubation and Box B: airway control after induction of anesthesia.*
[b]*Awake tracheostomy.*

to yield an "airway grade" that determines whether the patient should be intubated conscious, have the airway controlled after induction, or undergo an awake tracheostomy (**Table 2.6**). A surgical airway is indicated when ventilation becomes inadequate despite utilization of a nonsurgical airway ventilation device [jet ventilation, LMA, Combitube (Tyco-Kendall, Mansfield, MA)] in a patient under general anesthesia.

If a difficult airway is suspected, instrumentation and plans for possible surgical airway should be available. Cricothyroidotomy is the preferred method in adults. Briefly, the neck is extended, and the cricothyroid membrane is palpated and incised with a scalpel. The airway is entered and an endotracheal or tracheotomy tube is placed to ventilate the patient. Details on cricothyroidotomy are given subsequently.

Clinical situations involving a patient with a difficult airway can be divided into two categories. The first is the acute or urgent problem, the second an elective situation with a suspected or known difficult airway. Both of these scenarios are to be handled differently. The ASA Difficult Airway Algorithm (**Fig. 2.1**) is a good educational and planning tool, but it is designed neither for making decisions in a high-risk, high-stress environment where a situation of "Cannot Intubate, Cannot Ventilate" develops nor for organizing the team resuscitating the airway at the pace of an airway code. For these, the use of a cognitive aid, such as the Vortex Approach to the unanticipated difficult airway, seems to be more appropriate (vortexapproach.com). It would address issues such as limitations of attempts at airway interventions (mask ventilation, tracheal intubation, supraglottic airway placement) before proceeding to an emergency surgical airway, identifying the most experienced practitioner and maneuvers for optimal attempts at each of these, and the psychological and practical preparation for an emergency surgical airway. The otolaryngologist—head and neck surgeon should have particular expertise in ensuring an adequate airway and should be skilled in the use of laryngoscopy, bronchoscopy, and surgical approaches to the airway.

Specific techniques to be discussed here include cricothyroidotomy and awake tracheotomy.

Cricothyroidotomy

For a patient with impending or complete obstruction, rapid establishment of an airway is required—the OR is the safest place for this airway control, though this is not always possible. If the situation requires establishment of an emergency surgical airway, a cricothyroidotomy is generally the preferred procedure (**Fig. 2.6**). This is because it is simpler and faster than a tracheotomy and has a lower complication rate, especially in less experienced hands. If it is impossible to mask-ventilate, intubate, or control the airway by any other technique such as a laryngeal mask or jet ventilation, or if these are not readily available, cricothyroidotomy should be performed by the most trained and skilled physician in attendance.

Contraindications to cricothyroidotomy include subglottic stenosis or mass and laryngeal trauma with an inability to identify landmarks; in general, it should be avoided in the pediatric population. A cricothyroidotomy should be revised to a tracheotomy in the OR within 24 hours to prevent subsequent development of subglottic stenosis and to facilitate adequate ventilation.

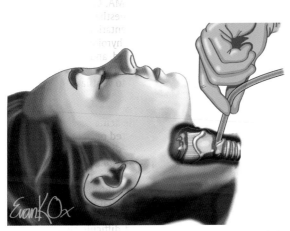

Fig. 2.6 Cricothyoidotomy. The tracheotomy tube is inserted through the cricothyroid membrane. The tracheal hook can be redirected to facilitate entry of the tracheotomy tube into position (see also **Appendix A7**).

Table 2.7   Indications for tracheotomy

Upper airway obstruction with any of the signs or symptoms at right	Air hunger, stridor, retractions, obstructive sleep apnea, bilateral vocal fold paralysis, previous neck surgery or throat trauma, previous neck irradiation, prolonged or expected prolonged intubation
Pulmonary toilet	Inability of patient to manage secretions, including the following: aspirations and excessive bronchopulmonary secretions
Ventilatory support	Where prolonged ventilation or ventilatory problems are anticipated

For needle cricothyroidotomy, a catheter is placed over a needle that penetrates the cricothyroid membrane, allowing ventilation by a pressurized stream of oxygen. Needle cricothyroidotomy is the preferred method of establishing an emergency airway in children younger than 10 to 12 years. (See the Cricothyroidotomy section, A7, in **Appendix A**.)

Stable but Compromised Airway

A patient with supraglottitis, angioedema, or a laryngeal mass may have a stable but compromised airway. These patients maintain their oxygen saturation and do not require an emergency airway; however, the stability of the situation requires clinical judgment. In some cases, the patient can be managed with medical management and close monitoring. In other cases, it may be prudent to secure a surgical airway.

Tracheotomy is a surgical procedure in which the tracheocutaneous airway is created through the anterior neck and the trachea. It may be reversible (**Table 2.7**). (For details on open surgical tracheotomy, see A6 in **Appendix A**.)

Awake Tracheotomy

In the unstable, poorly ventilated patient, an airway must be secured. If intubation is deemed impractical or dangerous, an awake tracheotomy can be performed. It is important to note that this is best done in a controlled environment, in the OR, or in the intensive care unit (ICU) with local anesthetic and a patient who can maintain spontaneous adequate ventilation. Clear communication between the otolaryngologist—head and neck surgeon, anesthetist, nurses, and technicians is vital. It is important to note that a life-threatening emergency may arise, and this will necessitate close collaboration. All equipment should be open and ready.

For the awake tracheotomy, the patient should be placed in the semi-Fowler position, allowing the anesthesiologist ready access to the airway. Every effort should be made to keep the patient comfortable, and the general atmosphere should be as calm as possible. The patient is typically only minimally sedated and should not be paralyzed, maintaining spontaneous adequate ventilation.

Note that in the elective (nonurgent) tracheotomy, the patient is intubated prior to the start of surgery.

Awake Tracheotomy Technique

Surgical landmarks are palpated, and a horizontal or vertical skin incision is made between the cricoid and suprasternal notch. Subcutaneous tissue is bluntly spread. Next, lateral retraction of the strap musculature is performed. The thyroid isthmus is encountered and either retracted caudad, retracted cephalad, or divided using a monopolar cautery. Once the trachea is in view, a tracheal hook may be used to provide superior retraction on the cricoid ring; next, the trachea is entered, usually below the second ring, and a window or inferiorly based (Björk) flap is created.

An appropriate tracheotomy tube is then placed while the anesthesiologist withdraws the ETT under direct visualization. After the tracheotomy tube is in place, the cuff is inflated, the patient is ventilated, and CO_2 return and appropriate rise in oxygenation are confirmed. Then the tracheotomy tube is sutured at four corners with suture, and a tracheotomy tie should be placed to secure the tracheotomy tube around the neck.

Complications of tracheotomy include bleeding, infection, crusting or mucus plugging, pneumothorax, and accidental dislodgement of the tracheotomy tube. Late postoperative complications include tracheoesophageal fistula, tracheal stenosis, tracheocutaneous fistula, and airway stenosis. A rare but deadly complication is a trachea–innominate artery fistula.

Percutaneous Dilation Tracheotomy

A percutaneous dilation tracheotomy (PDT) is *not* to be used in an emergent airway situation: this procedure is to be performed *only* on patients who are already intubated. Bedside PDT has become a safe alternative to elective open tracheotomy in many ICUs. There are several different techniques, all widely based on the Seldinger technique (needle and catheter over guidewire). Indications for a PDT are identical to those used for a routine open operative tracheotomy. The most common indication is prolonged intubation, mechanical ventilation. However, particular attention should be paid to potential contraindications. Some absolute contraindications for the performance of a PDT are the need for emergency tracheotomy (i.e., an emergent airway) or a population of infants and children. Relative contraindications include poor neck landmarks, morbid obesity, previous neck surgery, limited neck extension, and severe coagulopathy that is not correctable. Other relative anesthetic contraindications include high positive end expiration pressure (PEEP; > 18 cm), high airway pressure (> 45 cm), high fraction of inspired oxygen (FiO_2) requirement (> 80%), retrognathic mandible with limited view of the larynx, and an inability to reintubate.

An appropriate percutaneous tracheotomy kit (i.e., Ciaglia or Griggs kit) and a video bronchoscope are needed to perform this procedure. At least two persons are needed: one to perform the tracheotomy, the other to manage the ETT and video bronchoscope.

Percutaneous Dilation Tracheotomy Technique

A shoulder roll is placed beneath the patient's shoulders, and a bronchoscopist should perform simultaneous bronchoscopy through the ETT during the procedure. An incision is made either horizontally or vertically between the cricoid and the suprasternal notch, and an introducer needle is placed into the trachea at about the second ring; this is confirmed with bubbling of air and with simultaneous video bronchoscopy. In addition, transillumination of light from the bronchoscope can be used to help demarcate the best site for the introducer needle. The needle is withdrawn, and the overlying plastic cannula is left in place. A J-tipped guidewire is then placed under direct visualization through the cannula into the trachea. Again, every step should be bronchoscopically visualized on the video monitor during the procedure. Dilation is then performed using the provided dilator over the guidewire. This is removed, and once dilation of the anterior tracheal wall has been performed, a percutaneous tracheotomy appliance is placed over the guidewire and positioned in the airway. Following this, the bronchoscope should be withdrawn from the endotracheal tube and introduced via the tracheotomy tube to confirm placement in the airway. The placement is confirmed by visualization of the carina. The tracheotomy tube is connected to the anesthesia circuit to confirm bilateral breath sounds and end-tidal CO_2. It is then secured using a suture on each corner of the flange, and a tracheotomy tie is also used to secure the appliance around the neck. Only then can the orotracheal tube be fully removed.

For percutaneous tracheotomy, the first tracheotomy tube change should *not* be performed sooner than 10 days postoperatively, to allow for formation of a safe tract.

Criteria for Extubation

- Respiratory rate (RR) < 30 per minute
- Tidal volume (TV) > 5 mL/kg
- Vital capacity (VC) > 10 mL/kg
- Negative inspiratory force (NIF) > −20 cm H_2O
- Tidal volume/respiratory rate (TV/RR) > 10
- PaO_2 > 70 mm Hg (40% fraction of inspired oxygen [FiO_2])
- $PaCO_2$ < 50 mm Hg
- Level of consciousness (LOC) stable or improving
- Ventilation, dead space/tidal volume ratio (Vd/Vt) < 0.6

2.2 Anesthesia

2.2.1 Principles of Anesthesia

◆ Modes of Anesthesia

General anesthesia: This mode is characterized by total loss of consciousness with blunted (or absent) protective upper airway reflexes and the use of an endotracheal tube (ETT) or supraglottic device (e.g., laryngeal mask airway).

Sedation: This mode aims to maintain protective upper airway reflexes in patients with iatrogenically altered levels of consciousness. Supplemental oxygen is often required (e.g., nasal cannula), with or without the assistance of an oral/nasopharyngeal airway. It can range from minimal (i.e., patient is responsive to verbal command) to deep (i.e., no response to procedural stimulation).

Regional anesthesia: This mode involves the use of local anesthetics in conjunction with sedation or general anesthesia to improve analgesia, expedite recovery, and reduce overall IV/inhalational anesthetic requirements. It can be used as a sole anesthetic for minor or superficial procedures.

◆ Factors of Anesthesia

An ideal anesthetic strikes a balance between the following four essential factors, which in turn are influenced by independent patient risk factors, unique surgical requirements, and circumstances under which recovery is to occur.

Amnesia/anxiolysis: Management of preoperative anxiety and control of intraoperative awareness is a cornerstone of anesthetic care. Various oral, IV, and/or inhalational agents may be used, depending on the desired effect.

Analgesia: Multimodal therapy is the preferred method of achieving intra- and postoperative pain control with a combination of opioids, COX-2 selective and nonselective nonsteroidal antiinflammatory drugs (NSAIDs), and local anesthetics, and/or adjuvants, especially in patients suffering from chronic pain (e.g., the calcium channel $\alpha_2\delta$ antagonists gabapentin and pregabalin, the N-methyl-D-aspartate [NMDA] receptor antagonist ketamine, or α_2 agonists such as clonidine).

Muscle relaxation: Depolarizing and/or nondepolarizing muscle relaxants facilitate optimal airway conditions for laryngoscopy and surgical manipulation.

Antiemetics: Postoperative nausea and vomiting (PONV) is a strongly undesirable complication in patients following head and neck surgery. High-risk procedures include otology surgery, adenotonsillectomy, and thyroidectomy as well as head and neck cancer surgery. PONV influences patient satisfaction, length of stay, recovery, and surgical outcome. Multimodal and prophylactic therapy improves outcomes. Emesis may predispose development of wound hematoma, which can become an airway emergency in the presence of a neck wound.

◆ Phases of Anesthesia

Preinduction: This phase begins in the preoperative area and continues to the point where a patient is positioned on the operating room (OR) table with standard monitors (electrocardiogram [ECG], noninvasive blood pressure, pulse oximetry, capnography) and has been adequately preoxygenated.

Induction: General anesthesia in patients with established IV access is initiated with rapid-acting parenteral drugs to facilitate airway control. Otherwise, inhalational anesthetics are administered via a face mask; once an adequate depth of anesthesia is achieved, IV access is established and is followed by the placement of an ETT or supraglottic device (unless a very brief procedure is planned). For sedation cases, IV agents are titrated to effect while maintaining spontaneous ventilation. For difficult airway situations, awake fiberoptic nasotracheal intubation or awake tracheotomy may be indicated to secure the airway, prior to induction of general anesthesia.

Maintenance: Global amnesia is maintained during surgery with inhalational agents and/or parenteral drug infusions. Surgical analgesia is maintained either with a well-established regional block, generous local anesthetic infiltration, intermittent opioid boluses, and/or IV narcotic infusion. Duration of required muscle paralysis depends on several factors and may be just long enough to facilitate ETT placement. In some instances (e.g., cases involving extensive neuromonitoring), anesthesia may be maintained through the predominant or exclusive use of parenteral infusions (total intravenous anesthesia, TIVA). TIVA is sometimes useful to reduce vasodilation and bleeding (e.g., in endoscopic sinus surgery).

Emergence: Extubation is performed upon the patient's meeting the criteria of spontaneous ventilation, reversal of neuromuscular blockade, suctioning of airway.

Table 2.8 provides an overview of the key aspects of each phase of anesthesia.

◆ Stages of Anesthesia

Stage 1: The period between initial delivery of induction agents and loss of consciousness. Patients experience analgesia without amnesia and can often carry on a conversation during this time.

Stage 2: More commonly known as the "excitement stage," this stage follows loss of consciousness and is characterized by delirious, uninhibited, and often spastic activity. Cardiovascular and respiratory patterns are erratic.

Table 2.8   Key areas in each phase of anesthesia

Preinduction	Induction	Maintenance	Emergence
Airway assessment Intravenous access Anxiolysis Aspiration precautions Positioning for safety and patient comfort Baseline vital signs Preoxygenation	Adequate depth of anesthesia (to prevent awareness or laryngospasm) Aspiration precaution (cricoid pressure, rapid sequence induction) Positioning for optimal view of the airway upon direct laryngoscopy Securing the airway (confirmed by auscultation, inspection, and capnography)	Maintenance of end organ perfusion Adequate fluid administration Normothermia Appropriate anesthetic depth Procedural analgesia Facilitation of optimal surgical field (e.g., controlled hypotension)	Extubation upon meeting criteria (spontaneous ventilation, reversal of neuromuscular blockade, suctioning of airway)

There is also an increased risk for aspiration. The goal of any anesthetic induction is thus to minimize time spent in this stage.

Stage 3: In this stage, also known as "surgical plane," procedural stimulation causes minimal, if any, cardiovascular and/or respiratory changes.

Stage 4: This stage occurs when a massive anesthetic overdose causes severe depression of brainstem activity, leading to respiratory and/or cardiovascular collapse. This stage should never be reached, as it may be lethal even with appropriate cardiovascular and/or respiratory support.

2.2.2 Regional Anesthesia Techniques

◆ Benefits of Regional Anesthesia

When combined with a general anesthetic, regional nerve blocks reduce narcotic requirements and their subsequent side effects, such as nausea, vomiting, somnolence, and respiratory depression. Time to discharge is reduced.

◆ Contraindications to Regional Anesthesia

Contraindications to regional anesthesia include lack of patient consent and interference with surgical field/technique. Relative contraindications include coagulopathy, infection at the skin site, and presence of neurologic disease.

◆ Complications Common to All Nerve Blocks

Complications common to all nerve blocks include local anesthetic complications (intravascular injection, overdose, and allergic reaction), nerve damage (needle trauma, intraneural injection), infection, and hematoma.

◆ Blocks of the Scalp and Face

Supraorbital and Supratrochlear Nerve

Indications: Closure of lacerations, forehead and ear procedures

The forehead and anterior scalp can be rendered insensate by blocking the supraorbital and supratrochlear nerves, branches of the ophthalmic division of the trigeminal nerve (CN V_1), where they exit from their respective foramina along the brow line.

A skin wheal is placed over the glabella. A 25-gauge needle, bent to aid in superficial placement, is inserted through the anesthetizing wheal and advanced laterally along the brow. A total of 8 mL of local anesthetic is applied from the glabella to the lateral edge of each brow.

Greater and Lesser Occipital Nerves

Indications: Closure of lacerations

By blocking the greater and lesser occipital nerves, the posterior scalp can be anesthetized. By placing a track of local anesthetic from the mastoid process to the inion (i.e., external occipital protuberance) along the highest nuchal line from each side, both the greater and lesser occipital nerves will receive a dose of local anesthetic, and the posterior scalp will become anesthetized.

A large skin wheal is placed over the mastoid process on each side using a 27-gauge needle. Then, through this wheal, a wheal is placed from the mastoid process to the inion using a 25-gauge Quincke needle that is bent to facilitate a superficial injection.

Infraorbital Nerve

Indications: Closure of lacerations, facial surgery

The maxillary division of the trigeminal nerve (CN V_2) innervates the midface, from the inferior portion of the orbit to the mandible. This area includes the area overlying the zygoma, the maxilla, and most of the nose, as well as the philtrum and the hard and soft palate.

The infraorbital foramen is palpable 2 to 3 mm below the rim of the orbit, just medial to the equator of the orbit. A small-gauge needle is used to inject local anesthesia just outside the foramen. Avoid injection into the foramen, as the nerve is located in a confined space.

A small amount (2–4 mL) of local anesthetic is sufficient, and it should be injected based on which area is to be anesthetized. Specifically, emphasize *above* the foramen for lower lid work, *medial* to the foramen for lateral nasal work, and *inferomedial* to the foramen for work on the philtrum.

◆ Blocks of the Neck

Superficial Cervical Plexus

The cervical plexus is composed of four nerve roots, C_1–C_4, and terminates in four branches: the lesser occipital, great auricular, transverse cervical, and supraclavicular nerves. The terminal branches emerge superficially at the posterior border of the sternocleidomastoid (SCM) muscle along the midportion of the muscle.

This is a purely cutaneous nerve block; there is no motor block with the superficial cervical plexus block. Neuromonitoring and stimulation of the recurrent laryngeal nerve are not compromised when using this block.

The patient is positioned in the seated position. A line connecting the insertion of the SCM at the midpoint of the clavicle to the mastoid process along the posterior muscle border designates the path in which subcutaneous local anesthetic should be injected. Initially, 3 to 5 mL of local anesthetic is injected at the midpoint of the SCM using a 27-gauge needle. Using a 25-gauge Quincke point spinal needle, subcutaneous injections are then performed from this initial injection site in caudad and cephalad directions along the posterior edge of the SCM. Infiltration along these paths should require 6 to 8 mL of anesthetic in each direction. Aspiration prior to injection is important to avoid intravascular injection.

Deep Cervical Plexus

The deep cervical plexus (DCP) is the collection of the C_2–C_4 nerve roots as they exit the "gutter" formed by the transverse processes of the respective vertebrae. By injecting proximal to the division of the cervical roots into dorsal and ventral rami, a more complete blockade of the ipsilateral neck is achieved—including both sensory and motor elements (including the phrenic nerve, paralyzing the ipsilateral diaphragm). This is not commonly used for otolaryngology procedures.

The patient is seated upright in a high Fowler position with a small towel behind the shoulders. The above-mentioned line is drawn between the mastoid process and the anterior tubercle of C_6, which is palpable in the vast majority of patients. A line parallel to this is drawn 1.5 cm behind the first, and the posterior tubercle is palpated on C_2, C_3, and C_4. Deep palpation can be uncomfortable, and a light touch is indicated. After a small skin wheal is placed with a 27-gauge needle, a short (2.5-cm) blunt needle is advanced to the posterior process of each of the three vertebrae and then "walked" laterally and anterior to the posterior tubercle. An advance of 1 mm beyond the bony tubercle will suffice. It is not uncommon for the patient to describe a light paresthesia in the dermatome of the root being blocked. After careful aspiration, 4 to 5 mL of local anesthetic (with epinephrine) is injected at each of the three levels (C_2, C_3, C_4). The proximity to the spinal column and major vascular structures increases the risk of intrathecal or intravascular injection.

Specific Nerve Blocks for the Upper Airway

Maxillary Division of the Trigeminal Nerve (Pterygopalatine Ganglion)

- The transnasal topical approach to the pterygopalatine (sphenopalatine) ganglion involves application of local anesthetic to the mucous membranes surrounding the ganglion.

- Position the patient supine with neck extension. A local anesthetic (typically 80 mg of 4% cocaine) is applied to each nostril. Cotton-tipped applicators soaked in 4% cocaine are gently swirled and advanced into the nares. Each applicator is advanced a little further than the one prior, and once placed, the applicator is left there as successive applicators are introduced. Each nostril should receive four to seven applicators as the opening allows. The applicators should remain in the nares for at least 20 minutes, allowing the local anesthetic to diffuse through the mucosa overlying the ganglion.

- The pterygopalatine ganglion can also be approached through the greater palatine foramen, located at the posterior portion of the hard palate. In this approach, the patient is positioned in the supine position with the neck extended. The foramina can be palpated medial to the gumline of the third molar. A small-gauge needle is advanced < 2.5 cm through the foramen in a superior and slightly posterior direction. To avoid an intravascular injection, aspirate prior to injection.

Glossopharyngeal Nerve

- The glossopharyngeal nerve (CN IX) exits the skull at the jugular foramen and passes between the internal jugular vein and the internal carotid artery. It descends just dorsal to the styloid process before curving forward and anterior to innervate the palatine tonsil, the mucous membranes of the fauces, and the base of the tongue. This nerve has motor, sensory, and autonomic components and supplies lower motor neurons to the stylopharyngeus and parasympathetic innervation of the parotid and mucous glands.

Superior Laryngeal Branch of the Vagus Nerve

- The superior laryngeal nerve can be blocked as it passes into the thyrohyoid membrane inferior to the greater cornu of the hyoid bone and superior to the greater cornu of the thyroid cartilage. This block will provide anesthesia to the glottis above the vocal folds.

- With the patient seated in an upright (high Fowler) position with a towel roll transversely laid behind the shoulders, the thyroid cartilage is palpated. It can be helpful to lightly displace the thyroid cartilage toward the side of the block. Using a small-gauge needle, 2 to 3 mL of local anesthetic is injected near the cartilaginous greater cornu. Aspiration prior to injection will confirm that the needle has not entered the supraglottic air column. This procedure is then repeated on the other side.

Topical Anesthesia of the Subglottic Airway

- The recurrent laryngeal branch of the vagus nerve pierces the subglottic trachea to innervate all the laryngeal muscles other than the cricothyroid muscle as well as provide sensory innervation to the subglottic mucosa.

- The patient is positioned in a high Fowler position with a towel roll laid transversely behind the shoulders. Moderate neck extension is helpful. After skin disinfection, the thyroid cartilage is identified. The next palpable cartilage inferiorly is the cricoid cartilage. The palpable gap between these two structures overlies the cricothyroid membrane. A 22-gauge needle containing local anesthetic (2 to 4 mL 3% chloroprocaine or 2 to 4 mL 4% lidocaine) is advanced perpendicular to the skin while gentle aspiration is applied to the syringe plunger. Air will be freely aspirated when the needle penetrates the cricothyroid membrane, entering the trachea. The patient should be alerted that the injection will induce coughing. The local anesthetic should be rapidly administered and the needle withdrawn. The patient will cough and should be encouraged to do so several times to enhance spread of the anesthetic.

2.2.3   Anesthesia Drugs

◆ Opioids

Opioids work by binding to specific receptors located throughout the central nervous system (CNS) and other tissues (**Table 2.9**). The pharmacodynamic effect of an administered opioid depends on which receptor is bound, the affinity of the binding, and whether the receptor is activated or inhibited. There are four opioid receptors: mu, delta, kappa, and sigma (**Table 2.10**).

Table 2.9 Opioid effects on organ systems

Organ system	Physiologic response
Cardiovascular	In general, opioids do not impair cardiovascular function. At high doses opioids can lead to bradycardia. Meperidine, structurally similar to atropine, can cause tachycardia. Hypotension seen with opioid use is secondary to bradycardia and, in the case of morphine and meperidine, histamine-induced vasodilation.
Respiratory	Opioids depress ventilation, particularly respiratory rate. The hypoxic drive, the body's ventilatory response to CO_2, is decreased. The result is an increase in $PaCO_2$ and decreased respiratory rate. The apneic threshold, the highest $PaCO_2$ at which a patient will remain apneic, is increased. In patients susceptible to histamine-induced reactive airway disease, morphine and meperidine can lead to bronchospasm. Chest wall rigidity, severe enough to prevent adequate ventilation, can be seen with fentanyl and remifentanil.
Central nervous	Opioids reduce cerebral oxygen consumption, cerebral blood flow, and intracranial pressure. Minimal changes are seen on EEG except for meperidine, which can cause an increase in EEG frequency. Even at high doses, opioids do not reliably produce amnesia. The high doses necessary to establish unconsciousness can lead to physical dependence.
Gastrointestinal	Opioids slow peristalsis, resulting in decreased gastric emptying and constipation. Contraction of the biliary sphincter, leading to biliary colic, is also common.
Endocrine	Opioids block the release of catecholamines, ADH, and cortisol associated with surgical stress.
Drug interactions	Barbiturates, benzodiazepines, and other CNS depressants have a synergistic effect on level of sedation and respiratory depression when combined with opioids.

Abbreviations: ADH, antidiuretic hormone; CNS, central nervous system; EEG, electroencephalogram.

Morphine

Because morphine is a hydrophilic compound, it has a slower onset with a longer clinical effect. Morphine can lead to hypotension secondary to histamine-induced vasodilation as well as decreased sympathetic tone. Morphine metabolites are excreted by the kidneys. Patients with renal failure can have prolonged duration of action given that between 5 and 10% of morphine is excreted unchanged in the urine. Morphine 6-glucuronide can lead to respiratory depression and narcosis.

Dosing: Preoperatively, postoperatively 5 to 15 mg intramuscular (IM)/IV; 0.05 to 0.2 mg/kg IV

Table 2.10   Opioid receptors

Receptor	Physiological characteristics
Mu	• μ_1 receptor is responsible for producing analgesia, miosis, nausea/vomiting, urinary retention, and pruritus. • The endogenous stimulus for μ_1 receptors are enkephalins. • μ_2 receptor activation leads to euphoria, respiratory depression, sedation, bradycardia, ileus, and physical dependence.
Delta	• Activation leads to analgesia and contributes to physical dependence. • These receptors are highly selective for endogenous enkephalins.
Kappa	• Activation leads to analgesia, sedation, dysphoria, and psychomimetic effects. • Pure κ agonists do not lead to respiratory depression. • Stimulation leads to vasopressin release and subsequent diuresis.
Sigma	Activation leads to dysphoria, hallucinations, tachypnea, and mydriasis.

Fentanyl

Fentanyl is a synthetic compound with higher lipid solubility than morphine; therefore, fentanyl has a rapid onset and short duration of action. It can accumulate in adipose tissue, creating a "reservoir." Prolonged respiratory depression is seen after large doses or prolonged fentanyl infusions.
Dosing: 0.5 to 1 µg/kg IV, 1 to 5 µg/kg per hour infusion. Larger doses may be used during general anesthesia.

Remifentanil

Remifentanil is an ultrafast-acting narcotic with an elimination half-life of less than 10 minutes. It is rapidly metabolized by plasma and tissue esterases and does not accumulate in adipose or other tissues. The length of infusion time therefore has no effect on wake-up time. Narcotic toxicity can, therefore, be avoided in patients with liver disease.
Dosing: 0.025 to 0.2 µg/kg per minute infusion

Meperidine

Meperidine (Demerol, Sanofi-Aventis Pharmaceuticals, Paris, France) is N-demethylated in the liver to normeperidine, an active metabolite that is associated with myoclonus and seizures. Patients with renal disease are particularly susceptible, as this metabolite is renally cleared. Meperidine is useful in the postanesthesia care unit (PACU) setting in the treatment of shivering. Note that postoperative oral meperidine use/prescription is discouraged due to adverse side effects.
Dosing: Preoperatively; postoperatively 50 to 150 mg IM/IV

◆ Reversal of Opioids

Naloxone

Naloxone is a competitive antagonist at opioid receptors, particularly the mu class. There is no significant agonist activity. Naloxone is indicated in cases of narcotic overdose. Respiratory depression secondary to narcotic overdosage is rapidly reversed with naloxone (1–2 minutes). Care should be taken to titrate low doses, as abrupt reversal of analgesia can result in abrupt sympathetic stimulation and acute withdrawal symptoms in those who are opioid dependent. Naloxone has a short duration of action (30–40 minutes), and redosing is usually required when reversing long-acting opioids.

Dosing: 0.5 to 1 µg/kg every 5 to 10 minutes; maximum total dose 10 mg

◆ Benzodiazepines

Benzodiazepines interact with specific receptors in the CNS that enhance the action of specific neurotransmitters (**Table 2.11**). In particular, the action of γ-aminobutyric acid (GABA), an inhibitory neurotransmitter, is enhanced. As a result, benzodiazepines produce amnesia, anxiolysis, and sedation and prevent seizures. Benzodiazepines have no direct analgesic properties. Like barbiturates, benzodiazepines are highly protein-bound and rely on redistribution for their offset of action. Biotransformation of benzodiazepines occurs in the liver, and metabolites are excreted mainly in the urine. Duration of action may be prolonged in patients with renal failure, as metabolites are pharmacologically active.

Table 2.11 Benzodiazepine effects on organ systems

Organ system	Physiologic response
Cardiovascular	• Depression of the cardiovascular system is minimal even at high doses. • Slight decreases in arterial blood pressure, cardiac output, and peripheral vascular resistance are often observed. • Midazolam decreases arterial blood pressure and peripheral vascular resistance more than lorazepam or diazepam. • Variability in heart rate during administration suggests that midazolam has vagolytic properties.
Respiratory	• Ventilatory response to CO_2 is reduced with benzodiazepine administration. This response is particularly pronounced when administered with other respiratory depressants, such as opioids.
Central nervous	• Benzodiazepines are very effective in seizure prophylaxis. • Cerebral oxygen consumption and cerebral blood flow are reduced.
Drug interactions	• When administered with opiates, benzodiazepines work synergistically to depress ventilation. • When administered with heparin, diazepam is displaced from its protein binding sites, causing an increased free drug concentration. • The MAC of volatile anesthetics is reduced up to 30%. CNS depressants such as alcohol and barbiturates potentiate the sedative effects of benzodiazepines.

Diazepam

Diazepam is insoluble in water and requires propylene glycol, which may cause venous irritation. Diazepam has a long duration of action secondary to slow hepatic extraction and a large volume of distribution. The elimination half-life is nearly 30 hours.

Dosing: 5 to 20 mg orally (PO), 2 to 10 mg IV

Midazolam

At low pH, midazolam is water-soluble. At physiologic pH, midazolam becomes more lipid soluble resulting in fast onset of action. Midazolam has the shortest elimination half-life (2 hours) because of a high hepatic extraction ratio. Midazolam's high potency and steep dose response curve require careful titration and close monitoring of respiration, as even small doses can lead to apnea.

Dosing: Adult 3 to 5 mg IM, 0.5 to 5 mg IV; pediatric 0.025 to 0.1 mg/kg IV; 0.25 to 0.5 mg/kg PO 30 minutes before procedure

Lorazepam

Like diazepam, lorazepam is insoluble in water and requires propylene glycol, which may cause venous irritation when administered. Because of its moderate lipid solubility, lorazepam has a slower onset of action secondary to slower brain uptake. The lower lipid solubility of lorazepam limits its volume of distribution and decreases its elimination half-life (15 hours) despite its having the same hepatic extraction ratio as diazepam.

Dosing: Adult 1 to 4 mg PO/IM/IV; pediatric 0.05 mg/kg PO/IM/IV preoperatively

◆ Benzodiazepine Reversal

Flumazenil

Flumazenil is a specific benzodiazepine receptor antagonist that reverses most of the effects of benzodiazepines. Onset is rapid (<1 minute) for the hypnotic effects of benzodiazepines. The amnestic effect is less reliably reversed. This agent is a competitive inhibitor at the benzodiazepine receptor. Elderly patients, in particular, are prone to resedation and should be observed for respiratory depression after flumazenil administration.

Dosing: 0.2 mg (titrate every minute until desired degree of sedation reversal is observed). Sedation reversal typically requires 0.6 to 1.0 mg. Infusions at 0.5 mg/h are indicated for overdoses of long-acting benzodiazepines.

◆ α_2 Agonists

Dexmedetomidine

Dexmedetomidine (brand name Precedex, Hospira, Inc., Lake Forest, IL) is an α_2 agonist with 8 to 10 times greater receptor affinity than clonidine. It has sympatholytic, analgesic, and sedating properties. The effect on the cardiovascular system is to lower heart rate and blood pressure, blunting the typical surgical response. α_2 agonists have minimal respiratory depression. Head and neck surgeons will find this drug useful for conscious sedation cases, augmented sleep studies, and fiberoptic intubations and tracheotomy placement. Also of interest to the otolaryngologist who employs the use of topical cocaine intraoperatively, recent research has suggested dexmedetomidine to be an effective treatment for the dangerous cardiovascular symptoms of cocaine intoxication.

Dosing: Loading dose of 1 µg/kg over 10 minutes followed by IV infusion at 0.2 to 0.7 µg/kg per hour

◆ Anesthesia Induction Medications

Propofol

Propofol is a rapidly acting induction agent that produces unconsciousness within 30 seconds of dosing, and effects last between 2 and 8 minutes (**Table 2.12**). Propofol enhances the inhibitory action of GABA. Propofol is metabolized in the liver; however, offset of action results from redistribution, which is rapid secondary to high lipid solubility. Compared with other induction agents, propofol provides a faster recovery with less "hangover" than barbiturates or etomidate. Additionally, this agent has antiemetic, antipruritic, and anticonvulsive properties. At low (subhypnotic) doses (10–15 mg), propofol can ameliorate nausea and vomiting. Propofol does not provide analgesia, but does enhance the analgesic effects of narcotics. Careful titration is advised in hypovolemia or coronary vascular disease, as propofol can lead to a profound decrease in blood pressure secondary to decreased systemic vascular resistance. Venous irritation with administration can be avoided with concomitant administration of lidocaine (20–80 mg). Because propofol is an emulsion, it should be avoided in patients with disorders in lipid metabolism.

Dosing: Induction 2 to 2.5 mg/kg IV (pediatric dosing: 2.5 to 3.5 mg/kg); infusion 100 to 200 µg/kg per minute; sedation 25 to 75 µg/kg per minute

Table 2.12   Effects of propofol on organ systems

Organ system	Physiologic response
Cardiovascular	• Decreased peripheral vasodilation; cardiac contractility and preload combine to cause hypotension. • The normal vagal response to hypotension is also impaired. • The hypotension with propofol is greater than that produced by barbiturates.
Respiratory	• Respiratory depression
Central nervous	• Reduced intracranial pressure by reducing cerebral blood flow

Table 2.13   Effects of etomidate on organ systems

Organ system	Physiologic response
Cardiovascular	Slight decrease in peripheral vascular resistance leads to slight decrease in arterial blood pressure. Myocardial contractility and cardiac output are unchanged.
Respiratory	Ventilation is reduced less than with other induction agents. Even at induction doses, apnea usually does not occur unless opioids are also administered.
Central nervous	Cerebral metabolic rate, cerebral blood flow, and intracranial pressure are reduced. Due to cardiovascular stability, cerebral perfusion pressure is maintained. Etomidate lacks analgesic properties.
Endocrine	Transient inhibition of enzymes responsible for cortisol and aldosterone synthesis occurs with intubation doses. Long-term infusions lead to adrenocortical suppression.

Table 2.14   Effect of ketamine on organ systems

Organ system	Physiologic response
Cardiovascular	Increased cardiac output, heart rate and blood pressure secondary to increased sympathetic outflow.
Respiratory	Minimally effects ventilatory drive. Ketamine is a potent bronchodilator and has benefits to patients with asthma. Increased salivation can be resolved by pretreatment with anticholinergic medications,
Central nervous	Increased cerebral blood flow, cerebral oxygen consumption, and intracranial pressure. Hallucinations, delirium, and disturbing dreams are decreased in children and those who receive benzodiazepines prior to ketamine. Ketamine produces analgesia, amnesia, and unconsciousness.

Etomidate

Etomidate depresses the reticular activation system by binding to the GABA receptors and enhancing the inhibitory effects of this neurotransmitter (**Table 2.13**). Etomidate is dissolved in propylene glycol, leading to pain on injection as with diazepam and lorazepam. This can be reduced by injecting lidocaine prior to induction. Myoclonic movements are common after etomidate induction. Etomidate is characterized by a rapid onset secondary to high lipid solubility at physiologic pH. Etomidate is metabolized into inactive end products by hepatic microsomal enzymes and plasma esterases. Metabolites are excreted in the urine. Etomidate has very little effect on the cardiovascular system and is therefore the induction agent of choice in cardiovascular disease and severe hypovolemia.

Dosing: induction 0.2 to 0.6 mg/kg

Ketamine

Ketamine has multiple effects through the CNS and has been demonstrated to be an N-methyl-D-aspartate (NMDA) antagonist (**Table 7.14**). By effectively "disconnecting" the thalamus from the limbic system, it causes a state of "dissociative anesthesia." In this state the patient appears conscious but is unable to process or respond to sensory stimulation. Ketamine is a structural analogue to phencyclidine (PCP), and as with PCP, hallucinations can ensue even at low doses. Ketamine is metabolized in the liver, resulting in pharmacologically active metabolites (norketamine). Products of hepatic metabolism are renally excreted.

Dosing: 1 to 2 mg/kg IV; 3 to 5 mg/kg IM

Barbiturates

Barbiturates have several sites of action, resulting in suppression of excitatory neurotransmitters and activation of the inhibitory effects of GABA. The result is inhibition of the reticular activation system. Methohexital and thiopental are the commonly used barbiturates used for induction. As more titratable induction agents have come into use, barbiturates have fallen out of favor. Barbiturates have no analgesic properties and cause dose-related depression of the respiratory, cardiac, and central nervous systems. Thiopental has a short duration of action secondary to a high rate of redistribution from the brain to inactive tissues, secondary in turn to a high lipid solubility. Barbiturates are contraindicated in patients with intermittent porphyria. Side effects include venous irritation, myoclonus, and hiccupping.

Dosing: Thiopental 3 to 6 mg/kg IV; methohexital 1 to 2 mg/kg IV

◆ Inhaled Anesthetics

In the OR, general anesthesia is commonly maintained with inhaled anesthetics. These agents also provide some analgesia, amnesia, and muscle relaxation. In pediatric patients in whom there is no IV access, anesthesia may be induced by inhalation. All of the inhaled anesthetics, with the exception of nitrous oxide, are bronchodilators and may be useful in those with reactive airways. Most inhaled agents reduce blood pressure. The onset of anesthetic induction, as well as emergence from anesthesia, is based on the lipid solubility characteristics of the inhaled anesthetic: the more lipid insoluble the anesthetic agent, the faster the induction of anesthesia. The agents with high lipid solubility prolong the emergence from anesthesia.

Minimum alveolar concentration (MAC) is defined as the alveolar concentration at which 50% of test subjects will not respond to a surgical stimulus. Dosing of inhaled agents is based on the MAC of each particular agent. The MAC of inhaled agents depends on the individual gas properties of each agent. MAC is additive, such that 0.5 MAC of isoflurane combined with 0.5 MAC nitrous oxide is equivalent to 1.0 MAC of sevoflurane.

Isoflurane

Compared with other inhaled anesthetics (sevoflurane, desflurane), isoflurane has a relatively high lipid solubility, leading to increased induction and emergence time. Isoflurane causes minimal cardiac depression and decreased blood pressure secondary to decreased systemic vascular resistance. Like other volatile anesthetics, isoflurane causes respiratory depression with a decrease in minute ventilation (**Table 2.15**). Despite its ability to cause airway irritation, isoflurane induces bronchodilation.

Desflurane

Other than the substitution of a fluorine atom for a chlorine atom, the molecular structure of desflurane is very similar to that of isoflurane. However, this composition makes desflurane highly lipid-insoluble. Because of its low lipid solubility, induction and emergence from anesthesia are rapid. The time required for patients to awaken is approximately half as long as that observed following isoflurane administration. Desflurane has cardiovascular and cerebral effects similar to those of isoflurane. Like isoflurane, this agent is irritating to the airway, making gas induction difficult.

Sevoflurane

Sevoflurane is the primary inhaled anesthetic agent used in anesthesia induction when an IV induction cannot be performed, such as in pediatric patients. Nonpungency and a rapid increase in alveolar anesthetic concentration make it an excellent choice where inhalational induction is necessary. The blood solubility of sevoflurane is slightly greater than that of desflurane. Sevoflurane mildly depresses myocardial contractility and systemic vascular resistance. Arterial blood pressure declines slightly less than with isoflurane or desflurane. Like isoflurane and desflurane, sevoflurane causes slight increases in cerebral blood flow and intracranial pressure.

Nitrous Oxide

The uptake and elimination of nitrous oxide are relatively rapid compared with other inhaled anesthetics. This is the result of its low blood–gas partition coefficient. Nitrous oxide produces analgesia, amnesia, mild myocardial depression, and mild sympathetic nervous system stimulation. It does not significantly affect heart rate or blood pressure. Nitrous oxide is a mild respiratory depressant, although less so than the volatile anesthetics. The elimination of nitrous oxide is via exhalation.

◆ Muscle Relaxation

Neuromuscular blocking agents are used most commonly for facilitation of endotracheal intubation and when patient movement is detrimental to the surgical procedure. Prior to administration, ventilation must be ensured by the anesthesiologist. Neuromuscular blockers have no intrinsic sedative or analgesic properties and must be used in concert with anesthetic agents. Inadequate sedation and hypnosis while using neuromuscular blockers can produce recall by patients, causing long-term side effects. There are two classifications of neuromuscular blocking agents: depolarizing and nondepolarizing.

Table 2.15 Physiologic effects of isoflurane

Organ system	Physiologic response
Cardiovascular	Decreased systemic vascular resistance leads to lower arterial blood pressure
Respiratory	Can cause airway irritation yet causes bronchodilation. Respiratory depression.
Central nervous	At high concentrations, increased cerebral blood flow and intracranial pressure can develop. Decreased cerebral metabolic oxygen requirements may provide cerebral protection.
Neuromuscular	Skeletal muscle blood flow is increased.
Renal	Decreases renal blood flow, glomerular filtration rate, and urinary output.

Table 2.16 Depolarizing muscle relaxant

Muscle relaxant	Intubating dose; onset; duration	Clinical considerations
Succinylcholine	Dose: 1–1.5 mg/kg Onset: 30–60 sec Duration: < 10 min Maximum: 150 mg total dose	• Succinylcholine is contraindicated for routine intubation in pediatric patients because of the risk of cardiac arrest with hyperkalemia in those with undiagnosed myopathies. • It is the agent of choice for rapid sequence induction. • Bradycardia can follow dosing, particularly in pediatric patients. • Fasciculations typically occur with receptor activation and can result in myalgias postop. • Potassium release with succinylcholine-induced depolarization can cause potassium to increase by 0.5 mEq/dL. Avoid in hyperkalemic patients. • Transient increases in intracranial and intraocular pressure are observed. • Avoid in patients with a history of malignant hyperthermia. • Agent is metabolized by pseudocholinesterase.

Depolarizing Muscle Relaxants

Depolarizing agents have a similar chemical structure to acetylcholine. They induce paralysis by binding to acetylcholine receptors at the skeletal muscle neuromuscular junction, causing depolarization. Paralysis ensues because these agents have a higher affinity for the postsynaptic receptor, preventing the reestablishment of its ionic gradient. Clinically, fasciculations are seen prior to relaxation after dosing. The only medication in this class that is still in use today is succinylcholine (**Table 2.16**).

Table 2.17   Commonly used nondepolarizing muscle relaxants

Muscle relaxant	Intubating dose; onset; offset	Clinical considerations
Rocuronium	Dose: 0.5–0.9 mg/kg Onset: 1–2 min Duration: 40–90 min	At doses of 0.9–1.2 mg/kg, rocuronium can have rapid onset (60–90 sec) and be substituted for succinylcholine for rapid sequence induction. Rocuronium undergoes no metabolism and is eliminated in the bile and slightly by the kidneys. Severe hepatic failure and pregnancy can prolong duration of action.
Vecuronium	Dose: 0.1 mg/kg Onset: 2–3 min Duration: 25–30 min	Vecuronium has a short duration of action. It has hepatic metabolism with renal excretion. It lacks hemodynamic side effects. It can be administered as an infusion (1–2 µg/kg/min).
Cisatracurium	Dose: 0.2 mg/kg Onset: 1–2 min Duration: 50–60 min	Cisatracurium undergoes organ-independent Hoffman degradation at physiologic pH and temperature. It may be safely administered to patients with renal or liver failure. It lacks hemodynamic side effects.
Pancuronium	Dose: 0.1 mg/kg Onset: 5 min Duration: 20–100 min	Pancuronium provides long duration of action. It has renal elimination. It has vagolytic effects causing tachycardia, particularly after bolus administration.

Nondepolarizing Muscle Relaxants

Nondepolarizing muscle relaxants induce paralysis by binding to the postsynaptic receptor at the skeletal muscle neuromuscular junction. Essentially, these medications compete with acetylcholine for binding sites at the receptor. In contrast to depolarizing blockade, the postsynaptic receptors are not activated, and fasciculations do not occur. Nondepolarizing blockade can be reversed by increasing the acetylcholine concentration at the neuromuscular junction. This is achieved by administration of medications such as neostigmine, which prevent the breakdown of acetylcholine. The commonly used nondepolarizing agents are summarized in **Table 2.17**.

2.2.4   Anesthetic Emergencies

Potential anesthetic emergencies are numerous. Emergencies related to management of the airway are covered in subsequent chapters. The importance of prevention, early recognition, and prompt, appropriate management is common to all potential anesthetic emergencies. In particular, airway fire and malignant hyperthermia are conditions with the potential for high morbidity or mortality and are thus reviewed here.

◆ Airway Fires

The prevention of airway fires is crucial. Every member of the surgical team and operating room (OR) staff should know about surgical fire protocols and where OR safety equipment resides, and a safety timeout should include fire risk assessment. Before approving cautery intraorally (e.g., tonsillectomy) or activation of a laser, reduce the delivered oxygen concentration to the minimum required to avoid hypoxia, stop the use of nitrous oxide, and wait a few minutes after reducing the oxidizer-enriched atmosphere. Laser precautions, such as the use of a laser-safe endotracheal tube (ETT) and packing and covering the surrounding field with wet gauze or towels, must be standard. The tracheal cuff of a laser tube must be inflated with saline and colored with an indicator dye such as methylene blue, according to the 2013 American Society of Anesthesiologists (ASA) practice advisory on the prevention of airway fires. Be sure there is no ETT cuff leak. Turn off oxygen temporarily when using cautery during facial procedures requiring sedation and nasal cannula. Communication between the anesthetist and the surgeon is crucial. If there is a fire, remove the ETT tube, stop flow of all airway gases, remove all flammable and burning materials from the airway, and pour saline or water into the

Table 2.18   Signs of malignant hyperthermia

Early signs
Metabolic
• Elevated end-tidal CO_2
• Increased O_2 consumption
• Hyperkalemia after succinylcholine
• Respiratory acidosis
• Concurrent or delayed metabolic acidosis
• Profuse sweating
• Mottling of skin
Cardiovascular
• Inappropriate tachycardia, cardiac arrhythmias, unstable arterial pressure
Muscular
• Masseter spasm if succinylcholine was used (may occur after hours of general anesthesia if succinylcholine was not given early)
• Generalized muscular rigidity
Later signs
• Hyperkalemia
• Rapid increase in body temperature
• Grossly elevated blood creatine phosphokinase and myoglobin levels
• Myoglobinuria
• Severe cardiac arrhythmias or cardiac arrest
• Disseminated intravascular coagulation

patient's airway. (It is a good idea to keep a 50 mL syringe filled with saline within reach during procedures where an airway fire is a possibility.) Once the airway or breathing circuit fire is extinguished, reestablish ventilation by mask, avoiding supplemental oxygen and nitrous oxygen if possible; examine the extinguished ETT for missing fragments; and consider rigid bronchoscopy to look for tracheal tube fragments, assess injury, and remove residual debris.

◆ Malignant Hyperthermia

Malignant hyperthermia (MH) is a hyperdynamic crisis caused by an uncontrolled increase in skeletal muscle metabolism (**Table 2.18**). The underlying pathophysiology is excessive calcium release from the sarcoplasmic reticulum, causing prolonged activation of muscle contractile units. This results in heat production, oxygen consumption, and acidosis. MH is an autosomal dominant myopathy that is triggered by inhalational anesthetics and depolarizing muscle relaxants (e.g., succinylcholine). "Triggers" should be avoided in those who have a history of MH or a family history of the disorder. Patients with a history of MH can be safely anesthetized

Table 2.19   Treatment of malignant hyperthermia

Immediately
• Stop all trigger agents.
• Hyperventilate.
• Declare an emergency.
• Change to nontrigger anesthesia (TIVA).
• Inform the surgeon and ask for termination/postponement of surgery.
• Disconnect the vaporizer.
• Give dantrolene 2 mg/kg every 5 min until cardiac and respiratory systems stabilize; the maximum dose of 10 mg/kg may need to be exceeded.
Monitoring
• Routine anesthetic monitoring
• Core temperature
• Establish well-functioning IV catheters with wide-bore cannulas.
• Consider arterial line and central venous line and bladder catheter.
• Potassium
• Creatine phosphokinase
• Arterial blood gases
• Myoglobin and glucose levels
• Renal and hepatic function
• Coagulation
• Signs of compartment syndrome; admit to ICU for 24 h
Symptomatic treatment
• For hyperthermia: chilled saline, surface cooling until temperature less than 39.5°C
• For hyperkalemia: dextrose with insulin, calcium, dialysis
• For acidosis: hyperventilate, sodium bicarbonate if pH less than 7.2
• For arrhythmias: amiodarone, lidocaine, β blockers
• For urinary output > 2 mL/kg/h: furosemide, mannitol, fluids

with a "nontriggering anesthetic," which includes IV agents (total intravenous anesthesia, TIVA), nitrous oxide, xenon, and nondepolarizing agents. Complications from MH are severe: they include cardiac arrest, cerebral or pulmonary edema, renal failure, diffuse intravascular coagulation (DIC), and death. Treatment is outlined in **Table 2.19**.

2.3 Fluids and Electrolytes

◆ Key Features

- Appropriate fluid balance perioperatively can be estimated from established formulas.
- Attention to fluids and electrolytes is especially important in the patient who is not capable of maintaining normal oral intake.

Surgical patients, especially head and neck cancer patients, may be incapable of adequate oral intake. Often, intravenous (IV) fluids are needed for a short period before postoperative oral intake can resume. In other cases, longer-term NPO (nothing by mouth) status is required, such as when a pharyngeal closure must heal or a fistula is resolving. An important rule is that if the gut is available and functional, it should be used; for example, if oral swallowing is not functional, intake should still be provided via a nasogastric (NG) tube or percutaneous endoscopic gastrostomy (PEG) tube rather than by total parenteral nutrition (TPN) or peripheral IV nutrients. A summary of important considerations for fluid management is provided here.

◆ Functional Compartments

Total Body Water (TBW)

Normal total body water is 60% (adult males), 50% (adult females) of ideal body weight (IBW).

Intracellular Fluid (ICF)

ICF comprises 35% of IBW or 60% of TBW. This is the principal *potassium*-containing space.

Extracellular Fluid (ECF)

ECF constitutes 25% of IBW or 40% of TBW; subdivided into interstitial fluid (ISF) and blood volume (BV is ~8% of total volume weight). This is the principal *sodium*-containing space.

Table 2.20 Electrolyte composition of commonly used perioperative fluids

Fluid	Glu (g)	Na⁺ (mEq)	Cl⁻ (mEq)	K⁺ (mEq)	Ca²⁺ (mEq)	HCO₃⁻ (mEq)	Kcal
D5W	50						170
NS		154	154				
D5¹/₄NS	50	38.5	38.5				170
LR		130	110	4	3	27	<10
Plasmalyte		140	98	5			

All quantities are per liter. Abbreviations: D5W, 5% dextrose in water; NS, normal saline; LR, lactated Ringer's solution; D51/4NS, 5% dextrose in 1/4 normal saline. (Data from Hamilton MA, Cecconi M, Rhodes A. A systematic review and meta-analysis in the use of preemptive hemodynamic intervention to improve postoperative outcomes in moderate and high-risk surgical patients. Anesthesia and Analgesia 2010; 112(6): 1392–1402.)

◆ Daily Electrolyte Requirements

- Sodium: 2 to 3 mEq/kg per day
- Potassium: 1 to 2 mEq/kg per day
- Chloride: 2 to 3 mEq/kg per day

See **Table 2.20**.

◆ Perioperative Fluid Management

The modern approach to fluid management is based on the concept of goal-directed fluid therapy (GDT), where interventions are performed specifically to affect a meaningful clinical variable. Fluids can be harmful and should be given only when they can be expected to benefit the patient. Hypervolemia is one of the stimuli, along with surgical trauma, for the release of atrial natriuretic peptide (ANP), which damages the delicate glycocalyx lining of capillaries and leads to interstitial edema.

Management of fluid guided such that flow-based parameters such as stroke volume index (normal = 35 mL/m² of body surface area [BSA]) and stroke volume variation (normal = 9–13%) are optimized is a well-validated approach that has been shown to reduce morbidity. These flow-based parameters can be monitored by means of arterial pressure–based cardiac output measurements such as the FloTrac (Edwards Lifesciences, Irvine, CA, USA). There is essentially no place for "maintenance" IV fluids in modern fluid management—rather, fluids are given as targeted boluses when they are expected to lead to a hemodynamic improvement.

GDT is an integral component in the current emphasis in surgical services on enhanced recovery after surgery (ERAS) programs, including head and neck surgery.

The classic third space, previously thought to reflect an ill-defined compartment reflecting an otherwise unexplainable perioperative fluid shift, quantitatively does not exist.

Blood Loss (see also Chapter 1.2)

Below a hemoglobin of 7 mg/dL, cardiac output has to increase substantially in order to maintain oxygen transport. Therefore, hemoglobin should be maintained above that value (consider 10.0 in patients with a cardiac history).

◆ Calcium Disturbances

- Normal plasma concentration of Ca is 8.5 to 10 mg/dL with 50% free ionized and 40% protein-bound.
- Normal free ionized concentration is 4.5 to 5 mg/dL.
- Corrected calcium = measured calcium/[0.6 + (total protein)/8.5].
- Ionized calcium increases 0.16 mg/dL for each decrease of 0.1 unit in plasma pH.

2.4 Common Postoperative Problems

A deviation from expected recovery requires prompt and appropriate evaluation. Such deviations may present with a change in exam findings, a subjective complaint from the patient, or laboratory test or vital sign anomalies. Commonly encountered postoperative problems are reviewed here.

◆ Fever

Generally, an elevated temperature ≥ 38.5°C requires work-up. Timing is important, as postoperative fever within the first 24 hours suggests atelectasis (unexpanded lung), possibly an early wound infection, or a urinary tract infection (UTI). Other considerations for fevers, especially after 24 hours postoperatively, include drug reactions, wound abscess, sepsis, pneumonia, an IV or central line infection, or deep venous thrombosis. In appropriate circumstances, transfusion reaction or an infected decubitus ulcer should be considered.

Work-up

A bedside examination includes taking vitals with pulse oximetry and checking the wound for erythema, edema, fluctuance, drainage, and warmth. Auscultate for rales or diminished breath sounds, examine IV sites for redness, and check the patient's legs for calf tenderness. If the patient has a tracheotomy, look for increased and discolored sputum. Consider ordering a chest X-ray, blood cultures, sputum cultures, and/or a urinalysis with cultures.

Fever is a prominent sign of systemic illness in the postoperative patient. Clarifying whether patients have an isolated fever versus systemic inflammation response syndrome (SIRS; **Table 2.21**) and sepsis is important in reducing morbidity and mortality. SIRS and sepsis require urgent

Table 2.21   SIRS

SIRS (Systemic Inflammatory Response Syndrome)

• *Two or more of:*
  o Temperature >38°C or <36°C
  o Heart rate >90/min
  o Respiratory rate >20/min or $Paco_2$ <32 mm Hg (4.3 kPa)
  o White blood cell count >12 000/mm³ or <4000/mm³ or >10% immature bands

(Data from *Bone RC, Balk RA, Cerra FB, et al. American College of Chest Physicians/Society of Critical Care Medicine Consensus Conference:* definitions for sepsis and organ failure and guidelines for the use of innovative therapies in sepsis. *Crit Care Med* 1992;20(6):864–874.)

intervention to improve patient outcome. *Sepsis* is defined as SIRS with a known or suspected infectious source, with evidence of end organ dysfunction (e.g., mental status change, hypotension, decreased urine output/ elevated creatinine). *Septic shock* is sepsis which requires vasopressor agents to maintain mean arterial blood pressure > 65 mm Hg and lactate level > 2 mmol/L (18 mg/dL) despite adequate fluid resuscitation.

For atelectasis/pneumonia, empiric treatment may include a chest physical therapy, supplemental oxygen, and respiratory therapy with incentive spirometry, mucolytics, nebulized bronchodilators, and empiric antibiotics (determined after the results of culture specimens have been received). For the treatment of pneumonia, cephalosporin and clindamycin are recommended, and for a suspected UTI, treat the patient with sulfa or fluoroquinolone. Adjust antibiotics based on culture results. Gentle IV hydration may be useful. Treat with an antipyretic, such as acetaminophen 650 mg for adults (15 mg/kg for children). A wound abscess will require opening the wound, draining it, initiating a Gram stain with culture, and changing the packing. If other vital signs are abnormal, consider transferring the patient to a monitored bed, with continuous pulse oximetry and arterial blood gas assessment.

◆ Confusion (Mental Status Change)

This is one of the most common calls in otolaryngology—head and neck surgery regarding postoperative patients. Although the possible causes for a mental status change are many, it is prudent to consider the cause to be hypoxia until proven otherwise.

Resist the request for a benzodiazepine to "calm the patient down"; instead instruct the nurse to obtain a full set of vitals, including pulse oximetry. Personally visit the patient.

The differential diagnosis includes hypoxia (which can be due to tracheostoma occlusion, crusting, mucus plugging, underlying severe chronic obstructive pulmonary disease [COPD, common in heavy smokers], atelectasis, pneumonia, aspiration, overmedication with narcotics, pneumothorax, pulmonary embolism, or acute postoperative pulmonary edema); cardiac arrhythmia; alcohol withdrawal; delirium from medications; stroke; meningitis; hypoglycemia or severe hyperglycemia; sepsis; anxiety; or psychosis.

Work-up

The bedside exam should include taking a full set of vitals with pulse oximetry, lung auscultation, an examination of the tracheostoma, if present, and a focused neurologic exam looking for focal deficits and the patient's orientation to person, place, and time. For ancillary tests, start with arterial blood gases (ABGs), a 12-lead electrocardiogram (ECG), a fingerstick glucose test, and a portable chest X-ray. A full metabolic panel may be of use to identify electrolyte aberrations or end organ dysfunction. Acute respiratory insufficiency in the head and neck patient often presents with a low PaO_2 and elevated PCO_2; however, a PCO_2 below 40 may be seen with compensatory overventilation. Typically, the patient has an underlying chronic lung disease and has had inadequate tracheopulmonary toilet, allowing secretions to accumulate and mucus plugging to form. Thus, treat with humidified supplemental oxygen and aggressive suctioning. If there is an inadequate response and other tests are normal, consider testing the patient for a pulmonary embolism (PE).

Pulmonary Embolism

In the case of a possible PE, currently spiral chest computed tomography (CT) imaging is obtained, although ventilation/perfusion (V/Q) scans can be performed and laboratory testing for D-dimer may be useful. Patients with proven PE and an otherwise stable cardiovascular status are often managed with supplemental oxygen and anticoagulation, using an IV heparin bolus of 10,000 units with a drip at 800 to 1200 units per hour, maintaining an activated partial thromboplastin time (aPTT) at 1.5 to 2.0 times normal. The patient is transferred to the intensive care unit (ICU) with continuous monitoring; if the patient becomes unstable with cyanosis, low PaO_2, cardiac arrhythmia, hypotension, and low urine output, consider intubation with ventilatory support as well as prescribing an inotropic agent. Thrombolytics may be indicated in certain cases, although they may not be feasible in the postoperative state. Consideration for consultation with pulmonary or critical care services should be considered in these cases.

Acute Postobstructive Pulmonary Edema

Acute postobstructive pulmonary edema (APOPE) should be suspected in patients with postoperative acute respiratory failure. The development of hypoxia, bradycardia, and pink frothy sputum is characteristic in patients with APOPE. Type I APOPE occurs with acute airway compromise usually following extubation. This develops from inspiration against a closed glottis due to laryngospasm or other obstruction. Type II APOPE develops after relief of chronic upper airway obstruction. This may occur in children or adults following surgery to correct severe obstructive sleep apnea, airway stenosis, or neoplasm. In both cases, a sudden decrease in intrathoracic pressure leads to increased pulmonary venous return and transudation from the capillary bed into the interstitium.

The treatment of APOPE includes intensive care monitoring and a low threshold for immediate reintubation. Positive end expiratory pressure may be necessary for adequate ventilation. Diuretics and steroids should be considered. In patients who are stable, medical management with oxygen supplementation, diuretics, and close observation may be appropriate. Careful restriction of intravenous crystalloids may also be an option.

Other Causes of Mental Status Change

If the hypoxia work-up is normal, other testing may reveal an obvious cause. The ECG should rule out the possibility of cardiac arrhythmia, ST changes, or signs of cardiac ischemia or infarction. If the ECG is positive, transfer of the patient to the ICU and a consult with cardiology is mandatory. The fingerstick glucose test is a rapid way to exclude a common cause for mental status change, especially in known diabetics. Glucose below 40 mg/dL should be treated with an ampoule of IV D50 and repeated. If the neurologic exam suggests focal deficit, a brain CT scan to screen for stroke should be considered, although a magnetic resonance imaging (MRI) scan is much more sensitive. Mental status change in a patient with a high fever should prompt consideration of meningitis, especially if the patient has had skull base or otologic surgery. Work-up includes a lumbar puncture, then treatment with empiric antibiotics followed by the transfer of the patient to an ICU setting (see **Chapter 3.2.3** for further details regarding meningitis).

Alcohol Withdrawal

Many head and neck patients have a history of alcohol abuse, which is often underreported. Thus, in the absence of other obvious causes for mental status change, attempting to obtain an honest alcohol use history is important. Unrecognized delirium tremens can have up to an 8% mortality rate. Thus, the postoperative alcoholic patient must be handled properly. Typically, diazepam 5 to 10 mg every 4 hours may be needed, although initially much more frequent doses may be needed to achieve adequate control of the withdrawal. Some patient may require much higher doses. Patients with moderate to severe withdrawal, age over 40, respiratory depression, or refractory symptoms to initial therapy may require ICU admission. IV fluids may contain D10, instead of the typical D5, and also should be supplemented with a 10 mL multivitamin solution per bag. The patient should also be given thiamine daily. Check serum magnesium levels, which are typically low, and replete.

Psychiatric Disorders

Severe anxiety, delirium, or psychosis can be seen in the postoperative patient. There are many predisposing factors, such as sleep deprivation, elderly state, ICU stay, drug dependency, or metabolic alterations. It is important to exclude hypoxia or other obvious medical causes for mental status change or agitation. Psychiatric consultation, if available, may be helpful. Haloperidol 5 mg IV as needed is a reasonably safe drug to use short term, as it will decrease agitation while having little to no influence on cardiovascular status.

◆ Wound Problems

A variety of wound problems can arise following head and neck surgery, including hematoma, seroma, infection, dehiscence, development of a pharyngocutaneous fistula, exposure of the carotid artery leading to rupture or "carotid artery blowout," chyle leak, or reconstructive flap complications such as venous edema or arterial ischemia. As with most situations, prevention is helpful: proper preoperative assessment, management of identified risk factors such as malnutrition or coagulopathy, and meticulous surgical technique. Preoperative radiation therapy is a common issue that greatly increases the risk of healing problems.

Assessment and Management of Wound Problems

Hematoma and Seroma

In cases of hematoma and seroma, the wound will be swollen, usually fluctuant but possibly tense or discolored. A fluid collection can lead to infection or dehiscence or decrease skin flap viability. A small fluid collection may resorb, or it may be simply aspirated. With a rapidly expanding or large fluid collection, the patient should be taken to the OR and the wound opened, irrigated, and explored to maintain hemostasis. *A hematoma following thyroid surgery is an emergency.* Most commonly, this is seen the day of surgery and presents with an expanding mass and discomfort that may progress to dyspnea, stridor, and severe airway compromise. This is due to venous back-pressure causing the rapid development of laryngeal edema. The wound is opened immediately at the bedside and the patient is then taken to the OR to wash out the wound and establish hemostasis. Intubation may be difficult, but opening the wound should facilitate intubation. If this remains difficult, a tracheotomy should be simple to perform, because the thyroidectomy procedure has exposed the subglottic trachea.

Wound Infection

An infected neck wound is typically warm, red, swollen, and tender; it may present with purulent drainage, a fluctuant collection, or abscess formation. Complications may lead to fistula, flap necrosis, or carotid exposure. Management includes opening the wound, culture of drainage, appropriate antibiotics, and packing change. Empiric antibiotic coverage should be broad-spectrum, such as Unasyn (Pfizer Pharmaceuticals, New York, NY), or cefuroxime and clindamycin. Simple wet to dry saline gauze changes twice a day may be sufficient. Sodium oxychlorosene (Clorpactin, United-Guardian, Hauppauge, NY) or acetic acid gauze packing have antimicrobial properties and promote granulation tissue formation. However, if there is carotid exposure, it is prudent to perform surgery to cover the carotid with vascularized tissue, such as a pectoralis flap.

Pharyngocutaneous Fistula

Salivary drainage increasing in suction drains or draining via an incision indicates development of a fistula. One can test drainage for amylase to confirm; salivary secretions will have amylase levels far higher than levels in serum. Most commonly, poor wound healing leads to a fistula following salvage surgery in a patient with persistent or recurrent disease after radiation therapy. Again, this is managed with packing changes, antibiotics, NPO (nothing by mouth) status, and consideration of surgery to bring in vascularized tissue if this fails to heal. Check prealbumin and thyroid-stimulating hormone (TSH) levels to assess for malnutrition and hypothyroidism, and correct. Using the gut when it works is a sound principle, so the patient who must be kept NPO to reduce fistula output should be fed via a nasogastric (NG) or percutaneous endoscopic gastrostomy (PEG) tube. Only if this cannot be accomplished should total parenteral nutrition (TPN) be used.

Chylous Fistula

The incidence of chylous fistula after neck dissection is reported to be between 1% and 5.8%. Chylous fistula results from injury to the thoracic duct, which is encountered in level 4 on the left. However, 25% of chyle leaks occur on the right. This complication is best treated if recognized intraoperatively with suture ligature or oversewing local muscle flaps. Chylous fistula is suspected postoperatively in the face of increased drain outputs. The quality of output may change from serosanguineous to a more milky/turbid consistency. This may occur with the onset of oral intake. High-output chyle loss may lead to electrolyte disturbances, hypovolemia, hypoalbuminemia, immunosuppression, chylothorax, peripheral edema, and local skin breakdown. If there is a question about the diagnosis of a chylous fistula, obtain a drain output analysis for triglycerides and chylomicrons. First-line treatment involves conservative management. This is aimed at reducing chyle flow. The patient may be started on a medium-chain fatty acid diet. If there is no improvement, a trial of NPO with TPN should be considered. Local pressure dressing should be placed. Surgical management is indicated in chylous drainage in excess of 600 mL per day, persistent low-output drainage for an extended period of time, or electrolyte disturbances. Treatment involves wound reexploration and ligation of lymphatic channels. Alternatively, thorascopic ligation or percutaneous lymphangiography-guided embolization of the thoracic duct may be useful.

◆ Carotid Artery Blowout

A carotid artery blowout is a devastating complication, and efforts are aimed at prevention. If postoperative wound problems result in exposure of the carotid, it can rapidly desiccate and then rupture, either externally or into the trachea, depending upon the wound situation. Maintaining healthy vascularized tissue between the carotid and the external environment can generally prevent the problem. Preoperatively, correcting malnutrition, hypothyroidism, and stopping tobacco use are important, especially in the previously irradiated neck. Surgically, if the sternocleidomastoid muscle can be preserved without oncologic compromise, this will help cover and protect the carotid. Avoiding placement of an incision trifurcation directly over the carotid is best. If there is postoperative wound breakdown that may threaten the carotid, prompt management with packing and prevention of desiccation is critical. It is prudent to consider "carotid precautions": maintain large-bore IV access, have a type and crossmatch order in place with the blood bank, and keep an emergency instrument kit in the room. Moreover, if there appears to be any evidence of carotid exposure, one should proceed with surgery to bring in vascularized tissue coverage, rather than hope for healing. A pectoralis flap is ideal; a microvascular free flap is another option.

If a carotid artery blowout occurs, this can present first with a relatively minor sentinel bleed, which stops. Again, one should proceed with flap coverage if there has been a sentinel bleed. If there is a true blowout, there will be a profuse hemorrhage. One should establish direct, firm pressure, treat with bolus IV fluids, and proceed directly to the operating room (OR) for hemostasis. This will involve establishment of proximal and distal control of the vessel, with a risk of stroke. Transfusion will likely be necessary, and if the patient can be saved, wound coverage should be performed. If the blowout occurs into a tracheotomy stoma in a patient who has had a laryngectomy, one may use an endotracheal tube (ETT) to intubate a mainstem bronchus distal to the site of rupture, tightly inflate the cuff, and then tightly pack the stoma opening to achieve tamponade while ventilating on one lung on the way to the OR.

◆ Gastrointestinal and Genitourinary Problems

Renal Failure

Low urine output is a common postoperative issue. The problem may be considered as prerenal, renal, or postrenal. Low urine output is generally defined as less than 30 mL per hour for a 70-kg patient. A prerenal problem means the kidney is underperfused. Usually, this is from hypotension and/or hypovolemia. One should treat with IV hydration. If there is no cardiac failure, give 500 mL of normal saline as an IV bolus. If cardiac failure exists, this must be treated to correct renal perfusion. Diuretics should be used carefully, as these will exacerbate a prerenal situation. Acute renal failure of parenchymal cause may be due to glomerulonephritis, nephrotoxicities, or acute tubular necrosis. Urine may show casts, urine osmolality is equal to that of plasma, and urine sodium is elevated. Follow daily fluid intake and output carefully, and follow laboratory results closely. Electrolytes and creatinine will guide the need for dialysis. Postrenal problems consist of obstructive uropathy. One must identify and correct the source of obstruction. The placement of a Foley catheter may be all that is needed, or imaging studies such as an IV pyelogram may be indicated. In any patient with low urine output or possible renal failure, one must be cautious administering potassium. If hyperkalemia exists, watch for ECG changes. Potassium > 6 should be lowered. A Kayexalate (Sanofi-Aventis Pharmaceuticals, Paris, France) 15 g enema may be given; also IV glucose can be given, along with 10 units of regular insulin, to rapidly lower plasma potassium.

Diarrhea

The main concern in hospitalized patients with diarrhea is the possibility of *Clostridium difficile* colitis, also known as pseudomembranous colitis. This is an anaerobic spore-forming bacterium that is highly transmissible, especially by health care workers with poor hand washing. Stool samples should be sent for the *C. difficile* toxin assay in triplicate. Typically, colonic flora has been reduced by antibiotic use, leading to the *C. difficile* overgrowth and infection. Thus, it is important to stop antibiotics whenever possible and to use them appropriately. Patients with *C. difficile* are treated with metronidazole (Flagyl, Pfizer Pharmaceuticals, New York, NY) 500 mg orally or IV three times per day (TID). There are resistant strains that may require the use of vancomycin given orally. Proper handwashing is critical. New highly virulent strains of *C. difficile* have resulted in fatal infections, and other cases have been treated with colectomy. This is a problem to be taken seriously.

Electrolytes

Hypocalcemia may be seen on the head and neck service, following thyroid or parathyroid surgery. Inadequate parathyroid gland function rapidly results in low serum calcium. One may follow total serum calcium, correlated to albumin level, or may follow ionized calcium. As total calcium drops below ~7.5 to 8.0, the patient may become symptomatic with tingling hands or twitching; with severe hypocalcemia, tetany may ensue. Chvostek sign is twitching of the corner of the mouth in response to tapping over the facial nerve trunk; a positive sign tends to correlate with a calcium level lower than ~8.0. For mild hypocalcemia, the patient may be treated with oral calcium carbonate, 1 g TID, along with calcitriol (Rocaltrol, Validus Pharmaceuticals, Parsippany, NY) 0.25 to 0.5 µg orally daily. In more symptomatic patients, IV correction is necessary using 10% calcium gluconate given 20 mL IV over 15 to 30 minutes. For severe hypercalcemia, a rare condition, treat with massive IV hydration.

For further information on hypercalcemia and hypocalcemia, see **Chapter 7.12**.

Magnesium and phosphate levels should be monitored, especially in the malnourished head and neck oncology patient. Hypomagnesemia may present similarly to hypocalcemia, with neuromuscular manifestations. It may lead to hypocalcemia as well through inhibition of parathyroid hormone action. Repletion of these essential elements should be considered, based on symptoms and degree of the deficit.

3 Otology and Neurotology

Section Editor

Christine T. Dinh

Contributors

Christine T. Dinh

David Goldenberg

Bradley J. Goldstein

Jon E. Isaacson

Gregory T. Lesnik

Adam J. Levy

Elias M. Michaelides

Kari Morgenstein

Stuart A. Ort

Daniel I. Plosky

Julie A. Rhoades

3.0 Embryology and Anatomy of the Ear

◆ Embryology

Auricle

Week 6: Hillocks of His form from condensations of the first and second branchial arches. The first three hillocks are attributed to the first arch, and the second three hillocks are attributed to the second arch (**Table 3.1**).
Week 20: Adult configuration is achieved.
The auricle continues to grow and reaches 85% of adult size by 5 years of age.

External Auditory Canal

Week 8: Ectoderm of the first pharyngeal groove (branchial cleft) invaginates. Epithelial cells then grow as a solid core (meatal plug) toward the middle ear. The core begins to dissolve at ~21 weeks to create the external auditory canal (EAC). The lateral epithelium forms the skin of the bony EAC, while the medial epithelium forms the lateral surface of the tympanic cavity—particularly, the lateral layer of the tympanic membrane (TM). The EAC may not reach final adult size and shape until the early teenage years.

Tympanic Membrane

The tympanic membrane (TM) forms as the **ectoderm** of the first pharyngeal groove (EAC) medializes, thins the **mesenchyme** of the first branchial arch (fibrous middle layer of the TM or the "tympanic ring"), and abuts the **endoderm** of the first pharyngeal pouch (tubotympanic recess or middle ear). The **tympanic notch** (notch of Rivinus) lacks the fibrous middle layer.

Middle Ear

Week 3: Endoderm from the first pharyngeal pouch forms the tubotympanic recess. Pneumatization begins at 10 weeks to form the middle ear and auditory tube (eustachian tube, ET).
Week 4: Mesenchyme from the first and second pharyngeal arches fuses and begins to form the malleus and incus. The first **pharyngeal arch cartilage** is also referred to as Meckel's cartilage, and the **second pharyngeal arch cartilage** is also referred to as Reichert's cartilage. The cartilaginous ossicles

Table 3.1 Embryology of the auricle

Hillock	Arch	Auricular structure
1	1	Tragus
2	1	Crus of helix
3	1	Helix
4	2	Crus of antihelix
5	2	Antihelix
6	2	Antitragus and lobule

Note: There remains some controversy regarding the final contributions of hillocks 4, 5, and 6.

Table 3.2   Embryology of the Meckel and Reichert cartilages

Cartilage	Arch	Ossicular structure
Meckel	1	Head and neck of malleus, body and short process of incus
Reichert	2	Manubrium of malleus, long process of incus, stapes suprastructure

Note: The manubrium of the malleus never completely ossifies.

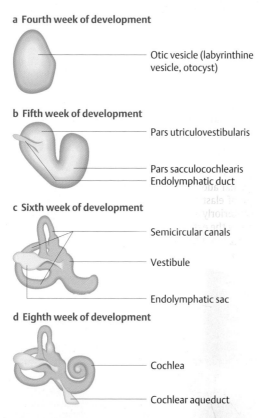

a **Fourth week of development**

Otic vesicle (labyrinthine vesicle, otocyst)

b **Fifth week of development**

Pars utriculovestibularis

Pars sacculocochlearis
Endolymphatic duct

c **Sixth week of development**

Semicircular canals

Vestibule

Endolymphatic sac

d **Eighth week of development**

Cochlea

Cochlear aqueduct

Fig. 3.1   Embryology of the inner ear. The otocyst forms from an epithelial thickening between the cutaneous ectoderm and neural groove in the third and fourth weeks of embryonic development. **(a)** This thickening invaginates and closes off to form a separate vesicle. **(b)** In the fifth week, the otocyst becomes infolded, forming the upper pars utriculovestibularis and the lower pars sacculocochlearis. **(c)** In the sixth week, the three semicircular canals form from the pars utriculovestibularis. **(d)** In the seventh to ninth weeks, the cochlear duct forms as a tubular extension of the pars sacculocochlearis and becomes coiled. (Used with permission from Probst R, Grevers G, Iro H. *Basic Otorhinolaryngology: A Step-by-Step Learning Guide.* Stuttgart/New York: Thieme; 2006:158.)

form at adult size and shape by week 16. Subsequently, ossification occurs by endochondral bone formation (**Table 3.2**). The second pharyngeal arch cartilage also goes on to form the stapes blastema between weeks 4 and 5, which gives rise to the stapes suprastructure. The footplate is of otic capsule origin.

In general, the second pharyngeal arch cartilage forms the ossicular portions seen through the TM on otoscopy (manubrium of the malleus, long process of the incus, stapes superstructure). The first pharyngeal arch cartilage forms the ossicular portions superior to the TM (head of the malleus, body and short process of the incus). In addition, the tensor tympani is formed from the first pharyngeal arch, while the stapedial muscle is formed from the second pharyngeal arch.

Inner Ear

Week 3: The otic placode forms from ectoderm of the first pharyngeal groove. It invaginates and is completely encircled in mesoderm and termed the otocyst by week 4. The pars superior (semicircular canals and utricle) develops prior to the pars inferior (saccule and cochlea). The membranous labyrinth is complete by week 15 or 16. Ossification occurs between weeks 20 and 25 (**Fig. 3.1**).

◆ Anatomy

Auricle

The auricle and the external auditory canal are referred to as the external ear. The auricle is made of elastic cartilage with perichondrium and skin that is tightly adherent anteriorly and loosely adherent posteriorly (**Fig. 3.2**). It is attached to the head by the extension of cartilage into the ear canal and anterior, superior, and posterior ligaments and muscles.

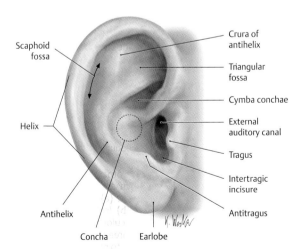

Fig. 3.2 Anatomy of the auricle. (From Gilroy AM, MacPherson BR, Ross LM. *Thieme Atlas of Anatomy, Head and Neuroanatomy*. 1st ed. Stuttgart/New York: Thieme; 2007. Illustration by Karl Wesker.)

External Auditory Canal

The EAC is one-third cartilaginous (lateral) and two-thirds osseous (medial). The EAC contains fibrocartilage, not elastic cartilage. The skin lining the cartilaginous EAC is thick with hair follicles and sebaceous and ceruminous glands. The medial skin is thin without any adnexal structures or subcutaneous tissue, is extremely pain-sensitive, and is the only site in the entire body with skin lying directly on periosteum. The EAC is innervated by contributions from the trigeminal nerve (cranial nerve [CN] V_3, auriculotemporal branch), the cervical plexus (C3, great auricular nerve), the vagus nerve (CN X, Arnold's nerve), and the facial nerve (CN VII). C2 and C3 contributions from the lesser occipital nerve innervate the inferior auricle, but not the EAC.

Arnold's reflex occurs when manipulation of the ear canal produces coughing. **Hitzelberger sign** is numbness over the posterior aspect of the EAC due to impaired facial nerve function from a cerebellopontine angle tumor. The **fissures of Santorini** are two vertical fissures in the anteroinferior aspect of the cartilaginous EAC, while the **foramen of Huschke** (foramen tympanicum) is a developmental defect in the anteroinferior aspect of the bony EAC. Infection and malignancies can travel through these channels to the temporomandibular joint, parotid gland, and infratemporal fossa.

Tympanic Membrane

The TM is made up of three layers. From lateral to medial, they are the squamous epithelium, a radiating and circular fibrous layer, and an inner mucosal layer. The TM is ~10 mm in height and 9 mm in width. Circumferentially, the fibrous anulus sits within the bony anulus but is discontinuous superiorly at the **tympanic notch**. Inferiorly to the tympanic notch, the TM has a well-organized fibrous middle layer and is known as the **pars tensa.** At the level of the tympanic notch and above, the middle fibrous layer is less organized and is known as the **pars flaccida**. **Prussak's space** is at the level of the pars flaccida, bounded laterally by the TM and medially by the neck of the malleus. It is a frequent site of retraction and cholesteatoma formation.

Middle Ear

The middle ear is divided into three pneumatized spaces. The epitympanum is the middle ear space above the TM, the mesotympanum is the middle ear space medial to the TM, and the hypotympanum is the middle ear space below the TM. The protympanum is the anterior portion of the mesotympanum, where the entrance of the ET is located. The boundaries of the middle ear space are:

- Lateral: tympanic membrane
- Superior: tegmen
- Inferior: jugular bulb
- Anterior: carotid canal, ET
- Posterior: mastoid via facial recess or retrofacial cells
- Medial: cochlear promontory and labyrinthine wall

Ossicles

● *Malleus.* The **malleus** (hammer) consists of a manubrium (handle), anterior and lateral processes, neck, and head. It is incorporated into the TM from the lateral process to the tip of the manubrium (at the umbo of the TM). The tensor tendon runs from the cochleariform process of the middle ear to the medial surface of the neck and manubrium of the malleus.

● *Incus.* The **incus** (anvil) is the largest ossicle and articulates with the malleus head in the epitympanum. It has a body and short, long, and lenticular processes. The short process is held in place by the posterior incudal ligament. Both the incudomalleolar and incudostapedial joints are synovial diarthrodial joints.

● *Stapes.* The **stapes** (stirrup) is the smallest ossicle and articulates with the lenticular process of the incus. It has a capitulum, an anterior and a posterior crus, and a footplate. The stapedial tendon runs from the pyramidal eminence to the posterior surface of the capitulum or the posterior crus. The footplate is kept in position by the annular ligament.

See **Fig. 3.3**. *Note:* The tensor tympani muscle is innervated by CN V$_3$, while the stapedius muscle is innervated by CN VII.

Eustachian Tube

The ET measures ~18 mm at birth and 35 mm in adulthood. The lateral one-third is bony, is located at the anterior mesotympanum (protympanum), and is lined with ciliated cuboidal epithelium. The medial two-thirds is cartilaginous, terminates at the torus tubarius of the nasopharynx, and is lined with pseudostratified columnar epithelium. The ET

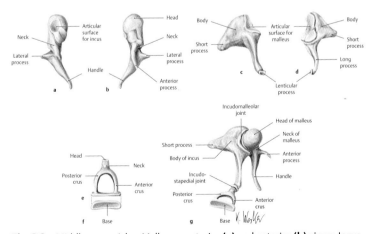

Fig. 3.3 Middle ear ossicles. Malleus, posterior **(a)** and anterior **(b)** views. Incus, medial **(c)** and anterolateral **(d)** views. **(e)** Stapes, superior and medial views. **(f)** Medial view of the ossicular chain. (From Gilroy AM, MacPherson BR, Ross LM. *Thieme Atlas of Anatomy, Head and Neuroanatomy.* 1st ed. Stuttgart/New York: Thieme; 2007. Illustration by Karl Wesker.)

functions to ventilate, clear secretions from, and protect the middle ear. It is closed at rest, and its primary dilator is the tensor veli palatini muscle (CN V$_3$).

Inner Ear

Bony Labyrinth

The cochlea is the auditory portion of the inner ear. It is shaped like a spiral around its central axis, called the modiolus. It has $2^1/_2$ turns and is divided in the basal, middle, and apical turns. The perilymphatic fluid of the basal turn of the cochlea communicates with the subarachnoid space through the **cochlear aqueduct** (a bony channel that houses the periotic duct).

The vestibular system consists of the otolith organs of the vestibule (utricle and saccule), the endolymphatic sac, and the semicircular canals (SCCs). The vestibule is the central chamber of the vestibular portion of the inner ear. Its medial wall has two depressions. The **elliptical recess** is located posterosuperior and contains the macula of the utricle, while the **spherical recess** is located anteroinferior and contains the macule of the saccule. The **vestibular aqueduct** is the bony channel that contains the **endolymphatic sac**; it communicates with the vestibule posteroinferiorly via the **endolymphatic duct**.

The SCCs are three paired canals that lie at ~90° angles to one another. The canals are referred to as the horizontal (or lateral) SCC, the superior (or anterior) SCC, and the posterior SCC. Each SCC has ampullated and nonampullated ends that communicate with the vestibule. All ends connect to the vestibule separately except the nonampullated ends of the posterior and superior SCCs, which fuse and join the vestibule together as the common crus. The horizontal canal lies ~30° from the true horizontal.

Membranous Labyrinth

The membranous labyrinth is the fluid-filled chamber within the bony labyrinth. The membranous labyrinth contains endolymph, which has similar consistency to intracellular fluid (high potassium, low sodium). The membranous labyrinth is surrounded by perilymph, which has similar consistency to extracellular fluid (high sodium, low potassium).

The cochlear duct (or scala media) is the membranous portion of the cochlea, contains endolymph, and houses the auditory hair cells of the spiral organ (organ of Corti; **Fig. 3.4**). The scala media is flanked by two fluid-filled spaces called the scala vestibuli and scala tympani. The perilymph of the scala vestibuli and scala tympani communicate at the helicotrema of the apex of the cochlea. The endolymphatic fluid of the scala media connects to the saccule through the ductus reuniens. It also connects to the subarachnoid space through the periotic duct of the cochlear aqueduct.

The utricle and the saccule are the membranous portions of the vestibule. They contain endolymph but are surrounded by perilymph. The utricle and saccule are otolith organs that contain gelatinous membranes coated with otoconia and sense linear acceleration. The utricle senses movement in the horizontal plane, and the saccule senses motion in the vertical plane as well as gravitational force.

The semicircular ducts are the membranous channels within the SCCs. The semicircular ducts contain endolymph and are surrounded by perilymph. Each duct has an ampullated end, which houses the crista ampullaris, a cone-shaped organ containing hair cells that detect angular acceleration.

The endolymphatic sac contains endolymph and is located in the vestibular aqueduct within the dura of the posterior fossa. The endolymphatic sac communicates with the saccule via the endolymphatic duct.

Internal Auditory Canal

The internal auditory canal (internal acoustic meatus) is the bony channel of the posterior fossa that houses the facial nerve (CN VII) and vestibulocochlear nerve (CN VIII). It begins medially at as the porus acusticus internus and runs laterally to end at the fundus. At the fundus, it is split horizontally by the falciform or transverse crest. The superior portion of the canal above the falciform crest is then split again into an anterior and posterior compartment by the vertical crest or Bill's bar. In the fundus, the facial nerve is located anterosuperior, the cochlear nerve is located anteroinferior, the superior part of the vestibular nerve is located posterosuperior, and the inferior part of the vestibular nerve is located posteroinferior.

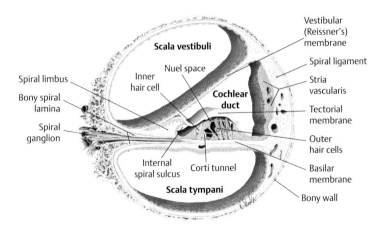

Fig. 3.4 The cochlear duct. (From Gilroy AM, MacPherson BR, Ross LM. *Thieme Atlas of Anatomy, Head and Neuroanatomy*. 1st ed. Stuttgart/New York: Thieme; 2007. Illustration by Karl Wesker.)

3.1   Otologic Emergencies

3.1.1   Sudden Hearing Loss

◆ Key Features

- Sudden hearing loss can be sensorineural or conductive in nature.
- Audiogram is performed to differentiate between sensorineural and conductive hearing loss.
- Idiopathic sudden sensorineural hearing loss is diagnosed when other causes have been excluded.
- Early treatment of idiopathic sudden sensorineural hearing loss with oral and/or intratympanic steroids is commonly recommended.

Sudden hearing loss is the rapid onset of subjective hearing impairment over 72 hours or less. Sudden sensorineural hearing loss (SSNHL) is one type of sudden hearing loss. The potential causes of SSNHL are broad: infection, vascular insult, trauma, autoimmune, neoplasm, acoustic trauma, drug-related, iatrogenic, and idiopathic. One common criterion used to define SSNHL is at least a 30-decibel (dB) reduction in sensorineural thresholds in at least three consecutive frequencies compared to baseline. Early implementation of high-dose systemic and/or intratympanic steroids is commonly recommended.

◆ Epidemiology

SSNHL affects 5 to 20 per 100,000 people in the United States. Men and women are affected equally. Most commonly it affects middle-aged people.

◆ Clinical

Signs and Symptoms

Patients may report sudden subjective hearing loss, ear fullness, and/or tinnitus in one or both ears. Dysequilibrium or vertigo can also occur. A history of upper respiratory tract infection, head trauma, cardiac surgery, ototoxic drug intake, otologic surgery, barotrauma, and loud noise exposure may precede onset of symptoms. Preexisting history or family history of autoimmune disorder may be ascertained.

Differential Diagnosis

Idiopathic SSNHL is diagnosed when other causes have been excluded. The potential causes of SSNHL are broad and include viral infections, syphilis, vascular insult, trauma, autoimmune disease, internal auditory canal or cerebellopontine angle neoplasm, acoustic trauma, ototoxic drugs, barotrauma, perilymphatic fistula, endolymphatic hydrops, Menière's disease, and iatrogenic injury. Middle ear or external auditory causes such as middle ear effusion and cerumen impaction are causes of conductive hearing loss and should be excluded.

◆ Evaluation

Physical Exam

A complete head and neck examination, including cranial nerve assessment, should be performed. External and middle ear disorders should be assessed on otoscopy. Neurologic exam can identify signs of central or systemic disorders. Vestibular exam can demonstrate any associated vestibular weakness. A tuning fork and fistula test are important as well.

Audiometry

Pure tone and speech audiometry and tympanogram are required. Causes of conductive hearing loss can be excluded on these examinations. A poor word recognition score out of proportion to pure tone thresholds and rollover should raise suspicion for a retrocochlear lesion. A low-frequency sensorineural hearing loss is suspicious for endolymphatic hydrops or Ménière's disease. A notch at 3 to 4 kHz suggests acoustic trauma. A commonly accepted definition for SSNHL is a reduction in sensorineural hearing of at least 30 dB in at least three contiguous frequencies compared to baseline; however, in clinical practice, SSNHL includes hearing loss of lesser degrees.

Imaging

Magnetic resonance imaging (MRI) of the brain with and without gadolinium enhancement is obtained to rule out retrocochlear or cerebellopontine angle tumor.

Intracranial disorders can also be excluded on MRI. Auditory brainstem response (ABR) testing and follow-up audiometry are acceptable alternatives to MRI if appropriate counseling regarding limitations is performed. In patients with a presenting history of head trauma, computed tomography (CT) of the temporal bone without contrast is considered to assess for temporal bone fractures and pneumolabyrinth causing SSNHL.

Labs

Routine ordering of laboratory tests in patients with unilateral idiopathic SSNHL is not recommended. In patients with fluctuating and bilateral SSNHL, additional testing is suggested: (1) rapid plasma reagin (RPR) test or a fluorescent treponemal antibody absorption (FTA-ABS) test to rule out syphilis, (2) erythrocyte sedimentation rate (ESR) to screen for inflammatory disorder, (3) rheumatoid factor, antinuclear antibody, and antineutrophil cytoplasmic antibodies to assess for autoimmune etiology, (4) Lyme serology if risk factors are present, (5) thyroid function tests, (6) and (7) glucose testing for diabetes.

◆ Treatment Options

Treatment is tailored to the etiology of SSNHL. However, approximately 85% of cases are considered idiopathic. SSNHL may resolve spontaneously in up to 65% of patients. Early treatment with oral and/or intratympanic steroids is commonly recommended as initial therapy for SSNHL, as prolonged delay in treatment may result in permanent hearing loss. Most clinicians prescribe oral prednisone (1 mg/kg daily) for 1 week with 1 week additional taper. Intratympanic dexamethasone has been used in various concentrations but usually requires at least three injections. Routine use of antivirals, thrombolytics, vasodilators, vaso-active substance, and antioxidants is not recommended. Hyperbaric oxygen therapy may be offered within three months of onset of idiopathic SSNHL.

◆ Outcome and Follow-Up

Although approximately two-thirds of patients with idiopathic SSNHL experience some recovery without treatment, early treatment is associated with better hearing outcomes. Follow-up audiograms to assess for recovery or progression are performed within 6 months of diagnosis and treatment of idiopathic SNHL. Hearing rehabilitation is offered to patients with incomplete recovery. Tinnitus associated with hearing impairment should also be addressed and treated appropriately.

3.1.2   Ear and Temporal Bone Trauma

◆ Key Features

> - Auricular injuries include lacerations, avulsions, blunt injury with hematoma, thermal injury, and frostbite. Treatment depends on etiology.
> - Penetrating and blunt trauma to the temporal bone can cause hearing loss, dizziness, facial paralysis, cerebrospinal fluid leak, and life-threatening hemorrhage. Early recognition and treatment of complications can reduce morbidity and mortality.

Penetrating and blunt trauma can affect all aspects of the ear and temporal bone, including the auricle, external auditory canal (EAC), tympanic membrane, ossicles, inner ear, carotid artery, venous sinuses, tegmen, and facial nerve. High suspicion and prompt recognition and treatment of associated temporal bone injuries is important in reducing trauma-related complications.

◆ Epidemiology

The most common cause of temporal bone fractures is motor vehicle accidents. Assault is the second most common cause; males are more commonly affected. Approximately 20% of skull fractures involve the temporal bone. Soft tissue injuries to the auricle are common.

◆ Clinical

Signs and Symptoms

Presentation depends upon the type of trauma and the location and extent of injury. Trauma to the auricle can be due to laceration, avulsion, blunt injury, thermal injury, or frostbite. Trauma to the temporal bone can be from acoustic trauma, barotrauma (e.g., diving), penetrating trauma (e.g., cotton tip applicator, gunshot wound), or blunt trauma (e.g., motor vehicle accident, assault). Thermal injury can also injure the tympanic membrane; for example, hot slag from a blast.

Auricular Injury

Blunt injury to the auricle may result in auricular pain, edema, erythema, and hematoma. Localized pain and bleeding are common after lacerations and avulsions of the auricle. Burn injuries can cause blistering, skin de-epithelialization, and cartilage exposure. The auricle is a common site of frostbite injury, which may present as a spectrum of findings over several weeks, from clear blistering, hemorrhagic blisters, or a dry insensate wound to blackened tissue demarcation and necrosis.

External, Middle, and Inner Ear Injuries

EAC trauma and traumatic tympanic membrane perforations can present with pain, bloody otorrhea, and conductive hearing loss. Injuries affecting the middle ear present as hemotympanum (blood in the middle ear) and/or conductive hearing loss and can involve ossicular fracture or discontinuity. Trauma involving the inner ear can cause sensorineural hearing loss (e.g., cochlear concussion, otic capsule violating fracture) and vertigo (e.g., benign paroxysmal positional vertigo, labyrinthine concussion, perilymphatic fistula, vestibular loss).

Other Injuries

Penetrating trauma and temporal bone fractures can involve the facial (fallopian) canal and cause immediate and delayed facial palsies. The perigeniculate area is the most common site of facial nerve injury in temporal bone fractures. Blunt trauma to the extratemporal facial nerve can also cause facial paralysis. Penetrating trauma and temporal bone fractures involving the middle cranial fossa plate, posterior cranial fossa plate, or otic capsule can cause leakage of cerebrospinal fluid (CSF) into the temporal bone, which can manifest as clear middle ear effusion, otorrhea, or rhinorrhea. Injuries to the horizontal and vertical petrous internal carotid artery, sigmoid sinus, or jugular bulb can cause life-threatening hemorrhage and hemodynamic instability.

Temporal Bone Fractures

Temporal bone fractures are most often seen in patients with severe head trauma. Additional injuries requiring resuscitation and multi-team care are common. ENT findings may include otorrhea, hearing loss, nystagmus, and facial paralysis. A bruise over the mastoid (**Battle sign**) is an indication of fracture of the middle cranial fossa and injury of the posterior auricular artery. Periorbital ecchymosis (**raccoon eyes**) suggests a basal skull fracture.

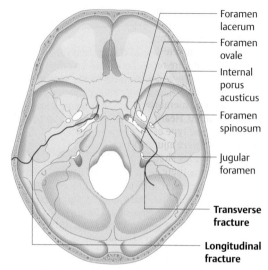

Fig. 3.5   Temporal bone fractures: a typical longitudinal temporal bone fracture (left) and transverse temporal bone fracture (right). (Used with permission from Probst R, Grevers G, Iro H. *Basic Otorhinolaryngology: A Step-by-Step Learning Guide*. Stuttgart/New York: Thieme; 2006:303.)

Temporal bone fractures are classified as either **otic-sparing or otic-violating fractures**. Otic-violating fractures are more commonly associated with sensorineural hearing loss. Older classifications divide temporal bone fractures with respect to the long axis of the petrous pyramid (**Fig. 3.5**): (1) **longitudinal fracture** (oriented along the petrous axis, parallel to the petrotympanic fissure), (2) **transverse fracture** (oriented perpendicular to the petrous axis), (3) **oblique** (oriented along the petrous axis, crossing the petrotympanic fissure), or (4) **mixed** fractures.

Oblique/longitudinal fractures represent 80% of all temporal bone fractures (~25% associated with facial nerve injury). Transverse fractures are less common; however, 40 to 50% are associated with facial palsy. Transverse fractures more commonly affect the otic capsule and cause sensorineural hearing loss.

Differential Diagnosis

There is a broad range of causes of trauma and associated injuries, some of which have been listed in preceding paragraphs.

◆ Evaluation

Physical Exam

Soft tissue injuries isolated to the auricle are evaluated with a focused otologic exam. Exposed cartilage, auricular hematoma, and auricular viability should be noted.

Patients with severe head or multisystem injury should receive standard trauma and resuscitation. Life-threatening injuries (e.g., cervical spine trauma, intracranial bleeding) must be treated emergently, and the patient should be stabilized. Complete head and neck, otologic, neurologic, and cranial nerve examinations are recommended.

When feasible, immediate or delayed facial paralysis should be assessed early and prior to intubation. The ear canal should be cleaned, and injuries to the EAC and tympanic membrane should be assessed. Presence of CSF leak should be ascertained. Hearing can be evaluated with a 512-Hz tuning fork, and the presence and type of nystagmus should be noted.

In patients with less severe injury, a more focused exam is feasible. Foreign body or penetrating injuries should be evaluated with an oto-microscope. In uncooperative children, there should be a low threshold for exam under anesthesia.

Imaging

High-resolution computed tomography (CT) of the temporal bone is recommended to assess for temporal bone fractures and integrity of the EAC, ossicles, otic capsule, middle and posterior cranial fossa plates, carotid canal, jugular bulb, and sigmoid sinus. Fractures involving the carotid canal and penetrating traumas (e.g., gunshot wounds) to the temporal bone require angiography to rule out vascular injury.

Other Tests

Pure tone and speech audiometry should be obtained when feasible. Electrophysiologic testing of the facial nerve (e.g., electroneuronography [ENoG] and electromyography [EMG]) may be helpful in terms of predicting recovery and guiding treatment decisions in patients with complete facial paralysis.

◆ Treatment Options

Soft Tissue Injuries

Auricular lacerations must be cleaned thoroughly. Cartilage may be reapproximated. When possible, soft tissue should be closed over exposed cartilage. If tissue is devitalized, wet-to-dry dressing coverage can be provided and surgical reconstruction planned in a delayed fashion. Antibiotics with adequate *Pseudomonas* coverage are prescribed.

Auricular hematomas must be drained to prevent a cauliflower deformity. To prevent reaccumulation, a pressure bolster is applied. Dental rolls or rolled Xeroform (Kendall Company, Mansfield, MA) are placed on the anterior and posterior surface of the auricle and secured with 2–0 nylon in a through-and-through mattress stitch for 5 days. Antibiotics are generally prescribed.

Auricular burns are treated topically with mafenide acetate. This sulfonamide-type medication can penetrate eschar and prevent cartilage loss. Infected cartilage is débrided. Treatment for frostbite injury is focused on rapid rewarming; avoidance of thawing and refreezing are critical for auricular viability. Anti-inflammatories are also important for pain control and reducing inflammation. Prophylactic antibiotics are not routinely recommended. However, ongoing local wound care is often required as the injury demarcates.

Microsurgical revascularization and surgical reattachment of avulsions should be performed; however, there is a high failure rate, requiring delayed débridement and reconstruction. Most animal and human bites to the face or auricle can be thoroughly irrigated, débrided, sutured closed, and treated with antibiotics. Human bites have a higher risk of infection, and some clinicians advocate healing by secondary intention.

Tetanus vaccination, tetanus immunoglobulin, and rabies vaccination should be administered in the appropriate scenarios.

Penetrating Trauma to the External Auditory Canal and Middle Ear

Ear canal injuries should be cleaned under the microscope and stented if there is circumferential injury, to prevent stenosis. When stenting is performed with Oto-Wick (Medtronic Xomed, Inc., Jacksonville, FL) or Gelfoam (Pfizer Pharmaceuticals, New York, NY), antibiotic-and-steroid otic drops are prescribed.

Most traumatic tympanic membrane perforations can be observed for spontaneous resolution, because approximately 90% of small perforations resolves without treatment. Nonhealing tympanic membrane perforations can be treated with myringoplasty or tympanoplasty. Prophylactic antibiotic ear drops are prescribed for contaminated wounds. Dry ear precautions and avoidance of nose blowing are discussed.

Exploratory tympanotomy (myringotomy) and perilymphatic fistula repair is recommended if the injury is located in the posterosuperior quadrant of the tympanic membrane, severe vertigo is present, and stapes dislocation and perilymphatic fistula are suspected. Treatment of hearing loss and vertigo related to perilymphatic fistula may also require bed rest, systemic steroids, antiemetics, and short-term vestibulosuppressants.

Follow-up audiogram within three months of injury is recommended. Tympanoplasty and ossiculoplasty can be performed for persistent tympanic membrane perforation and ossicular discontinuity or fracture.

Temporal Bone Fracture and Other Injuries

Uncomplicated temporal bone fractures can be managed conservatively with wound care and follow-up audiograms. Otic-violating fractures or inner ear concussion causing sensorineural hearing loss should be treated with systemic steroids unless there is a medical contraindication. Vestibular dysfunction should be treated symptomatically with bed rest, antiemetics, and short-term vestibulosuppressants. Follow-up audiograms are recommended, and vestibular testing can be obtained for prolonged dizziness.

Immediate-onset facial paralysis after temporal bone fracture is thought to be from nerve transection, while incomplete facial palsy and delayed-onset facial paralysis may be due to nerve compression from edema or hematoma. High-dose steroids are recommended for facial nerve impairment. The prognosis for incomplete or delayed-onset facial paralysis is excellent, and surgical intervention is rarely indicated. Immediate-onset paralysis has a worse prognosis. Surgical decompression or nerve repair is considered if there is > 90% degeneration on ENoG between 3 and 14 days after onset. EMG is performed if ENoG shows absent responses (phase cancellation can occur from simultaneous degeneration and regeneration). On EMG, no voluntary action potentials indicates a poor prognosis.

Gunshot wounds may involve widespread injury, carrying a high incidence of severe vascular injury and high mortality rate. Endovascular stenting may be necessary to prevent life-threatening hemorrhage from vascular injury. Most cases of CSF otorrhea or rhinorrhea resolve spontaneously with bed rest and stool softeners. Lumbar drain is considered if the CSF leak does not resolve in 5 to 7 days. Surgical intervention with removal of epithelial elements, closure of the ear canal, and auditory tube and mastoid obliteration with abdominal fat can be performed if lumbar drain fails to resolve the CSF leak. Antibiotic prophylaxis is controversial.

◆ Outcome and Follow-Up

Aural rehabilitation for permanent hearing loss can be offered. Treatment can include conventional hearing aid, bone-anchored hearing aid, contralateral routing of sound (CROS) hearing aids, and in extreme cases, cochlear implantation. Persistent vestibular complaints can be evaluated with vestibular testing and treated appropriately with particle repositioning for canalolithiasis and vestibular therapy for uncompensated vestibulopathy. In patients with facial paralysis, frequent wetting or lubrication of the eye is recommended; gold or platinum weight implants can be performed to assist in eye closure. Dynamic and static facial reanimation, nerve transfer (e.g., hypoglossal-to-facial nerve transposition, masseteric-to-facial nerve transposition), and free flap (e.g., gracilis free flap) reanimation can be discussed for poor nerve regeneration outcomes.

3.1.3 Acute Facial Paresis and Paralysis

◆ Key Features

- Facial paralysis in Bell's palsy occurs rapidly, usually within 24 to 48 hours.
- Treatment consists of high-dose oral steroids and antiviral medication.
- Eye care is essential and should not be overlooked.
- Spontaneous recovery to normal or near-normal function occurs in ~85%.

Bell's palsy, or acute idiopathic facial nerve palsy, accounts for 60 to 75% of all acute facial palsies. Bell's palsy is characterized by rapid-onset (24 to 48 hours) facial weakness that may progress to complete paralysis. A facial

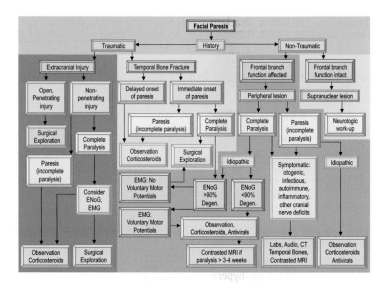

Fig. 3.6 Algorithm for the differential diagnosis of facial paresis. Many advocate surgical decompression only for cases of complete paralysis, and, although not specifically indicated on this algorithm, facial nerve decompression may be useful in cases of nontraumatic paralysis. (Modified with permission from Probst R, Grevers G, Iro H. *Basic Otorhinolaryngology: A Step-by-Step Learning Guide.* Stuttgart/New York: Thieme; 2006:293.)

weakness that progresses slowly over weeks to months is suspicious for a neoplasm. Treatment for Bell's palsy consists of a prednisone taper (~ 1 mg/kg orally daily) plus an antiviral medication for at least one week. Eye lubrication is recommend if eye closure is compromised (see also **Chapter 9.2**). If there is little to no recovery of facial function after 2 to 3 months, then imaging is recommended to rule out neoplastic etiology.

◆ Epidemiology

The incidence of Bell's palsy is 20 to 30 cases per 100,000 people per year. It accounts for almost 75% of all unilateral facial palsy; 40,000 cases occur in the United States each year. Median age of onset is 40 years, but the incidence is highest over age 70. Men and women, and right and left sides, are affected equally. Pregnant women and patients with diabetes and hypertension are at increased risk.

Table 3.3 The House–Brackmann Facial Nerve Grading Scale

Grade	Facial nerve findings
I. Normal	Normal
II. Mild dysfunction	Slight weakness on close inspection
III. Moderate dysfunction	Appears normal at rest; weakness with effort but still full eye closure
IV. Moderately severe dysfunction	Weakness visible at rest; incomplete eye closure
V. Severe dysfunction	Only barely perceptible motion
VI. Total paralysis	Complete paralysis

Data from House JW, Brackmann DE. Facial nerve grading system. Otolaryngol Head Neck Surg 1985;93(2):146–147.

◆ Clinical

Signs and Symptoms

Patients usually present with rapid-onset (24–48 hours) facial nerve weakness that may progress to complete paralysis. Patients often report pain and numbness around the ear, hyperacusis, and dysgeusia; 70% of patients will have a preceding viral illness.

Differential Diagnosis

Idiopathic facial nerve palsy is a diagnosis of exclusion (**Fig. 3.6**). Herpes zoster oticus (Ramsay-Hunt) is characterized by severe otalgia and vesicular lesions involving the ear and accounts for 10 to 15% of acute facial palsies. Melkersson-Rosenthal's syndrome consists of recurrent bouts of unilateral facial palsy in association with facial edema and a fissured tongue. Facial palsy occurs in 11% of patients with Lyme disease and may be bilateral. Acute and chronic otitis media with or without cholesteatoma can also cause acute facial palsy, as can necrotizing or malignant otitis externa. Neoplasms need to be ruled out if there is no symptomatic improvement after 2 to 3 months or if the palsy is characterized by slow onset or relapse. Temporal bone trauma can also result in acute facial paralysis.

◆ Evaluation

History

The most important information is the history. Time of onset and history of previous episodes are paramount. Hearing loss and vertigo are also important to note. Patients with herpes zoster oticus are likely to experience involvement of the vestibulocochlear nerve (CN VIII).

Physical Exam

A complete head and neck examination is required. Determination is made whether facial nerve function is weak or completely absent. The House–Brackmann scale for facial function is often used for charting and physician communication (**Table 3.3**). If the upper face is spared, then a central etiology is suspected. The eardrum is carefully inspected to rule out acute or chronic middle ear disease, cholesteatoma, or a temporal bone neoplasm, either benign or malignant. The skin is evaluated for signs of vesicular lesions. Vesicular lesions may be periauricular, auricular, in the ear canal, or even on the palate. They are generally tender and present in various stages of healing. Palpation of the neck and parotid gland is crucial in ruling out an extratemporal process. The remaining cranial nerves are also examined, looking for evidence for polyneuropathy.

Ancillary Tests

An audiogram is recommended when there are otologic complaints or prolonged facial paralysis. Asymmetry in hearing may suggest cochlear, retrocochlear, or cerebellopontine angle process contributing to facial weakness.

Imaging

Imaging is not routinely obtained at presentation if the history is consistent with acute idiopathic palsy. If the history is suspicious for neoplasm or otologic symptoms are present, then a magnetic resonance imaging (MRI) scan of the head with and without gadolinium enhancement is obtained to visualize the entire course of the facial nerve. If there is any enhancement along the intratemporal course of the nerve, a noncontrast fine-cut temporal bone computed tomography (CT) scan will help to delineate the facial (fallopian) canal looking for dilation or erosion. If the palsy shows no signs of improvement within 3 months, imaging is recommended.

Labs

Labs are not routinely ordered. If the clinical picture does not follow that of an idiopathic palsy or there are risk factors for other disorders, then labs are ordered as indicated. Systemic disorders causing facial weakness include autoimmune syndromes, Wegener's granulomatosis, sarcoidosis, Lyme disease, and syphilis.

Electrical Testing

Electrical testing continues to be controversial. If a patient is evaluated within the first 2 weeks of the onset, an electroneuronography (ENoG) can be obtained. It is useful when performed within 3 to 14 days of onset of total paralysis and when the contralateral face is unaffected. A stimulating surface electrode is placed at the stylomastoid foramen, and a recording surface electrode is placed at the nasolabial fold. A compound muscle action potential is then recorded and compared with that recorded from the unaffected side. Changes in amplitude are calculated and interpreted as a percentage of nerve fiber dysfunction. If serial ENoGs are performed starting after day 3, and the amplitude on the affected side indicates > 90% loss of function, then surgical decompression may be an option. Electromyography (EMG) is also recommended in this circumstance, and surgical candidates are expected to demonstrate no voluntary action potentials within 2 weeks of paralysis.

Pathology

Similar to idiopathic SNHL, idiopathic facial nerve palsy as a symptom is likely secondary to multiple insults. Theories focus on virally mediated inflammation followed by ischemia, neural blockade, and degeneration. The inflammation leads to physical compression as the facial nerve enters the fundus of the temporal bone and forms the labyrinthine segment. This region is known as the meatal foramen and is the narrowest portion of the facial canal, forming a bottleneck area. Nerve conduction studies on patients undergoing decompression surgery for Bell's palsy have consistently demonstrated decreased electrical responses distal to the meatal foramen. Histopathologic studies obtained from autopsy of patients who died shortly after onset of Bell's palsy have been reported. The findings are similar though not uniform. Inflammatory neuritis consistent with a viral infection is most often reported, but intraneural vascular congestion and hemorrhage have also been identified. Viral studies have shown evidence implicating herpes simplex virus (HSV) as the offending agent. Herpes virus has been harvested from nasal and oral secretions of patients experiencing an acute facial palsy. Animal models have also been used to demonstrate acute facial paralysis after intraoral and periauricular inoculation with HSV. All of these studies are persuasive but as yet not conclusive.

◆ Treatment Options

Medical

Management of Bell's palsy consists of high-dose oral steroids (e.g., prednisone ~1 mg/kg start dose) with a 2- to 3-week taper and a concurrent 7 to 10 days of an oral antiviral (e.g., valacyclovir 500 mg orally three times daily). The natural history of the disorder suggests that almost 85% of patients will recover normal or near-normal function without treatment, but there is no test to determine outcomes at the time of presentation. Therefore, all patients are treated with this medical regimen.

Patients must also be evaluated for the need for eye care. If paralysis is complete and facial tone is poor, there will be corneal exposure throughout the day and night. Patients receive frequent doses of artificial tears to that eye and use a nighttime lubricant to protect the cornea while they sleep. They can also wear a clear moisture chamber over the eye.

Surgical

Surgery for these patients remains controversial. Centers that see large volumes of these patients have developed algorithms that include serial ENoG testing in conjunction with EMG. If patients present within 2 weeks of onset of paralysis, and reach > 90% facial nerve degeneration without evidence of EMG action potentials, they are offered middle fossa facial nerve decompression. The middle fossa route enables complete decompression of the labyrinthine portion of the facial nerve, including the meatal foramen, without sacrificing hearing. Small series have shown that patients choosing decompression have a 91% chance of good recovery (House–Brackmann I or II). Patients who refuse surgery have a 58% chance of poor recovery (House–Brackmann III or IV).

Patients who experience poor recovery often require facial enhancement or reanimation procedures. Tarsorrhaphy, spring, or gold weight should be recommended to prevent or treat corneal abrasions. Refer to **Chapter 9.2** for more details. Botulinum toxin A has been used to help with bothersome blepharospasm due to synkinesis.

◆ Outcome and Follow-Up

Patients are followed longitudinally to assess final recovery. Final recovery from a facial nerve injury may not be seen until 18 to 24 months after insult. According to Peiterson's article charting the natural history of untreated Bell's palsy, 71% of patients will recover completely, and an additional 13% will achieve near normal recovery (House–Brackmann I or II). Anyone with poor recovery or at risk for corneal abrasion should be considered for surgical reanimation or surgical management of the paralyzed eye. Patients with herpes zoster oticus are at a much higher risk (almost 50%) to experience poor recovery (House–Brackmann III or worse). Patients who recover but then experience a recurrence of symptoms should be evaluated for a neoplasm, Melkersson-Rosenthal's syndrome, or inflammatory/autoimmune conditions.

3.1.4   Ear Foreign Bodies

◆ Key Features

- Ear foreign bodies are commonly found in young children.
- The injury may be acute or chronic, with associated infection.
- Foreign bodies often consist of insects, small batteries, food, beads, pencil erasers, and other inert objects.
- Injury to the tympanic membrane, ossicles, facial nerve, or inner ear must be considered.

Foreign bodies in the external auditory canal are a common problem, especially in pediatric patients. The otolaryngologist often becomes involved after unsuccessful attempts at removal by the patient, parent, emergency room providers, and/or pediatricians. With children, one should have a low threshold for removal under anesthesia in the operating room.

◆ Epidemiology

An ear foreign body is most commonly seen in children under 12 years of age.

◆ Clinical

Signs and Symptoms

An acute foreign body may cause otalgia due to pressure on thin skin of the medial ear canal. Insects are extremely bothersome if alive. Obstruction may cause conductive hearing loss. Chronic foreign bodies, especially organic material such as food, may present with foul otorrhea or purulence.

Pronounced hearing loss, vertigo, or facial weakness suggests injury to the middle ear (see **Chapter 3.1.2**).

Differential Diagnosis

The differential diagnosis includes a foreign body, otitis externa, otitis media, middle ear trauma, or a tumor.

◆ Evaluation

History

When taking the patient's history, you should inquire about the time course and possible nature of foreign body, if unclear. The previous level of hearing is important, as is a history of known tympanic membrane perforation. Injury involving an only-hearing ear mandates careful and experienced management.

Physical Exam

The examination should include a full head and neck exam to evaluate for other foreign bodies. Document facial nerve function and perform a 512-Hz tuning fork exam if the patient is old enough and cooperative. The ear should be examined with the otomicroscope. Any purulence or drainage is suctioned with #3 or #5 Frazier tip suction to enable visualization of the foreign body, canal skin, and tympanic membrane, if possible.

Imaging

High-resolution CT scanning of the temporal bone is the most useful imaging study if there is concern for a middle or inner ear injury.

Other Tests

Perform an audiologic assessment if there is any concern of a middle or inner ear injury.

◆ Treatment Options

Most foreign bodies do not constitute an emergency and can be removed within a reasonable time period (i.e., days). Exceptions requiring prompt treatment include batteries (which can cause tissue necrosis due to alkaline or acid leakage), insects, or objects associated with additional trauma to the middle ear or temporal bone. In the adult or cooperative child, one may be able to remove a foreign body easily in the office. If a child is at all uncooperative, it is preferable to proceed with removal under anesthesia in the operating room in an elective setting. Live insects are first treated by instillation of 1% lidocaine to the canal, which promptly drowns/paralyzes the insect and anesthetizes the canal skin. The most useful instrument is a blunt otologic right angle hook, which may be positioned medial to the foreign body, enabling removal. This is especially helpful for smooth objects, such as beads. An object that can be grasped and is intact may be amenable to the use of alligator forceps. Longstanding decaying organic material associated with infection requires suctioning. Gravel or sand against an intact tympanic membrane is best removed with irrigation. Following removal of a foreign body, careful inspection of the canal skin and tympanic membrane is important. Topical antibiotic and steroid drops for a few days are often helpful in treating or preventing local infection. Oral antibiotics are added for cellulitis, chondritis, and otitis media, as well as for the diabetic or immunosuppressed patient.

The presence of canal skin edema may require the placement of an ear wick (e.g., Merocel Pope Oto-Wick, Medtronic, Inc., Minneapolis, MN). Necrotic tissue secondary to acid or alkaline battery leakage or thermal burns from slag foreign bodies (e.g., due to welding) are managed with serial débridement and antibiotic steroid drops; wicks or stenting are required for a circumferential canal injury. Management of injuries to the tympanic membrane and the middle ear, as well as temporal bone penetrating trauma, are discussed in **Chapter 3.1.2.**

◆ Outcome and Follow-Up

Uncomplicated removal of a foreign body usually does not require follow-up. If there is any associated infection, follow-up within a few weeks to document resolution following topical therapy is routine.

3.2 Otitis Media

3.2.1 Acute Otitis Media

◆ Key Features

- Acute otitis media occurs when there is a bulging tympanic membrane with middle ear fluid.
- It is one of the most common childhood illnesses.
- It may be accompanied by hearing loss, nausea, vomiting, otorrhea, and fever.
- First-line treatment is amoxicillin. Watchful waiting is advocated in some patients.

Acute otitis media (AOM) is defined as middle ear inflammation lasting up to 3 weeks, accompanied by pain and bulging tympanic membrane (TM). Severe cases of AOM can be associated with high fever (≤ 39°C). The TM can spontaneously rupture, and purulent otorrhea can occur. AOM should be differentiated from otitis media with effusion (also known as serous otitis media), mucoid otitis media ("glue" ear), and chronic otitis media. The mainstay of treatment is oral antibiotics, but some children with recurrent AOM or complications associated with AOM may require surgical management with tympanostomy tubes.

✦ Epidemiology

Sixty percent of all children under the age of one year will suffer at least one episode of AOM. That percentage increases to 85% by age 3. In children less than 10 years, AOM accounts for up to 20% of all clinic visits. Risk factors associated with AOM are daycare attendance, exposure to secondhand smoke, food or environmental allergies, and chronic rhinitis. Children between 3 and 18 months of age are the most susceptible.

✦ Clinical

Signs

The most important diagnostic feature for AOM is a bulging or full and opaque TM associated with middle ear effusion. A ruptured TM can present with purulent otorrhea. If acute mastoiditis is present, the postauricular region may also be erythematous and edematous; the auricle may also protrude anteriorly. Fever can also occur.

Symptoms

AOM is more common in children than in adults. It can present with otalgia, otorrhea, irritability, fever, nausea, vomiting, and feeding difficulties. Children may also tug on the ear. Hearing loss, ear fullness, and tinnitus can also be present. An upper respiratory tract infection may precede onset of AOM.

Differential Diagnosis

The differential diagnosis of AOM is a differential diagnosis for ear pain. Temporomandibular joint disease is a common cause of referred otalgia in adults. Other conditions include herpes zoster oticus, primary temporal bone malignancy, referred pain from other head and neck malignancies, nasopharyngeal mass causing auditory (eustachian) tube obstruction, cerumen impaction, cholesteatoma, otitis externa, mastoiditis, and foreign body. A common cause of otalgia in children is AOM; however, other pediatric causes include otitis externa, ear canal trauma, mastoiditis, and ear canal foreign body. It is important to differentiate AOM with otitis media with effusion (middle ear fluid without infection).

✦ Evaluation

Physical Exam

The most important portion of the physical exam is inspecting the TM. The auricle and the external canal remain normal in appearance and are not tender to palpation.

The appearance of the TM will change as the disease process follows its usual course. Initially, the TM is engorged and hyperemic. The hyperemia is most prominent along the manubrium of the malleus and the periphery of the drum. The TM is sluggish to pneumatic otoscopy, but all normal topographic landmarks are visible. As the infection progresses and the middle ear fills with purulence, the TM thickens, bulges, and loses normal landmarks. There may be erythema, tenderness, and edema in the postauricular region, especially in small children. A tuning fork examination can demonstrate conductive hearing loss pattern.

If the infection progresses, the TM perforates in the pars tensa, and the patient experiences a resolution of pain and fever. If purulence is seen in the external canal, then cultures should be obtained. If the perforation heals and purulence reaccumulates, the infection may spread through the antrum into the mastoid; the mastoid trabeculae may begin to decalcify, leading to coalescent mastoiditis along with other complications. At this stage, the auricle displaces from the skull as postauricular edema increases. It is important to differentiate this from a severe otitis externa with painful cellulitis and swelling of the auricle.

Imaging

Imaging is usually not indicated unless coalescent mastoiditis or another complication of AOM is suspected. If a complication is suspected, a fine-cut temporal bone computed tomography (CT) scan is indicated.

Labs

Labs are rarely needed to treat routine AOM. Leukocytosis may be seen on complete blood count (CBC). Cultures can be obtained if the ear is draining, especially in infants less than 6 weeks of age. Routine tympanocentesis is not indicated in AOM but may be informative in patients who are immuno-compromised or when suspicion for resistant or atypical pathogen is high.

Other Tests

An audiogram is not needed in the acute phase but can be helpful in evaluating children with recurrent AOM, especially in light of other cognitive delays. In cases where the presence of an effusion is in question, tympanograms will show low-volume flat (type B) or negative pressure (type C). Occasionally, the combination of a good pneumatic exam and an accurate tympanogram are needed to determine the presence of an effusion, even for an experienced otologist. Nasopharyngoscopy to evaluate for nasopharyngeal mass and auditory tube obstruction should be performed in adults with persistent unilateral middle ear effusion.

Pathology

Most commonly, AOM is caused by bacteria that gain entry into the middle ear cleft through the auditory tube. Infants are at higher risk for developing AOM because the auditory tubes are short and horizontal and feeding often occurs in the reclined position. As children grow, the auditory tubes become longer and more vertical, and the incidence of AOM declines. Other factors that contribute to AOM include allergic rhinitis, recurrent adenoiditis, adenoid (pharyngeal tonsil) hypertrophy, cleft palate, and immunodeficiency.

AOM in adults, especially if unilateral, may be ominous. The nasopharynx must be fully evaluated to identify the cause of the auditory tube blockage or dysfunction. A nasopharyngeal mass must be ruled out prior to attributing the cause to upper respiratory tract infection, allergic rhinitis, or recent flight.

Historically, the most common bacterial pathogens causing AOM have been *Streptococcus pneumoniae* (40–50%), nontypeable *Haemophilus influenzae* (20–30%), and *Moraxella catarrhalis* (10–15%). Vaccination with pneumococcal 13-valent conjugate vaccination (PCV13) can protect against many strains causing AOM. However, alterations in penicillin-binding proteins in *S. pneumoniae* and *H. influenzae* have increased the incidence of antibiotic resistance.

Histologically, middle ears display signs of inflammation and edema. The TM and middle ear mucosa are thickened and engorged with an inflammatory infiltrate. There is often frank purulence in the middle ear space.

◆ Treatment Options

Medical

There has been a trend toward withholding antibiotic treatment and advocating "watchful waiting" for 72 hours in children with uncomplicated AOM (< 24 months with unilateral AOM or ≥ 24 months with unilateral or bilateral disease). Pain is treated symptomatically. If AOM persists for more than 72 hours, the first-line antibiotic is amoxicillin (80 to 90 mg/kg/day) because it is effective, well tolerated, and inexpensive. A beta-lactamase antibiotic should be prescribed if there is a history of AOM within the last month, failed amoxicillin initial therapy, or conjunctivitis. If patients are penicillin-allergic, second- or third-generation cephalosporins, macrolides, or clindamycin are all options. Breastfeeding for initial 6 months of life, pneumococcal conjugate vaccine, and annual influenza vaccination can help prevent AOM. Reducing risk factors such as secondhand smoke exposure and daycare may also prevent AOM.

Otitis media with effusion (OME, also referred to as serous otitis media and nonsuppurative otitis media) is defined as the presence of middle ear fluid without signs or symptoms of acute ear infection. OME can occur after an episode of AOM; 75% of children with OME following AOM resolve by 3 months. When OME does not resolve spontaneously within 3 months, tympanostomy tubes should be offered.

Surgical

In patients in whom empiric therapy has failed, diagnostic tympanocentesis may be done for culture. Removing the fluid from the middle ear may also relieve pain. Tympanostomy tube placement may be offered if AOM is recurrent, which is defined as 3 episodes of AOM in the last 6 months or >4 episodes of AOM in the past 1 year. Tympanostomy tubes with adenoidectomy are recommended in children ≥ 4 years of age for OME lasting more than 3 months. For children < 4 years of age, adenoidectomy is performed only when there is nasal obstruction and chronic adenoiditis.

◆ Complications

Complications of tube placement include otorrhea, conductive hearing loss, retained tubes, cholesteatoma, and postextrusion TM perforations. Posttympanostomy otorrhea occurs in 10% of patients and is treated with appropriate ototopical drops (i.e., fluoroquinolones, as they are not ototoxic). Most tubes will extrude spontaneously; however, removal of the tube may be necessary. TM perforations are estimated to occur 3 to 5% of the time and are followed conservatively. If they persist or cause considerable hearing loss, tympanoplasty may be recommended.

◆ Outcome and Follow-Up

Children with tympanostomy tubes require little postoperative care, and physician preference is usually the driving force determining postoperative recommendations. Many otolaryngologists advocate the use of 5 days of antibiotic topical drops twice daily, such as Ciprodex (Alcon Laboratories, Fort Worth, TX) or Floxin Otic (Daiichi Pharmaceutical Corporation, Montvale, NJ), postoperatively only to children with mucoid or purulent effusions found at the time of tube placement. Many otolaryngologists also recommend ear plugs for children only when swimming in fresh water and not during bath or shower time. The children are otherwise followed with a postoperative audiogram and interval visits at 6 to 12 months until the tubes extrude.

3.2.2 Chronic Otitis Media

◆ Key Features

- Chronic otitis media is long-term inflammation or infection affecting the middle ear space.
- Chronic otitis media may present with tympanic membrane perforation with otorrhea, retracted tympanic membrane with middle ear fluid, and cholesteatoma.
- The goal of medical and surgical treatment is to create a dry, safe ear.

Chronic otitis media (COM) comprises several long-term inflammatory or infectious disease processes that affect the middle ear. It can occur with or without a tympanic membrane perforation, cholesteatoma, and active drainage. When middle ear fluid exists, it may be serous ("chronic serous otitis media" or "chronic otitis media with effusion") or thick ("chronic mucoid otitis media"). Purulent drainage through a tympanic membrane (TM) perforation is often referred to as "chronic suppurative otitis media." COM can also be associated with retracted TM, granulation tissue, polyps, and ossicular erosion. Conductive hearing and otorrhea are common occurrences. Chronic auditory (eustachian) tube dysfunction can be the underlying cause in many patients. Treatment can include medical and surgical options.

◆ Epidemiology

The epidemiology of COM is not well defined. It affects males and females equally; however, there is a preference for certain populations: Native Americans, American Eskimos, and Australian Aborigines.

◆ Clinical

Signs

Signs of COM include perforated or retracted tympanic membrane, middle ear fluid, otorrhea, polypoid granulation tissue, ossicular erosion, and cholesteatoma. In patients with severe infection or cholesteatoma, facial palsy, nystagmus, or signs of meningitis can be seen in severe cases.

Symptoms

Symptomatology is broad and depends on the nature of the COM. Common symptoms include chronic or intermittent painless otorrhea and hearing loss. When COM is associated with cholesteatoma or severe infection, the otic capsule may be breached and sensorineural hearing loss, tinnitus, vertigo, dizziness, and imbalance can occur. The facial nerve can be involved, and facial droop may be reported. In severe cases, meningitis can occur and patients will present with altered mental status, fever, headache, and stiff neck. A chronic history of sinus disease and auditory tube dysfunction may also be elicited.

Differential Diagnosis

The differential diagnoses for chronic otorrhea and TM perforation are foreign body, temporal bone malignancy, Wegener's granulomatosis, and tuberculosis. Persistent polypoid tissue after medical treatment necessitates a biopsy. Wegener's granulomatosis may present as COM with fluctuating hearing loss and cranial nerve palsy without a previous history of OM. Tuberculous otitis media should be considered in a draining ear that does not improve despite maximal medical and surgical treatment. The classic description of tuberculous otitis media is painless otorrhea with multiple TM perforations.

◆ Evaluation

Physical Exam

A focused head and neck examination is performed, concentrating primarily on the otologic exam. The external auditory canal may be filled with moist debris that requires meticulous cleaning; at times, medical treatment of an inflamed ear canal is necessary to be able to visualize the TM. The TM should be inspected for retraction (e.g., myringoincudostapediopexy), bulging, perforation, cholesteatoma, and granulation tissue. Debris and granulation tissue should be cleaned thoroughly with an otomicroscope. Abnormal tissue can be sent to pathology for review. The presence of middle ear fluid should be evaluated with pneumatic otoscopy. A tuning fork exam can indicate presence of conductive hearing loss. Cranial nerve examination, particularly the facial nerve (CN VII), should be performed. A nasopharyngoscopy is recommended when there is unilateral COM with effusion in an adult patient in order to rule out nasopharyngeal mass.

Imaging

When COM is associated with cholesteatoma or intracranial or intratemporal complications, high-resolution computed tomography (CT) imaging of the temporal bones is recommended. Additional imaging such as magnetic resonance imaging (MRI) of the brain with and without gadolinium contrast is necessary when there are intracranial complications of COM. Uncomplicated COM may not require imaging.

Labs

Otorrhea, especially if recalcitrant to empiric therapy, should be cultured. Aerobic and fungal cultures are routinely sent. Additional blood work is rarely indicated. If the onset of symptoms is bilateral, recent, and accompanied by fluctuating hearing loss or cranial nerve palsy, then c-ANCA (cytoplasmic anti–neutrophil cytoplasmic autoantibody) is ordered to rule out Wegener's granulomatosis.

Other Tests

An audiogram is obtained once the ear is dry and prior to any surgical intervention. A conductive hearing loss is expected, and a mixed loss is not uncommon. Any granulation retrieved from the ear is sent to pathology to rule out malignancy.

Pathology

Historically, the most common pathogens were *Pseudomonas aeruginosa* and *Proteus*. Today, the most common pathogen is methicillin-resistant *Staphylococcus aureus* (MRSA). Pathogens gain access to the middle ear through the perforated TM. They then spread from the middle ear to the mastoid process. These same pathogens can also colonize the avascular debris collecting within a cholesteatoma. The middle ear mucosa becomes thick, fibrotic, and infiltrated with inflammatory cells. Mucosal edema leads to polyp formation and granulation. Bony vascular channels embolize secondary to chronic inflammation, leading to bone erosion, particularly involving the ossicular chain. Cholesteatoma may erode bone by additional local inflammatory response and osteolytic enzymes.

◆ Treatment Options

The goals of treatment are elimination of infection and restoration of function. The primary goal is to restore a "safe and dry ear."

Medical

COM may be initially treated with empiric ototopical antibiotic drops. Awareness of ototoxicity has made fluoroquinolone drops the preferred method of treatment. Ototopical drops reach the middle ear in such high

Table 3.4 Topical therapy for chronic otitis media

Topical agent	Typical dose regimen
2% acetic acid	5 drops 2–3 times daily
2% acetic acid/1% hydrocortisone solution	5 drops 2–3 times daily
Burow solution (13% aluminum acetate)	Drops or soaked pledget
Floxin (ofloxacin)* otic	10 drops twice daily
Ciprodex (ciprofloxacin/dexamethasone)† or Cipro HC (ciprofloxacin/hydrocortisone)† otic	5 drops twice daily
Cortisporin (neomycin/polymyxin B/hydrocortisone)‡ otic suspension	5 drops 3 times daily
CSF powder (chloramphenicol 50 mg, p-aminobenzenesulfonamide 50 mg, and amphotericin 5 mg, with or without hydrocortisone 1 mg)	2 puffs twice daily
Gentian violet (aqueous)	Physician applies topically under microscope in office as needed
Boric acid powder	2 puffs twice daily

*Daiichi-Sankyo Co., Ltd., Tokyo, Japan.
†Alcon Pharmaceuticals, Inc., Fribourg, Switzerland.
‡Endo International, Dublin, Ireland.

concentrations that resistance is rarely an issue. See **Table 3.4** for topical treatment options. If the drainage does not respond, then cultures are indicated to rule out a resistant strain such as MRSA or a fungal infection. Vinegar washes or 2% acetic acid drops may be effective. There are several topical powders that also may periodically be applied if drops do not work. One such mixture includes ciprofloxacin, boric acid, dexamethasone, and fluconazole. Appropriate long-term IV antibiotics may also be indicated if an osteitis is suspected. Another effective topical powder preparation to help dry the chronically draining ear that is unresponsive to drops consists of chloramphenicol 50 mg, p-aminobenzenesulfonamide 50 mg, and amphotericin 5 mg, with or without hydrocortisone 1 mg; this is mixed and delivered in 1 or 2 puffs via a powder insufflator (e.g., Sheehy–House insufflator Otomed, Grace Medical, Memphis, TN) twice daily. Another option for office management is aqueous gentian violet, which has antifungal properties and may be "painted" over inflamed areas under the otomicroscope.

Surgical

The goals of surgery for COM are to eradicate the infection, improve hearing, prevent otorrhea, and remove cholesteatoma. Medical intervention with systemic or topical antibiotic preparations may be necessary to dry the ear prior to surgery. Surgical algorithms vary by preference, training, and experience. The following is a general list of options (not exhaustive) with definitions.

1. *Myringotomy* with tube placement is performed to remove middle ear fluid.

2. *Tympanoplasty without mastoidectomy* is performed to eradicate disease limited to the middle ear. Middle ear cholesteatoma can be removed through this technique, and the TM can be grafted if there is a TM perforation. TM grafting material includes loose areolar tissue, temporalis fascia, perichondrium, vein, or cartilage. The graft can be placed either medial or lateral to the TM.

3. *Atticotomy* can be performed in addition to tympanoplasty by removing the posterior bony anulus and scutum to better visualize the epitympanum and posterior mesotympanum. Through this approach, the entire ossicular chain can be visualized and cleaned, as well as the tympanic portion of the facial nerve. This can facilitate removal of granulation, retractions, and small cholesteatomas, especially for disease lateral to the ossicles. This is ideal for pars flaccida cholesteatoma that is lateral to the ossicular chain. Cartilage is used to reconstruct the scutum to prevent future retraction, and a formal mastoidectomy can be avoided.

4. *Tympanomastoidectomy with an intact canal wall* requires mastoidectomy and tympanoplasty to remove cholesteatoma or disease in the middle ear and antrum. A partial transcanal atticotomy may be performed if additional exposure is needed in the epitympanum. A facial recess approach can aid in removing disease in the sinus tympani and improve aeration. Microsurgical techniques are required to exenterate all involved air cell tracts. Removal of the malleus head is often required for disease extending into the anterior epitympanum or supratubal recess. A second look operation is often planned in cases of cholesteatoma, to assess for recurrent disease and/or perform ossicular reconstruction.

5. *Tympanomastoidectomy with canal wall down* is a technique that is employed for extensive cholesteatoma and rarely necessary in uncomplicated COM without cholesteatoma. This technique is also indicated in otherwise unresectable disease, noncompliant patients, only hearing or deaf ears, and patients with small or contracted/sclerotic mastoids prior to surgery. Removing the posterior canal wall increases visualization of the anterior epitympanum and the posterior mesotympanum and provides access to remove disease more effectively from the sinus tympani. Postmastoidectomy cavities may fail, harbor cholesteatoma, or chronically drain if a high facial ridge is left, there is a dependent mastoid tip, the TM graft fails, or the meatoplasty is inadequate. Surgeons must carefully attend to these fine details to ensure success.

◆ Complications

Complications of COM itself are divided into intratemporal and intracranial subcategories, and are covered in **Chapter 3.2.3**. Complications from surgery for COM are covered here. Postoperative complications are rare if surgery is performed meticulously. Postoperative pain is usually mild, and all patients calling with severe pain need to be evaluated. *Pseudomonas* is the most common offending organism in COM, and empiric treatment with fluoroquinolones is often effective. *Staphylococcus* is also a common pathogen for COM. When possible, wound infections are treated with culture-directed antibiotics. Postoperative hematomas at the site of graft harvesting are rare but need to be drained when encountered.

Facial nerve injuries are rare. The use of facial nerve monitoring during even routine ear surgery is becoming widely accepted. Intraoperative injury needs to be addressed immediately with appropriate nerve exploration, decompression, and grafting if indicated. Getting the advice of a partner or a more experienced otologic surgeon can be helpful in these cases. Facial function that is normal initially and worsens over time is usually the result of edema; this is commonly treated with a two-week course of systemic steroids. When a patient awakens from a mastoid procedure with an unexpected facial weakness, it is prudent to observe the patient for a few hours to allow for the reversal of local anesthetic effects on the facial nerve prior to reexploration.

Cerebrospinal fluid (CSF) leak can be encountered intraoperatively and should be repaired intraoperatively. This can be done with a combination of fascia, cartilage, and/or bone cement. A neurosurgical consultation with lumbar drain placement is rarely required for small CSF leaks.

Mild vertigo is common following any middle ear procedure, but intraoperative labyrinthine injury results in severe postoperative vertigo and sensorineural hearing loss. Addressing the defect immediately with bone wax or fascia is recommended when the semicircular canal has been violated; patients may require hospitalization for symptomatic control of severe vertigo. Perilymphatic fistula may also present similarly. Oral or parenteral vestibular suppressants and antinausea medications are administered short term. Vestibular exercises can hasten recovery.

Granulations and synechiae in the ear canal or canal-wall-down mastoidectomy cavity are removed when encountered. Meatoplasties may require revision.

◆ Outcome and Follow-Up

Perioperative antibiotics are commonly administered prior to surgery for COM. The use of postoperative systemic antibiotics is controversial; however, active infection at the time of surgery necessitates systemic antibiotics, preferably culture-directed antibiotics. Surgery for COM is predominantly outpatient unless intracranial complications of COM are present. A variety of packing materials are utilized in the ear canal and canal-wall-down mastoidectomy cavities. Ototopical drops are prescribed to be administered twice a day. Although some packing can be removed 1 to 2 weeks postoperatively, the entirety of the packing is generally not removed for 4 to 6 weeks postoperatively to allow healing of graft. Routine postoperative audiometry is performed at 8 to 12 weeks. Success rates of surgical management for COM range from 78% to over 90% and likely are affected by disease severity and surgical technique. Cholesteatoma recurrence occurs 3 to 50% of the time. With these percentages in mind, patients are usually followed for several years.

3.2.3   Complications of Acute and Chronic Otitis Media

◆ Key Features

- Complications of acute and chronic otitis media may be intracranial, intratemporal, and extracranial.
- A decline in the incidence of otitis media complications is seen in the era of antibiotics.
- The most common extracranial complication is subperiosteal abscess; the most common intracranial complication is meningitis.
- Culture-directed antibiotics should be initiated when possible.

Complications of acute otitis media (AOM) and chronic otitis media (COM) are subdivided by site (extratemporal, intratemporal, and intracranial). When otitis media is associated with cholesteatoma, complications from cholesteatoma can also occur.

◆ Extratemporal Complications

Subperiosteal Abscess

Mastoiditis either directly erodes the bone of the lateral wall of the mastoid or traverses mastoid emissary veins into the subperiosteal space adjacent to the mastoid.

Signs and Symptoms

Fever, malaise, and otalgia are associated with a subperiosteal abscess.

Physical Exam

Otorrhea and an anteriorly and laterally displaced auricle can be seen on exam. The postauricular space can be erythematous, edematous, and fluctuant with fluid collection.

Imaging

Computed tomography (CT) of the temporal bones with contrast is recommended.

Treatment Options

Treatment is wide-field myringotomy or myringotomy with tube placement. The subperiosteal abscess should be incised and drained. A cortical mastoidectomy can be performed carefully if the mastoid is not severely inflamed. Culture should be obtained and empiric intravenous (IV) antibiotics started. Culture-directed antibiotics should be initiated when possible.

Bezold Abscess

Mastoiditis leads to bone erosion of the mastoid tip deep to the digastric ridge. Purulent material tracks into the neck, deep to the sternocleidomastoid muscle.

Signs and Symptoms

Fever, malaise, and neck pain are associated with a Bezold abscess.

Physical Exam

The patient may present with otalgia, otorrhea, postauricular tenderness, and a tender upper cervical mass.

Imaging

Contrast-enhanced CT will confirm the presence of a rim-enhancing cervical abscess in combination with mastoiditis.

Treatment Options

Recommended treatment includes IV antibiotics, wide-field myringotomy or myringotomy with tube placement, cortical mastoidectomy, and incision and drainage of the neck abscess. Culture-directed antibiotics should be initiated when possible.

◆ Intratemporal Complications

Labyrinthine Fistula

A labyrinthine fistula is caused by an erosion of otic capsule bone and exposure of the membranous labyrinth. This occurs in 7% of patients with cholesteatoma. Ninety percent of fistulas occur in the horizontal semicircular canal.

Signs and Symptoms

Most patients (62%) report periodic vertigo or imbalance. Patients may experience the Tullio phenomenon (dizziness induced by loud sounds) and sensorineural hearing loss. However, a significant number of patients will be asymptomatic.

Physical Exam

Fistula testing (nystagmus with pneumatoscopy) is positive in ~50% of patients. A tuning fork test may demonstrate sensorineural hearing loss.

Imaging

Thin-cut temporal bone CT is preferred; however, small fistulas may still be missed.

Treatment Options

Treatment of labyrinthine fistula is controversial because violation of the membranous labyrinth may result in a dead ear. Many authors recommend canal-wall-down mastoidectomy, leaving cholesteatoma matrix overlying the fistula to form the lining of the exteriorized mastoid cavity. In cases of small fistulas that have not violated the membranous labyrinth, some authors advocate complete matrix removal and semicircular canal resurfacing with bone paste, fascia, or a similar sealant. Others recommend leaving the matrix in place, leaving the canal wall up, and coming back to remove the matrix and resurface the labyrinth at a second stage.

Coalescent Mastoiditis

Coalescent mastoiditis can occur in untreated or inadequately treated acute otitis media. Suppurative progression leads to erosion of the trabecular bone of the mastoid cavity. Time course of progression is typically 2 to 4 weeks.

Signs and Symptoms

Symptoms include fever, malaise, and otalgia.

Physical Exam

On the physical examination, purulent otorrhea or a bulging tympanic membrane (TM) can be seen. Postauricular erythema and edema, with displacement of the auricle anteriorly and laterally, is typical.

Imaging

A CT scan of the temporal bones demonstrates middle ear and mastoid opacification with erosion of trabecular mastoid bone. Erosion of the sigmoid sinus plate is not uncommon.

Treatment Options

Recommended treatment includes wide-field myringotomy or myringotomy with tube placement, IV antibiotics, and cortical mastoidectomy. Some advocate myringotomy with IV antibiotics for 3 to 6 weeks with follow-up CT scan to confirm resolution of infection. Culture-directed antibiotics should be initiated when possible.

Petrous Apicitis

Petrous apicitis is a rare complication resulting from the spread of infection into air cells within a pneumatized petrous apex (the prevalence of pneumatization is 30%).

Signs and Symptoms

The classic triad of deep retroorbital pain, purulent otorrhea, and ipsilateral abducens palsy (Gradenigo's syndrome) is seen. CN VII and VIII dysfunction also may occur.

Imaging

A CT scan of the temporal bones will show opacification of a pneumatized petrous apex. The trabeculae of the petrous apex may also be eroded. Contrast administration can demonstrate some rim enhancement consistent with abscess.

Other Tests

Magnetic resonance imaging (MRI) of the brain with and without gadolinium and lumbar puncture (LP) are helpful to assess concurrent intracranial processes.

Treatment Options

Empiric IV antibiotics should be initiated. Abscess, bone erosion, or failed medical therapy requires surgical drainage. Hearing status determines the choice of approach. Hearing preservation may be attempted by infracochlear, infralabyrinthine, retrolabyrinthine, subarcuate, and middle fossa approaches. Translabyrinthine or transcochlear approaches may be used for nonserviceable ears.

Facial Paralysis

Facial paralysis results from inflammation of dehiscent segments of the facial nerve secondary to infection.

Signs and Symptoms

Facial weakness may be sudden, progressive, complete, or partial.

Imaging

CT scan of the temporal bone to evaluate the integrity of the intratemporal facial (fallopian) canal and extent of cholesteatoma can be performed.

Pathology

In the setting of children with AOM, a congenitally dehiscent tympanic segment of the facial nerve is suspected. The paralysis is usually incomplete and resolves within 3 weeks. In the face of COM and cholesteatoma, dehiscence is typically due to facial canal erosion secondary to disease. Onset may be slow and progressive. The prognosis is poorer and recovery slower.

Treatment Options

Facial paralysis due to AOM is treated with wide-field myringotomy or myringotomy with tube placement, IV antibiotics, and systemic steroids. Cholesteatoma-associated paralysis requires mastoidectomy, nerve decompression proximal and distal to the diseased segment, and débridement of inflammatory tissue.

Acute Suppurative Labyrinthitis

Acute suppurative labyrinthitis results from direct bacterial invasion of the labyrinth, resulting in total auditory and vestibular loss. Acute suppurative labyrinthitis may lead to meningitis and vice versa.

Signs and Symptoms

Acute-onset total sensorineural deafness and severe vertigo are signs of acute suppurative labyrinthitis. Nausea and vomiting are common. Nystagmus can be seen on exam.

Pathology

Predisposing factors include congenital inner ear malformations and otic capsule erosion secondary to cholesteatoma.

Treatment Options

IV antibiotics are initiated and vertigo is treated symptomatically. Systemic steroid treatment is controversial. Residual dizziness and imbalance can be treated with vestibular therapy to promote central compensation. Wide-field myringotomy or myringotomy with tube placement is considered. Culture-directed antibiotics should be initiated when possible.

◆ Intracranial Complications

Meningitis

Meningitis is the most common intracranial complication of otitis media.

Signs and Symptoms

Fever, headache, nausea, vomiting, photophobia, and nuchal rigidity are symptoms of meningitis. Seizures, ataxia, and other focal neurologic signs are ominous findings.

Imaging

CT or MRI of the brain with and without contrast is essential to rule out other intracranial processes mimicking meningitis and to establish the safety of LP.

Other Testing

LP is diagnostic. Cerebrospinal fluid (CSF) can demonstrate increased pressure, increased protein, decreased glucose, inflammatory cells, or bacteria present. CSF culture is obtained.

Pathology

The potential routes of bacterial spread from the ear to the CSF space include hematogenous seeding, bony erosion with direct spread, and through bony channels (e.g., suppurative labyrinthitis, Hyrtl fissures, congenital inner ear defects, cochlear aqueduct, and traumatic defects).

Treatment Options

Because meningitis is the most common complication seen with otitis media, detailed antibiotic guidelines are listed in **Table 3.5**. First-line therapy is IV antibiotics and wide-field myringotomy or myringotomy with tube placement. Mastoidectomy is considered when medical therapy fails, there is radiographic confirmation of coalescent mastoiditis, or cholesteatoma is present. Use of systemic steroids is controversial but may reduce neurologic sequelae of meningitis and brain edema. Culture-directed antibiotics should be initiated when possible.

Table 3.5 Intravenous antibiotic treatment for meningitis*†

Neonate (<1 month) Ampicillin + gentamicin; or ampicillin + third-generation cephalosporin
Newborn (1–3 months) First choice: Ampicillin + (cefotaxime or ceftriaxone) + dexamethasone (0.15 mg/kg every 6 h × 4 d)
Alternative: Chloramphenicol + gentamicin
Infant or child (>3 months) First choice: (Cefotaxime or ceftriaxone) + dexamethasone
Alternative: Ampicillin
Older child or adult (Cefotaxime 2 g IV every 6 h or ceftriaxone 2 g IV every 12 h) + ampicillin 2 g IV every 4 h + dexamethasone 0.4 mg/kg every 12 h × 2 d + vancomycin (child 15 to 22.5 mg/kg IV every 6 h; adult 1 g IV every 12 h)
If *Pseudomonas* suspected: Cefepime 2 g IV every 8 h instead of cefotaxime or ceftriaxone
For a penicillin-allergic patient in whom cephalosporin cannot be used: Vancomycin 15–22.5 mg/kg IV every 12 h + trimethoprim/sulfamethoxazole 15 to 20 mg/kg/day IV divided every 6 h *or*
Vancomycin 15 to 22.5 mg/kg IV every 12 h + chloramphenicol 1 g IV every 6 h ± rifampin 600 mg once daily

*Other regimens may be indicated for certain situations, such as an alcoholic patient, a patient with a CSF leak or a debilitating condition such as acquired immunodeficiency syndrome (AIDS), or a postneurosurgical patient.
†Length of treatment is generally at least 14 days.
(Data from Johns Hopkins Online Antibiotic Guide, http://hopkins-abxguide.org; and Greenberg MS. Handbook of Neurosurgery. 7th ed. Stuttgart/New York: Thieme, 2010.)

Brain Abscess

The most frequently lethal intracranial complication of OM is a brain abscess.

Signs and Symptoms

The clinical course is multistage, starting with fever, malaise, nausea, vomiting, headache, altered mental status, and seizures. This may be followed by a quiescent phase with moderate clinical improvement. The third stage, thought to represent abscess growth and ultimate rupture, is a rapid and fulminant return of symptoms with sudden clinical decline.

Imaging

CT brain or MRI brain with and without contrast is recommended. These studies can also aid in surgical planning.

Pathology

Infection spreads secondary to thrombophlebitis of venous channels leading from the mastoid to brain parenchyma. The temporal lobe and cerebellum are the most common sites of abscess.

Treatment Options

Treatment is IV antibiotics, neurosurgical consultation, and urgent craniotomy with drainage of abscess when medically stable. Wide-field myringotomy or myringotomy with tube placement should be performed. Mastoidectomy is typically recommended at the same time but may be delayed if the patient is medically unstable. Systemic steroids are controversial but may reduce brain edema and prevent neurological sequelae. Anticonvulsants are given if seizure risk is high. Frequent neurological checks and placement in the neurological intensive care unit are recommended. Culture-directed antibiotics should be initiated when possible.

Lateral Sinus Thrombosis

Bone overlying the sigmoid is eroded by infection, and perisinus inflammation leads to vessel wall necrosis and mural thrombus formation. Thrombus may propagate proximally to the confluence of sinuses and superior sagittal sinus, resulting in life-threatening hydrocephalus. Clot may also propagate distally into the internal jugular vein, leading to possible pulmonary embolus. Additionally, the infected thrombus may release septic emboli, leading to septicemia or deeper intracranial infections.

Signs and Symptoms

Patients report headache, malaise, and "picket-fence" pattern of diurnal spiking fevers. Neck pain may imply clot propagation distally into the neck. A Tobey-Ayer or Queckenstedt test (lack of CSF pressure elevation with occlusion of the internal jugular vein ipsilateral to the thrombosis) is suggestive of the diagnosis. Signs suggestive of hydrocephalus include papilledema on ophthalmologic exam and obtundation.

Imaging

Contrasted CT may show the "delta sign" resulting from sinus wall enhancement with a central filling defect. MRI and magnetic resonance venography (MRV) are very sensitive.

Treatment Options

Treatment is IV antibiotics, wide-field myringotomy or myringotomy with tube placement, and mastoidectomy. The sigmoid sinus and lateral sinus are surgically decompressed at the time of mastoidectomy. Inspection of the patency of the sigmoid sinus can be performed with a small-gauge needle and syringe. Incision into the thrombosed sigmoid sinus and removal of the infected thrombus can be considered. Ligation of the internal jugular vein should be performed if there is significant distal propagation and cervical infection. Anticoagulation is controversial but advocated when there is propagation of the thrombus towards the confluence of sinuses, cavernous sinus, or distally into the internal jugular vein. Culture-directed antibiotics should be initiated when possible.

Epidural Abscess

Granulation tissue and abscess form between the inner cortical bone of the skull base and adjacent dura.

Signs and Symptoms

Symptoms include headache, fever, and malaise. There are no specific symptoms or signs on exam; however, many patients report a deep mastoid pain.

Imaging

Contrast-enhanced MRI or CT of the brain will demonstrate a biconvex peripherally enhancing epidural collection adjacent to the temporal bone.

Treatment Options

IV antibiotics are initiated, and a wide-field myringotomy or myringotomy with tube placement in addition to mastoidectomy are performed. Depending on the location of the epidural abscess, decompression of the middle or posterior cranial fossa bony plate will drain the abscess. Granulation tissue can be débrided off of bone and intact dura. Neurosurgical consultation for burr hole placement or craniotomy to drain the abscess is recommended for collections that cannot be approached with a mastoidectomy. Culture-directed antibiotics should be initiated when possible.

Subdural Empyema

A subdural empyema is a rapidly progressive, fulminant bacterial infection between the dura and arachnoid layers. Infection spreads rapidly, resulting in significant brain edema, herniation, and death.

Signs and Symptoms

Presentation is similar to meningitis. Patient can present with fever, headache, altered mental status, seizures, and rapid deterioration. Progression of the empyema may result in more focal neurologic signs.

Imaging

Contrast-enhanced MRI or CT of the brain will demonstrate a crescent-shaped, peripherally enhancing collection adjacent to the bone.

Other Tests

LP is contraindicated because associated brain edema puts patients at high risk of tonsillar herniation.

Treatment Options

Treatment includes IV antibiotics, wide-field myringotomy or myringotomy with tube placement, neurosurgical consultation, and urgent neurosurgical drainage of the purulent collection. Mastoidectomy can be performed in conjunction with the craniotomy if the patient is hemodynamically stable. Culture-directed antibiotics should be initiated when possible.

Otitic Hydrocephalus

Otitic hydrocephalus is a condition of increased intracranial pressure associated with temporal bone infection.

Signs and Symptoms

The symptoms include headache, nausea, vomiting, blurry vision, diplopia, and lethargy. Papilledema or abducens palsy may be observed on eye exam.

Imaging

MRI or MRV will detect dural sinus thrombosis, rule out other intracranial causes, and confirm the safety of LP. In contrast to typical hydrocephalus, the ventricles are not dilated.

Pathology

The pathophysiology is controversial and is thought to be secondary to clot propagation into the confluence of sinuses and ultimate blockage of CSF flow through the arachnoid villi of the superior sagittal sinus.

Treatment Options

Treatment of lateral sinus thrombosis is imperative and was discussed. The otitic hydrocephalus is treated medically with acetazolamide, fluid restriction, and steroids. If medical management fails, lumbar drainage or long-term ventriculoperitoneal shunting may be considered. Culture-directed antibiotics should be initiated when possible.

3.2.4   Cholesteatoma

◆ Key Features

- A cholesteatoma is a slow-growing destructive lesion of the middle ear and mastoid.
- It consists of trapped and frequently infected desquamated keratin.
- A cholesteatoma requires definitive surgical management to avoid complications.

A cholesteatoma is a slow growing and destructive cystic lesion composed of desquamating keratin. It is accurately referred to as a keratoma. There are two types: acquired and congenital cholesteatoma. Acquired cholesteatoma is generally located superiorly or posteriorly in the middle ear and extends over time into the mastoid. A congenital cholesteatoma is generally found in the anterosuperior portion of the middle ear. Growth and infections of cholesteatomas can lead to intratemporal, extratemporal, and intracranial complications. Routine débridement of a dry and limited cholesteatoma pocket can be performed; however, definitive surgical resection is advocated for most patients who tolerate general anesthesia.

◆ Epidemiology

The prevalence or incidence of acquired cholesteatoma in the general population is unclear. The incidence of congenital cholesteatoma is 0.12 per 100,000 population. One to three percent of children with chronically draining ears have cholesteatoma.

◆ Clinical

Signs

Signs of a congenital cholesteatoma include conductive hearing loss and a white pearl in the anterosuperior quadrant of the middle ear behind an intact tympanic membrane (TM). Signs of an acquired cholesteatoma include conductive hearing loss and a posterior superior retraction pocket with a keratinaceous crust or desquamating debris. An aural polyp, granulation, or purulent otorrhea can also be seen. There may also be erosion of the ossicles, scutum, and posterior bony wall of the external auditory canal.

Symptoms

The symptoms of cholesteatoma are similar to that of chronic otitis media (COM). The most common presenting symptoms are painless chronic otorrhea and hearing loss. The otorrhea may be bloody or purulent. Patients may also present with complications of cholesteatoma, including dizziness secondary to a labyrinthine fistula, facial nerve paralysis, or fever, malaise, and altered mental status suggesting an intracranial process.

Differential Diagnosis

Cholesteatoma frequently presents with signs of COM, but not all patients with COM harbor cholesteatoma. The symptoms and the complications of both diseases are similar, and the two sometimes can be differentiated only in the operating room (OR). The differential diagnosis also includes benign and malignant neoplasms of the temporal bone and foreign body.

◆ Evaluation

Physical Exam

A general head and neck exam is performed, paying particular attention to the otologic exam and cranial nerves (particularly the facial nerve). An otomicroscope aids in meticulous cleaning and examination of the ear. Frequently, a large attic or posterior TM retraction with keratin debris is encountered. The retraction may be covered by a crust, which must be removed to complete the exam. Occasionally, a polyp may be encountered, covering the retraction and debris. The polyp should be manipulated with suction to see around it or debulk it. Polyps should *not* be aggressively removed with cup forceps, as ossicular injury can result. A congenital cholesteatoma will slowly grow undetected, but may be seen as a white "pearl" anterosuperiorly behind an intact TM. Nystagmus (Tullio phenomenon) can be seen with pneumatic otoscopy if a labyrinthine fistula is present. A tuning fork can indicate conductive or sensorineural hearing loss.

Imaging

Computed tomography (CT) is the initial imaging modality to evaluate the extent of cholesteatoma and the state of the bony structures of the temporal bone. A thin-section (1-mm) CT with true axial and coronal cuts is best. The cholesteatoma appears as a homogeneous soft tissue density that is frequently difficult to differentiate from soft tissue edema or fluid. Therefore, it is imperative to combine physical exam findings with CT results to diagnose cholesteatoma. In certain circumstances, magnetic resonance imaging (MRI) can be obtained with diffusion-weighted sequences to differentiate between cholesteatoma and other temporal bone pathology. Cholesteatomas restrict (hyperintense) on diffusion-weighted images.

Potential findings on coronal CT imaging:

1. Scutum erosion
2. Ossicular erosion
3. Tegmen dehiscence
4. Semicircular canal dehiscence or fistula
5. Dehiscence of the facial (fallopian) canal

Potential findings on axial CT imaging:

1. Ossicular erosion
2. Soft tissue opacification of antrum and air cells
3. Semicircular canal dehiscence or fistula
4. Dehiscence of the sigmoid sinus
5. Dehiscence of the facial canal

Other Tests

An audiogram with tympanogram is essential in determining the degree and nature of the hearing loss. Conductive hearing loss may suggest involvement of the TM and ossicular erosion/discontinuity.

Pathology

The pathophysiology of both congenital and acquired cholesteatoma remains controversial.

Pathology of Congenital Cholesteatoma

Congenital cholesteatoma is initially defined as a pearly mass behind an intact TM in the absence of otitis media (OM). The absence of otitis media was removed from the definition, as there is a high prevalence of OM in children. Two competing theories of formation are:

1. Epithelial rest: There is a localized epithelial rest that has been identified in fetal temporal bones at the lateral wall of the auditory (eustachian) tube in the anterosuperior quadrant of the middle ear that disappears at 33 weeks gestation. Persistence of this rest into childhood can account for congenital cholesteatoma.

2. Acquired inclusion: The speculation is that a microinjury and retraction occurs to the pediatric TM, allowing small foci of epithelial tissue to invade the middle ear and proliferate just anterior to the malleus manubrium.

Pathology of Acquired Cholesteatoma

There are four theories for acquired cholesteatoma.

1. TM retraction (primary acquired): There is retraction of the TM secondary to negative middle ear pressure from auditory tube dysfunction. This most commonly involves the pars flaccida retracting up into the attic, collecting keratinaceous debris, and forming a cholesteatoma.
2. Epithelial migration (secondary acquired): Migration of canal and TM epithelium through a TM perforation. This occurs most commonly with a marginal perforation. The epithelium then proliferates within the middle ear.
3. Implantation (secondary acquired): Similar to migration except that epithelium is actively implanted into the middle ear secondary to either trauma or surgery (e.g. myringotomy tube placement).
4. Metaplasia (historical theory): COM is believed to trigger metaplastic change of middle ear mucosa from cuboidal to keratinizing squamous cells.

In an actively growing cholesteatoma, there is local inflammation and infection. This inflammation causes fibroblasts and leukocytes to release enzymes that erode bone. Inflammatory cytokines also act as osteoclastic-activating factors that stimulate osteoclasts to erode bone. Persistent pressure by an expanding cholesteatoma may also erode adjacent bone.

◆ Treatment Options

Medical

There is no definitive medical therapy for cholesteatoma; however, the ear should be débrided with the aid of an otomicroscope, and coexisting infections should be treated with appropriate antibiotic/steroid ototopical preparations. Having a dry ear with low bacterial burden and granulation will aid in surgical treatment.

Surgical

The goals of surgery are to remove the disease, make a dry and safe ear, and restore hearing. Surgeons will differ on their methods of achieving these goals. Some surgeons prefer a staged method with ossicular chain reconstruction at a later stage; others prefer to do everything at a single stage (reexplore ears only with signs of persistent or recurrent disease). Surgical options follow. Postoperative antibiotics are usually recommended when infection is present at the time of surgery.

1. Tympanoplasty alone is performed to eradicate small cholesteatomas that are limited to the middle ear. The TM can be grafted if there is a TM perforation.

2. Atticotomy can be performed in addition to tympanoplasty by removing the posterior bony anulus and scutum to visualize the epitympanum and posterior mesotympanum better. Through this approach, the entire ossicular chain can be visualized and cleaned, as well as the tympanic portion of the facial nerve. This can facilitate removal of granulation, retractions, and small cholesteatomas, especially for disease *lateral* to the ossicles. This is ideal for pars flaccida cholesteatoma that is lateral to the ossicular chain. Cartilage is used to reconstruct the scutum to prevent future retraction, and a formal mastoidectomy can be avoided.

3. Tympanomastoidectomy with an intact canal wall requires mastoidectomy and tympanoplasty to remove cholesteatoma or disease in the middle ear and antrum. The bony ear canal is preserved. A partial transcanal atticotomy may be performed if additional exposure is needed in the epitympanum. A facial recess approach can aid in removing disease in the sinus tympani and improving aeration. A second-look operation can be performed to look for recurrent disease and perform a delayed ossicular reconstruction.

4. Tympanomastoidectomy with canal wall down (CWD) is a technique that is employed for extensive cholesteatoma, unresectable disease, noncompliant patients, disease in only hearing ears, largely eroded bony ear canals, cholesteatoma matrix adhering to a dehiscent facial nerve, contracted/sclerotic mastoids, and labyrinthine fistulas. Once the facial nerve is identified, the posterior wall of the ear canal is removed down to the level of the facial ridge. A low facial ridge will aid in postoperative mastoid débridement. All air cells are removed and all edges are saucerized. If there is a dependent mastoid tip, it can be amputated above the digastric ridge. The TM is grafted and ossicular chain reconstruction and meatoplasty are performed. Some of the mastoid cavity dead space can be obliterated with soft tissue from the postauricular region. Cholesteatoma recurrence rates are lower for CWD procedures, but patients require lifelong mastoid cavity care.

5. Radical mastoidectomy is a techniques that involves a CWD mastoidectomy, removing the TM and middle ear contents, and obliterating the auditory tube to render it nonfunctional.

◆ Complications

Complications from cholesteatoma and COM are addressed in a separate chapter (**Chapter 3.2.3**). Intraoperative complications in otologic surgery are prevented using careful technique with avoidance of any operative misadventures. Identifying solid landmarks such as the tegmen or lateral semicircular canal are important in preventing complications.

◆ Outcome and Follow-Up

Surgery is primarily outpatient; however, patients with suspected labyrinthine or cochlear fistulas remain overnight to monitor them for dizziness. Patients return for an office visit at either 1 or 2 weeks. At that visit, most of the reachable packing is removed, and the patient is placed on ototopical antibiotic drops. CWD cavities are filled with dissolving packing or an antibiotic/steroid ointment, and ototopical drops are prescribed.

Patients are then seen at 4- to 6-week intervals to inspect the graft and clean any granulations. Water is kept out of the ears until complete epithelialization occurs. CWU ears can return to full preoperative activities once healed. CWD ears can engage in water-related activities with caution, knowing that they are at risk for infection secondary to retained moisture and dizziness from exposure to cold water. Cholesteatoma patients are followed for several years to monitor for recurrence. This involves yearly or twice-yearly visits for inspection and mastoid cavity cleaning if needed.

For surgeons who prefer a staged CWU technique, patients undergo a second-look operation within 6 to 12 months to rule out and manage recurrent or residual disease, and reconstruct the ossicular chain if indicated. If moderate disease is encountered, then a third look may be indicated; if extensive disease is encountered, a CWD procedure may be performed.

3.3 Otitis Externa

3.3.1 Uncomplicated Otitis Externa

◆ Key Features

- Otitis externa (OE) is an infectious process of the external auditory canal.
- The most common pathogens are *Pseudomonas aeruginosa* and *Staphylococcus aureus*.
- Otomycosis is less common and caused by *Aspergillus* and *Candida*.
- Treatment involves meticulous cleaning and topical preparations.
- Systemic therapy is required if the infection spreads out of the confines of the canal, or the patient is immunocompromised or a poorly controlled diabetic.

Otitis externa is a localized infection of the skin of the external auditory canal (EAC). The EAC contains varying amounts of cerumen and desquamated skin. Acute OE, called "swimmer's ear," is most common after water exposure but may also follow EAC trauma. Retained moisture will alkalize the canal, making it prone to bacterial infection. As long as the infection is confined to the ear canal, local aural toilet and topical drops will be curative. If the infection extends outside the confines of the canal to become a periauricular cellulitis or the patient has a complicating factor that may impede the effectiveness of topical antibiotics, then oral and occasionally IV antibiotics are required.

◆ Epidemiology

Acute otitis externa affects from 1:100 to 1:250 of the general population. A lifetime incidence may be as high as 10%. The disorder is more common in warm environments with high humidity and increased water exposure.

◆ Clinical

Signs

Otorrhea, conductive hearing loss, and EAC swelling are all common. As the skin of the EAC swells, the periosteum is irritated and becomes very painful. Pressing on the tragus or pulling the auricle may lead to significant pain. The auricle and periauricular tissues may also become edematous and tender if the condition becomes a periauricular cellulitis. If the infection has spread to a cellulitis, then the ear may be prominent with an increased auriculocephalic angle similar to that seen with acute mastoiditis. Signs of otomycosis include itching and visible hyphae on inspection.

Symptoms

Usually present with a 48- to 72-hour history of progressive pain, itching, discharge, and aural fullness. Patients may also complain of jaw pain. If the ear canal fills with debris or swells completely, then hearing loss will also occur.

Differential Diagnosis

The differential diagnosis includes foreign body of the EAC, otitis media, malignant or necrotizing OE in a diabetic, coalescent mastoiditis, malignancy, chronic OE, and other inflammatory lesions (e.g., eosinophilic granuloma). Dermatological conditions (eczema, contact dermatitis), allergic reaction to ototopical drops, and herpes zoster oticus with painful EAC vesicles need to be excluded. A localized furuncle may also mimic OE, as can chronic otitis media or acute otitis media with otorrhea. The presence of inflammation of the TM with formation of bullae and severe pain indicates bullous myringitis; this is rare, may be associated with influenza, and may be superinfected with bacteria. The best treatment for bullous myringitis is controversial but can include pain medications, oral antibiotics (e.g., macrolides), and ototopical antibiotic preparations.

◆ Evaluation

Physical Exam

A head and neck examination, concentrating on the otologic exam, is performed. When possible, the EAC should be débrided with an otomicroscope. Inspection may reveal eczema, otorrhea, edematous canal skin, erythema, moist cerumen, debris, or hyphae. One classic finding is pain with palpation or manipulation of the auricle or the tragus. Frequently, the skin is so swollen that the TM cannot be seen. If visible, the TM may appear inflamed but mobile (differentiating it from acute otitis media). The skin of the auricle and periauricular region may also demonstrate erythema, edema, and tenderness.

Imaging

Imaging is not needed for uncomplicated OE. However, when there is auricular or periauricular involvement with protruded auricle, a computed tomography (CT) scan of the temporal bones can help differentiate a coalescent mastoiditis from severe OE with postauricular cellulitis.

Labs

Labs are rarely indicated for uncomplicated OE. In patients with suspected uncontrolled diabetes, a blood glucose level may be helpful.

Other Tests

Cultures are recommended for recurrent, chronic, or recalcitrant OE. Cultures should be sent for routine culture and sensitivity as well as fungus. Any abnormal-appearing tissue or polyp that does not respond to medical management should be biopsied to exclude malignancy.

Pathology

The infection usually begins with moisture buildup in the EAC. The acidic and hydrophobic qualities of cerumen make it bacteriostatic. A warm, moist EAC with decreased cerumen favors bacterial overgrowth. The bacteria will readily invade the skin. Although > 90% of OE cases are bacterial, a moist alkaline environment also favors fungal growth. *Pseudomonas aeruginosa* and *Staphylococcus aureus* are most common bacteria, and *Aspergillus* and *Candida* are the most common fungi.

◆ Treatment Options

Medical

The ear must be meticulously cleaned with an otomicroscope with complete removal of debris. This may need to be repeated in a few days. Once the ear is cleaned, otic drops should be placed. There are several preparations available, including nonantibiotic, antibiotic alone, and antibiotic plus steroid therapies (**Table 3.6**). They may be used two or three times per day for 7 to 14 days. Dry ear precautions are recommended until the infection clears.

Placement of a wick (e.g., Pope Oto-Wick; Medtronic, Inc., Minneapolis, MN) to carry drops medially may be required, especially in canals so swollen that the TM is not easily visible. Keep in mind that placing a wick can be a very uncomfortable experience for the patient. Analgesics, even those with narcotic, may be required to control the pain. As edema regresses, the wick will usually fall out or may be removed. OE due to a foreign body will not resolve without removal of the foreign body.

Relevant Pharmacology

Topical preparations are superior to systemic medications in cost and side effect profile. The medication concentration is significantly higher with topical medications than with systemic drugs. The efficacy of ototopical drugs depends on drug delivery; therefore, ear débridement is critical and wicks are placed when appropriate.

Table 3.6 Topical preparations useful for management of otitis externa

Topical agent	Typical dose regimen
Antibacterial agents	
2% acetic acid	5 drops 3–4 times daily
2% acetic acid/1% hydrocortisone solution	5 drops 3–4 times daily
Burow solution (13% aluminum acetate)	Drops of soaked pledget
Floxin Otic (ofloxacin otic)*	5 drops twice daily
Ciprodex (ciprofloxacin/ dexamethasone)† or Cipro HC (ciprofloxacin/hydrocortisone)† otic	5 drops twice daily
Cortisporin otic suspension (neomycin/ polymyxin B/hydrocortisone)‡	3–5 drops 3 times daily
Antifungal agents	
Clotrimazole (1%)	4 drops 3–4 times daily
Gentian violet (aqueous)	Physician applies topically under microscope in office as needed
Boric acid solution (3%)	5 drops twice daily
Boric acid powder	1–2 puffs 1–2 times daily
CSF powder (chloramphenicol, p-aminobenzenesulfonamide, amphotericin ± hydrocortisone)	1–2 puffs 1–2 times daily

*Daiichi Pharmaceuticals, Montvale, NJ.
†Alcon Pharmaceuticals, Inc., Fribourg, Switzerland.
‡Endo International, Dublin, Ireland.
Note: Use in combination with serial débridement; may require Oto-Wick placement if canal is severely swollen.

Ototopical antibiotic drops include Cortisporin (neomycin/polymyxin B/ hydrocortisone), ofloxacin, and ciprofloxacin. There is a 10 to 15% sensitization rate with neomycin containing products. Acidifying solutions such as Domeboro (2% acetic acid; Bayer Consumer Health, Morristown, NJ) or VoSoL (2% acetic acid and propylene glycol) can be used. Currently, U.S. Food and Drug Administration (FDA)-approved preparations for patients with tympanic membrane perforations and exposed middle ear are ofloxacin and ciprofloxacin/dexamethasone.

Surgical

There is no specific role for surgery in acute OE. Patients may occasionally require a general anesthetic to carry out the canal cleaning and wick placement if the ear is too tender to instrument in the office. If a foreign body is suspected, especially in a child, then a general anesthetic may be needed to remove it.

Chronic OE results after fibrosis thickens the skin of the EAC, sometimes to the point of completely obliterating the canal. In some of these cases, a canalplasty with meatoplasty and skin grafting may be necessary.

◆ Outcome and Follow-Up

Most cases resolve within 7 to 10 days of treatment. Causative factors such as eczema, swimming, or cotton swab (Q-tip) use need to be addressed to promote resolution and prevent recurrence. Patients may need to be seen frequently in the office for repeated cleanings until the infection resolves. Patients should keep the ears dry for 7 to 10 days. Swimmers can return to the water with waterproof ear plugs in 3 days. Hearing aids can be replaced after pain and discharge resolve.

3.3.2   Malignant Otitis Externa

◆ Key Features

- Malignant otitis externa (MOE) is most frequently caused by *Pseudomonas aeruginosa*.
- Patients are immunocompromised, most commonly with diabetes.
- It is characterized by severe deep aural pain, especially at night.
- The facial nerve is the most common cranial nerve involved.

Malignant otitis externa (MOE) is a severe and serious form of infective otitis externa (OE). It is also referred to as necrotizing otitis externa. Diagnostic criteria include pain, edema, exudate, granulation at the bony-cartilaginous junction, failed local medical treatment > 1 week, abnormal culture, and abnormal bone imaging studies. When diagnosis and treatment are delayed, MOE can progress to skull base osteomyelitis, cranial nerve palsies, and death. Medical treatment with long-term systemic antipseudomonal antibiotics is the mainstay of treatment. Surgical management has little role in treating MOE.

◆ Epidemiology

Ninety percent of patients are diabetic, and most are over 60 years old. Other predisposing factors include immunosuppression (e.g., human immunodeficiency virus [HIV], transplant patients, chemotherapy).

◆ Clinical

Signs

Patients will have external auditory canal (EAC) and periauricular tissue edema and tenderness. The tympanic membrane (TM) may be normal or inflamed with a middle ear effusion. There is granulation tissue along the floor of the canal at the bony-cartilaginous junction. Palsy of cranial nerves (CN) VII, IX, X, XI and XII may be present. Visual disturbance from CN III, IV, and VI palsies and facial paresthesias can also occur during the progression of skull base osteomyelitis.

Symptoms

Aural pain and discharge are not responsive to the usual measures. Pain is often severe at night and may awaken patients from sleep. Also, headache and temporomandibular joint (TMJ) pain are common. Symptoms typically persist for more than a week. As the disease progresses, patients may complain of facial weakness, dysphagia, hoarseness, shoulder/tongue weakness, lethargy, nausea, blurred vision, and mental confusion.

Differential Diagnosis

MOE must be differentiated from routine OE or acute otitis media with mastoiditis. Fungal MOE must also be considered. Granulation tissue should be biopsied to rule out a malignancy. The differential diagnosis also includes EAC foreign body, infected cholesteatoma, other inflammatory disorders (e.g., Wegener's granulomatosis), and other infectious disorders (e.g., tuberculosis).

◆ Evaluation

History

The history should focus on elucidation of predisposing factors, such as diabetes and immunosuppressive disorders (e.g., HIV, leukemia, chemotherapy, transplant, malnutrition, alcoholism). If the patient is diabetic, information regarding recent glucose levels and hemoglobin A1c (HbA1c) is useful.

Physical Exam

A complete head and neck examination concentrating on the cranial nerve and otologic exam is warranted. The ear canal is débrided and examined carefully using an otomicroscope. This may require general anesthetic if pain is severe. Parotid palpation and TMJ mobility are noted.

Imaging

High-resolution computed tomography (CT) of the temporal bone is recommended. Findings on CT can include bony EAC or skull base erosion, soft tissue thickening of the EAC, and opacification of the middle ear and mastoid. CT is not as useful for determining intracranial and soft tissue involvement nor for determining the endpoint of treatment (bony erosion persists on CT despite resolution of infection). Magnetic resonance imaging (MRI) of the skull base with and without gadolinium contrast is helpful in detecting the progression of disease and is superior to CT in detecting intracranial, dural, and soft tissue involvement.

Technetium-99m (^{99m}Tc) nuclear scanning highlights areas of osteoblastic activity seen in osteomyelitis. Increased uptake, indicative of skull base osteomyelitis, is seen a few hours after ^{99m}Tc administration. This modality may be positive prior to bony changes seen on CT but cannot be used to determine the end point of treatment (can remain positive for months to years as a sign of bony repair and remodeling). It is very helpful in confirming an early diagnosis.

Table 3.7 A consideration of key diagnostic tests for malignant otitis externa

Labs
• CBC with differential (follow ANC level if neutropenic) • Blood glucose level (serially) • HbA1c, ESR (serially)

Pathology
Histopathologic exam of granulation tissue to exclude neoplasm

Microbiology
Bacterial and fungal culture and sensitivities of ear canal debris

Imaging
• Temporal bone CT to assess for extent of disease, bone erosion • MRI with gadolinium may be helpful to assess dural, intracranial, and soft tissue involvement. • Nuclear scanning: ^{99m}Tc scan is better for early diagnosis of MOE and determining extent of skull base osteomyelitis; ^{67}Ga and ^{111}In nuclear scanning are preferred for follow-up and assessment of disease resolution.

Abbreviations: HbA1c, hemoglobin A1c; ANC, absolute neutrophil count; CBC, complete blood count; CT, computed tomography; ESR, erythrocyte sedimentation rate; MRI, magnetic resonance imaging.

Gallium-67 (^{67}Ga) or indium-111 (^{111}In) nuclear scanning highlights areas of inflammation by binding to leukocytes. Increased uptake, indicative of skull-base osteomyelitis, can be seen on imaging 24 to 72 hours after administration of the radioactive tracer. It is a good test for end point treatment because it reverts to normal once the infectious response has resolved. It may be repeated several times throughout the treatment course to monitor response.

Labs

Routine laboratory testing will display an increased white blood cell (WBC) count, an increased erythrocyte sedimentation rate (ESR), and elevated blood glucose (in diabetics). Serial ESR levels can be used to monitor treatment response.

Other Tests

The ear canal should be swabbed for culture and sensitivity. Granulation tissue should be biopsied to rule out malignancy. A baseline audiogram is important, especially when utilizing potentially ototoxic antibiotic medications and determining the effects of skull base osteomyelitis on the otic capsule. See **Table 3.7** for a consideration of diagnostic tests.

Pathology

Pseudomonas aeruginosa is the causative bacteria in a majority of cases; however, the incidence of methicillin-resistant *Staphylococcus aureus* (MRSA) has increased. Infection begins at the skin of the EAC and spreads into the mastoid and temporal bone directly or through venous channels and fascial planes. Infection can also spread to the parotid gland, infratemporal fossa, and skull base via the fissures of Santorini and the tympanomastoid suture line. Infection and inflammation involving adjacent bone can cause cranial nerve palsies.

Patients are immunocompromised; the most common reason for immunosuppression is uncontrolled diabetes mellitus. Their cerumen is neutral pH, which promotes bacterial overgrowth and infection. MOE from fungal etiology can be seen in HIV with acquired immune deficiency syndrome (AIDS), hematologic malignancies, and immunosuppression after transplantation. *Aspergillus* is usually the culprit.

◆ Treatment Options

Medical

Medical therapy is the mainstay of treatment; however, there are no established guidelines for treatment. Early, uncomplicated MOE from nonresistant *Pseudomonas aeruginosa* may be treated with oral fluoroquinolone in an outpatient setting with close follow-up. However, severe and complicated MOE require parenteral therapy with good bone penetration. Prior to the development of a third-generation antipseudomonal cephalosporin, empiric treatment with intravenous antipseudomonal penicillin *and* aminoglycoside was commonly recommended. Systemic therapies for MOE are described in **Table 3.8.** Culture-directed antibiotics are used when possible. Some advocate two systemic medications over monotherapy in order to prevent drug resistance.

Ototopical treatments are also initiated early in the disease process (e.g., fluoroquinolones ± steroid, neomycin/polymyxin B/hydrocortisone, tobramycin, gentamicin). When possible, nonototoxic drops should be prescribed when a TM perforation exists. Wick placement may be necessary when the EAC is narrow or completely stenosed.

Long-term oral or systemic therapy is recommended and can range from 4 weeks to 6 months. The end point of therapy for MOE is controversial, varies from institution to institution, and may rely on availability of resources. In general, treatment has been stopped when serial ^{67}Ga/^{111}In scan obtained every 4 to 6 weeks returns to normal. Alternatively, normalization of serial ESRs and three negative ear cultures has also been argued. Patients with skull base osteomyelitis may need to be on lifelong therapy, especially to prevent relapse. Failure of therapy may indicate development of multi-drug-resistant pathogens or surge of other pathogens; new cultures should be performed.

In addition, immunosuppression is reversed when possible (e.g., correcting diabetes, halting chemotherapy, initiating antiretroviral therapy for HIV). Hyperbaric oxygen is considered in patients with extensive skull

Table 3.8   Empiric antibiotic therapy for malignant otitis externa

Antibiotic	Class	Dosage
Ciprofloxacin	Fluoroquinolone	750 mg orally every 12 hours 400 mg IV every 12 hours
Ceftazidime	Third-generation cephalosporin	2 g IV every 8 hours
Cefepime	Fourth-generation cephalosporin	2 g IV every 12 hours
Piperacillin-tazobactam	Antipseudomonal penicillin	3.375 or 4.5 g IV every 6 hours
Ticarcillin-clavulanate	Antipseudomonal penicillin	3 g IV every 4 hours
Gentamicin	Aminoglycoside	1–1.66 mg/kg IV every 8 hours
Tobramycin	Aminoglycoside	1–2 mg/kg IV every 8 hours

Note: Aminoglycosides are usually prescribed along with an antipseudomonal antibiotic. Aminoglycosides require peak and trough monitoring and observation for renal failure and hearing loss. Therapy should be culture-directed whenever possible.

base osteomyelitis or progressive disease despite aggressive medical management.

Surgical

Traditionally, surgical management is limited to initial and serial canal débridement. A myringotomy tube is considered if there is middle ear fluid.

◆ Complications

Progressive MOE becomes osteomyelitis of the skull base. With spreading infection, CNs VII, IX, X, XI, and XII may become involved. Consequences include aspiration with difficulties in speech and swallowing. CNs III, V, and VI may also be involved. Meningitis, lateral sinus thrombosis, cerebral abscess, and death may all occur.

◆ Outcome and Follow-Up

With proper diagnosis and treatment, cure rates are over 80%. Mortality rates have significantly declined in the antibiotic era. Serial examinations and débridements in follow-up may be necessary. Topical and systemic treatment is generally completed when the TM and EAC return to normal appearance, pain resolves, cultures are negative, ESR normalizes, and there is a negative ^{67}Ga/^{111}In scan. Treating the underlying immunosuppression is an important factor in the management of MOE and skull base osteomyelitis.

3.4 Audiology

3.4.1 Basic Audiologic Assessments

◆ Key Features

- Pure tone testing—air and bone conduction thresholds
- Speech testing—speech reception thresholds (SRT) and word recognition ability
- Immittance battery—tympanometry, acoustic reflex thresholds, acoustic reflex decay, auditory tube function assessment

Air and bone conduction pure tone testing determines the type, degree, and configuration of hearing loss. Thresholds represent the softest sound audible at least 50% of the time, measured in decibels (dB). Speech reception thresholds (SRT) serve to verify pure tone thresholds. Word recognition ability represents an individual's ability to discriminate speech. Immittance testing assesses the status of the tympanic membrane, middle ear, and acoustic reflex pathways.

◆ Epidemiology

Approximately 28 million Americans have hearing loss. Approximately 314 in 1,000 people over age 65 have hearing loss. Forty to fifty percent of people over the age of 75 suffer from hearing loss.

◆ Clinical

Signs and Symptoms

Persons with hearing loss frequently report difficulty hearing in background noise. They mistakenly feel others around them are mumbling. They often need the television volume louder than is comfortable for others and ask for things to be repeated. Many experience tinnitus.

Differential Diagnosis

Results of audiometric testing are typically plotted on an audiogram (**Fig. 3.7**). An audiogram is a graph with frequency (in Hz) plotted on the x axis and intensity (in dB) plotted on the y axis. It is necessary to employ masking (a static type of noise) in certain situations to prevent the nontest ear from detecting the test signal.

Results of the audiogram and tympanogram (**Fig. 3.8**) may suggest various forms of otologic disease. Red flags should prompt referral to an otolaryngologist (discussed below). Otologic disease may be categorized as conductive hearing loss, sensorineural loss (SNHL), or mixed hearing loss. In a conductive loss, there is an air–bone gap on the audiogram, with better bone conduction thresholds, with appropriate masking. The loss may be due to dysfunction involving the external canal, tympanic membrane, or ossicular chain or to middle ear fluid. In a sensorineural loss, bone conduction thresholds typically equal air conduction, and the loss may be due to dysfunction at the level of the cochlea, CN VIII, or central pathways. A poor word-recognition score, especially out of proportion to pure tone thresholds, suggests possible retrocochlear pathology, such as an acoustic tumor.

Patterns of SNHL may be suggestive of certain etiologies, taken together with clinical history and exam. For example, acoustic trauma (noise-induced loss) often results in a loss centered around 4 kHz with recovery at higher frequency (i.e., a 4-kHz notch); presbycusis often involves symmetric downsloping loss, worse at higher frequency; a fluctuating low-frequency loss is often seen with Ménière's disease.

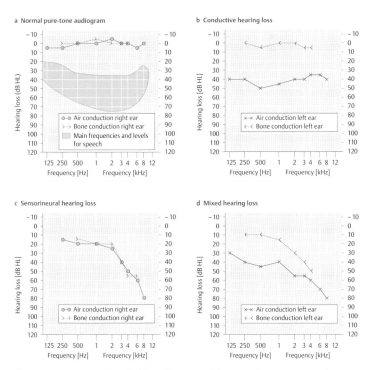

Fig. 3.7 Pure-tone threshold audiometry. **(a)** Normal pure-tone audiogram. **(b)** Audiogram showing conductive hearing loss. **(c)** Audiogram showing sensorineural hearing loss. **(d)** Audiogram showing mixed hearing loss. (Used with permission from Probst R, Grevers G, Iro H. *Basic Otorhinolaryngology: A Step-by-Step Learning Guide.* Stuttgart/New York: Thieme; 2006:179.)

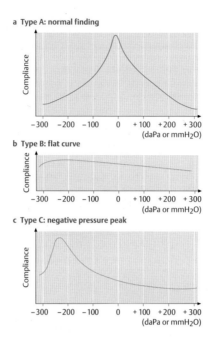

Fig. 3.8 Normal and abnormal tympanogram patterns. **(a)** The normal tympanogram has a prominent, sharp peak between +100 and –100 daPa. **(b)** The type B tympanogram is flat or has a very low, rounded peak. This indicates immobility of the tympanic membrane, which may be due to fluid in the middle ear or tympanic atelectasis. A type B tympanogram with large volume is seen with the perforation. **(c)** The type C tympanogram has a peak in the negative pressure region below –100 daPa, consistent with impaired middle ear ventilation. (From Probst R, Grevers G, Iro H. *Basic Otorhinolaryngology: A Step-by-Step Learning Guide*. Stuttgart/New York: Thieme; 2006:185.)

The Jerger system is commonly used to classify tympanometric results:

- Type A: Normal
  - Pressure peak +100 to –100 daPa
  - Immittance 0.3 to 1.7 mL
- Type As: Shallow
  - Pressure peak +100 to –100 daPa
  - Immittance < 0.3 mL
- Type Ad: Deep
  - Pressure peak +100 to –100 daPa
  - Immittance > 1.7 mL
- Type C: Negative pressure
  - Pressure peak ≤ 100 daPa
  - Immittance normal or shallow

- Type B: Flat
  - ○ No pressure peak or immittance
  - ○ Small ear canal volume suggests ear canal occlusion.
  - ○ Normal volume suggests otitis media.
  - ○ Large ear canal volume suggests patent pressure equalization tube or perforated eardrum.

◆ Evaluation

Tuning Fork Tests

The goal of these tests, including the Weber test (**Fig. 3.9**), is to differentiate between conductive and SNHL. The tuning forks vibrate at a fixed frequency between 256 and 1024 Hz. To test bone conduction, the fork is placed firmly on the skull bone. Typically, a 512-Hz tuning fork is used.

Weber Test

The Weber test will lateralize to the ear with worse conductive loss if sensory hearing is equal in both ears (**Fig. 3.9**). Alternatively, the Weber test will lateralize to the ear with better sensory hearing if there is no conductive hearing loss in either ear.

Rinne Test

The Rinne test (**Fig. 3.10**) compares the level of air conduction and bone conduction in the same ear. In a normal ear, air conduction is greater. It usually takes about a 30-dB conductive loss to flip the tuning fork response to bone conduction greater than air.

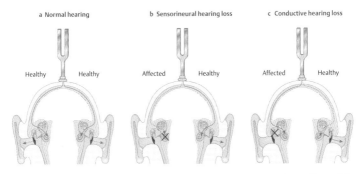

Fig. 3.9   The Weber test. A vibrating tuning fork is placed on the midline of the skull. **(a)** When hearing is normal, the sound is perceived with equal loudness in or between both ears. **(b)** With unilateral sensorineural hearing loss, the sound is lateralized to the better ear. **(c)** With unilateral conductive hearing loss, the sound is lateralized to the affected side. (Used with permission from Probst R, Grevers G, Iro H. *Basic Otorhinolaryngology: A Step-by-Step Learning Guide*. Stuttgart/ New York: Thieme; 2006:168.)

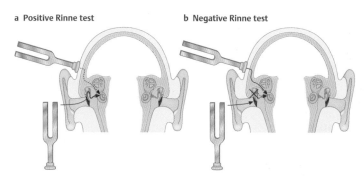

a Positive Rinne test **b Negative Rinne test**

Fig. 3.10 The Rinne test. Air and bone conduction are compared in the same ear to determine the auditory threshold for the tuning fork and/or its loudness. **(a)** In the absence of conductive hearing loss, air conduction is perceived as being louder and/or of longer duration than bone conduction. **(b)** When conductive hearing loss is present, bone conduction is perceived as being louder and/or more prolonged than air conduction. (Used with permission from Probst R, Grevers G, Iro H. *Basic Otorhinolaryngology: A Step-by-Step Learning Guide.* Stuttgart/New York: Thieme; 2006:69.)

Physical Exam

Test results are best obtained in a sound-treated booth. Insert earphones placed in the ear canal are the transducer of choice in assessing air conduction thresholds due to infection control, increased interaural attenuation, and prevention of collapsed ear canals. Supra- and circumaural headphones are options as well in certain situations. Bone conduction is assessed by placing an oscillator on a mastoid bone. Forehead placement is another option in special situations.

Conventional behavioral audiometry is conducted by having a person respond to pure tones (e.g., raising a hand, pushing a button). SRTs are obtained by repeating spondees (two-syllable words with equal weight on both syllables; e.g., hotdog, baseball). Word recognition is assessed by repeating phonetically balanced lists of monosyllabic words at suprathreshold intensity (approximately 30–40 dB above the SRT).

In tympanometry, the maximum compliance peak is determined by presenting a probe tone (typically 1,000 Hz in infants up through 6 months of age, 226 Hz in all others) in the sealed ear canal while varying air pressure (+200 to –400 daPa). Maximum compliance occurs when the middle and external ear air pressures are equal.

Other Tests

Acoustic reflex thresholds and acoustic reflex decay can be measured both ipsilaterally and contralaterally and across different frequencies. A probe tone is presented in either ear while a change in immittance is monitored.

This assesses the acoustic pathways by measuring the contraction of the stapedius muscle in response to acoustic stimulation. Auditory (eustachian) tube function testing reveals how well middle ear pressure is equalized. Testing occurs in the same manner as basic tympanometric testing, but with a person pinching the nose and swallowing in between artificial changes in ear canal air pressure (Toynbee test).

Pathology

Hearing loss may be congenital, acquired (e.g., exogenous sources such as perinatal infection) or genetic (hereditary). Genetic hearing loss may be syndromic or nonsyndromic. Acquired hearing loss is frequently related to the aging of the auditory system (presbycusis). It can also occur from trauma, infection, excessive noise exposure, and ototoxic medications. Hearing loss may remain stable over time, sudden, progressive, or fluctuating.

◆ Treatment Options

Patients with unilateral or conductive hearing losses should be referred for medical evaluation. Other red flags should prompt otolaryngology referral, such as evidence of a sudden hearing loss, rapidly progressing or fluctuating sensorineural loss, word recognition score poorer than expected based on pure tone thresholds, word recognition score asymmetry greater than 10%, evidence of middle ear dysfunction, evidence of otorrhea, or any hearing loss in a child.

◆ Outcome and Follow-Up

Following medical clearance, a variety of amplification devices are available and appropriate for most persons with hearing loss.

3.4.2 Pediatric Audiologic Assessments

◆ Key Features

- The goal of universal newborn hearing screening is to have all infants screened by 1 month, comprehensive audiologic evaluation when needed by 3 months, and intervention in infants with confirmed hearing loss by 6 months.
- There are more stringent cutoffs for normal hearing thresholds in pediatric patients: 15- to 20-decibel (dB) hearing loss, as opposed to 25-dB hearing loss in adults.
- Children require specialized testing that is administered by a well-trained pediatric audiologist. It is essential to use the cross-check principle when evaluating children in order to ensure a proper diagnosis.
- Testing protocols often need to be modified to obtain the same audiologic information readily acquired from cooperative adults.

Prior to the implementation of newborn hearing screenings, children with hearing loss were often misdiagnosed or identified later in life. When the diagnosis and treatment are delayed, the impact of hearing loss in children can result in speech, language, cognitive, social, and academic delays. Early Hearing Detection and Intervention (EHDI) programs have become the standard of care in the United States, and screening for hearing loss occurs in 95% of infants born in the United States. Screening of neonates for hearing loss should be performed with automated distortion product otoacoustic emissions (DPOAE) or auditory brainstem response testing (ABR) prior to discharge from hospital.

The goal of universal newborn hearing screening is to have all infants screened by 1 month of age, comprehensive audiologic evaluation when needed before 3 months of age, and early intervention in infants with confirmed hearing loss by 6 months of age.

◆ Epidemiology

The prevalence of congenital hearing loss in newborns is about two to three infants per 1,000, or approximately 13,000 babies born in the United States each year with some degree of permanent hearing loss. Most of these babies are otherwise healthy and have no family history of hearing loss.

◆ Clinical

Even mild, untreated hearing loss in infants and young children can significantly impact their speech, language, social, cognitive, and academic development. As children develop, optimal learning and communication require hearing the speaker clearly, developmentally appropriate language, and speech levels that are at least 20 decibels (dB) above the background noise. Children with unidentified hearing loss will have considerable challenges, and as mentioned, these can greatly hinder a child from reaching his or her potential. Any concerns expressed by caregivers should be formally evaluated. Informal assessments are not adequate in evaluating a child's hearing.

A thorough birth history should be ascertained from parents, including history of prematurity, prenatal/postnatal infections, hyperbilirubinemia, exposure to ototoxic antibiotics, hypoxia, and encephalopathy. A developmental history is important to distinguish an isolated hearing loss from a more systemic problem causing speech delay. Syndromic causes and a family history of hearing loss should also be determined. A history of ear infections may indicated middle ear disease and conductive hearing loss. Further information can be found in **Chapter 8.11**.

◆ Evaluation

Physical Exam

A full head and neck physical exam concentrating on the otologic exam should be performed. When possible, an otomicroscope should be used to remove any cerumen or debris from the ear canal. The external auditory canal, tympanic membrane, and associated landmarks are assessed. Pneumatic otoscopy should be performed to determine mobility of the tympanic membrane and presence of tympanic membrane perforation or middle ear fluid. Craniofacial abnormalities may indicate a syndromic cause of hearing loss.

Testing

Depending on the developmental age of the child, behavioral observation, visual reinforcement audiometry, conditioned play audiometry, and conventional audiometry are utilized to obtain pure tone thresholds. Behavioral observation testing is performed in infants up to 6 months of age. Visual reinforcement audiometry is done in children between 6 months and ~3 years of age. Conditioned play audiometry can be performed in children between the ages of 3 and 6. Last, conventional audiometry is performed in children that are older than 6 years of age.

With any of these tests, results are most reliable when testing is conducted with two people (i.e., one person performing the test protocol and one person in the booth to redirect the child—it is typically not advantageous to use a child's parent for this role). Testing with insert earphones is preferred so that ear-specific information can be obtained (headphones may also be used in some instances, but caution is needed to avoid collapsing young ear canals). Testing can also be conducted in the sound field; however, ear-specific information will not be known. Warbled tones and narrowband noise are frequently used in testing children in addition to pure tones.

In behavioral observation testing, examiners look for any physical changes in a child in response to sound (i.e., blinking or other eye movement, cessation of sucking). In visual reinforcement audiometry, children are rewarded (e.g., a lighted box with an animated character) by turning their head in response to sound. In play audiometry, children are conditioned to perform a task (e.g., drop blocks in a bucket, put pegs on a board) in response to pure tones. Conventional audiometry requires the patient to raise a hand or press a button when a sound is heard.

Speech awareness thresholds may be obtained in place of speech reception thresholds. Picture boards or body part pointing can also help in obtaining speech information. High-frequency probe tone (1,000 Hz) testing is needed in tympanometry to appropriately assess the middle ear function in children who have a developmental age of 6 months or younger. In some children, behavioral information should be confirmed through objective/electrophysiological testing. If the child has severe cognitive impairment or is otherwise unable or too young to cooperate for behavioral testing, objective testing should be obtained via otoacoustic emissions (OAE) and auditory brainstem response (ABR) evaluations.

OAE is an objective test to determine functional capacity of the outer hair cells of the cochlea. When sound is delivered to the cochlea, it produces a low-intensity sound called otoacoustic emissions. There are several types of otoacoustic emissions, however. Distortion product OAE (DPOAE) testing is widely used due to the ability to test at different frequencies. A probe is placed in the ear canal and two simultaneous pure tones at two different frequencies and intensities are delivered to the ear. Emissions are recorded at different frequency levels. DPOAEs should be interpreted with caution, as results are affected by obstructed external auditory canal, positioning and seal of the probe, tympanic membrane perforations, and middle ear disease.

ABR testing is an objective test that evaluates the function of the auditory nerve and brainstem elicited after an auditory stimulus. The interpeak latency (time between peaks) and interaural latency (difference between ears) are also assessed. Each waveform in ABR correlates to a structure on the auditory pathway. In general, waves correspond to the eighth cranial nerve, cochlear nucleus, olivary complex (superior), lateral lemniscus, and inferior colliculus (mnemonic: ECOLI). Different frequencies and intensities are tested until a reproducible waveform is identified. Further information regarding DPOAEs and ABRs is found in **Chapter 3.4.3**.

◆ Treatment Options

The priority in children is to obtain appropriate auditory rehabilitation as soon as the problem is identified. Because plasticity within the auditory cortex is finite and diminishes dramatically after the first few years, a failure to obtain auditory input within this critical period will result in cortical deafness: an inability of the brain to process auditory input adequately later in life if aided or implanted. Thus, if hearing loss cannot be corrected by treating obvious causes, such as a myringotomy tube for middle ear fluid, amplification should be obtained. If there is minimal or no benefit from appropriate amplification, cochlear implant (CI) evaluation should be sought as soon as possible.

There are many modifications available to assist in the fitting of hearing aids to even very young infants and children. To accommodate ear growth, children are fitted with behind-the-ear hearing aids, and their earmolds need to be replaced frequently. In addition to hearing aids, children may benefit from the use of hearing assistive technology (e.g., FM system) in classrooms to improve the signal-to-noise ratio. Hearing assistive technology provides a handheld microphone for teachers to talk into, which transmits the sound of the teacher's voice directly to child's hearing aid.

◆ Outcome and Follow-Up

Children diagnosed with hearing loss should receive an otologic consult, an ophthalmologic consult, possibly genetic counseling, and routine monitoring of their hearing abilities. Depending on the origin of the hearing loss, siblings of diagnosed children should also have their hearing assessed. Children with high risk factors for hearing loss should receive periodic reevaluations as well. Infants who pass the newborn hearing screening but have risk factors for hearing loss should have at least one diagnostic audiology assessment by 24 to 30 months of age.

3.4.3   Objective/Electrophysiologic Audiologic Assessments

◆ Key Features

- Otoacoustic emissions (OAEs)
- Auditory brainstem responses (ABRs; aka BAER, BSER)
- Auditory steady-state responses (ASSRs)
- Electrocochleography (ECoG)
- Electroneuronography (ENoG)

Otoacoustic emissions (OAE) test the functional integrity of the outer hair cells in the cochlea. Auditory brainstem response (ABR) and auditory steady-state responses (ASSR) test the function of the auditory nerve and brainstem. Electrocochleography (ECoG) measures the summation and action potential to determine the presence of endolymphatic hydrops or elevated inner ear pressure, a finding in Ménière's disease. Electroneuronography (ENoG) is not an audiologic test, but it is presented in this section because it is an objective, electrophysiological test often performed by audiologists to assess distal facial nerve function.

◆ Evaluation

OAEs test the functional integrity of the outer hair cells in the cochlea. OAEs represent a low-intensity sound emitted from the outer hair cells in response to sound stimulation. They are valuable in newborn hearing screenings, difficult-to-test patients, assessing auditory neuropathy, and in chemotherapy monitoring. There are several types of OAEs: spontaneous, transient, sustained frequency, and distortion product otoacoustic emissions (DPOAE). Transient evoked and distortion product OAEs are present in > 99% of persons with normal hearing. Clinically, DPOAEs are more widely used, as different frequencies can be evaluated. A probe is placed in the ear canal, and two simultaneous pure tones at two different frequencies and intensities are delivered to the ear. The outer hair cell response is recorded from the same probe placed in the ear canal. Emissions are recorded at different frequency levels. DPOAE should be interpreted with caution, as results are affected by obstructed external auditory canal, positioning and seal of the probe, tympanic membrane perforations, and middle ear disease.

ABR testing is an objective test that evaluates the amplitude and latency of auditory nerve and brainstem waves elicited after an auditory stimulus. The interpeak latency (time between peaks) and interaural latency (difference between ears) are also assessed. ABRs are also used in newborn hearing screenings, neurodiagnostics (e.g., retrocochlear or cerebellopontine angle pathology such as vestibular schwannomas; auditory neuropathy/dyssynchrony) and intraoperative monitoring. In general, the five waves seen on ABR can be recalled using the mnemonic "ECOLI": eighth cranial nerve (wave I), cochlear nucleus (wave II), olivary complex (superior) (wave III), lateral lemniscus (wave IV), and inferior colliculus (wave V). When used as a screening tool for retrocochlear pathology, an interaural wave I to V latency difference > 0.2 ms or prolonged wave V are abnormal. When hearing thresholds are desired, different frequencies and intensities are tested until a reproducible waveform is identified. ABR relies on an examiner reviewing the waveforms obtained from low-repetition brief sound bursts. ASSR is similar to ABR, but high-repetition sounds are used and a sophisticated and statistical mathematical detection algorithm is used to determine hearing thresholds. ABR normative data vary with age in children under 2 years. Results are affected by level of hearing loss, test parameters (stimulus rate and intensity), patient factors (movement, body temperature), and environmental factors (ambient noise, electrical interference).

ECoG is used in assessing endolymphatic hydrops and in intraoperative monitoring. Similarly to ABR, electrical potentials are generated from the auditory nerve and brainstem in response to sound. An electrode is placed on the tympanic membrane, and the amplitude of the cochlear summating potential (SP) and auditory nerve action potential (AP) are recorded. An SP/AP ratio > 45 to 50% is abnormal and suggests endolymphatic hydrops. It is not routinely used in the diagnosis of Ménière's disease. Limitations in testing are similar to those of ABR. Electrical potentials in ECOG, ABR, and ASSR are recorded through electrodes on the mastoids, earlobes, forehead, and/or tympanic membranes.

ENoG testing is used when there is complete facial paralysis with normal contralateral facial nerve function. A brief electrical stimulus is delivered to the facial nerve near the stylomastoid foramen, while the compound action potential of terminal nerves is recorded near the nasolabial fold. The results are compared to the normal contralateral facial nerve. It has the most clinical value when performed between 3 and 14 days of onset of complete facial paralysis. It has been used to determine percentage of nerve degeneration in patients with acute facial paralysis, such as with Bell's palsy and temporal bone fracture. Surgical decompression of the facial nerve has been recommended when serial ENoGs demonstrating > 90% facial nerve degeneration without evidence of action potentials on electromyography (EMG). This topic is further addressed in **Chapter 3.1.3**.

3.5 Hearing Loss

3.5.1 Conductive Hearing Loss

◆ Key Features

- Conductive hearing loss (CHL) occurs when sound is not efficiently transmitted through the external auditory canal, tympanic membrane, and ossicles to a functioning cochlea.
- CHL can occur due to dysfunction of the external auditory canal (EAC), the tympanic membrane, or the ossicles.
- Most cases of CHL can be surgically corrected.

Disorders of the external auditory canal (EAC), tympanic membrane (TM), middle ear, and ossicles can impair sound transmission to a functioning cochlea, resulting in conductive hearing loss (CHL).

◆ Clinical

Signs

Various forms of obstruction can occur at the level of the EAC (e.g., cerumen, foreign body, congenital canal atresia, inflammatory stenosis with acquired atresia, bony exostosis, canal cholesteatoma). Blockage of the EAC can cause up to a 40-dB hearing loss. The TM may be thickened from scarring or tympanosclerosis; it can be retracted from negative middle ear pressure and drape on the incus and stapes (e.g., myringoincudostapediopexy) or even onto the cochlear promontory. In addition, perforations of any size and middle ear effusion may interfere with the proper vibration of the ear drum and cause hearing loss. Interruption of the continuity or mobility of the ossicular chain can also cause CHL; ossicles may be eroded or missing.

Symptoms

Patients will report hearing loss, difficulty understanding speech in noisy environments, and occasionally tinnitus. Disorders of the EAC and TM (e.g., cholesteatoma, chronic otitis media) may also cause otorrhea and recurrent infections. Inciting events may be elicited, such as head trauma, recent upper respiratory tract infection, or flight. Causes of potential auditory (eustachian) tube dysfunction should be elicited, such as chronic sinusitis, allergic rhinitis, or cleft palate.

Differential Diagnosis

The differential diagnosis of CHL is broad and can involve disorders of the EAC, TM, middle ear, and ossicles. Disorders of the EAC include congenital atresia, cerumen, foreign body, exostosis, osteoma, and neoplasm. Disorders of the TM include scarring, tympanosclerosis, retraction, and perforation. Disorders of the middle ear can include adhesions and effusions and may stem from underlying auditory tube dysfunction. Disorders that can cause ossicular discontinuity or ossicular erosion are trauma, cholesteatoma, chronic otitis media, and neoplasm. Otosclerosis and malleus fixation can also impair the vibratory potential of the ossicular chain. Third window disorders such as semicircular canal dehiscence can also cause CHL.

◆ Evaluation

Physical Exam

A full head and neck examination should be performed to elicit signs of underlying sinonasal disease, auditory tube dysfunction, or neoplasm. In an adult with persistent unilateral middle ear effusion, nasopharyngoscopy is performed to rule out nasopharyngeal mass causing auditory tube dysfunction. Binocular microscopic evaluation of the EAC and TM is extremely helpful in identifying pathology of CHL, which may otherwise be missed with a handheld otoscopy. Complete removal of cerumen aids in visualization. Pneumatic otoscopy can assist in determining TM mobility and should always be documented. The integrity of the manubrium of the malleus, long process of the incus, and stapes can also be seen on exam. In general, the Weber test with a 512-Hz tuning fork generally lateralizes to the ear with CHL. Depending on the degree of CHL, the Rinne test will demonstrate bone conduction greater than air conduction ("negative Rinne").

Imaging

High-resolution computed tomography (CT) of the temporal bones is not necessary in all cases of CHL. CT scan is obtained when there is a chronically draining ear (e.g., chronic otitis media), evidence of cholesteatoma, or mass lesion of the EAC or middle ear or when the cause of CHL is unclear. CT can also be done for surgical planning (e.g., atresia repair). Otosclerotic foci can be demonstrated on CT, although imaging is not necessary in all cases.

Other Tests

Comprehensive audiometry with both air conduction and bone conduction testing should be performed to determine air–bone gap (ABG), which represents the amount of hearing loss attributed to the conductive mechanism. Tympanometry can be performed to determine the mobility of the drum, detecting perforations and middle ear effusions. Acoustic reflexes should be absent. If acoustic reflexes are present in a patient with a conductive hearing loss, superior semicircular canal dehiscence should be suspected. In this case, cervical vestibular evoked myogenic potential (cVEMP) testing can be helpful, as superior semicircular canal dehiscence syndrome patients typically demonstrate larger amplitudes and lower thresholds on cVEMP testing at 500 Hz.

◆ Treatment Options

Medical

Amplification and observation should be offered to patients as a treatment option. Amplification can include hearing aids and soft band (bone conducting hearing aid). Certain conditions may require surgical intervention prior to amplification (e.g., neoplasm, chronic otitis media, cholesteatoma).

Surgical

Surgical intervention can potentially improve hearing when there is a significant ABG. The surgery depends on the etiology of the CHL. Osseointegrated implants (see **Chapter 3.5.5**) are an alternative treatment for CHL that should be considered when surgery for the underlying disorder may carry high risk to sensorineural component of hearing or facial nerve (e.g., atresia).

Outer Ear

- Cerumen removal
- Foreign body removal
- Canalplasty with or without skin graft (for exostosis or stenosis)
- Meatoplasty
- Atresia repair

Tympanic Membrane

- Myringotomy with or without tympanostomy tube for middle ear effusion
- Paper patch or fat myringoplasty for small perforation (often office procedures)
- Tympanoplasty

Middle Ear

- Ossicular chain reconstruction using remodeled incus or synthetic prosthesis
- Stapedectomy/stapedotomy
- Exploratory tympanotomy with or without mastoidectomy
  - Lysis of middle ear adhesions
  - Removal of tympanosclerosis
  - Repair of malleus fixation
  - Removal of cholesteatoma
  - Treat chronic otitis media
  - Removal of neoplasm

◆ Typical Clinical Pictures

Otosclerosis

Otosclerosis is a process in which the stapes loses mobility by excessive bony growth at the oval window. It typically causes a CHL with a distinctive dip in sensorineural levels at 2 kHz, known as Carhart notch. Patients may have tinnitus and progressive hearing loss in one or both ears. Otosclerosis has a bimodal age epidemiology; it usually presents in the early twenties or later in the fifties. Early otosclerosis can be managed with fluoride supplementation, but often the CHL will progress and patients will need to consider amplification or stapes surgery. Stapedectomy or stapedotomy involves removing the superstructure of the stapes, and entering into the inner ear, either by making a fenestration in the footplate (stapedotomy), or partially removing it (stapedectomy). A synthetic prosthesis is then placed into the oval window and attached to the incus to reestablish ossicular transmission of sound waves.

Ossicular Disease

Cholesteatoma, chronic ear infections, and trauma can all cause erosion or disruption of the ossicular chain. After appropriately treating the aforementioned causes, one may evaluate the remaining middle ear structures to determine the appropriate surgical repair. Once the current ossicular status (anatomic and functional integrity of each ossicle) is determined, the appropriate prosthesis can be selected. Prostheses exist for nearly every situation of ossicular disease. Common prostheses include a partial ossicular reconstruction prosthesis (replaces incus and malleus), incus struts (replace incus only), and a total ossicular reconstruction prosthesis (replaces all ossicles).

◆ Complications

Obstructive EAC stenosis after canalplasty may require revision canalplasty. Tympanoplasty has a failure rate of ~15%, and revision tympanoplasty may be necessary; factors that may affect success rate is the size of the TM perforation (e.g., subtotal or total), location (e.g., anterior, marginal), and etiology (e.g., chronic otitis media). Revision surgery may be necessary after ossicular chain reconstruction if the prosthesis shifts and no longer conducts sound effectively. Six months is generally considered the earliest time point at which revision surgery should be considered. Progressive hearing loss 10 to 14 days after stapes surgery may indicate reparative granuloma, and middle ear exploration should be considered.

◆ Outcome and Follow-Up

Water precautions should be observed in the postoperative period. If the TM is grafted or a stapedotomy is performed, caution regarding airline flight should be considered in the immediate postoperative period to avoid TM movement. A postoperative audiogram to determine level of hearing restoration should be performed 6 to 8 weeks after procedure (adequate time for gelatin packing in the middle ear to absorb).

3.5.2 Sensorineural Hearing Loss

◆ Key Features

> - Sensorineural hearing loss (SNHL) is caused by the dysfunction of the sensory (cochlea) or neural components of the auditory system.
> - Asymmetric SNHL may need to be evaluated by MRI or ABR to rule out retrocochlear pathology.
> - Treatment may include amplification, osseointegrated implants, and cochlear implantation

Sensorineural hearing loss (SNHL) can stem from disorders of the cochlea, cochlear nerve, and central auditory processing. It can affect one or both ears. Asymmetrical SNHL is often described as a 10-dB difference in three consecutive pure tone frequencies, a 15-dB difference in two consecutive frequencies, and/or a ≥ 12% point difference in speech recognition.

◆ Clinical

Signs and Symptoms

Patients typically notice difficulty in crowds or with background noise. They may report having to increase the volume of the television or radio to understand. Patients with high-frequency hearing loss may notice difficulty with understanding women or children's voices. Many patients will not realize they have hearing loss until it has progressed significantly, as the hearing loss is usually very gradual. Often, tinnitus is associated with hearing loss and may be the presenting symptom. Other otologic symptoms, such as otorrhea, aural fullness, and vertigo, may also help identify the etiology of the hearing loss. Inciting events or risk factors for hearing may be present, such as head trauma, acoustic trauma, chronic loud noise exposure, family history of hearing loss, ototoxic drug use, prematurity, prenatal/postnatal infection, barotrauma, and autoimmune disease. A full review of systems concentrating on neurologic or rheumatologic symptoms may also imply the cause.

Differential Diagnosis for Symmetric SNHL

Presbycusis

Slowly progressive bilateral SNHL in the older population (presbycusis) is widely prevalent and is the most common form of SNHL. It is often a familial condition. However, a detailed otologic history may find other factors that may contribute to SNHL.

Noise-Induced Hearing Loss

Exposure to loud noise can lead to permanent hearing threshold shifts. This may happen immediately with extreme exposure (nearby explosion or gunfire) but more commonly occurs slowly over time with repeated exposure to industrial or environmental noise. Patients will often have a typical 4-kHz

Table 3.9   Common ototoxic drugs

Aminoglycoside antibiotics (e.g., streptomycin, gentamicin, neomycin)
Platinum-based chemotherapy (especially cisplatin)
Loop diuretics
Vinca alkaloids (especially vincristine)
Quinine
Salicylates

notch in their audiograms. Patients should be counseled to prevent further noise damage by wearing appropriate hearing protection and minimizing exposure.

Ototoxicity

Exposure to a variety of medications may induce permanent hearing loss (**Table 3.9**). This hearing loss is typically first noted in the highest frequencies and then progresses to lower pitches. Common agents include aminoglycoside antibiotics, vinca alkaloids, and platinum-based chemotherapeutic agents. Careful monitoring of audiograms during therapy allow for early identification of hearing loss. Prolonged use of high-dose loop diuretics (e.g., furosemide) may also lead to hearing loss. Of note, many ototoxic drugs are also nephrotoxic; therefore, renal function studies should be obtained as well.

Hearing Loss Present at Birth

See **Fig. 3.11** for a classification overview of hearing loss at birth. About 50% of cases are nonhereditary, from prematurity, sepsis, or TORCH infections (toxoplasmosis, rubella, cytomegalovirus, herpes simplex encephalitis, and otosyphilis). Of the 50% that are congenital hereditary cases, these may be syndromic (one-third of cases) or nonsyndromic (two-thirds of cases); see **Table 3.10**. Of the nonsyndromic cases, ~80% are autosomal recessive.

Hearing loss may be present at birth due to congenital defects in either the structure or the physiology of the inner ear. Cochlear malformations

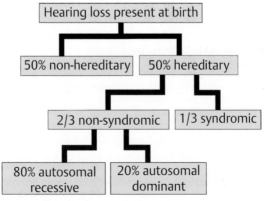

Fig. 3.11   Hearing loss present at birth: a classification overview.

Table 3.10 Hereditary syndromic hearing loss

Autosomal dominant	Autosomal recessive	Sex-linked
Treacher Collins	Usher	Alport
Goldenhar	Pendred	
Waardenberg	Jervell-Lange-Nielsen	
Branchio-oto-renal		
Stickler		

(e.g., Mondini malformation, common cavity, cochlear hypoplasia, cochlear aplasia) may be associated with various syndromes. Many cases of nonsyndromic congenital hearing loss have been attributed to chromosomal defects in the hair cell protein connexin 26 (Cx 26). Most congenital cases are now discovered early due to universal newborn screening programs. However, certain types, such as enlarged vestibular aqueduct syndrome, may not manifest until later in life. Auditory neuropathy can also cause unilateral or bilateral SNHL.

Metabolic

Symmetric bilateral rapidly progressive hearing loss may be caused by a variety of systemic diseases, including autoimmune disease, thyroid disease, or vitamin B_{12} or folate deficiencies.

Other

Cochlear otosclerosis, primary autoimmune inner ear disease, barotrauma, perilymph fistula, migraine, vertebrobasilar occlusion, Ménière's disease, labyrinthitis ossificans from meningitis, and a variety of autoimmune disorders may all be associated with SNHL.

Differential Diagnosis for Asymmetric Hearing Loss

Tumors

Neoplasms of the cerebellopontine angle and/or internal auditory canal, such as vestibular schwannomas and meningiomas, may cause unilateral SNHL. Endolymphatic sac tumors, especially in patients with a history suggestive of Von Hippel–Lindau's syndrome, can also cause unilateral SNHL. Disorders of the otic capsule bone (e.g. fibrous dysplasia, Paget's disease, osteogenesis imperfecta) may also cause a sensory component to an asymmetric hearing loss that more commonly is associated with conductive hearing loss. Metastasis to the temporal bone should be considered in patients with a history of malignancy such as breast, prostate, thyroid, lung, and renal cancer.

Ménière's Disease

Active Ménière's disease typically causes a fluctuating low-frequency hearing loss. As the disease progresses, higher frequencies are affected and can progress to severe levels. Bilateral Ménière can also occur, but onset of symptoms in the second ear is generally years after the first.

Infectious

Meningitis may lead to the spread of bacteria to the inner ear through the cochlear aqueduct, which can lead to cochlear fibrosis and ossification. Congenital TORCH infections can cause early-onset SNHL. Viral labyrinthitis can also cause SNHL. Infectious causes may lead to symmetric or asymmetric losses.

Traumatic

Fractures of the temporal bone involving the otic capsule usually lead to profound hearing loss. Leakage of perilymph from the oval or round windows can cause progressive hearing loss and dizziness. Strong Valsalva during heavy lifting, head trauma, or barotrauma may initiate these perilymphatic fistulas.

Neurologic Disease

Multiple sclerosis is well known for causing a myriad of neurologic symptoms, including hearing loss. Cerebrovascular disease leading to brainstem stroke or impaired blood supply to the cochlea can also cause hearing loss.

◆ Evaluation

Physical Exam

A thorough head and neck examination should be performed. The ear should be examined for any potential cause of CHL, such as cerumen, tympanic perforation, middle ear effusion, and ossicular chain disorder. Tuning fork tests may be done to document laterality and nature of hearing loss. In general, the Weber test using a 512-Hz tuning fork will lateralize toward the better hearing ear (in the absence of conductive hearing loss). Rinne test is positive (air conduction > bone conduction).

Imaging

Temporal bone computed tomography (CT) is helpful in identifying inner ear abnormalities associated with hearing loss in children (e.g., enlarged vestibular aqueduct, inner ear malformation). Both magnetic resonance imaging (MRI) and CT can identify labyrinthitis ossificans. CT is helpful in identifying temporal fracture as an etiology for disorders of the otic capsule bone. To assess for retrocochlear pathology in asymmetric hearing loss, MRI scanning of the brain with fine cuts through the internal auditory canals can be performed with and without contrast media. Heavily weighted T2 fast spin echo series has also been used to screen for retrocochlear pathology.

Labs

There is controversy regarding laboratory testing. For pediatric hearing loss, consider urinalysis (for Alport and branchio-oto-renal syndrome), electrocardiogram (ECG, for Jervell-Lange-Nielsen's syndrome), and referral for ophthalmology exam (to rule out retinitis pigmentosa). Additional testing can include rapid plasma reagin (RPR) or fluorescent treponemal antibody absorption (FTA-ABS), toxoplasmosis, cytomegalovirus-related tests, thyroid function testing, erythrocyte sedimentation rate (ESR), antinuclear antibody testing, rheumatoid factor, liver function tests, and complete blood count (CBC).

In adults with bilateral progressive or fluctuating hearing loss, consider antinuclear antibody, rheumatoid factor, anti–neutrophil cytoplasmic antibody (ANCA), ESR, and syphilis testing (RPR or FTA-ABS). Lyme serology can be ordered if suspected as well. The utility of a 68-kD antibody testing for diagnosing autoimmune inner ear disease is controversial.

Other Tests

Pure tone audiometry is the standard for documentation of hearing loss. Speech reception thresholds and word discrimination testing should also be performed. Patients may also be screened with otoacoustic emission testing and auditory brainstem response (ABR) testing when audiometry cannot be performed. ABR can also be used as an alternative to MRI for evaluating asymmetric hearing loss. Referral for genetic testing can be considered. Hearing loss can be classified by its severity:

- Mild (15–40 dB)
- Moderate (41–55 dB)
- Moderate to severe (56–70 dB)
- Severe (70–90 dB)
- Profound (> 90 dB)

◆ Treatment Options

Medical

Bilateral symmetric SNHL with >50% speech discrimination should be offered hearing aid amplification. Depending on the pattern of hearing loss, middle ear implants or implantable hearing aids are alternative therapies. When patients have profound SNHL or word discrimination is very poor, hearing aid trial and cochlear implant evaluation should be considered.

Patients with asymmetric SNHL can benefit from standard hearing aids. Contralateral routing of sound (CROS), Bi-CROS (if the good ear requires amplification), and osseointegrated implants are treatment options for single-sided deafness.

Medical treatment of the underlying etiology (when known) may be important in controlling disease progression. Treatment of sudden hearing loss can include oral and/or intratympanic steroid administrations. Treatment of associated tinnitus is discussed in **Chapter 3.7**.

Surgical

Patients with profound bilateral loss that is not helped by hearing aids may be candidates for cochlear implantation (see **Chapter 3.5.4**). Patients with profound unilateral loss can be candidates for osseointegrated bone-anchored hearing devices (see **Chapter 3.5.5**).

◆ Outcome and Follow-Up

Frequent adjustments and cleaning of hearing aids will ensure better patient compliance and satisfaction. Yearly audiograms should be performed on patients with identified SNHL to monitor for progression.

3.5.3 Hearing Aids

◆ Key Features

> - Amplification of sound can improve hearing in many hearing-impaired patients.
> - Most hearing aids today are digital and programmable. They can be adjusted to accommodate different levels of hearing loss and improve situational hearing.
> - There are several types of hearing aids that vary in size, discreetness, programmability, and strength.

Hearing aids amplify sound to improve auditory perception in many hearing-impaired patients; however, they cannot restore normal hearing. Hearing aid technology has changed dramatically in the past two decades to allow advanced programming and wireless applications to improve hearing in different environments.

◆ Epidemiology

Hearing aids are worn by approximately five million people in the United States, representing only one in five people with hearing loss who could benefit from sound amplification.

◆ Clinical

Hearing-impaired patients may complain of difficulty understanding in quiet and noisy environments, asking people to repeat themselves frequently, and turning up the volume on the TV or radio to be able to hear. Untreated hearing loss can lead to anxiety, stress, depression, social isolation, and dementia. In children, hearing loss can present with speech, language, and learning delays. A thorough history identifying risk factors for hearing loss, progression and onset of hearing impairment, and associated otologic symptoms can aid in identifying individuals who can benefit from hearing aids.

◆ Evaluation

Physical Exam

A head and neck examination, concentrating on the otologic exam, can help identify disorders of the external auditory canal, tympanic membrane, middle ear, and auditory (eustachian) tube that can contribute to hearing impairment. Tuning fork tests can be performed to assess for conductive or sensorineural hearing loss. The size and patency of the external auditory canal is particularly important in choosing an appropriate hearing aid.

Testing

Audiometry and tympanometry are performed to determine the type of hearing loss (conductive, sensorineural, or mixed), the degree of hearing impairment (mild, moderate, severe, or profound), and the configuration of hearing loss (low-, middle-, and/or high-frequency). Evidence of congenital, pediatric, conductive, asymmetric, sudden, rapidly progressing, or fluctuating hearing loss will require evaluation and treatment by an otolaryngologist prior to obtaining medical clearance for hearing aids. Additional audiologic, laboratory, and imaging tests may be required to ascertain the cause and type of the hearing loss before hearing aids can be considered or recommended.

◆ Treatment Options

Medical Clearance

Active inner ear disease and disorders of the external auditory canal, tympanic membrane, middle ear, and auditory tube may need to be treated prior to consideration for hearing aids. Once the patient is medically optimized, a referral to audiology for hearing aid evaluation can be ordered. Cerumen removal is beneficial prior to hearing aid evaluation and fitting.

Hearing Aid Devices

Hearing aids can amplify sound to improve hearing perception in patients with conductive, sensorineural, and mixed hearing loss; however, the benefit from hearing aids is reduced when word discrimination declines. In particular, individuals with poor word discrimination (< 40% on speech discrimination tests) do not perform as well with hearing aids. Hearing aid amplification will not restore clarity in these patients but may provide sound awareness and assist in lip reading.

Most hearing aids today are digital and programmable. They can be adjusted to accommodate different levels of hearing loss and improve situational hearing. There are several types of hearing aids that vary in size, discreetness, programmability, and strength. The main types of hearing aids include the behind-the-ear (BTE), receiver-in-canal (RIC), in-the-ear (ITE), in-the-canal (ITC), and completely-in-the canal (CIC) hearing aids. Miniature-size options for BTE and RIC hearing aids are also available.

In general, individuals with severe to profound hearing loss require larger hearing aids, such as the BTE and ITE devices, to provide adequate amplification. Furthermore, patients with narrow external auditory canals may have difficulty wearing hearing aids that are inserted deep in the ear canal. Noise reduction algorithms can be employed in hearing aids with dual microphones to filter and minimize amplification of background noise. Dual microphones are standard in BTE and RIC hearing aids; however, they are not available in CIC hearing aids and are optional in ITE and ITC hearing aids. Most hearing aids have a wireless feature that allows the hearing aids to pick up a signal from a compatible telephone or closed system, connect to an external microphone through FM or Bluetooth technology, and project sound received by one hearing aid to both ears automatically. In addition, hearing aids can be programmed to improve hearing in different noisy environments, enhance hearing in different directions, reduce feedback, and mask tinnitus.

Contralateral routing of signal (CROS) hearing aids are specialized hearing devices that can be prescribed when one ear has unserviceable hearing loss, as in single-sided deafness. A transmitter is worn on the poor ear and a receiver is worn on the normally hearing ear. Sound presented to the poor ear is detected by the transmitter and routed to the receiver that delivers the sound to the normally hearing ear. BiCROS hearing aids have an additional feature that allows the receiver to amplify the sound that it delivers to the better ear as well; this device is recommended when the better ear has hearing loss.

Patients with significant conductive hearing loss may also benefit from bone-conducting hearing aids fitted using a soft band. They are particularly suitable for infants, toddlers, and children with severe external auditory canal stenosis or atresia or chronic otitis externa, otitis media, or otorrhea that precludes use of a traditional hearing aid that amplifies sound through air.

Surgical Options

Individuals with severely reduced word discrimination and/or hearing thresholds that are unaidable with a hearing aid may benefit from cochlear implantation. Patients with a significant conductive component in their hearing loss or who have single-sided deafness may benefit from an implantable bone-anchored hearing device.

◆ Complications

Hearing aids can cause cerumen impaction, pressure ulcers, and infections of the external auditory canal. Regular cerumen removal may be necessary to treat or prevent cerumen buildup. Ear molds and inserts may need to be adjusted to prevent pain, erythema, and ulceration of the skin of the external auditory canal and conchal bowl. Patients with infective otitis externa or otorrhea should refrain from using hearing aids until the infection is properly treated.

◆ Outcome and Follow-Up

Hearing aids require routine maintenance to continue functioning optimally. They must be cleaned regularly and kept dry. Batteries will usually need to be changed every few days, depending on the severity of hearing loss, the size of the battery, and the type of hearing aid. Hearing aids need to be worn routinely for the wearer to receive the most benefit. Patients with bilateral hearing loss perform best when aided binaurally. There is generally an adjustment period for the ear to accommodate to the hearing aid and the brain to adapt to the new sound input. Hearing aids will need to be reprogrammed routinely, especially when hearing loss continues to progress over time.

3.5.4 Cochlear Implants

◆ Key Features

- Cochlear implantation can restore the perception of sound to patients with profound hearing loss.
- Cochlear implants are approved for patients as young as 12 months.
- Careful preoperative evaluation is vital for appropriate patient selection.

Cochlear implants (CI) have an internal and an external component. The internal component consists of the receiver-stimulator attached to the cochlear electrode array. The external component is the speech processor and transmitter. CIs can deliver electrical stimulation to the cochlear nerve to enable sound perception. These impulses are transmitted transcutaneously from the speech processor to the receiver-stimulator via magnet. Electrical signals are sent to the cochlea through the electrode array. Depolarization of cochlear nerve fibers in the cochlea initiates the perception of sound. CIs should be approached as a team effort among surgeons, audiologists, and speech pathologists to ensure comprehensive care and maximize benefit to the patient.

◆ Clinical

CI candidacy in adults requires moderate to profound bilateral sensorineural hearing loss (SNHL) with ≤ 50% open set sentence recognition (e.g., hearing in noise test, HINT) in the ear to be implanted and ≤ 60% in the best aided condition. However, Medicare and Medicaid have stringent criteria (≤ 40% open set sentence recognition).

CI candidacy in pediatric patients requires bilateral profound SNHL with minimal or no benefit from binaural hearing aids during a 3- to 6-month trial. In certain situations (e.g., known history of genetic hearing loss in patient and family), cochlear implantation performed at less than 12 months of age can be advocated. Testing in children can include auditory brainstem response (ABR) testing and age-appropriate audiometry. A contraindication to CI is cochlear aplasia.

Several factors may contribute to CI outcomes, including prelingual versus postlingual deafness, age at implant, etiology and duration of deafness, cognitive ability, family support, proper motivation, realistic expectations, and rehabilitation/educational support for speech and language. Special considerations are given to children with auditory neuropathy spectrum disorder ("auditory dyssynchrony"), who can benefit from CI in the absence of central nervous system pathology.

◆ Evaluation

History

Etiology of the hearing loss may be elicited in the history. The potential causes of pediatric and adult sensorineural hearing loss are discussed in (**Chapter 3.5.2**). For identifying good CI candidates, it is important to elicit the timing and onset of hearing loss, whether it was prelingual or postlingual deafness, the duration of deafness, and the etiology of the hearing loss. Although there are many factors associated with CI outcome, postlingual deafness is associated with better postimplantation hearing outcomes than prelingual deafness. In children with prelingual deafness, implantation should occur as soon as possible, and certainly before 4 to 6 years of age, when the brain begins to lose its plasticity. In postlingual children or adults, a longer duration of deafness may be associated with poorer outcomes. A history of meningitis may indicate labyrinthitis ossificans.

Physical Exam

A full head and neck examination with cranial nerve and otologic exam is performed. Using an otomicroscope, the external auditory canal, tympanic membrane, and middle ear contents should be examined. Active middle ear disease should be treated concurrently, but treatment may precede cochlear implantation.

Imaging

Imaging should be obtained prior to cochlear implantation: either high-resolution computed tomography (CT) scan of the temporal bone or magnetic resonance imaging (MRI). There are advantages and disadvantages to both tests. A CT scan can assess inner ear morphology, cochlear patency, the position of the facial nerve, the size of the facial recess, the height of the jugular bulb, internal auditory canal volume, and the thickness of parietal bone (especially in young children); however, it does not provide information on the presence or absence of the cochlear nerve. MRI is superior because it can also be used to assess the contents of the temporal bone similarly to the CT, but the presence of a cochlear nerve can be visualized on sagittal scans. In addition, MRI can better rule out intracranial disorders that may coexist; however, it is more costly and time-consuming.

Congenital cochlear malformations should be carefully identified on imaging. Mondini malformation may not allow a full insertion of electrodes, but this is not an absolute contraindication for implantation. Prior history of meningitis can indicate possible cochlear fibrosis and ossification, making electrode insertion difficult to impossible.

Other Tests

A comprehensive audiogram is the initial study for evaluating the hearing loss. CI evaluation includes open set sentence recognition in the unaided and best aided condition. Complete CI evaluation should be performed by a qualified audiologist. In children who do not tolerate age-appropriate audiometry, ABR is performed. Otoacoustic emissions are helpful in diagnosing auditory dyssynchrony.

✦ Treatment Options

Hearing aid trial is recommended in children and adults who are being considered for cochlear implantation. Patients who meet CI criteria and who have appropriate expectations, good family/social support, and an implant-able cochlea are identified. Medical clearance for general anesthesia should be obtained. Alternative therapies to CI can include hearing aids, lip reading, and American Sign Language. Children who are marginal or not candidates for CI should be enrolled in a total communications program. Evaluation and treatment of hearing loss in children require a multidisciplinary approach that includes an otolaryngologist, diagnostic pediatric audiologist, hearing aid specialist, cochlear implant audiologist, speech pathologist, and psychol-ogist. Pneumococcal 13-valent conjugate, pneumococcal polysaccharide 23, and annual influenza vaccines are recommended.

Typically, implantation is performed via a transmastoid approach. A simple mastoidectomy is performed and the vertical facial nerve is identified. The facial recess is then opened, allowing good visualization of the round window niche. A cochleostomy is performed near the round window, and the electrode array is then inserted via this opening. The receiver-stimulator is typically secured to a shallow bony seat developed posterior to the mastoid, and the wound is closed. After a few weeks of healing, the external magnet can be placed, activated, and adjusted. Approximately 40 hours of therapy is to be expected.

✦ Complications

The incision and flap complication rate is ~ 2 to 3%. The risk of postoperative facial paralysis is 0.4%. Electrodes are delicate and can be damaged intra-operatively; the incidence of damaged or misplaced electrodes is 1.2%. In case of implant extrusion, local flaps to cover the implant can be employed. Explantation with replacement may be necessary if cochlear electrodes migrate out of the cochleostomy or there is a device failure. Tinnitus and dizziness typically subside slowly after implantation. Scalp flaps may have to be thinned to ensure good magnet contact in obese patients.

If postoperative acute otitis media occurs, aggressive treatment with intravenous antibiotics and myringotomy with tube placement should be considered, especially in children who have cochlear malformations or complicated acute otitis media (e.g., meningitis) or who don't respond to oral medications. Recurrent postauricular swelling may be due to aggressive autoinsufflation, and the patient should be counseled. CI infection may be associated with biofilm colonization; when systemic antibiotics fail, CI explantation with delayed reimplantation should be considered. The Advanced Bionics Clarion with Positioner has been associated with higher rates of meningitis and has been removed from the market.

✦ Outcome and Follow-Up

An anteroposterior skull X-ray can be obtained postoperatively to ensure appropriate placement of electrodes within the cochlea, although this is not typically necessary. Mastoid dressing should remain in place for 24 hours. Inspection of the wound should be performed to rule out hematoma formation. Facial nerve function should be documented. Once implanted, patients may not have monopolar electrocautery used during any subsequent surgeries. Caution should be used when considering MRI scans, as the receivers that are not MRI-compatible may need to have their internal magnets removed.

Mapping of the electrodes and programming can begin as early as 2 weeks postoperatively, but more commonly, patients begin programming 4 to 5 weeks postoperatively to ensure adequate wound healing. The external processor can be updated when the technology becomes available. Younger patients may develop excellent speech discrimination; however, prelingual deafened adults may only gain sound awareness and limited speech ability. Currently, data are accruing regarding the results of bilateral implantation, both simultaneous and sequential. Outcomes are very promising.

3.5.5 Other Implantable Hearing Devices

◆ Key Features

- Auditory brainstem implant (ABI)
- Osseointegrated bone conducting implant
- Middle ear implant (MEI)

Alternative implantable hearing devices are auditory brainstem implants (ABI), osseointegrated bone conducting implants (e.g., Baha, Cochlear Bone Anchored Solutions AB, Mölnlycke, Sweden), and middle ear implants (MEI).

◆ Epidemiology

Several hundred people worldwide have ABIs. More than 30,000 people worldwide use the Baha system. A few MEI devices have received Food and Drug Administration (FDA) approval in the United States; however, their use has not become widespread.

◆ Clinical

ABIs are for persons who cannot benefit from a CI because there has been damage to both auditory nerves (e.g., neurofibromatosis type II [NF2]). Osseointegrated implants are used in cases of conductive or mixed hearing loss where fitting of traditional hearing aids is not feasible (i.e., atresia, chronic drainage) and in single-sided deafness. MEIs are indicated for adults greater than 18 years of age with stable bilateral moderate to severe sensorineural hearing loss with > 50% speech discrimination. MEIs may not be suitable for patients with chronic middle ear disease.

◆ Treatment Options

Auditory Brainstem Implants

An ABI is an implantable device that is placed in the lateral recess of the fourth ventricle. Electrodes deliver electrical stimulus to the ventral cochlear nucleus to activate the central auditory pathway. Candidacy criteria includes bilateral vestibular schwannomas in neurofibromatosis 2 patients greater than 12 years of age who are undergoing vestibular schwannoma excision. ABI in children with bilateral cochlear malformations or cochlear nerve deficiency has also been done in the research setting. Vestibular schwannoma resection and ABI placement can be performed through a translabyrinthine or retrosigmoid approach. Postoperative complications can include meningitis, device failure, and cerebrospinal fluid (CSF) leak. Activation generally occurs 4 to 6 weeks after implantation. Postoperative hearing outcomes depend on a variety of factors that include surgical experience, patient motivation, and duration of use.

Osseointegrated Bone Conduction Implants

Osseointegrated bone conduction implants are implantable devices that can protrude through the skin ("percutaneous") or may be hidden under the skin ("transcutaneous"). In general, they are indicated in moderate to severe conductive hearing loss as well as single-sided deafness. The benefits of bone conduction implants for conductive hearing loss are well documented; in single-sided deafness, however, unilateral bone conduction implants improve speech in noise hearing outcomes.

- In the percutaneous osseointegrated implants, a titanium screw is placed into the mastoid bone and allowed to osseointegrate; a titanium abutment can be attached to the osseointegrated implant simultaneously or in a delayed fashion (e.g., in young children with thin bone). The abutment protrudes through an incision made in the overlying skin. After several weeks of healing (some advocate more than 6 weeks), the sound processor is attached to the abutment and enables sound transmission. In children, at least two sleeper implants are placed and allowed to osseointegrate for ~6 months; a second surgery is necessary to place the percutaneous abutment. Percutaneous devices include Baha, including the Cordelle II Sound Processor, and Ponto (Oticon Medical, Askim, Sweden).
- A transcutaneous bone conduction implant is also placed into the mastoid bone but does not come through the skin; sound transmission occurs through an implantable magnet. In transcutaneous implants, the overlying skin may need to be thinned; these implants may have attenuation of the high frequencies due to soft tissue dampening. Programming generally occurs ~6 weeks after surgery to allow enough time for osseointegration to occur. Transcutaneous implants are the Baha Attract, Sophono (Medtronic, Minneapolis, MN), and Bonebridge (MED-EL Corp., Barnsley, UK) and in general are magnetic resonance imaging (MRI) conditional.
- The cortical bone should be more than 3 mm thick on computed tomography (CT). Complications include flap necrosis, hypertrophic skin, infection, failure to osseointegrate, and disintegration. Single-incision placement has significantly reduced the soft tissue complication rate compared to the flap technique.

Middle Ear Implants

MEIs are implantable devices that are attach directly to the ossicular chain. They can be totally implantable or may have a component of the device that is implantable. These devices have not gained much popularity and are not in wide use in the United States. FDA-approved devices are the Esteem (Envoy Medical Corp., White Bear Lake, MN), Maxum (Ototronix, St. Paul, MN), and Vibrant Soundbridge (MED-EL Corp., Barnsley, UK). Devices differ in type of transducer and ossicular coupler. The Esteem and the Vibrant Soundbridge require a formal mastoidectomy, while the Maxum can be inserted transcanal. Complications can include ossicular erosion, device extrusion, taste disturbance, and facial palsy; rates vary with each device. Totally implantable devices require revision surgery to replace the battery every 4 to 6 years. These devices are not compatible with MRI.

3.6 Vertigo

3.6.1 Balance Assessment

◆ Key Features

- Electronystagmography (ENG)
- Rotational chair
- Dynamic post urography
- Vestibular evoked myogenic potential (VEMP)

Balance involves three components: (1) sensory input from the visual, vestibular, and proprioceptive systems; (2) central nervous system integration of these sensory signals with the subsequent generation of appropriate motor commands; and (3) adequate musculoskeletal abilities to perform the motor tasks. Proper assessment of balance/vertigo issues involves looking at all three of these components.

◆ Epidemiology

Dizziness is a common symptom in ~30% of people over the age of 65. Approximately 615,000 persons in the United States have been diagnosed with Ménière's disease. Between 10 and 64 persons per 100,000 are affected by benign paroxysmal positional vertigo (BPPV) each year. Hundreds of thousands of hospital days are incurred every year in the United States due to vertiginous symptoms.

◆ Clinical

Persons with vestibular disorders report a variety of symptoms. They can include, but are not limited to, vertigo (i.e., spinning sensation), dysequilibrium (i.e., subjective sense of falling), imbalance (i.e., observable unsteadiness), lightheadedness (i.e., feeling of faintness), oscillopsia (i.e., vision instability with head movement), nausea, and vomiting. Dizziness can also be accompanied by hearing loss, tinnitus, and hyperacusis (sound sensitivity). Dizziness can be brief (lasting seconds to minutes) or prolonged (lasting hours to days). Patients may report episodic or positional dizziness. Precipitating factors such as recent upper respiratory tract infection, head trauma, vestibulotoxic drug exposure, and migraine can be ascertained.

◆ Evaluation

Physical Exam

A full head and neck with otologic and cranial nerve exam is performed. Neurologic exam can also give insight into central causes of dizziness. Use of Frenzel goggles can help accentuate nystagmus on exam by removing visual fixation. Physical exam should include evaluation of spontaneous, gaze, and headshake nystagmus. Gait is assessed for ataxia and wide stance. Romberg and Fukuda stepping tests are done to evaluate for sway. A Dix-Hallpike test will assess presence of posterior canalolithiasis. Cerebellar testing (such as finger-to-nose) can test for dysmetria and tremor. A head impulse test can demonstrate catch-up saccades. Proprioception of upper and lower extremities can be assessed with a tuning fork. Mobility of the neck (e.g., cervicogenic dizziness) and vertebral artery (e.g., vertebral artery stenosis) should be tested as well.

Basic Balance Testing

ENG/VNG

Electronystagmography (ENG) and videonystagmography (VNG) test peripheral and central vestibular function. During ENG, electrodes are placed above and below the eyes, at the outside corner of the eye, and on the forehead. Electrical potentials during testing reflect direction and velocity of eye movements. VNG does not rely on electrical potentials but rather on video analysis of eye motion. VNG measures the movements of the eyes directly through infrared cameras and may be more accurate, more consistent, and more comfortable for the patient than traditional ENG. One advantage to VNG is the ability to test torsional nystagmus in addition to vertical and horizontal nystagmus. There are four main components to ENG/VNG:

1. Oculomotor activity: Smooth pursuit tracking, saccade analysis, gaze fixation, spontaneous nystagmus, and optokinetic stimulation
2. Positioning tests: Such as Dix-Hallpike
3. Positional tests: Nystagmus on head supine, head left and right, body left and right, and 30° incline

4. Caloric irrigation: Warm and cold air or water

Rotary Chair

Rotational chair testing expands the evaluation of the peripheral vestibular system beyond the frequency and intensity limitations of the ENG/VNG evaluation. The phase, gain, and symmetry of the vestibular ocular reflex are assessed. The patient is then subjected to various rotations through sinusoidal harmonic acceleration tests and step tests with the head restrained to a chair with a computer-controlled motor in a darkened enclosure. Off-axis rotation provides ear-specific information and tests the utricle and superior vestibular nerve function. Standard rotational chair tests the horizontal semicircular canal function and stimulates the otoliths. Utricular function can specifically be assessed through subjective visual vertical or horizontal testing. The patient attempts to set an illuminated light to true vertical or horizontal in the absence of a visual reference and ambient light.

Posturography

Dynamic posturography assesses the functional relative use of vision, vestibular, and somatosensory cues. Sensory organization is assessed by measuring a patient's ability to maintain balance while disrupting somatosensory and/or visual input. The patient is exposed to six conditions using a combination of normal, eyes closed, and the tilting of the support surface and/or the visual surround. Instability or fall on conditions 5 (eyes closed, moving platform, stable visual surround) and 6 (eyes open, moving platform and visual surround) suggest peripheral vestibulopathy.

VEMP

Cervical vestibular evoked myogenic potentials (cVEMP) are recorded by electrodes placed on the ipsilateral sternocleidomastoid muscle in response to click stimuli. This assesses saccular function and the integrity of the inferior division of the vestibular portion of the eighth cranial nerve. Lower thresholds and increased peak-to-peak amplitudes suggest superior semicircular canal dehiscence. Asymmetry ratios > 40% suggest a saccular or inferior vestibular nerve weakness.

Ocular vestibular evoked potentials (oVEMP) are recorded by electrodes placed on the contralateral inferior oblique muscle in response to sound stimulus. This test assesses utricular function and the integrity of the superior division of the vestibular nerve. Lower thresholds and increased peak-to-peak amplitudes suggest superior semicircular canal dehiscence. Asymmetry ratios > 40% suggest a utricular or superior vestibular nerve weakness.

Other Tests

An audiologic evaluation should be conducted when a balance disorder is suspected to be vestibular in origin.

Pathology

Balance disorders can be caused by disorders of the peripheral vestibular system or the central vestibular system, systemic issues with parts of the body other than the head and brain, and vascular disorders. Peripheral vestibular system issues can be caused by Ménière's disease, labyrinthitis, BPPV, perilymphatic fistula, vestibular neuritis (VN), ototoxicity, vestibular schwannomas, superior canal dehiscence syndrome (SCDS), autoimmune disease, and other disorders. Central vestibular system issues can be caused by migraine, hydrocephalus, brain tumors, multiple sclerosis, cerebrovascular disease including transient ischemic attack or stroke, stress, tension, fatigue, vision disturbances, and other disorders. Systemic issues can include peripheral neuropathies, hyperventilation, and dehydration. Vascular disorders can include orthostatic hypotension, arteriosclerosis, vertebral artery stenosis, and vasovagal syndrome. Cervicogenic dizziness can occur after neck injury or in association with neck pain.

◆ Treatment Options

Treatment for the underlying cause of dizziness should be initiated. Factors that contribute to dizziness (e.g., migraine, visual disturbance) should be addressed and treated. In cases of BPPV, canalith repositioning is highly effective (e.g., the Epley maneuver for posterior canalolithiasis). Ablation of the vestibular organ through vestibulotoxic injections (e.g., intratympanic gentamicin) or surgery (e.g., labyrinthectomy or vestibular nerve section) may be appropriate in certain situations to allow symptom reduction through compensation. In cases of superior semicircular canal dehiscence or a perilymphatic fistula, surgery to repair the defect may alleviate the patient's symptoms. Neurology consultation is ordered when central vestibulopathy or complex vestibular migraine is suspected.

Vestibular therapy is helpful in a number of vestibular disorders. Adaptation, habituation, substitution, and particle repositioning exercises are addressed during vestibular therapy. Vestibulosuppressants can be prescribed for severe vertigo; however, this may prolong time to recovery.

◆ Complications

Vision problems and limitations in physical mobility can influence the ability to conduct accurately some components of ENG/VNG, rotary chair, posturography, and VEMP testing. Results can also be influenced by a variety of medications and alcohol.

3.6.2 Benign Paroxysmal Positional Vertigo

◆ Key Features

- Transient, episodic vertigo is induced by head position changes.
- Benign paroxysmal positional vertigo (BPPV) is most commonly caused by otoliths displaced into the posterior semicircular canal.
- Posterior canalolithiasis produces a latent geotropic upbeating torsional nystagmus that fatigues with time on Dix-Hallpike test.
- Repositioning maneuvers depend on canal involved.

Benign paroxysmal positional vertigo (BPPV) is the most common form of vertigo reported by multidisciplinary balance centers. Displaced otoconia settle in the lowest part of the inner ear, the posterior semicircular canal. Head motion moves these crystalline masses, stimulating the neuroepithelium of the posterior semicircular canal. This causes patients to experience brief episodes of vertigo. Vertigo with latent and fatigable geotropic upbeating rotary nystagmus elicited by the Dix-Hallpike maneuver is diagnostic of posterior canalolithiasis, and most cases are treated successfully with the Epley repositioning maneuver. The horizontal canal is the second most commonly affected semicircular canal; anterior (or superior) canalolithiasis is rare.

◆ Epidemiology

BPPV is the most common form of dizziness. Typically, it occurs spontaneously in elderly patients; in younger patients, BPPV often presents after head trauma or viral labyrinthitis. Symptoms can resolve without treatment.

◆ Clinical

Signs

In posterior canalolithiais, upbeating, geotropic rotatory nystagmus is noted when a patient is placed in the Dix-Hallpike position. There may be a short latency (delay) in the onset of nystagmus, and the duration is brief (less than 1 minute). Nystagmus reverses upon sitting upright (i.e., downbeating, ageotropic rotary nystagmus). The response fatigues with repetition. In horizontal canalolithiasis, geotropic or ageotropic nystagmus is demonstrated on supine roll test. In anterior canalolithiasis, downbeating torsional nystagmus toward the affected ear can be seen during Dix-Hallpike; it is controversial whether anterior canalolithiasis is a true entity.

Symptoms

The patient experiences a spinning sensation that lasts less than a minute, which is associated with head movement, most often when bending forward, looking upward, or lying down and rolling from one side to another. Patients may also have mild, generalized imbalance. Symptoms may also include nausea and vomiting.

Differential Diagnosis

Most diagnoses can be eliminated on history alone. The differential diagnosis for dizziness lasting seconds includes perilymphatic fistula, BPPV, vertebrobasilar insufficiency, superior semicircular canal dehiscence, and cervicogenic dizziness. Dizziness lasting hours can suggest endolymphatic hydrops, Ménière's disease, and vestibular migraine. When symptoms last for days, labyrinthine concussion, labyrinthitis, and vestibular neuritis are suspected. Dizziness lasting months may indicated a retrocochlear mass, vestibulotoxicity, or cerebellar disorder. Central etiologies such as stroke and multiple sclerosis can also present with dizziness.

◆ Evaluation

Physical Exam

A full neurotologic exam should be performed. A basic vestibular exam is described in **Chapter 3.6.1**.

Imaging

Patients with positioning nystagmus suggestive of canalolithiasis do not typically require imaging. Computed tomography (CT) of the temporal bones may be useful in evaluating other causes of dizziness, such as superior semicircular canal dehiscence or temporal bone trauma. Magnetic resonance imaging (MRI) of the brain with and without gadolinium may be useful in ruling out intracranial process or retrocochlear mass.

Labs

Laboratory evaluation is not useful in the diagnosis of BPPV.

Other Tests

Other causes of vertigo may be evaluated with electronystagmography or videonystagmography, vestibular evoked myogenic potentials, rotary chair, and posturography. Tullio phenomenon and Hennebert sign for fistula can also be performed. Audiologic testing is obtained in vestibular symptoms other than BPPV.

Pathology

Cadaveric temporal bone dissections and labyrinthine operations performed in patients with symptoms of BPPV have demonstrated the presence of small calcium crystals (thought to be displaced otoconia from the saccule or utricle) within the posterior semicircular canal. Changing head position causes movement of otoliths within the canal, inducing motion of the cupula. There has also been speculation that cupulolithiasis (presence of otolithic crystals trapped on the cupula) plays a role in some cases. The most common canal affected is the posterior semicircular canal. The second most common canal is the horizontal canal.

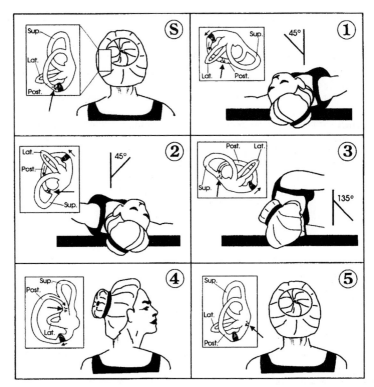

Fig. 3.12 The Epley repositioning maneuver. Positioning sequence for left posterior semicircular canal, as viewed by operator (behind patient). The inset boxes show exposed views of labyrinth, with migration of particles (large arrows). S, Start, patient seated. 1. Place head over end of table, 45° to the left. 2. Keeping head tilted downward, rotate 45° to the right. 3. Rotate head and body until facing downward 135° degrees from supine. 4. Keeping head turned right, bring patient to a sitting position. 5. Turn head forward, chin down 20°. Pause at each position until induced nystagmus approaches termination, or for *T* (latency + duration) seconds if no nystagmus. Keep repeating entire series (1 through 5) until there is no nystagmus in any position. (Used with permission from Epley JM. Particle repositioning for benign paroxysmal positional vertigo. *Otolaryngol Clin North Am* 1996;29:327.)

◆ Treatment Options

Medical

For posterior canal BPPV, the Epley repositioning maneuver is the mainstay of treatment, with success rates exceeding 90% (**Fig. 3.12**). This maneuver entails performing a Dix-Hallpike maneuver to elicit vertigo. Following cessation of vertigo, the patient's head is rotated 90° to the unaffected side. After 45 to 60 seconds, the head is then turned 90° further by having the patient lie on his or her side, such that the face is toward the floor. The patient is then brought back to the upright position with his or her chin tucked to the chest. Each of these positions can be kept for approximately one minute. The canaliths are ultimately repositioned in the vestibule away from sensory epithelium. This procedure may be repeated as needed for relapses or refractory cases. Following the Epley, patients are instructed not to lie flat or assume any provoking position for a few days. Habituation exercises such as Brandt-Daroff exercises can be prescribed for relapsing cases or patients who cannot tolerate the Epley maneuver in the office. The Semont maneuver is an alternative repositioning maneuver for posterior canal BPPV.

Lateral canal BPPV can be treated with the barbecue roll (logroll), Gufoni, or Vannucci maneuvers. Anterior canal BPPV can be treated with an Epley maneuver on the opposite ear or modifications of the Semont maneuver. Habituation exercises can also be prescribed. Referral to vestibular therapy may be necessary when maneuvers cannot be performed in the office (e.g., cervical disease or reduced mobility).

Surgical

Two surgical procedures can be performed for refractory cases of posterior canal BPPV: singular neurectomy and posterior canal occlusion. Singular neurectomy entails sectioning the singular nerve (posterior ampullary nerve) as it courses from the ampulla of the posterior canal to join the saccular nerve to form the inferior part of the vestibular nerve. This procedure is technically difficult, carries a high risk of postoperative sensorineural hearing loss (SNHL), and is not often performed. Posterior canal occlusion involves identifying the posterior canal via a transmastoid approach and packing the canal with bone dust, fascia, or bone wax to create a barrier preventing the flow of endolymph and stimulation of neuroepithelium. Canal plugging can also be done in refractory cases of horizontal and anterior canal BPPV. When performed bilaterally, there is hypofunction of both canals that may cause oscillopsia.

◆ Outcome and Follow-Up

Following the Epley maneuver, patients are instructed not to lie flat or assume any provoking position for the next week, to allow canaliths to settle. Patients with persistent symptoms may have the Epley maneuver repeated or may benefit from Brandt-Daroff exercises or treatment with a trained vestibular physical therapist. BPPV after head trauma often affects multiple canals and is more difficult to treat; vestibular therapy referral is commonly obtained in these patients.

3.6.3 Ménière's disease

◆ Key Features

- Ménière's disease is classified into two categories: definite Ménière's disease and probable Ménière's disease (2015 Diagnostic Criteria).
- The classical presentation is episodic vertigo associated with low- to medium-frequency sensorineural hearing loss and fluctuating aural symptoms lasting 20 minutes to 12 hours.
- Ménière's disease is caused by excess endolymph within the labyrinth ("endolymphatic hydrops").
- Conservative, non-vestibular-destructive treatments are considered prior to invasive, vestibular-destructive procedures for controlling vertigo.

Ménière's disease, or endolymphatic hydrops, is a common cause of recurrent vertigo. The diagnostic criteria of Ménière's disease was revised in 2015. Ménière's disease is classified into two categories: definite Ménière's disease and probable Ménière's disease.

Definite Ménière's disease is defined as (1) two or more spontaneous episodes of vertigo each lasting 20 minutes to 12 hours, (2) audiometrically documented low- to medium-frequency sensorineural hearing loss in one ear, at least on one occasion, and (3) fluctuating aural symptoms in the affected ear (hearing, tinnitus, or fullness), with (4) no better vestibular diagnosis.

Probable Ménière's disease is defined as (1) two or more episodes of vertigo or dizziness each lasting 20 minutes to 24 hours and, (2) fluctuating aural symptoms in the affected ear (hearing, tinnitus, or fullness), with (3) no better vestibular diagnosis.

◆ Epidemiology

The prevalence of Ménière's disease is approximately 34 to 190 per 100,000 population. There is a slight female predominance, and age of onset ranges from the third to seventh decade. Bilateral Ménière's disease rarely presents simultaneously; one ear precedes the other by several years. Progression to bilateral Ménière's disease occurs in 5 to 33% of affected patients.

◆ Clinical

Signs and Symptoms

A classic presentation of Ménière's disease is episodic vertigo lasting minutes to hours, associated with fluctuating hearing loss, tinnitus, and aural fullness. Patients often report nausea and vomiting, which may be followed by severe fatigue. Between episodes, patients will commonly have resolution

Table 3.11 Diagnostic guidelines for Ménière's disease

Definite Ménière's disease
(1) Two or more spontaneous episodes of vertigo each lasting 20 minutes to 12 hours
(2) Audiometrically documented low- to medium-frequency sensorineural hearing loss in one ear, at least on one occasion
(3) Fluctuating aural symptoms in the affected ear (hearing, tinnitus, or fullness)
(4) No better vestibular diagnosis

Probable Ménière's disease
(1) Two or more episodes of vertigo or dizziness each lasting 20 minutes to 24 hours
(2) Fluctuating aural symptoms in the affected ear (hearing, tinnitus, or fullness)
(3) No better vestibular diagnosis

Data from American Academy of Otolaryngology—Head and Neck Foundation Inc. Guidelines for the diagnosis and evaluation of therapy in Meniere's disease. Otolaryngol Head Neck Surg 1995;113)3): 181–185.

of symptoms. Occasionally, imbalance is reported. Familial Ménière's disease should be considered if at least one first- or second-degree relative has definite or probable Ménière's disease. Patients may report drop attack, also known as Tumarkin crisis, which presents as sudden spontaneous falls without loss of consciousness (patient remembers the episode).

Differential Diagnosis

The differential diagnosis for episodic vertigo is benign paroxysmal positional vertigo (BPPV), superior semicircular canal dehiscence syndrome (SCDS), perilymphatic fistula, autoimmune inner ear disease, vestibular schwannoma, endolymphatic sac neoplasm, other intracranial neoplasm, migraine-related vestibulopathy, and transient ischemic attacks (**Table 3.11**).

◆ Evaluation

Physical Exam

A complete neurotologic examination should be performed. A physical examination may demonstrate the presence of low-frequency hearing loss via tuning fork exam. A basic vestibular exam with Tullio and Hennebert tests is performed to evaluate other causes of dizziness (described in **Chapter 3.6.1**). Nystagmus may be present during an acute attack; however, most patients with Ménière's disease will have a normal exam at the time of an office visit.

Imaging

Patients with unilateral or asymmetric sensorineural hearing loss and dizziness should have a magnetic resonance imaging (MRI) study of the brain with and without contrast, including thin cuts of the internal auditory canals to rule out vestibular schwannoma or other retrocochlear pathology.

Labs

Autoimmune serology (e.g. antinuclear antibody [ANA], anti–neutrophil cytoplasmic antibodies [ANCA], rheumatoid factor [RF]), erythrocyte sedimentation rate (ESR), syphilis testing (rapid plasma reagin [RPR] or fluorescent treponemal antibody absorption [FTA-ABS]), diabetic testing, thyroid function tests, and Lyme titers (when appropriate) should be considered for patients exhibiting symptoms of bilateral Ménière's disease.

Other Tests

Audiograms are routinely used in the diagnosis and monitoring of Ménière's disease. Audiograms classically reveal hearing loss that is more severe in the low frequencies. Fluctuation may occur rapidly during acute episodes. Electrocochleography may aid in the diagnosis when the summating potential to action potential ratio is greater than 0.5. Electronystagmography or videonystagmography may demonstrate a significant vestibular weakness in the affected ear. Caloric testing is essential prior to consideration of ablative management.

Pathology

Ménière's disease is hypothesized to be caused by excess endolymph, which causes dilation of the stria vascularis and resultant ischemia. Ischemia then results in weakness in the walls of the scala media, causing rupture and mixing of endolymph with perilymph. Cadaveric temporal bone studies on patients with Ménière's disease demonstrate these findings.

◆ Treatment Options

Medical

Conservative and nondestructive approaches are initially tried in the treatment of Ménière's disease and include short-term vestibulosuppressants, instituting a low-salt diet (< 1500 mg of sodium daily), and potassium-sparing diuretics (Dyazide). Systemic steroids may be used in the short term to control acute attacks; intratympanic steroids have also been utilized for management of vertigo and associated sensorineural hearing loss (efficacy difficult to establish). Betahistine has also shown efficacy in managing vertigo episodes. Other nondestructive therapies include the Meniett device (Medtronic, Inc., Minneapolis, MN) for vertigo prevention.

Intratympanic gentamicin injection to medically ablate the labyrinth (40 mg/mL of buffered gentamicin solution) is a highly effective alternative to surgical ablation in patients with Ménière's disease who have debilitating vertigo. Gentamicin is toxic to dark cells as well as hair cells within the inner ear but preferentially affects vestibular cells. Hearing loss may occur in as many as 15% of patients. Multiple gentamicin injections may be required to ablate vestibular function completely in the affected ear; functional reserve can be monitored with caloric testing. Patients will report worse sensation of dizziness prior to improvement of symptoms. Vestibular training exercises may be helpful to improve balance following medical labyrinthectomy.

Surgical

Refractory Ménièr disease may require more invasive treatments. The treatment algorithm depends on degree of residual hearing. Surgical procedures done in patients with serviceable hearing are endolymphatic sac decompression, with or without shunt placement, and vestibular nerve section with preservation of the cochlear nerve. When hearing is not serviceable, a labyrinthectomy or vestibulocochlear nerve section can be performed.

Endolymphatic sac surgery is performed via a transmastoid approach where the sac is identified and subsequently either decompressed or shunted into the mastoid cavity or arachnoid space. Vestibular nerve sectioning may be performed via a middle cranial fossa, retrosigmoid, or retrolabyrinthine approach. Labyrinthectomy may be performed via a transmastoid approach but results in hearing destruction. Vestibular nerve section and/ or labyrinthectomy (medical or surgical) should not be done bilaterally, as the patient will experience debilitating profound vestibular hypofunction and oscillopsia.

◆ Outcome and Follow-Up

The natural history of the disease appears to involve a gradual resolution of active symptoms in most patients over 5 years. Patients are generally followed clinically as needed. Serial audiometry to monitor stability of hearing is helpful, especially in patients with substantial fluctuation, and in patients who have been treated with aminoglycosides. Sudden hearing loss should be treated appropriately. Hearing loss is progressive over time.

3.6.4   Vestibular Neuritis

◆ Key Features

- In vestibular neuritis (VN), severe vertigo may last days to weeks.
- VN must be distinguished from acute intracranial pathology.
- Recovery may take several weeks.

Vestibular neuritis (VN) is a fairly common cause of acute-onset nonrecurring vertigo. The vertiginous episode is often preceded by viral upper respiratory tract infection. Inflammation of the vestibular nerve results in hypofunction of the affected side and causes vertigo. VN typically has no associated hearing loss.

◆ Epidemiology

Vestibular neuritis primarily affects the middle aged to the elderly but can occur at any age. No gender predominance has been noted.

◆ Clinical

Signs and Symptoms

Some cases of VN may be preceded by upper respiratory infection symptoms. Severe nausea and vomiting with dehydration may warrant hospital admission. Spontaneous and headshake nystagmus is usually present and can be more easily noted by using Frenzel goggles. Episodes usually last several days to weeks. Full compensation from a severe vestibular loss can sometimes take months. Interestingly, it is not unusual for some patients to develop benign paroxysmal positional vertigo (BPPV) several months after their VN symptoms resolve.

Differential Diagnosis

The differential diagnosis includes pathologies of both central and peripheral etiology. Cerebellar or brainstem infarction can cause sudden-onset vertigo. Peripheral causes of sudden-onset vertigo include perilymphatic fistula, Ménière's disease, BPPV, or lesions of the cerebellopontine angle. Bacterial or viral labyrinthitis can also mimic VN; however, in labyrinthitis patients generally report hearing loss as well and require additional treatment.

◆ Evaluation

Physical Exam

A complete neurotologic exam should be performed with Frenzel goggles. Spontaneous, gaze, and headshake nystagmus is generally present, is directed away from the affected ear and is suppressible. Due to a hypofunctioning labyrinth, patients will sway or fall to the affected side on Romberg testing or Fukuda stepping test. Patients will often present their heads tilted to one side, which often lessens their symptoms. A head thrust test will often be abnormal and indicates loss of the vestibuloocular reflex.

Imaging

Imaging is warranted to rule out intracranial infarction, hemorrhage, or other retrocochlear pathology. Magnetic resonance imaging (MRI) is the preferred study to identify infarction, but computed tomography (CT) can be used initially to rule out hemorrhage.

Labs

Lyme disease titers may be of value depending on geographic location.

Other Tests

An audiogram should also be performed to determine baseline hearing and assess for sensorineural hearing loss that may indicate another diagnosis. Electronystagmography or videonystagmography is not necessary but may be performed to confirm the unilateral vestibular weakness on the affected side, especially in patients with persistent dizziness and imbalance.

Pathology

No conclusive evidence of the exact etiology of VN exists. Cadaveric temporal bones have demonstrated inflammation and degeneration of primarily the superior vestibular nerve and the vestibular ganglion (Scarpa's ganglion). Herpes virus has been demonstrated as a cause in some cases.

◆ Treatment Options

See **Table 3.12** for management options. As a rule, VN resolves spontaneously. The vertigo induced by the hypofunctioning vestibular nerve can resolve spontaneously through central compensation. Admission for severe vertigo and dehydration from persistent vomiting is sometimes required for rehydration and intravenous (IV) medication administration. Nausea may be symptomatically treated most effectively with vestibular suppressants: promethazine (25 mg parenterally–intramuscular or rectal suppository preferred; an IV route is discouraged because of severe reactions from inadvertent intraarterial infusion), meclizine (25 mg orally [PO]), or benzodiazepines such as diazepam (5 mg PO). Patients should be cautioned about using vestibular suppressants for long periods, as they can slow down central compensation.

Corticosteroids can be administered as methylprednisolone tablets (Medrol Dosepak, Pfizer, New York, NY) or a dexamethasone IV taper (Decadron 10 mg; Merck & Co., Inc., Whitehouse Station, NJ) and may improve long-term recovery. Acyclovir or valacyclovir (Valtrex; GlaxoSmithKline, Brentford, Middlesex, UK) may be utilized due to the association with

Table 3.12   Management options for vestibular neuritis

Vestibular suppressants
Promethazine (Phenergan, Pfizer, New York, NY) 25 mg IM, PR, PO every 6 hours as needed Diazepam (Valium; Roche Pharmaceuticals, Nutley, NJ) 2–10 mg IM, IV, PO two to three times daily as needed Clonazepam (Klonopin; Roche Pharmaceuticals, Nutley, NJ) 0.5–1 mg PO three times daily as needed
IV hydration
Lactated Ringer solution bolus or maintenance infusion
Steroids
Consider taper, e.g., methylprednisolone tablets (Medrol DosePak, Pfizer, New York, NY) 4-mg tabs PO, start 24 mg/day and taper by 4 mg daily over 6 days
Consider antivirals
Acyclovir 800 mg PO 5x daily x 1 week
Valacyclovir (Valtrex, GlaxoSmithKline, Brentford, Middlesex, UK) 1,000 mg PO twice daily × 1 week
Vestibular physical therapy

Abbreviations: IM, intramuscularly; IV, intravenously; PR, per rectum; PO, orally.

herpes virus, but their efficacy is yet to be determined. Patients should be encouraged to perform at-home vestibular exercises. Vestibular rehabilitation can be helpful for patients with slow compensation.

◆ Outcomes and Follow-Up

Most patients never have recurrence of symptoms. Unsteadiness and dizziness may be experienced for months after an event. Some patients may go on to develop BPPV months later.

3.6.5 Migraine-Associated Vertigo

◆ Key Features

- Over a quarter of patients with migraine will report vestibular symptoms.
- The pathophysiology of vestibular migraine is poorly understood.
- Many patients do not experience headache in conjunction with attacks.
- Management focuses on treatment and prevention of migrainous attacks.

Migraine is among the most common central disorders that produce vestibular symptoms ranging from head motion intolerance to spontaneous vertigo. Although the association between migraine and vertigo has been well documented, a causal relationship has not been elucidated. The classification of this disorder includes vestibular migraine and probable vestibular migraines. Treatment is aimed at migraine control.

Vestibular migraine is defined as (1) at least 5 episodes with vestibular symptoms of moderate or severe intensity, lasting 5 minutes to 72 hours, (2) current or previous history of migraine with or without aura, and (3) one or more migraine features with at least 50% of the vestibular episodes (headache, photophobia/phonophobia, and visual aura), with (4) no better vestibular or International Classification of Headache Disorders (ICHD) diagnosis. Headaches should demonstrate at least two characteristics: one-sided location, pulsating quality, moderate or severe pain intensity, and aggravation by routine physical activity.

Probable vestibular migraine is defined as (1) at least 5 episodes with vestibular symptoms of moderate or severe intensity, lasting 5 minutes to 72 hours, and (2) history of migraine or migraine features during episodes, with (3) no better diagnosis.

◆ Epidemiology

Migraine is a common disorder that affects 18 to 29% of women and 6 to 14% of men. Vestibular migraine affects up to 1% of the general population. Familial occurrence of vestibular migraine with autosomal dominance has been documented in several families.

◆ Clinical

Signs and Symptoms

The typical migraine headache is unilateral, throbbing, moderate to severe, exacerbated by physical activity, and accompanied by sensitivity to light and noise. Migraines are classified with or without aura. Several vestibular symptoms can accompany migraine, including dizziness, head motion intolerance, and spontaneous vertigo. The attacks of vertigo can last minutes to days. Nausea and vomiting can also occur. Most patients are symptom-free between attacks, which can occur several times a month. Some patients will also experience other otoneurologic symptoms such as aural fullness. The attacks of vertigo are not temporally associated with headache symptoms during all episodes. In some women, there is an association with menstruation (i.e., perimenstrual migraine with vertigo). Benign paroxysmal vertigo of childhood is regarded as a precursor to migraine syndrome.

Differential Diagnosis

The differential diagnosis of episodic vertigo is broad and includes peripheral conductions such as benign paroxysmal positional vertigo, perilymphatic fistula, superior semicircular canal dehiscence, autoimmune inner ear disease, otosyphilis, and Ménière's disease. Central causes of recurrent vestibulopathy include basilar migraine, vertebrobasilar insufficiency, hydrocephalus, retrocochlear mass, and stroke. Anxiety, depression, and other underlying psychiatric disorder may cause dizziness as well; more than 50% of patients with vestibular migraine have comorbid psychiatric disorder.

◆ Evaluation

History

A thorough history focusing on vestibular and migrainous symptoms is critical. The definitions of vestibular migraine and probable vestibular migraines are as previously described. International Headache Society diagnostic criteria for migraine are described in **Table 3.13.** Migraine triggers

Table 3.13   International Headache Society (IHS) Diagnostic Criteria for Migraines

Recurrent headaches separated by symptom-free intervals and accompanied by any three of the following:
• Abdominal pain
• Complete relief after sleep
• Nausea and/or vomiting
• Aura
• Hemicrania
• Throbbing, pulsatile quality
• Family history of migraine

Data from International Headache Society. The International Classification of Headache Disorders. 2nd ed. *Cephalalgia* 2004;24 (Suppl 1).

are also important to identify. Other otologic symptoms, such as hearing loss, tinnitus, and aural fullness, may suggest a different or additional etiology for dizziness.

Physical Exam

The physical exam in patients with migraine-associated vertigo is usually normal. However, thorough head and neck examinations, including neurologic and vestibular exams, should be completed to exclude other causes of vertigo.

Other Tests

Vestibular testing can be helpful in separating peripheral from central causes of vertigo. Patients with migrainous vertigo usually have normal electronystagmography or videonystagmography tracings; however, abnormalities may be seen on rotary chair (e.g., increased vestibulo-ocular reflex time constant). Complete audiologic assessment should be obtained; low-frequency loss may be found as an early sign of Ménière's disease (a condition that can coexist with vestibular migraine).

Imaging

Magnetic resonance imaging (MRI) and computed tomography (CT) of the brain are usually normal in cases of migraine-associated vertigo but are useful in excluding other serious neurologic conditions. There is often considerable value in offering patients reassurance that MRI results are normal.

◆ Treatment Options

Treatment for migraine-associated vertigo centers on control of migrainous attacks by prophylactic or abortive medical management (**Table 3.14**). The choice of medications depends on the side effect profile and comorbidities of patients. Prophylactic treatment includes the avoidance of dietary triggers, β-blockers in patients with hypertension without asthma (propranolol 40 mg twice daily or metoprolol), calcium channel blockers (verapamil 80 mg three times daily or flunarizine), and anticonvulsants (topiramate, valproic acid, lamotrigine). If patients have anxiety, antidepressants (amitriptyline, nortriptyline, selective serotonin reuptake inhibitors) and anxiolytics (clonazepam) are considered. Acetazolamide is an effect in rare genetic disorders related to migraine-like episodic ataxia. Triptans (sumatriptan 25 mg PO at onset of symptoms) and analgesics (ibuprofen 600 mg) can be used to abort or reduce symptoms when they do occur.

Few studies have evaluated the effects of these management strategies on vestibular symptoms; however, there is some evidence that the same prophylactic drugs can be effective. For acute vertiginous episodes,

Table 3.14 Management strategies for migraine-associated vertigo

Prophylaxis	Treatments to abort acute attack
Avoidance of dietary triggers (e.g., aged cheeses, chocolate, beer, red wine, excessive caffeine, aspartame, monosodium glutamate, high salt)	Nonsteroidal anti-inflammatories: Ibuprofen 600 mg PO at onset
β-blockers: Propranolol 40 mg PO twice daily	For perimenstrual migraine with vertigo: Clonazepam (Klonopin; Roche Pharmaceuticals, Nutley, NJ) 0.5–1 mg PO every 8 hours as needed
Calcium channel blockers: Verapamil 80 mg three times daily	Triptans: Sumatriptan (Imitrex, GlaxoSmithKline, Brentford, Middlesex, UK) 25–100 mg PO at onset of symptoms, or 4–6 mg SC × 1, or 5 or 20 mg nasal spray × 1
	Rizatriptan (Maxalt, Merck, Kenilworth, NJ) 5–10 mg PO × 1
	Naratriptan (Amerge, GlaxoSmithKline, Brentford, Middlesex, UK) 1–2.5 mg PO × 1
	Others
Tricyclic antidepressants: Amitriptyline 25–150 mg PO qhs, Nortriptyline (Pamelor, Mallinckrodt, Dublin, Ireland) 25–150 mg PO qhs, Protriptyline (Vivactil, Merck, Kenilworth, NJ) 5–10 mg PO three times daily	Combination: Single-tablet combination of sumatriptan and naproxen sodium (Treximet, Pernix Therapeutics, Morristown, NJ) 1 tab PO × 1

Abbreviations: PO, orally; qhs, before bedtime; SC, subcutaneously.

sumatriptan is helpful in some patients, but only for attacks lasting longer than one hour. Patients who develop chronic dysequilibrium may also benefit from vestibular rehabilitation therapy. Patients with perimenstrual migraine with vertigo often respond well to clonazepam (Klonopin; Roche Pharmaceuticals, Nutley, NJ) 0.5 to 1 mg PO every 8 hours as needed.

◆ Outcome and Follow-Up

Avoidance of identifiable triggers is highly successful. If pharmacotherapy is needed, the majority of patients respond favorably to prophylactic medications or triptans.

3.7 Tinnitus

◆ Key Features

- Tinnitus is the perception of sound without an unrelated external source of sound.
- Retrocochlear pathology in unilateral tinnitus must be excluded.
- Vascular anomalies and neoplasms should be excluded in pulsatile tinnitus.

Tinnitus is a common but poorly understood disorder. Its severity can range from insignificant to disabling. Tinnitus is a nonspecific symptom characterized by the sensation of buzzing, ringing, clicking, pulsations, and other noises in the ear. Objective tinnitus, or somatosounds, refers to noises generated from within the ear or adjacent structures. The term "subjective tinnitus" is used when the sound is audible only to the affected patient.

◆ Epidemiology

Fifty million Americans report tinnitus, representing an estimated prevalence of 10 to 15% of adults in the United States. Twelve million will seek medical attention. Males report it more frequently than females.

◆ Clinical

A targeted history at the initial evaluation of the patient, including risk factors for hearing loss, should be obtained to identify conditions that, if promptly identified and managed, can relieve tinnitus. It is important to determine whether the tinnitus is unilateral, pulsatile, new onset, or sudden onset with hearing loss. A history of hearing loss (unilateral, bilateral, asymmetric), noise exposure, ototoxic exposure, and head trauma should be elicited. Additional neurotologic symptoms such as vertigo, imbalance, dizziness, and even otalgia and otorrhea may help determine the etiology of the tinnitus. Depression, anxiety, and cognitive impairment often coexist with tinnitus. Tinnitus can also impair concentration, memory, and sleep. It is also important to elicit whether the tinnitus is mild, moderate, or severed based on effect on quality of life (i.e., how bothersome it is to the patient). Duration of tinnitus may facilitate discussion about natural history, treatment, and follow-up care. Persistent tinnitus occurs when symptoms last for ≥ 6 months.

Differential Diagnosis

Subjective (Nonpulsatile)

- Otologic: Hearing loss, otosclerosis, Ménière's disease
- Neurologic: Multiple sclerosis, trauma, vestibular schwannoma
- Infectious: Lyme disease, syphilis, otitis, meningitis

- Drug-induced: Aspirin, nonsteroidal anti-inflammatory drugs (NSAIDs), aminoglycosides, furosemide, vincristine, platinum-based chemotherapeutics
- Miscellaneous: TMJ or myofascial, dental, depression, idiopathic

Objective (Pulsatile)

- Turbulent flow: Glomus tumors, carotid atherosclerosis, benign intracranial hypertension, dural arteriovenous malformations, cerebral aneurysms
- Muscle contractions: Palatal myoclonus—stapedial, tensor tympani
- Spontaneous otoacoustic emissions

◆ Evaluation

Physical Exam

A complete otoneurologic exam should be performed. The mastoid, neck, and heart should be auscultated for vascular causes of tinnitus (e.g., heart murmurs, carotid bruits, vascular sounds). Focal neurologic signs, such as cranial nerve palsy, may suggest neoplastic cause, and additional evaluation and treatment are recommended. Otologic exam should include inspection of the external auditory canal, tympanic membrane, and middle ear for causes of conductive hearing loss that contributes to tinnitus. Otorrhea may be a sign of middle ear or external ear infection. The head and neck should be inspected and palpated for neoplasm. Occlusion of the ipsilateral internal jugular vein may alleviate pulsatile tinnitus in patients with venous sinus stenosis or diverticulum.

Imaging

Imaging of the head and neck should be considered in patients with unilateral tinnitus, pulsatile tinnitus, focal neurologic abnormalities, or asymmetric sensorineural hearing loss. Computed tomography (CT) or CT angiography (CTA) of the brain or temporal bone, or magnetic resonance imaging (MRI)/angiography of the brain or internal auditory canals are common choices for initial imaging studies for pulsatile tinnitus. When asymmetric sensorineural hearing loss or unilateral tinnitus is present, MRI of the internal auditory canal with and without contrast is considered to evaluate retrocochlear pathology as well as to rule out intracranial pathology.

Labs

Laboratory tests are not routinely ordered.

Other Tests

Comprehensive audiologic examination in patients is recommended. Auditory brainstem response (ABR) testing my be used to assess retrocochlear pathology. Tinnitus questionnaires (e.g., tinnitus handicap inventory, tinnitus functional index, tinnitus reaction questionnaire) may provide insight on how tinnitus affects quality-of-life measures.

Pathology

The pathophysiology of tinnitus is controversial. It is likely due to compensatory adaptation of the central auditory system to hearing loss. Although there is a clear association of tinnitus with hearing loss, many people with hearing loss do report tinnitus. Alterations in neurotransmitters along the auditory pathway have been linked to tinnitus.

◆ Treatment Options

The definition of tinnitus, its relationship to hearing loss, its association with ototoxic drugs, and the current pathophysiology of the disease should be explained to the patient. The management strategies should be discussed with patients with persistent, bothersome tinnitus. Additional approaches that can inform and educate patients include providing brochures, suggesting self-help books, describing counseling and sound therapy options, and discussing availability and limitations of pharmacologic and complementary and alternative medicines. Referral to support organizations (such as the American Tinnitus Association) and tinnitus specialists may also be helpful. It is important for patients to understand that there is no cure for tinnitus, but there are several treatments that can relieve the effects of tinnitus on concentration and sleep and improve hearing.

Medical

Hearing aid evaluation is recommended for patients with hearing loss and persistent, bothersome tinnitus. Sound therapy to mask tinnitus should be offered to patients with tinnitus that is bothersome and prolonged. Sound therapy device options include environmental enrichment devices (e.g., fans, TV, radio, tabletop sound generators) and hearing aids fitted with tinnitus maskers. The goal of sound therapy is tinnitus habituation, which is the adaptation of the auditory system that results in reduced intensity of perceived tinnitus. Tinnitus retraining therapy utilizes sound therapy for habituation but also incorporates simultaneous counseling. Identifying the frequency and intensity of the tinnitus may help tinnitus specialists individualize sound therapy for patients with more severe forms of tinnitus. Reassurance and noise precautions should also be provided.

Cognitive/behavioral therapy (CBT) has demonstrated effectiveness in treatment of tinnitus-related distress. It is usually performed by a mental health specialist. CBT teaches patients ways to identify negative thought patterns related to tinnitus and restructure to emphasize positive thought patterns. Treatment also includes behavioral interventions such as relaxation techniques, sleep hygiene, and auditory enrichment.

Antidepressants, anticonvulsants, anxiolytics, intratympanic medications, or dietary supplements (e.g., melatonin, zinc, *Ginkgo biloba*) should not be routinely recommended for persistent and bothersome tinnitus. Acupuncture may be considered as an alternative therapy in recalcitrant, bothersome tinnitus; however, its effectiveness has not been proven in clinical trial. Currently, there is no conclusive evidence that transcranial magnetic stimulation improves tinnitus, and therefore, it should not be recommended at this time.

Surgical

Where appropriate, surgery can be considered for some objective sources of tinnitus. Sigmoid sinus diverticula can be cauterized and dehiscences resurfaced via transmastoid approach. Vascular lesions (e.g., glomus tympanicum, glomus jugulare) causing tinnitus can be addressed with surgery and, in some cases, radiation or stereotactic radiosurgery. Tegmen dehiscences, meningoceles, and encephaloceles can be repaired through a middle cranial fossa and/or transmastoid approach. Arteriovenous malformations can be embolized or surgically resected.

◆ Outcome and Follow-Up

Healthcare professionals have the opportunity to help tinnitus patients learn how to cope with and manage their tinnitus. Realistic expectations and treatments should be provided to the patient. Annual audiograms should be performed to determine progression of hearing loss.

3.8   Cerebellopontine Angle Tumors

◆ Key Features

- The most common tumors of the cerebellopontine angle are vestibular schwannomas, followed by meningiomas and epidermoids.
- Treatment options depend on the etiology but may include observation, stereotactic radiosurgery, and surgical excision.
- Surgical approaches to the cerebellopontine angle are the middle fossa, retrosigmoid, and translabyrinthine approaches.

The cerebellopontine angle (CPA) is a cerebrospinal fluid (CSF)-filled space found at the ventral aspect of the junction between the cerebellum and the pons. Most neoplasms found in this location are benign. Vestibular schwannomas (also known as acoustic neuromas) are the most common, followed by meningioma, and epidermoids. Presenting symptoms usually include unilateral sensorineural hearing loss, tinnitus, and dizziness/imbalance.

◆ Epidemiology

Vestibular schwannomas are the most common CPA neoplasm. These most commonly arise from the inferior vestibular division of CN VIII. Spontaneous yearly occurrence is ~1 in 100,000, or roughly 2,280 new cases annually in the United States. Most tumors grow slowly (average is 1–2 mm per year). Bilateral tumors can be seen in patients with neurofibromatosis 2 (NF2).

◆ Clinical

Signs and Symptoms

Presenting symptoms can include unilateral hearing loss, unilateral tinnitus, or progressive imbalance or vertigo. Difficulty talking on the phone with one ear is a common complaint. Sudden hearing loss may be the presentation in ~10% of cases. Large tumors can cause brainstem compression and cranial nerve (CN) V, VI, VII, VIII, IX, X, and XI palsies. Compression of the fourth ventricle may cause hydrocephalus, typically with giant tumors measuring more than 4 cm. Ataxia, altered mental status, headache, nausea, vomiting, diplopia, respiratory depression, and coma can also occur.

Differential Diagnosis

The differential diagnosis may include vestibular schwannoma, meningioma, epidermoid, arachnoid cysts, facial nerve schwannoma, trigeminal schwannomas, endolymphatic sac tumors, chondrosarcoma, and metastatic tumor.

◆ Evaluation

Physical Exam

A complete otoneurologic, head and neck, and full cranial nerve exam should be performed. Cranial nerve deficits should be documented. The corneal reflex (CN V_1) and blink reflex (CN VII) can be assessed using a wisp of cotton. Hoarseness and dysphagia warrant fiberoptic laryngoscopy for evaluation. Spontaneous, gaze, and headshake nystagmus tests may indicate unilateral vestibular weakness (fast phase to the opposite side). Fall or sway may be seen with Romberg, Fukuda stepping, and tandem gait tests. Dysmetria may be seen on cerebellar tests such as the finger-to-nose test. Hitzelberger sign may also be elicited (reduced sensation of the posterior ear canal from tumor compression of the facial nerve).

Imaging

Magnetic resonance imaging (MRI) of the brain with and without contrast with thin cuts through the internal auditory canals is the gold standard for diagnosis. Vestibular schwannomas and meningiomas are slightly hypointense to isointense on T1-weighted images, are heterogeneously hyperintense with cystic areas on T2, and enhance with contrast. Meningiomas are more sessile, broad-based, and may display a dural tail. They are rarely centered within the internal auditory canal. Diffuse and extensive dural involvement can occur ("en plaque meningioma"). Computed tomography (CT) scan of a meningioma may demonstrate calcifications and adjacent hyperostosis. Epidermoids are usually hypointense on T1 and hyperintense on T2. They do not enhance with contrast but they may be hyperintense on fluid-attenuated inversion recovery (FLAIR).

Other Tests

- Audiogram: Unilateral pure-tone sensorineural loss is usually seen. Decreases in speech discrimination are common and usually greater than

Table 3.15 Management of non–neurofibromatosis Type 2 vestibular schwannomas (acoustic neuromas)

Tumor size	Options
Small (≤ 2 cm diameter), noncystic	Observation
	o MRI every 6–12 mo until stable, then annually
	o Annual audiometry
	o Treat if > 2 mm interval growth
	Radiotherapy
	Surgery
	o Translabyrinthine approach if no useful hearing
	o Suboccipital or middle fossa approach if good discrimination score
Large (> 2 cm diameter)	Treat (consider age comorbidities to determine best modality)

expected considering pure tones. Decay in speech discrimination may be demonstrated at higher test stimuli (rollover).

- Auditory brainstem response (ABR) test: The sensitivity of ABR is approximately 95%; however, this percentage drops to 67% for smaller, intracanalicular tumors. Interaural difference in wave V of > 0.2 ms is abnormal.

- Vestibular testing: Tumors may cause weakness of the superior and/or inferior vestibular nerves. Peripheral vestibular weakness may be demonstrated on caloric testing (function of horizontal canal and its afferent pathway through the superior vestibular nerve) and vestibular evoked myogenic potentials (VEMP). Cervical VEMP may detect dysfunction of the saccule or inferior vestibular nerve; ocular VEMP may detect dysfunction of the utricle or superior vestibular nerve.

Pathology

On pathology, vestibular schwannomas demonstrate Antoni A (hypercellular) and Antoni B (hypocellular) areas. Verocay bodies are fusiform cells arranged in palisades, characteristic of Antoni A areas. Meningiomas demonstrate round uniform nuclei with intranuclear pseudoinclusions and eosinophilic cytoplasm. Psammoma bodies may also be present. Epidermoid cysts demonstrate squamous epithelium.

◆ Treatment Options

See **Table 3.15** for treatment options for a vestibular schwannoma. Tumor size, growth rate, severity of symptoms, hearing levels, anesthetic risk, patient age, and other factors must be evaluated for the individual patient to determine the best option for treatment. The average growth rate of a vestibular schwannoma is ~1 to 2 mm per year, although this can vary. Treatment options include observation with serial MRI scans every 6 to 12 months (to determine growth rate), radiotherapy (e.g., stereotactic radiosurgery), and microsurgical resection.

Stereotactic radiosurgery, as by Gamma Knife (Elekta, Stockholm, Sweden) or CyberKnife (Accuray, Inc., Sunnyvale, CA), can deliver a high dose of radiation to a small area of the body with excellent precision. Radiation injury to surrounding normal tissue is reduced compared to conventional fractionated radiation. Facial nerve palsy occurs in ~3% of patients. The hearing preservation rate is ~23% at 10 years. MRI scans are obtained at 6- or 12-month intervals to assess for tumor growth. Stereotactic radiosurgery is generally reserved for tumors that are < 2.5 cm, although indications may still be expanding.

Microsurgical approaches for resection of vestibular schwannoma are the middle cranial fossa, retrosigmoid, and translabyrinthine approaches (**Fig. 3.13**). The preference and experience of the surgeon will factor into the decision regarding the approach. Meningiomas have a slightly better chance of hearing preservation than vestibular schwannomas.

- The middle fossa approach is appropriate for small tumors less than 1.5 cm (mostly intracanalicular). Hearing preservation is possible, and the entire internal auditory canal (IAC) can be accessed. Air cells need to be obliterated with bone wax.

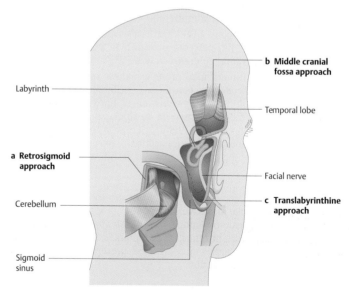

Fig. 3.13 Surgical approaches to the lateral skull base. The retrosigmoid approach requires a craniotomy posterior to the sigmoid sinus. The middle cranial fossa approach requires a transtemporal craniotomy and retraction of the temporal lobe. The translabyrinthine approach is a transmastoid approach that requires mastoidectomy and labyrinthectomy to expose the internal auditory canal and posterior cranial fossa. (Used with permission from Probst R, Grevers G, Iro H. *Basic Otorhinolaryngology: A Step-by-Step Learning Guide*. Stuttgart/New York: Thieme; 2006:301.)

- The retrosigmoid (suboccipital) approach can be performed for small and large tumors. Hearing preservation is possible; however, only the medial two-thirds of the IAC can be exposed safely. Cerebellar retraction may cause cerebellar edema and brainstem compression; however, decompression of CSF at the foramen magnum can reduce the need for cerebellar retraction. Air cells need to be obliterated with bone wax.
- The translabyrinthine approach can be used for any size tumor, but hearing preservation is not possible. Decompression of the labyrinthine segment of the facial nerve improves visualization and dissection of the meatal segment of the facial nerve. Cerebellar retraction is usually not necessary. The auditory (eustachian) tube is obliterated with fascia or bone wax. The surgical defect is generally packed with abdominal fat.

The management of vestibular schwannoma is continually evolving. Large vestibular schwannomas compressing the brainstem require surgical resection; patients who cannot tolerate general anesthesia may receive radiosurgery as the only alternative. Observation is offered for small to medium-sized vestibular schwannoma in all age groups. Microsurgical resection is generally preferred for growing small to medium-sized vestibular schwannomas in young, healthy patients (because of long-term complications of radiation exposure); radiosurgery may be a better alternative in older patients with medical comorbidities. Hearing preservation surgery can be performed through the middle cranial fossa or retrosigmoid approaches depending on the size and location of the tumor; however, the middle cranial fossa should be avoided in patients > 65 years due to higher complication rate from temporal lobe retraction. Translabyrinthine and retrosigmoid approaches can be performed in patients with small to large tumors; there is a potential for hearing preservation using the retrosigmoid approach with small to medium-sized tumors.

NF2 patients with bilateral vestibular schwannomas require special consideration and sometimes aggressive management to avoid eventual bilateral deafness. Enlarging tumors may impair function of the facial and cochlear nerves bilaterally. Unlike most sporadic acoustic tumors, NF2 tumors often infiltrate nerve fibers rather than displace them. Debulking procedures may not be feasible. Managing multiple cranial neuropathies can be challenging; lower cranial nerve involvement is common. Meningiomas have a slightly better chance of hearing preservation. NF2 patients require individualized evaluation and treatment planning. Hearing can potentially be aided with an auditory brainstem implant during vestibular schwannoma surgery.

◆ Complications

See **Table 3.16** for timetable and description of possible complications, as well as management issues. Initial postoperative facial weakness should be treated with steroids and eye protection in the short term. Appropriate eye

Table 3.16 Timetable of possible postoperative complications following craniotomy and cerebellopontine angle tumor resection

← ABCs →
Airway compromise: Mucus plugging, ventilator problems, vocal fold paralysis from lower cranial nerve dysfunction **B**leeding: Within the CPA from operative field—contralateral long-tract signs, ↑ICP **C**irculation: Normotension not maintained

| | ← **Intracranial hemorrhage** → |
(Parenchymal, epidural, subdural) |
| ← **Infarct** → |
(AICA, cerebellar, cerebral) |
| **CNS edema** |
| ← **SIADH/DI** → |
(Watch sodium; consider hydrocephalus; RAS suppression; medication effects) |
| ← **Emesis followed by change in mental status** → |
(Bleed, pneumocephalus, CSF leak. Could be prompted by movement, or disorientation in CT scanner) |
| ← **Fever, meningitis** → |
| ← **DVT, PE** → |
(TEDS, sequential compression stockings) |

TIME: →						
Postoperative day #						
0	1	2	3	4	5	+
	ICU	floor	Start PO intake Start PT			

Comments:

RAS suppression: Edema, increased pressure or displacement can inhibit brainstem reticular activating system function, causing, decreased consciousness in the early postoperative period. CPA surgery and cerebellar retraction predispose the patient to edema, *especially 24–72 hours postoperatively. Keep Na > 140; consider steroids.*

Increased intracranial pressure: Hemiparalysis with obtundation, a fixed dilated pupil and respiratory distress are the hallmarks of rapidly increasing ICP with peduncular herniation. If the patient does not recover properly from anesthesia or there is any unexpected neurologic abnormality, suspect hematoma, hydrocephalus with increased ICP, or cerebellar infarct. If deterioration is slow, obtain a CT scan; if rapid, go to OR.

Meningitis: Most common at postoperative day 4 or later; marked by postoperative fever, increased headache, malaise, photophobia, nausea. Promptly obtain LP with Gram stain, cell count, glucose, cultures. Treat with IV antibiotics and close monitoring.

CSF leak: There is a 5–17% incidence. Mastoid air cells may be opened intraoperatively during craniotomy or IAC drilling. If CSF rhinorrhea develops, treat with antibiotics, head of bed elevation, ± intermittent LP versus lumbar drain. If copious leakage, prompt mastoidectomy with fat obliteration is indicated.

Abbreviations: AICA, anterior inferior cerebellar artery; CNS, central nervous system; CPA, cerebellopontine angle; CSF, cerebrospinal fluid; CT, computed tomography; DI, diabetes insipidus; DVT, deep vein thrombosis; ICP, intracranial pressure; ICU, intensive care unit; LP, lumbar puncture; OR, operating room; PE, pulmonary embolus; PT, physical therapy; RAS, reticular activating system; SIADH, syndrome of inappropriate antidiuretic hormone; TEDS, thromboembolic deterrent stockings.

care is critical to avoid exposure keratitis, which is entirely preventable. A recommended regimen includes hourly artificial tears drops while awake and Lacri-Lube ointment when sleeping (Allergan, Inc., Irvine, CA). Some advocate use of a small square of Saran Wrap (SC Johnson, Racine, WI) taped over the eye while sleeping ("moisture chamber"). The ointment and wrap can also be used while awake if the patient is noncompliant with the drops regimen.

Moreover, in the setting of concurrent facial and trigeminal dysfunction, the patient will not feel the pain of the eye drying or abrading. Prolonged facial weakness may warrant an upper eyelid gold weight placement, as well as surgical reanimation. If no function returns after 18 to 24 months, then static or dynamic reanimation is recommended (see also **Chapter 9.2**). Gracilis free flap can be offered for facial reanimation in the appropriate patient.

CSF otorrhea, CSF rhinorrhea, or incisional CSF leaks may resolve with bed rest, stool softeners, lumbar drain placement, and pressure dressings. Persistent CSF leaks should be treated with reexploration, middle ear obliteration, and auditory tube closure/obliteration.

Unilateral complete hearing loss can be rehabilitated with a contralateral routing of signals (CROS) hearing aid or Bi-CROS hearing aids. Osseointegrated bone conducting hearing aids for single-sided deafness can improve speech understanding in noise (see **Chapter 3.5.5**). These techniques function on the principle of transferring sound from the deaf ear to the hearing ear.

◆ Outcome and Follow-Up

Patients may have significant vertigo following surgical treatment until adequate compensation occurs over several weeks. This is especially true of patients without preoperative vestibular hypofunction, who therefore have no previous compensation. Short-term vestibular suppressants and vestibular therapy can help improve symptoms. Careful monitoring of facial nerve function and observation for evidence of meningitis or CSF leak is critical. CSF leak rates run from 10% to 15%. Facial nerve preservation rates are dependent on both surgeon experience and tumor size. Facial nerve preservation can be more difficult for previously irradiated tumors.

Patients undergoing observation or radiation should have serial MRI scans every 6 to 12 months to watch for tumor growth. Surgical patients should have follow-up MRIs annually, which may become more infrequent with time if no growth or recurrence is identified.

3.9   Superior Semicircular Canal Dehiscence Syndrome

✦ Key Features

- Superior semicircular canal dehiscence (SSCD) occurs when there is an absence of intact bone overlying the superior semicircular canal.
- Presentation can include the Tullio phenomenon, autophony, and hyperacusis.
- A third mobile window leads to low-frequency conductive loss with intact acoustic reflex.
- Vestibular-evoked potentials (VEMP) can demonstrate reduced thresholds and large peak-to-peak amplitudes.
- Treatment is primarily surgical (resurfacing and/or canal plugging).

Superior semicircular canal dehiscence (SSCD), or semicircular canal dehiscence syndrome (SCDS), was first described by Minor in 1998 and is defined by the absence of bone overlying the superior semicircular canal, leading to vestibular and auditory symptoms. Patients with SSCD can present with conductive hearing loss (CHL) with intact acoustic reflexes, conductive hyperacusis, pulsatile tinnitus, and Tullio phenomenon.

✦ Epidemiology

The incidence of SCDS is unknown. However, temporal bone studies suggest that the anatomic incidence of dehiscence of the superior canal is 0.5%.

✦ Clinical

Signs and Symptoms

Clinically, signs and symptoms may range from very mild to severe. Patients with SSCD may exhibit some or all of the following:

- Tullio phenomenon: Vertigo or dizziness induced by loud sound, with oscillopsia and nystagmus
- Autophony: The person's own speech or other self-generated noises, such as chewing, are perceived as unusually loud in the affected ear.
- Dizziness, disequilibrium, or true vertigo
- Hyperacusis
- Conductive hearing loss, often in the low-frequency range
- Aural fullness
- Pulsatile tinnitus
- Headache

Differential Diagnosis

With a healthy or normal-appearing middle ear, the presence of normal acoustic reflex should help discriminate otosclerosis with stapes immobility from possible SSCD. Obviously, one must exclude other identifiable causes of CHL, such as tympanic membrane perforation, ossicular chain problems, or middle ear effusion. The differential diagnosis for dysequilibrium is broad. Noise-induced vertigo raises suspicion for SSCD. Perilymphatic fistula and an enlarged vestibular aqueduct are possible conditions associated with an inner ear third mobile window. Ménière's disease, patulous auditory (eustachian) tube, and migraine may have some overlapping findings.

◆ Evaluation

History

History should focus on complaints just described, including history of dizziness in loud noise, bothersome autophony, or aural fullness.

Physical Exam

An otoneurologic exam is performed to rule out other etiologies of conductive hearing loss and dizziness. Tullio phenomenon and Hennebert sign may be elicited. Tuning fork tests may indicate a conductive hearing loss. Conductive hyperacusis may be perceived when a tuning fork is placed on the medial malleolus of the ankle. Nystagmus may be elicited with Valsalva against a closed glottis or pinched nostrils or with tragal compression.

Imaging

High-resolution thin-cut computed tomography (CT) scanning (0.6-mm slice thickness or less) of the temporal bone is obtained and can suggest dehiscence of bone overlying the superior semicircular canal by examination of the coronal images. Dehiscence may be better appreciated if the images can be reformatted in the plane parallel to the superior canal (Pöschl) and in the plane perpendicular to the superior canal (Stenvers view).

Labs

Laboratory testing is not routinely ordered for SSCD.

Other Tests

Audiologic Assessment

Audiologic assessment should include pure tone testing for air conduction thresholds from 250 to 8,000 Hz, and bone conduction thresholds from 250 to 4,000 Hz. Conductive hyperacusis may be assessed by administering bone conduction testing at stimulus levels less than 0-dB hearing loss (e.g., –5 to –10 dB). Assessment should also include tympanograms, otoacoustic emissions, and acoustic reflexes.

Vestibular Evoked Myogenic Potential Testing

VEMP testing can be used to provide evidence of altered vestibular function; thus, it can help to determine if a suspected dehiscence of the superior canal, seen on CT scanning, is associated with an alteration of inner ear physiology. Patients with SSCD have larger peak-to-peak amplitudes and lower thresholds on VEMP testing. In cervical VEMP, sound is delivered via insert earphones, and activity is recorded from the ipsilateral sternocleidomastoid muscle. In ocular VEMP, activity is recorded from the contralateral inferior oblique muscle. Some studies suggest that ocular VEMP is more sensitive for detecting SSCD than cervical VEMP.

Pathology

A thinning of the bone overlying the superior semicircular canal leads to a third mobile window within the inner ear. This alters inner ear mechanics, leading to the clinical findings. The precise cause of the dehiscence is unknown.

◆ Treatment Options

Medical

Accurate diagnosis is important, as unnecessary stapes surgery (for the CHL) must be avoided. If the patient has mild symptoms, the identification of a source for the symptoms may provide reassurance, and ongoing observation may be all that is required.

Surgical

If the patient has severe symptoms, surgery to resurface or occlude the dehiscence may be warranted. The surgical candidate should have a correlation of symptoms, exam findings, VEMP, and imaging pointing to SSCD. The procedure can be performed via middle cranial fossa or transmastoid approaches. The middle cranial fossa allows for excellent exposure of the dehiscence; resurfacing and/or plugging can be performed under direct visualization. Hydroxyapatite cement and bone pate is subsequently placed. However, in the middle cranial fossa approach, the temporal lobe is retracted superiorly, which may cause temporal lobe edema and seizures. Dural tear, cerebrospinal fluid (CSF) leak, and injuries to the superficial middle cerebral vein (vein of Labbé) are additional risks. Facial nerve monitoring is performed, and intravenous steroids and mannitol are administered. Patients are admitted to the neuro-surgical ward for 2 or 3 days. Temporomandibular joint (TMJ) pain is common.

The dehiscence is not directly visualized with transmastoid approaches. A low-lying dura may preclude repair through this approach. The otic bone may need to be drilled to gain access to the superior semicircular canal; crura on either side of the dehiscence are plugged with bone wax, fascia, and/or bone dust/fragments. The superior aspect of the superior semicircular canal can be resurfaced using cartilage or cortical bone inserted through a bony window in the tegmen mastoideum; a tear in the membranous labyrinth of the superior semicircular canal can occur unnoticed due to limited visualization. Patients may be admitted for symptomatic control of dizziness and/or nausea.

◆ Complications

Global vestibular hypofunction and sensorineural hearing loss from perilymphatic fluid leak or labyrinthitis after the surgical intervention can be treated with systemic and/or intratympanic steroids. Facial weakness from inadvertent avulsion/injury to the greater superficial petrosal nerve in the middle cranial fossa approach should be treated with high-dose oral steroids. CSF leaks should be treated with bed rest, stool softeners, and lumbar drain; surgical intervention may be necessary if CSF leak persists.

◆ Outcome and Follow-Up

Most patients demonstrate improvement in autophony, conductive hearing loss, and dizziness. Vestibular therapy can be helpful postoperatively. Postoperative hearing testing is obtained several weeks after surgery. If symptoms return, reimaging and repeat VEMP testing should be considered.

3.10 Otologic Manifestations of Systemic Diseases

◆ Key Features

- Many systemic diseases may affect the vestibulocochlear system.
- Otologic manifestations can be the presenting signs of systemic disease.
- A high index of suspicion is required when evaluating otologic complaints.

A diverse group of systemic diseases affect the ear and produce otologic complaints. These conditions can be broadly characterized as infectious/granulomatous, autoimmune, neoplastic, metabolic, disorders of bone, and immunodeficiencies. Otologic manifestations can be part of the disease progression or the initial findings that can herald a diagnosis. A high index of suspicion is required, therefore, when investigating a patient's otologic complaints.

◆ Infectious/Granulomatous Processes

Tuberculosis

- *Mycobacterium tuberculosis* via blood vessels, lymphatic vessels, or direct through the auditory (eustachian) tube
- Chronic otorrhea, tympanic membrane (TM) perforations, granulation in middle ear, bone sequestra
- Diagnosis: acid-fast stain of exudates, culture (negative in 70%), polymerase chain reaction
- Treatment: standard antituberculosis therapies, surgery for refractory cases

Syphilis

- Spirochetal infection, *Treponema pallidum*, congenital and acquired forms
- Ossicular/temporal bone osteitis in latent syphilis
- Hearing loss abrupt, bilateral, and progressive in secondary/tertiary syphilis
- Granulomatous lesions (gummas) affect middle ear and cause TM perforation
- Treatment: benzathine penicillin 2.4 million units every week for 6 to 12 weeks, prednisone 60 mg every other day for 3 to 6 months, tapered slowly

Lyme Disease

- Spirochetal infection, *Borrelia burgdorferi*, transmitted by ticks
- Facial paralysis (especially bilateral), tinnitus, sensorineural hearing loss (SNHL), otalgia, vertigo
- Treatment: doxycycline 100 mg orally every day for 14 to 21 days

Mumps

- Paramyxovirus, an RNA virus
- Unilateral, high-frequency hearing loss, tinnitus. Hearing loss is usually permanent, vestibular symptoms resolve over weeks.
- Treatment: nonspecific; steroids may be of some benefit.

Measles (Rubeola)

- Paramyxovirus, an RNA virus
- Bilateral, high-frequency SNHL occurs acutely with onset of rash.
- 50% of patients have improvement in hearing loss.

Sarcoidosis

- Multisystem disorder characterized by noncaseating granulomas
- SNHL, vestibular dysfunction, facial nerve paralysis
- Uveoparotid fever (Heerfordt's syndrome): facial paralysis, parotitis, uveitis, pyrexia
- Treatment: nonspecific, corticosteroids, cytotoxic agents

Wegener's Granulomatosis

- Otologic involvement in 35% of cases, may be the first sign of disease
- Facial/postauricular pain, erythematous auricular swelling
- Otitis media (OM), conductive hearing loss (CHL), SNHL, vertigo, facial paralysis (rare presenting sign)
- Diagnosis: cytoplasmic anti–neutrophil cytoplasmic antibody (c-ANCA) present in 90% of patients with active disease
- Treatment: corticosteroids, cytotoxic agents

Eosinophilic Granuloma

- Also known as Langerhans cell histiocytosis
- Disorders characterized by proliferation of benign histiocytes
- Otologic manifestations in 15 to 61% of cases; may be presenting symptoms
- Otorrhea, postauricular swelling, hearing loss, vertigo, aural polyps, granulation tissue in external auditory canal (EAC), TM perforations
- Predilection for mastoid, erosion of posterior canal, secondary infection
- Treatment: corticosteroids, cytotoxic agents

◆ Autoimmune

Relapsing Polychondritis

- Recurrent inflammation of cartilaginous structures with eventual fibrosis
- Tender, red, edematous auricle with sparing of the lobule and external ear canal
- Diagnosis: mainly clinical, biopsy during acute phase is avoided
- Treatment: corticosteroids

Chronic Discoid Lupus Erythematosus

- Limited to skin of head, neck, and chest in 90% of cases
- Well-circumscribed, raised lesions on auricle that are pruritic and slowly enlarge
- Treatment: nonspecific, corticosteroids, immunosuppressants, antimalarial drugs

Polyarteritis Nodosa

- Necrotizing vasculitis of small and medium-diameter arteries
- CHL, SNHL, occasional facial paralysis with hearing loss
- Treatment: corticosteroids, cyclophosphamide

Rheumatoid Arthritis

- Affects ossicular articulations causing CHL
- Treatment: nonsteroidal anti-inflammatory drugs (NSAIDs), glucocorticoids, immunosuppressive therapy

◆ Neoplastic

Multiple Myeloma

- Malignancy of plasma cells, B cell derivatives
- Temporal bone frequently involved, may be only manifestation (plasmacytoma)
- Rounded, lytic lesions of the calvaria and temporal bone

Leukemia

- Leukemic infiltrates affect mastoid, middle ear, petrous apex.
- Hemorrhage can often accompany infiltrates in these areas.
- Sludging of cells in cochlea may cause ischemic hearing loss.

Metastatic Neoplasms

- In decreasing frequency: breast, lung, prostate, skin
- Lesions are usually osteolytic but can also be osteoblastic (e.g., breast, prostate).
- Most commonly involve internal auditory canal and petrous apex

◆ Metabolic Diseases

Gout

- Deposits of monosodium urate crystals in joints and cutaneous structures (tophi)
- Tophaceous deposits in helical rim are classic and are usually asymptomatic.

Ochronosis

- Lack of enzyme: homogentisic acid dehydrogenase
- Deposition of dark pigments in tissues rich in collagen
- Cartilage of ear is affected: blue, mottled brown macules on auricle

Mucopolysaccharidoses

- Characterized by deficiency of enzymes that degrade mucopolysaccharides
- CHL or SNHL (unknown mechanism)
- Auditory tube dysfunction and hypertrophy of middle ear mucosa are seen.

◆ Bone Diseases

Paget's Disease (Osteitis Deformans)

- Osteolytic and osteoblastic changes affecting axial skeleton in older individuals
- Mixed, progressive hearing loss, tinnitus, vestibular dysfunction
- Facial nerve not involved

Osteogenesis Imperfecta

- Genetic disorder of collagen synthesis manifested by fragile bones
- CHL and SNHL
- No correlation between hearing loss and severity or frequency of fractures
- Can mimic otosclerosis

Osteopetrosis

- Characterized by an increased bone density
- Affects the endochondral layer of otic capsule and ossicles; poorly pneumatized mastoid compartment
- Recurrent OM, mixed hearing loss, unilateral or bilateral facial nerve palsies

Fibrous Dysplasia

- Benign, chronic disease characterized by replacement of bone with fibrous tissue
- Temporal bone involvement most common in monostotic form
- Painless swelling in mastoid and squamous portions, narrowing of EAC, CHL
- Treatment is symptomatic.

◆ Immunodeficiencies

Primary/Congenital

- Results in recurrent OM often refractory to medical and surgical therapies
- DiGeorge's syndrome (cellular immunodeficiency) associated with Mondini deformity

Acquired Immunodeficiency Syndrome (AIDS)

- Human immunodeficiency virus (HIV)
- Kaposi sarcoma can affect outer ear.
- *Pneumocystis carinii* can cause middle and external ear disease.
- Otosyphilis, tuberculous otitis, fungal infections, and herpes zoster can also occur.

4 Rhinology

Section Editor

Bradley J. Goldstein

Contributors

David Goldenberg

Bradley J. Goldstein

Devyani Lal

4.0 Anatomy and Physiology of the Nose and Paranasal Sinuses

The external nose consists of the nasal pyramid (frontal process of the maxilla), with the paired nasal bones forming the dorsum and meeting the frontal bone superiorly at the glabella. Inferiorly are the upper lateral cartilages and lower lateral (alar) cartilages, which contribute to the nasal tip and nasal valves (**Fig. 4.1**).

The internal nasal and sinus anatomy is complex and variable. The midline nasal septum is composed of the quadrangular cartilage, the perpendicular plate of the ethmoid bone, the vomer bone, and the palatine bone, with an overlying mucosal covering. There are four paired sinuses: the maxillary sinus, frontal sinus, ethmoidal air cells, and sphenoidal sinus (**Fig. 4.2**). The lateral nasal wall consists of the inferior, middle, and superior conchae (turbinates); below each concha is its corresponding meatus. The nasolacrimal duct opens into the inferior meatus. The frontal and maxillary sinuses and anterior ethmoidal air cells drain via the middle meatus. The posterior ethmoidal air cells drain via the superior meatus. The sphenoidal ostia are near the level of the superior meatus on the anterior wall of the sphenoidal sinus. Clinically, the relation of the paranasal sinuses to adjacent anatomic structures is important, as it relates to the potential for the spread of infection or an iatrogenic injury. Specifically, the ethmoid roof may be an extremely thin bone along the lateral lamella of the cribriform plate and may vary in its height considerably; intracranial contents lie superiorly. The lamina papyracea is, as its name implies, a paper-thin sheet of bone that separates the orbit from the ethmoidal air cells.

The sphenoid sinus is bounded by the internal carotid artery, optic nerves, cavernous sinus, and sella turcica; an overriding posterior ethmoidal (Onodi) cell may risk critical structures. Dehiscence of the bone covering the internal carotid artery within the sphenoidal sinus is relatively common and should be routinely assessed for on a preoperative computed tomography

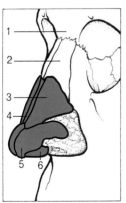

Fig. 4.1 Nasal skeleton. 1. Glabella. 2. Nasal bone. 3. Upper lateral cartilage. 4. Upper edge of the cartilaginous nasal septum. 5. Lower lateral cartilage. 6. Medial crus of lower lateral cartilage. (Used with permission from Becker W, Naumann HH, Pfaltz CR. *Ear, Nose, and Throat Diseases: A Pocket Reference*. 2nd ed. Stuttgart/New York: Thieme; 1994:170.)

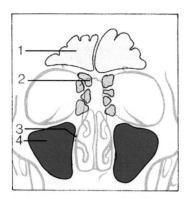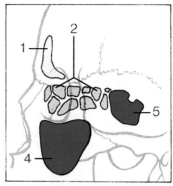

Fig. 4.2 Nasal sinuses: **(a)** frontal section, **(b)** sagittal section. 1. Frontal sinus. 2. Ethmoid sinus. 3. Maxillary ostium. 4. Antral cavity. 5. Sphenoid cavity. (Used with permission from Becker W, Naumann HH, Pfaltz CR. *Ear, Nose, and Throat Diseases: A Pocket Reference.* 2nd ed. Stuttgart/New York: Thieme; 1994:175.)

(CT) scan. The frontal sinus is bounded by the orbit and the anterior cranial fossa and may also be a source of spread of rhinogenic infection. A Haller cell is an anterior ethmoidal cell that pneumatizes laterally at the orbital floor and can contribute to maxillary sinus drainage problems. Agar nasi cells are anterior ethmoidal cells that pneumatize superiorly and can contribute to frontal sinus drainage problems.

◆ Blood Supply

There is abundant external and internal carotid supply (**Fig. 4.3**). Kiesselbach's area (also known as Little's area) of the anterior septum provides superficial anastomoses. External carotid branches supply the nose externally (via the facial artery), and the maxillary artery, including the sphenopalatine artery, does so internally. Internal carotid branches are supplied via the ophthalmic artery to the anterior and posterior ethmoidal arteries. Venous drainage occurs via facial veins as well as ophthalmic veins, which have valveless intracranial connections to the cavernous sinus and therefore relate to intracranial hematogenous spread of infection. Epistaxis (nosebleed) is discussed in **Chapter 4.1.5**.

◆ Innervation

General sensory supply is via the first and second divisions of the trigeminal nerve, cranial nerve (CN) V. Importantly, the nasal tip is supplied via CN V_1 (the first, ophthalmic, division of the trigeminal nerve). Thus, if possible herpetic lesions involve the nasal tip, ophthalmologic evaluation is indicated to rule out herpes zoster of the eye. Special sensory supply is via the olfactory (first cranial) nerve. Complex autonomic innervation is supplied to mucosa via the pterygopalatine ganglion, regulating vasomotor tone and secretion. The vidian nerve (nerve of the pterygoid canal) contains preganglionic

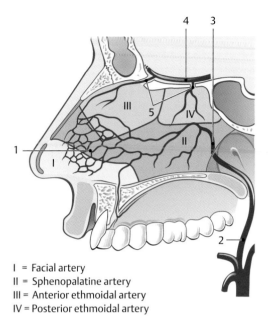

I   = Facial artery
II = Sphenopalatine artery
III = Anterior ethmoidal artery
IV = Posterior ethmoidal artery

Fig. 4.3   Vasculature of the nasal cavity. 1. Kiesselbach's area. 2. Internal maxillary artery. 3. Sphenopalatine artery. 4. Ophthalmic artery. 5. Anterior and posterior ethmoid arteries. I–IV: areas supplied by arteries to the nose. (Used with permission from Behrbohm H et al. *Ear, Nose, and Throat Diseases: With Head and Neck Surgery*. 3rd ed. Stuttgart/New York: Thieme; 2009:122.)

parasympathetic fibers from the greater superficial petrosal nerve (from the facial nerve, CN VII) and sympathetic fibers from the deep petrosal nerve (from the superior cervical ganglion) and synapses at the pterygopalatine ganglion prior to innervating the sinonasal mucosa.

◆ Physiology

Table 4.1 gives a summary of tests for the assessment of sinonasal physiology. Warming and humidification of inspired air, olfactory function, and immune function all are aspects of nasal physiology. The nose and paranasal sinuses play a role in host defenses. In general, mucociliary clearance is a key feature. Specific factors such as secretory immunoglobulin A (IgA), lactoferrin, lysozyme, cytokines, and the complex regulation of cells that mediate immunity are critical to the maintenance of normal sinus function. A detailed discussion of sinonasal physiology is beyond the scope of this book. The presence of infection, inflammation, allergy, neoplasm, or traumatic, iatrogenic, or congenital deformity may all perturb sinonasal physiology and must be considered in the evaluation of the patient with complaints related to the nose.

Table 4.1 Summary of tests for factors affecting sinonasal physiology

Lab test	Utility (tests for)
RPR; FTA-ABS	Syphilis
c-ANCA	Wegener's disease
ACE	Sarcoidosis
ANA	Autoimmune disease
ESR	Inflammation
Cultures of sinus drainage	Specific infectious organism
University of Pennsylvania (SIT)	Olfactory function
RAST (blood testing for allergen-specific IgE)	Allergy
Skin testing (prick test; SET)	Allergy
Acoustic rhinometry; rhinomanometry	Nasal obstruction; not currently widely used outside of research settings
Ciliary beat frequency; ciliary electron microscopy	Assess ciliary function and anatomy, e.g., for Kartagener's syndrome; typically tested on adenoid or mucosal biopsy

Abbreviations: ACE, angiotensin-converting enzyme; ANA, antinuclear antibody test; c-ANCA, cytoplasmic anti–neutrophil cytoplasmic antibody; ESR, erythrocyte sedimentation rate; FTA-ABS, fluorescent treponemal antibody absorbed; IgE, immunoglobulin E; RAST, radioallergosorbent test; RPR, rapid plasma reagin; SET, skin end point titration , SIT, smell identification test.

4.1   Rhinologic Emergencies

4.1.1   Acute Invasive Fungal Rhinosinusitis

◆ Key Features

- A rapidly progressive sinonasal fungal infection can be fatal.
- Acute invasive fungal infections occur almost exclusively in immuno-compromised or debilitated patients.
- Successful treatment requires early detection, wide surgical débridement, and correction of the underlying predisposing condition.

In the debilitated patient, certain fungal infections can become angioinvasive with tissue necrosis, cranial nerve involvement, and possible orbital or intracranial extension. The most common organisms are *Mucor* or *Aspergillus* species. High-risk patients include those with neutropenia from any cause (e.g., leukemia, bone marrow transplantation), other oncology patients undergoing chemotherapy, patients undergoing chronic immunosuppressive therapy or corticosteroid use, patients with diabetes mellitus and diabetic ketoacidosis, and patients with acquired immunodeficiency syndrome (AIDS). Acute invasive fungal rhinosinusitis is a distinct and rapidly aggressive disease process that is distinguished by its fulminant course from other forms of fungal sinusitis, such as mycetoma, allergic fungal rhinosinusitis, or chronic invasive (indolent) fungal rhinosinusitis.

◆ Epidemiology

Also known as rhinocerebral mucormycosis, acute invasive fungal rhinosinusitis occurs in the at-risk populations just described: patients with hematologic malignancies, patients post solid organ or bone marrow transplant, patients with diabetes, patients on chronic steroid therapy, neutropenic patients, and patients with AIDS.

◆ Clinical

Signs and Symptoms

A high index of suspicion in any at-risk patient is required, as early diagnosis improves prognosis. A fever of unknown origin should raise suspicion, as should any new sign or symptom of sinonasal disease. Facial edema, periorbital swelling, pain, or numbness are common findings. However, the leukopenic patient may be unable to mount a febrile response. Other findings may include epistaxis, headache, mental status change, or crusting/eschar at the naris that can be mistaken for dried blood. One should consider unilateral cranial neuropathy, acute visual change, or altered ocular motility in an immunocompromised patient to be acute invasive fungal rhinosinusitis until proven otherwise. A black intranasal eschar on exam is considered pathognomonic for invasive *Mucor*.

Differential Diagnosis

A noninvasive sinonasal infection, such as acute bacterial sinusitis, should be considered. An acute bacterial sinusitis complication, such as orbital cellulitis or intracranial suppurative spread, may present similarly. Radiographically similar processes may include squamous cell carcinoma, sinonasal lymphoma, and Wegener's granulomatosis.

◆ Evaluation

See **Fig. 4.4** for a diagnostic and treatment algorithm.

Physical Exam

The patient suspected to have acute invasive fungal rhinosinusitis should be seen without delay. The head and neck examination should focus on cranial nerve function and should include nasal endoscopy. Avoid tetracaine spray or other topical anesthetics. Insensate mucosa noted during an endoscopic exam is consistent with invasive fungal infection. Dark ulcers or pale, insensate mucosa may appear on the septum, conchae, palate, or nasopharynx. Early infection may appear as pale mucosa; the presence of dark eschar has been considered to be pathognomonic. Signs of cavernous sinus thrombosis

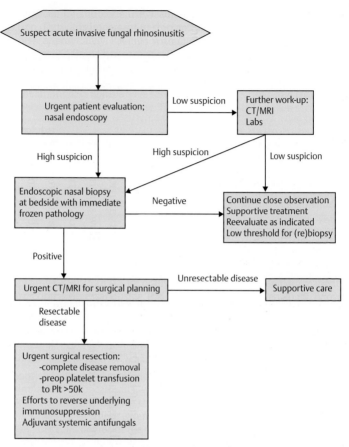

Fig. 4.4 Treatment algorithm for acute invasive fungal rhinosinusitis. Note that there should be a very low threshold to proceed with biopsy, as rapid diagnosis and treatment are critical to patient survival. CT, computed tomography; MRI, magnetic resonance imaging.

include ophthalmoplegia, exophthalmos, and decreased papillary responses. Biopsy of suspicious areas such as the middle concha or septal mucosa is required for diagnosis. It is important to obtain actual tissue at biopsy, not just overlying eschar or necrotic debris. These specimens should be sent fresh for immediate frozen-section analysis as well as silver stain. Patients may be thrombocytopenic, and although a low platelet count may lead to profuse bleeding after biopsy, the risk of this must be balanced with the high mortality associated with a delay in diagnosis. If necessary, platelet transfusion should be ordered early. As a rule, a platelet count of 50,000 is desired. Acceptable hemostasis can usually be obtained with chemical cautery and Avitene (Davol, Inc., Cranston, RI), Gelfoam (Pfizer Pharmaceuticals, New York, NY), or other hemostatic packing.

Imaging

Computed tomography (CT) findings may be nonspecific. However, the presence of bone erosion and adjacent soft tissue edema on contrast enhanced maxillofacial CT strongly suggests the diagnosis if clinical correlation is present. Unilateral edema of the nasal mucosa has also been associated with invasive fungal sinusitis, as well as obliteration of the retroantral fat planes. Both soft tissue and bone windows, as well as high-resolution axial and coronal views, are necessary. Magnetic resonance imaging (MRI) is useful for evaluating intracranial extension and extension beyond the paranasal sinuses.

Labs

Cultures are inadequate and play no role in the initial diagnosis and management of suspected acute invasive fungal rhinosinusitis. Positive culture results will most likely be available late in the course of the disease. Useful labs for assessing risk factors include a complete blood count (CBC), absolute neutrophil count, chemistries, blood glucose and hemoglobin A1C (HbA1c) in diabetics, and human immunodeficiency virus (HIV) testing with CD4 lymphocyte counts and viral load in AIDS patients.

Pathology

Biopsy of the middle concha or other suspicious lesions with immediate frozen-section analysis is the gold standard test to confirm the presence of tissue-invasive fungus. *Mucor* is identifiable within the mucosa as large, irregularly shaped nonseptate hyphae that branch at right angles. *Aspergillus* is identifiable as smaller hyphae that are septate and that branch at 45° angles. Methenamine silver stain is performed to confirm the diagnosis; however, these results may not be available for several hours.

◆ Treatment Options

This is a surgical emergency: complete surgical resection and the reversal of underlying immune dysfunction are critical. The diabetic patient can be successfully treated with early diagnosis, insulin drip, and wide surgical resection. In the oncology patient, if neutropenia cannot be reversed, mortality is high. Granulocyte-macrophage colony-stimulating factor (GM-CSF) may be useful. Surgical goal is resection of all involved tissue. This may be accomplished endoscopically in select cases. However, an extended total maxillectomy with orbital exenteration may be necessary in advanced disease. Systemic antifungals as well as intranasal nebulized amphotericin are administered, but these should be considered adjuvant therapy.

◆ Outcome and Follow-Up

Prognosis is very poor with intracranial involvement. A bone marrow transplant patient with uncorrectable neutropenia has a poor prognosis. Overall survival in diabetic patients may approach 80% if ketoacidosis is corrected.

4.1.2 Orbital Complications of Sinusitis

◆ Key Features

- Sinusitis is a common cause of orbital infection.
- Significant morbidity and even mortality can result.
- Orbital extension of sinusitis is most common in pediatric patients.
- Combined otolaryngology and ophthalmology care is required.

Orbital extension of sinonasal disease requires immediate attention, as rapid progression and blindness may occur. Anatomically, the orbit is bounded by all paranasal sinuses, and infection may spread to the orbit directly or via retrograde thrombophlebitis. The Chandler classification system is heuristically useful in staging and managing orbital complications of sinusitis (**Table 4.2**). Hospital admission and intravenous antibiotic therapy are required for treatment; surgical drainage is necessary in the event of abscess formation, vision compromise, or lack of improvement with medical therapy.

◆ Epidemiology

Orbital complications occur in ~3% of sinusitis cases. These are most common in children but can occur at any age. Subperiosteal abscess is present in ~20% of cases of orbital extension of sinusitis. Cavernous sinus thrombosis is rare. Immunosuppressed patients are at increased risk and require aggressive treatment.

◆ Clinical

Signs and Symptoms

The most common findings are orbital edema, pain, proptosis, and fever. Orbital disease may be the first sign of sinusitis in children. In more advanced cases, there may be gaze restriction and visual acuity change.

Differential Diagnosis

In the pediatric age group, orbital pseudotumor consists of painful proptosis without a fever or leukocytosis. Orbital rhabdomyosarcoma may present with inflammatory changes in 25% of patients. An ethmoid mucocele may

Table 4.2 Chandler Classification

Stage	Description
I	Preseptal cellulitis
II	Orbital cellulitis
III	Subperiosteal abscess
IV	Orbital abscess
V	Cavernous sinus septic thrombosis

present with proptosis, and CT will reveal an expanded sinus in this instance. Other sinonasal causes of proptosis or orbital edema include allergic fungal rhinosinusitis and neoplasm as well as iatrogenic injury. Abnormal thyroid state may cause ophthalmopathy.

◆ Evaluation

Physical Exam

Examination requires the combined input of the otolaryngologist and the ophthalmologist. In general, the patient will have a history of preceding sinusitis or current complaints consistent with acute sinusitis. Fever is usually present. Head and neck exam reveals lid or periorbital edema, erythema, and tenderness. In cases of preseptal (periorbital) cellulitis, the remainder of the eye exam is normal. The presence of proptosis, chemosis, extraocular muscle limitation, diplopia, or decreased visual acuity suggests orbital cellulitis or subperiosteal abscess. With cavernous thrombosis or intracranial extension, findings may include a frozen globe (ophthalmoplegia), papilledema, blindness, meningeal signs, or neurologic deficits secondary to brain abscess or cerebritis. Superior orbital fissure syndrome is a symptom complex consisting of retroorbital pain, paralysis of extraocular muscles, and impairment of first trigeminal branches. This is most often a result of trauma involving fracture at the superior orbital fissure, but dysfunction of these structures can arise secondary to compression. Orbital apex syndrome adds involvement of the optic nerve.

Imaging

Contrast-enhanced computed tomography (CT) scanning with coronal and axial views is the imaging study of choice if there is any suspicion of postseptal involvement (i.e., other than simple periorbital cellulitis). A subperiosteal abscess is identifiable as a lentiform, rim-enhancing hypodense collection in the medial orbit with adjacent sinusitis. The medial rectus is displaced. In the absence of abscess formation, there may be orbital fat stranding, solid enhancing phlegmon, or swollen and enhancing extraocular muscles, consistent with orbital cellulitis. A lid abscess may be present, less commonly. Suspicion of cavernous sinus thrombosis is better evaluated with magnetic resonance imaging (MRI).

Labs

A complete blood count (CBC) with differential may be useful. Preoperative labs should be ordered as indicated.

Pathology

In younger children, microbiology often consists of single aerobic species including alpha *Streptococcus*, *Haemophilus influenzae*, or coagulase-positive *Staphylococcus*. In those over 10 years old, organisms are often mixed and may include anaerobes.

◆ Treatment Options

Medical

All patients should be admitted and treated with serial ophthalmologic exams and intravenous (IV) antibiotics that have good cerebrospinal fluid (CSF) penetration. Generally, a third-generation cephalosporin is used. Oxacillin is often used in children. Older patients are often double-covered with clindamycin for anaerobes. Alternatives include ampicillin/sulbactam, vancomycin, or aztreonam. Antibiotics are adjusted according to cultures, if possible. Systemic steroids are not recommended. Topical nasal vasoconstrictors are useful (i.e., oxymetazoline).

Surgical

A majority of patients with orbital complications require surgery. This is an area of some controversy. Clearly, surgical drainage is required urgently for abscess formation or decreased visual acuity. If the clinical setting allows for close follow-up (i.e., frequent serial ophthalmologic assessment), many clinicians will observe certain cases of preseptal or early postseptal cellulitis. If there is any progression or lack of resolution with medical therapy over 48 hours, surgery is recommended. Surgical drainage may be accomplished endoscopically by experienced surgeons; however, consent for an external ethmoidectomy approach is recommended. Also, the location of certain abscesses may be amenable to external drainage by ophthalmologist. Regardless of approach, the abscess should be drained and the underlying sinus disease should be addressed. For cavernous thrombosis, involved sinuses, including the sphenoid, must be drained; systemic anticoagulation remains controversial.

◆ Outcome and Follow-Up

The natural history of untreated disease (all stages) results in blindness in at least 10%. Most cases of Chandler stage I–IV disease recover well with treatment. There remains up to an 80% mortality rate with cavernous sinus involvement, although new literature reports suggest this figure is high.

4.1.3   Intracranial Complications of Sinusitis

◆ Key Features

- Intracranial complications due to sinusitis are a life-threatening emergency.
- Management requires a multidisciplinary approach including neurosurgical consultation.
- Complications include meningitis, dural sinus thrombosis, and intracranial abscess.

Sinusitis may result in spread of infection intracranially. Extension may occur via osteomyelitic bone, trauma, or venous channels. The frontal sinus is commonly the source, although ethmoid or sphenoid sinusitis can lead to intracranial spread. Complications include meningitis, epidural abscess, subdural abscess, parenchymal brain abscess, and cavernous sinus thrombophlebitis.

◆ Epidemiology

Since the advent of antibiotics, the incidence has decreased dramatically. Currently, probably fewer than 1% of sinusitis cases are complicated by intracranial spread of infection.

◆ Clinical

Signs and Symptoms

The patient with meningitis of a rhinologic origin will manifest signs and symptoms typical of bacterial meningitis. These include high fever, photophobia, nausea and emesis, mental status change, nuchal rigidity, and pulse and blood pressure changes. However, epidural or subdural abscess without meningitis may be more subtle. Fever and headache may be present but are nonspecific. Usually focal signs are absent. Meningeal signs may develop gradually. A parenchymal brain abscess of rhinologic origin (frontal lobe abscess) may initially result in few signs or symptoms. However, this may progress from headache to signs of increased intracranial pressure, vomiting, papilledema, confusion, somnolence, bradycardia, and coma. Cavernous sinus thrombophlebitis results in spiking fevers, chills, proptosis, chemosis, decreased visual acuity and blindness, and extraocular muscle paresis. Infection can rapidly spread to the contralateral cavernous sinus via venous communications.

Differential Diagnosis

Meningitis of nonrhinologic origin must be considered. The incidental finding of paranasal sinus disease on imaging does not necessarily signify a causal relationship.

◆ Evaluation

Pathogenesis may involve several mechanisms. Extension may occur via osteomyelitic bone. Also, traumatic bone disruption may allow communication of infected sinus contents with dura, for example, after posterior table fracture of the frontal sinus. Also, infection may propagate via venous channels in bone or retrograde venous circulation to the cavernous sinus. General hematogenous spread is possible, especially in a severely immunocompromised host.

Physical Exam

Complete head and neck exam is required with careful assessment of all cranial nerves. Nasal endoscopy may reveal active sinonasal disease and provide mucopus for culture and sensitivities. A neurologic exam including orientation to person, place, and date will reveal any focal deficits and serve as a useful baseline to monitor for any deterioration. The presence of ocular findings or neurologic deficit should prompt ophthalmologic and neurosurgical consultations.

Imaging

Both computed tomography (CT) and magnetic resonance imaging (MRI) are usually obtained. Contrast-enhanced CT scanning will provide detail regarding paranasal sinus disease and will reveal evidence of bony dehiscence that may underlie intracranial spread of infection. Intravenous contrast will reveal an enhancing abscess. Gadolinium-enhanced MRI will provide a more sensitive assessment of dural enhancement and intracranial disease but lacks the bony detail necessary for planning sinus surgery.

Lumbar Puncture

Obtain cerebrospinal fluid (CSF) via lumbar puncture (LP) in the patient with possible meningitis, after obtaining a CT scan. There is a risk of acute tonsillar herniation following LP, almost always seen in patients with a noninfectious intracranial process causing a mass effect with localizing signs and papilledema. See **Table 4.3** for interpretation of CSF values. Cell count (tube 3), protein and glucose (tube 2), and Gram stain with culture and sensitivities (tube 1) are ordered. Cultures with sensitivity will guide antibiotic therapy.

Labs

In addition to CSF studies, other useful labs include blood cultures, complete blood count (CBC) with differential, chemistries, prothrombin time (PT), and partial thromboplastin time (PTT).

◆ Treatment Options

Medical

IV high-dose antibiotics are empirically started following LP and adjusted based on cultures. Broad-spectrum agents with good CSF penetration are

Table 4.3   Interpretation of cerebrospinal fluid findings

	Opening pressure (cm H_2O)	Appearance	Cells (per mL)	Protein (mg %)	Glucose (% serum)
Normal	7–18	Clear	0 PMNs 0 RBCs 0–5 monocytes	15–45	50
Acute purulent meningitis	Often elevated	Turbid	Few–20k (WBCs mostly PMNs)	100–1,000	< 20
Viral meningitis, encephalitis	Normal	Normal	Few–350 WBCs (mostly monocytes)	40–100	Normal

Abbreviations: PMNs, polymorphonuclear cells; RBCs, red blood cells; WBCs, white blood cells.

utilized, such as ceftriaxone or cefepime. Vancomycin is often added for double coverage and for possible methicillin resistance. Peak and trough levels must be monitored when vancomycin is used. The role of anticoagulation for cavernous thrombophlebitis remains controversial. Anticoagulation may interfere with the ability to perform intracranial pressure monitoring or craniotomy.

Surgical

The underlying sinus infection is drained by either endoscopic or open approach. If an intracranial abscess is present, it is drained by the neurosurgeon in conjunction with sinus drainage.

◆ Outcome and Follow-Up

Close observation in an intensive care unit (ICU) setting with serial neurologic exams is required postoperatively. Intracranial pressure monitoring may be required.

4.1.4 Cerebrospinal Fluid Rhinorrhea

◆ Key Features

- Cerebrospinal fluid (CSF) rhinorrhea may occur due to iatrogenic injury to the ethmoid roof or cribriform during sinus surgery, or it can be present as "spontaneous leak" due to increased intracranial pressure.
- Thin-cut computed tomography (CT) scan and β-2 transferrin assay are the most useful studies for evaluation, along with magnetic resonance imaging (MRI) for certain cases.
- The skull base can be repaired with endoscopic instruments from below or via neurosurgical approach from above.

Anterior skull base disruption can result in drainage of CSF via the nose. The underlying problem may be the result of trauma, iatrogenic injury, or congenital anomaly, or it may arise spontaneously (often seen with obesity). The management of CSF rhinorrhea related to skull base injury from endoscopic sinus surgery is highlighted. CSF leak from the temporal bone may present with rhinorrhea via the middle ear and auditory (eustachian) tube.

◆ Epidemiology

Although the exact incidence of complications is unclear currently, previous estimates suggest a ~0.5% rate of skull base injury with CSF leak following ethmoid surgery. Rising obesity incidence has resulted in increased recognition of "spontaneous" leak.

◆ Clinical

Signs and Symptoms

Patients present with watery rhinorrhea. Often, the drainage can be provoked by leaning the patient forward with the head lowered. Typically, the drainage has a salty or metallic taste. Headache may be reported. Anosmia and nasal congestion may accompany iatrogenic skull base injury with encephalocele.

Differential Diagnosis

The consideration for watery or clear rhinorrhea includes various forms of rhinitis versus CSF drainage. Vasomotor rhinitis typically is elicited by cold temperatures, physical activity, or other specific stimuli such as eating.

◆ Evaluation

History

The approach to the patient typically begins with a thorough history. A source of skull base damage may, of course, be quite obvious if there was a suspected iatrogenic injury during preceding endoscopic ethmoid surgery. One should note if the drainage is unilateral as well as its duration and severity. Associated complaints such as headache, visual disturbance, epistaxis, and anosmia should be noted. Details of any previous sinonasal surgery, neurosurgery, otologic surgery, or trauma are important. Any previous imaging studies of the head should be obtained, if possible. Previous history of meningitis should be sought. General past history, medication list, social and family history are obtained.

Physical Exam

A complete head and neck exam is performed. Cranial nerves (CNs) I to XII should be tested. A standard test for olfactory function such as the Smell Identification Test (SIT; Sensonics, Inc., Haddon Heights, NJ) is recommended, to document olfactory function prior to treatment. Nasal endoscopy is performed. A 4-mm rigid 30° endoscope is ideal. Drainage, masses, edema, purulence, and prior surgical changes are noted. If the injury is iatrogenic, it may be possible to assess the location and size of the skull base defect. Superior-based soft tissue mass should raise suspicion for encephalocele. Having the patient perform the Valsalva maneuver may result in visible enlargement of a meningocele or encephalocele.

Imaging

Identification of the site of leak may be straightforward or may be difficult. For a known iatrogenic injury, thin-cut axial CT with coronal views will typically verify the site of injury along the ethmoid roof or cribriform plate. Scanning with an image-guidance protocol may be helpful, by permitting the use of computer-assisted surgical navigation for endoscopic repair. For other situations, high-resolution CT is useful to study the bony detail of the anterior skull base and sphenoids. A bony dehiscence may be evident. For a patient presenting with a soft tissue mass, MRI is the study of choice to assess for possible meningocele or encephalocele, or for cerebritis.

Labs

If rhinorrhea fluid can be collected, this should be sent for β-2 transferrin assay. Usually, approximately 1 mL is required; the laboratory may require refrigeration or rapid handling of the specimen. The presence of β-2 transferrin suggests strongly that the fluid is indeed CSF.

Other Tests

See **Table 4.4** for a summary of available studies.

MR Cisternogram

Magnetic resonance (MR) cisternogram with intrathecal gadolinium can be highly useful for difficult-to-diagnose leaks, such as those in obese spontaneous-leak patients (idiopathic intracranial hypertension) who may have multiple sites of subtle skull base dehiscence, or patients with prior skull base surgery.

Radioactive Pledget Scanning

This study can be done to help confirm and localize the side of a leak site, although is rarely performed at present because of the success of thin-cut CT at identifying site of leak.

Intrathecal Fluorescein

The use of a dye to visualize the CSF leakage endoscopically is extremely helpful, both for endoscopic diagnosis and at the time of repair. For the procedure, a lumbar drain is placed and 10 mL of the patient's CSF is collected, after which 0.1 mL of 10% IV fluorescein is diluted into the 10 mL CSF sample. This is slowly reinjected intrathecally over 5 minutes. The fluorescein causes active CSF leakage to appear greenish endoscopically. Intrathecal fluorescein can cause seizures at higher dosage; however, the protocol described here is widely accepted as safe.

Table 4.4 Diagnostic studies for suspected cerebrospinal fluid (CSF) rhinorrhea

Study	Role
β-2 transferrin assay	Confirm that drainage is CSF
CT scan, thin cut	Assess bony detail of anterior skull base/identify site of leak; assess for intracranial hematoma or pneumocephalus following iatrogenic injury
MR cisternogram	Identify site(s) of leak, if difficult to identify
Radioactive pledget scanning	Confirm presence of CSF leak, provide localizing information
Intrathecal fluorescein	Localize site of leak during nasal endoscopy/endoscopic repair
MRI scan	Assess for anterior skull base encephalocele, meningocele, neoplasm

Abbreviations: CT, computed tomography; MR, magnetic resonance; MRI, magnetic resonance imaging.

◆ Treatment Options

Skull base disruption causing CSF rhinorrhea is managed with surgical repair. Repair of acute iatrogenic injury is discussed separately from other cases.

Repair of Acute Iatrogenic Injury

If the ethmoid roof is injured during sinus surgery, it may be possible to repair the injury. If there is extensive injury, severe bleeding, or obvious intradural injury, it is highly recommended that neurosurgical consultation be obtained, if possible. Concomitant injury to the anterior ethmoid artery can occur, so the orbit should be assessed for lid edema, ecchymosis, and proptosis. If this occurs, medial wall decompression and/or lateral canthotomy, IV mannitol, and IV steroids may be required. To repair the skull base defect, good visualization is required. Mucosa adjacent to the leak site is gently reflected away. Several graft materials have been described. Acellular dermis is widely used (e.g., AlloDerm [LifeCell Corp., Branchburg, NJ]); others prefer a bone graft placed intracranially, especially if the defect is larger than ~0.5 cm. For this graft, a portion of turbinate (nasal conchal) bone is ideal. After the acellular dermis or bone is placed on the intracranial side of the defect, fibrin glue (or similar material) and fascia or other soft tissue is layered on the nasal side of the defect, followed by several layers of absorbable packing material such as Gelfoam (Pfizer, Inc., New York, NY). Large defects may benefit from a pedicled mucosal flap. It is helpful if the patient can emerge from anesthesia smoothly, without "bucking" and straining, and without the need for high-pressure bag-mask ventilation following extubation, to minimize chances of causing pneumocephalus. Postoperatively, once the patient is stable, a head CT is recommended to evaluate for intracranial hematoma or pneumocephalus. If the scan reveals hematoma or significant pneumocephalus, neurosurgical consultation is necessary. Otherwise, postoperative management should include head of bed elevation, bed rest for 2 to 3 days, and stool softeners. Most surgeons recommend antibiotic prophylaxis with Ancef (GlaxoSmithKline, Brentford, Middlesex, UK) or clindamycin. The use of a lumbar drain is debated. For a large defect, lumbar drainage to reduce CSF pressure for 3 days can be helpful.

Elective Repair of Other Anterior Skull Base CSF Leaks

The management is individualized. Depending on surgeon experience, many ethmoid or sphenoid sinus leaks can be approached endoscopically. Intrathecal fluorescein used intraoperatively is very helpful; the lumbar drain may be used postoperatively to reduce CSF pressure. In other cases, neurosurgical colleagues may approach the skull base defect from above; a pericranial flap can be used to close the defect.

◆ Outcome and Follow-Up

Repair of anterior skull base CSF leaks has a good success rate. Complications can include repeat leakage, infection including meningitis or abscess, encephalocele, anosmia, postoperative intracranial bleeding, or pneumocephalus.

4.1.5 Epistaxis

♦ Key Features

- Management of epistaxis, as for other emergency situations, should begin with ABCs (airway, breathing, circulation) and follow standard protocols for resuscitation and treatment.
- Address predisposing conditions.
- Accurate localization of bleeding site is required for treatment.

The word "epistaxis" derives from the Greek *epi,* meaning on, and *stazo,* to fall in drops. A nosebleed may present as anterior (bleeding from the nostril), posterior (blood present in the posterior pharynx), or both. Accurate localization of the bleeding site is the key to treatment. It is estimated that > 90% of epistaxis cases arise from the anterior nasal septum at Kiesselbach's area (**Fig. 4.3**). However, the nasal blood supply involves both the internal and external carotid systems, and brisk bleeding can arise posteriorly. Major vessels include the anterior ethmoidal, posterior ethmoidal, sphenopalatine, greater palatine, and superior labial arteries.

♦ Epidemiology

Most nosebleeds are self-limited, not requiring medical intervention. An estimated 45 million Americans suffer from at least minor epistaxis. In children, nearly all cases are anterior, often due to digital trauma. Over age 40, the incidence of posterior bleeds rises.

♦ Clinical

Signs and Symptoms

Patients will report bleeding from the nares or the mouth. There may be an obvious antecedent nasal trauma, surgery, or foreign body reported. Hematemesis is common. On exam, blood may be fresh or clotted.

Differential Diagnosis

The existence of epistaxis is established on history and exam. A variety of underlying local and systemic conditions should be considered (**Table 4.5**). Most important to exclude is a neoplasm presenting with epistaxis. Consider juvenile nasopharyngeal angiofibroma in any teenage male with a unilateral sinonasal mass and epistaxis.

♦ Evaluation

History

In most cases, the approach to the patient begins with a thorough history. The exception to this rule is the patient with severe active bleeding or

Table 4.5 Causes of epistaxis

Trauma	Maxillofacial fractures Foreign body Nose picking
Neoplasm	Juvenile nasopharyngeal angiofibroma Squamous cell carcinoma Inverted papilloma Mucosal melanoma Other
Systemic disease	Hereditary hemorrhagic telangiectasia (Osler-Weber-Rendu disease) Wegener's granulomatosis Sarcoid Coagulopathies Thrombocytopenia
Drugs	Chemotherapy Warfarin, aspirin, clopidogrel, etc. Intranasal illicit drug use
Infection	Tuberculosis, syphilis, rhinoscleroma, viral Other

hemodynamic instability that must first be corrected. Important historical information should include how long nosebleeds have been occurring, their frequency, whether bleeding is typically left- or right-sided and whether it is typically anterior or posterior, how long nosebleeds last, and whether packing or cauterization has ever been required. Note any previous nasal or sinus surgeries. If recent sinonasal surgery has occurred, obtaining operative notes may be helpful. General information that is relevant includes a prior history of easy bruising or bleeding; a family history of such problems or known bleeding disorder; bleeding problems with previous surgeries or dental work; history of anemia, malignancy, leukemia, lymphoma, or chemotherapy; other systemic illnesses; or recent trauma. A complete, accurate medication list is needed. Specific attention is directed at any recent use of medications that can promote bleeding, such as aspirin, other nonsteroidal anti-inflammatory drugs (NSAIDs), warfarin, or clopidogrel (Plavix; Bristol-Myers Squibb, New York, NY). Also consider vitamins such as vitamin E and other supplements or herbs, many of which can promote bleeding. Social history is needed. Chronic alcohol abuse can be related to coagulation disorders from impaired liver synthetic function as well as malnutrition and vitamin deficiencies; illicit intranasal drug use may be causative. In summary, awareness and treatment of systemic conditions may be required to obtain definitive, effective management of epistaxis.

Physical Exam

Priorities with any severe epistaxis must focus on the ABCs and on resuscitation. The key to effective treatment is localization of the bleeding source. The head and neck exam should therefore focus on this goal. It is essential to have a nasal speculum and headlight, Frazier tip suctions, and oxymetazoline

(Afrin; Schering-Plough Healthcare Products Inc., Memphis, TN) or phenyl-ephrine (Neo Synephrine; Bayer Consumer Health, Morristown, NJ) spray (for decongestion and hemostasis). Topical 2% Pontocaine can be used for intranasal anesthetic, if needed. If topical 4% cocaine is available, this is a very effective decongestant and anesthetic, used sparingly. The availability of a 4-mm rigid nasal telescope (e.g., Karl Storz 7200B; Karl Storz, GmbH, Tuttlingen, Germany) and light source is ideal, especially to localize a posterior bleed. Often, the otolaryngologist will first need to remove improperly placed or ineffective packing materials. Removal of clots with suction will facilitate identification of bleeding sites, using the equipment just described.

Imaging

Profuse bleeding in a maxillofacial trauma patient should be managed with emergent angiography. An injury to the extradural portion of the internal carotid cannot be controlled with nasal packs; most of these injuries probably exsanguinate in the field. Also, in recurrent or difficult-to-treat epistaxis, angiography may be diagnostic (to localize a bleeding source and guide definitive therapy such as ethmoidal artery ligation) or therapeutic (to embolize an external carotid source).

Identification of an intranasal mass on exam should prompt computed tomography (CT) or magnetic resonance imaging (MRI) to evaluate a possible sinonasal neoplasm or inflammatory disease fully, prior to definitive therapy. However, this should not delay acute treatment of active epistaxis.

Labs

Blood work should include hemoglobin, hematocrit, platelet count, prothrombin time (PT) and partial thromboplastin time (PTT), as well as blood type and screening tests. Bear in mind that hemo-concentration in the under-resuscitated patient may yield laboratory results that do not initially reflect the degree of blood loss. Platelet function studies may be helpful, although results may not be rapidly available. Platelet dysfunction is seen with NSAID use and von Willebrand's disease.

◆ Treatment Options

A patient presenting to the emergency department with severe epistaxis or any suspicion of hypovolemia should have IV access, continuous cardiac monitoring, and aggressive fluid resuscitation.

Generalizations

Correction of severe clotting disturbances will facilitate the efficacy of local therapy for epistaxis (i.e., reversal of over-warfarinization with fresh frozen plasma [FFP] or IV vitamin K; platelet transfusion in the thrombocytopenic oncology patient). Spontaneous mucosal bleeding typically occurs in patients with platelet counts < 20,000. Control of hypertension is essential. Patients with underlying renal failure may need DDAVP (desamino-D-arginine vasopressin) to correct coagulopathy from underlying uremic platelet dysfunction. Some forms of von Willebrand's disease also respond to DDAVP or desmopressin.

Specifics

Localize the source, as previously described, using oxymetazoline spray, suction, a nasal speculum, and/or nasal endoscopy. Avoid removable packing unless other methods are ineffective. Most bleeds are anterior and can be treated effectively with topical vasoconstrictors and direct pressure and/or simple silver nitrate cautery sticks. A small piece of Gelfoam (Pfizer, Inc., New York, NY) or Surgicel (Johnson & Johnson, New Brunswick, NJ) placed over the cauterized area is helpful. If bleeding will not respond to this, nasal packing to place pressure over the bleeding site may be required. Gelfoam, Surgicel, with or without topical thrombin, or Floseal (Baxter, Deerfield, IL) are among the absorbable products available that will not require removal but will dissolve with nasal saline administration. Intranasal salt pork is a highly effective packing material.

For refractory bleeding, removable packing is placed. Many types are available, such as Merocel (Medtronic XOMED, Inc., Jacksonville, FL) sponges. Rapid Rhino (Brussels, Belgium) products, which are covered with a procoagulant and contain an inflatable balloon, are also effective. Experience has shown that an effective removable pack should be left in place about 4 days to enable healing prior to removal. Any patient with packing in the nose should be placed on systemic antibiotics with good gram-positive coverage, such as cephalexin or clindamycin, for prophylaxis against toxic shock syndrome. In the rare situation in which properly placed nasal packing results in ongoing hemorrhage via the posterior nares, an Epistat (Medtronic XOMED, Inc., Jacksonville, FL) balloon pack (or similar device) is very effective. This device has a balloon that is inflated in the nasopharynx and a second balloon that provides pressure intranasally, and it effectively tamponades a posterior bleeding vessel.

Other formal posterior packing techniques and devices are available as well. A patient with a formal posterior pack requires hospital admission with continuous pulse oximetry. A patient failing or rebleeding following these maneuvers is usually sent for angiography and possible embolization. If unavailable, and/or the surgeon is confident that the feeding vessel is identifiable, clipping or cauterization of the sphenopalatine artery can be performed endoscopically; ligation of the internal maxillary system can be performed via a Caldwell-Luc approach and takedown of the posterior wall of the maxillary sinus; or anterior or posterior ethmoidal artery ligation can be performed via an external incision. Recall the 24–12–6 mm rule to locate the anterior ethmoidal foramen, posterior ethmoidal foramen, and optic nerve canal along the orbital wall; however, there is substantial variation with these measurements.

Other Treatments

Therapy for the Osler-Weber-Rendu patient is a challenge. One should rule out pulmonary or intracranial vascular malformations, which may be life-threatening, with appropriate imaging. Avoid packing. Laser [Nd:YAG (neodymium:yttrium-aluminum-garnet), argon, KTP (potassium titanyl phosphate)] treatments at 1024 nm have been effective. Septodermoplasty remains an option in severe cases. Treatment with bevacizumab (Avastin, Genentech, South San Francisco, CA), a vascular endothelial growth factor (VEGF) inhibitor, has emerged as a highly effective therapy, although risks must be considered with this medication.

◆ Outcome and Follow-Up

Ongoing management of underlying medical disorders may be preventive. Moisture with nasal saline and humidification is helpful. Avoid blood-thinning medications while healing.

4.2 Rhinosinusitis

4.2.1 Acute Rhinosinusitis

◆ Key Features

- Rhinosinusitis is an inflammatory condition of the nose and sinuses.
- By definition of acute, signs and symptoms last less than one month.
- The condition resolves with treatment; inadequate treatment may lead to disabling chronic disease.

Acute bacterial rhinosinusitis is frequently managed by primary care providers. The otolaryngologist often sees patients who are inadequately treated or who have recurrent disease. Aggressive care is necessary with immunocompromised patients. Collection of mucopus during nasal endoscopy enables one to obtain data for culture-directed antibiotic therapy. Treatment is usually medical, in the absence of orbital or intracranial complications.

◆ Epidemiology

True incidence is difficult to establish because of some overlap with other complaints, such as upper respiratory infection or allergy. However, rhinosinusitis is among the most common of all healthcare complaints. Rhinosinusitis (all varieties) is reported to affect 31 million people in the United States. An estimated 20 million cases of acute bacterial rhinosinusitis occur annually in the United States. Annual U.S. expenditure related to the primary diagnosis of sinusitis totals approximately $3.5 billion.

◆ Clinical

Signs and Symptoms

Acute rhinosinusitis may be suspected based on signs and symptoms. Major factors include facial pain or pressure, congestion or fullness, nasal obstruction, nasal discharge, purulence, or discolored postnasal drainage, hyposmia/anosmia, purulence in nasal cavity on exam, and fever. Minor factors include headache, fatigue, halitosis, dental pain, cough, and ear pain or ear pressure/fullness.

Updated guidelines have simplified diagnostic criteria: purulent drainage with nasal obstruction and facial pain/fullness/pressure persisting 10 days, or worsening within 10 days after initial improvement. Fever is relatively specific to acute rhinosinusitis versus other forms of sinonasal disease. Localizing symptoms may suggest specific paranasal sinus involvement: cheek or upper dental pain with maxillary sinusitis, forehead pain, or frontal headaches with frontal sinusitis. Retro-orbital or occipital pain may be seen with sphenoid sinusitis. Pervasive sinus disease can, however, remain occult with nonspecific symptoms.

Differential Diagnosis

In the early phase of the disease (first 10 days), the etiology is presumed to be viral. Thus, a typical viral upper respiratory infection is the main alternative diagnosis in the patient with a history of symptoms of less than 2 weeks' duration. Other entities to be considered include allergic rhinitis exacerbation, unrecognized chronic rhinosinusitis, or rare nasal manifestations of systemic disease such as limited Wegener's granulomatosis or sarcoid. Other causes of localized symptoms include severe periodontal disease or recurrent migraine, which may include throbbing localized headache as well as nasal congestion. In the immunocompromised patient, a high index of suspicion for invasive fungal rhinosinusitis is critical.

◆ Evaluation

The diagnosis is generally made on the basis of signs and symptoms, by history in combination with objective exam findings. Occasionally, radiographic assessment is needed.

Physical Exam

A full head and neck examination is performed, including a cranial nerve exam. It is important to exclude evidence of complicated sinusitis, such as orbital or intracranial extension of disease. Therefore, note is made of proptosis, periorbital edema, extraocular motility, tenderness, and meningeal signs. Guidelines recommend anterior rhinoscopy or nasal endoscopy; nasal endoscopy is more informative. Assessment includes position of the septum; presence of mucosal edema; presence, location, and quality of mucus or purulence; and the presence and quality of polyps or masses. A calcium alginate swab (Calgiswab, Puritan Medical Products, Guilford, ME) or suction trap can be easily used to obtain a sample of any purulence endoscopically from the sinus ostia or middle meatus for culture and sensitivities, especially in recurrent sinusitis or previous antibiotic failure.

Imaging

The diagnosis of uncomplicated acute rhinosinusitis is generally made on history and exam. If complications or alternative diagnoses are suspected, thin-section noncontrast coronal and axial computed tomography (CT) scanning of the paranasal sinuses is the most useful study. The presence of fluid- or soft tissue–density opacification of a paranasal sinus is diagnostic. Mucosal thickening without obvious fluid suggests chronic disease. The bony detail of the skull base and orbits should be assessed. Bone erosion or thickening, or the presence of a sinonasal mass, suggests other than acute rhinosinusitis and will prompt additional work-up.

The utility of plain X-ray films is very limited. Disease of the middle meatus, infundibulum, frontal recess, anterior ethmoidal air cells, and superior nasal cavity is not identifiable. Furthermore, the radiation exposure from a screening sinus CT (i.e., limited cuts) is probably comparable to that from a plain film series.

Labs

Unless the patient is toxic or immunosuppressed, or one suspects complications of acute rhinosinusitis (orbital or intracranial extension), blood work such as a complete blood count (CBC) with differential is not helpful. Testing for allergy and immune function is considered with recurrent acute rhinosinusitis or chronic disease.

Microbiology

It is generally accepted that viral infection predominates for the first 10 to 14 days and then leads to sinus ostia obstruction. Inspissated mucus leads to bacterial infection. The most common organisms are *Streptococcus pneumoniae*, *Hemophilus influenzae*, and *Moraxella catarrhalis* as well as anaerobes and other *Streptococcus* species. Drug resistance is a growing problem.

♦ Treatment Options

Uncomplicated acute rhinosinusitis is observed or treated medically. If symptoms persist beyond 7 to 10 days, bacterial infection is more likely and antibiotics are indicated. The typical duration of therapy is 5 to 10 days. Adult empiric therapy published guidelines recommend (a) amoxicillin/clavulanate (1.75–4.0 g/250 mg per day, or 875 mg twice daily), (b) amoxicillin (1.5–4 g/d, or 500 mg three times daily), or (c) cefuroxime axetil (250 mg twice daily). In β-lactam-allergic patients, guidelines recommend (a) trimethoprim–sulfamethoxazole double-strength (twice daily); (b) doxycycline (100 mg twice daily); or (c) macrolide therapy (**Table 4.6**). If there is no improvement in 72 hours, or if there has been antibiotic use within the previous 4 to 6 weeks, the antibiotic should be switched; consider fluoroquinolone, ceftriaxone, or clindamycin. If possible, antibiotic therapy should be culture-directed at this point.

Table 4.6   Adult empiric antibiotic therapy for acute rhinosinusitis

Nonallergic	β-lactam-allergic
Amoxicillin (1.5–4 g/d) Amoxicillin–clavulanate (1.75–4.0 g/ 250 mg/d) Cefuroxime axetil (250 mg twice daily)	Trimethoprim–sulfamethoxazole double-strength (twice daily) Doxycycline (100 mg twice daily) Macrolide therapy (e.g., clarithromycin 500 mg twice daily)
If ineffective, or recent antibiotic use, consider fluoroquinolone; other alternatives include clindamycin and ceftriaxone.	

Note: Culture-directed treatment is highly recommended.

In pediatric patients, guidelines recommend (a) amoxicillin/clavulanate (90 mg/6.4 mg/kg per day), (b) amoxicillin (45–90 mg/kg per day), or (c) cefuroxime axetil (generally 30 mg/kg per day divided every 12 hours; maximum 1,000 mg daily). In β-lactam-allergic patients, guidelines recommend trimethoprim–sulfamethoxazole (6–10 mg trimethoprim per kg per day divided every 12 hours), or a macrolide such as clarithromycin (15 mg/ kg per day divided every 12 hours).

Additional medical therapy involves the use of oral decongestants such as pseudoephedrine (30–60 mg every 6 hours as needed). Caution should be used in patients with prostatic hypertrophy or poorly controlled hypertension. Topical decongestants such as oxymetazoline 0.05% (two sprays each nostril twice daily) can be used for 3 to 5 days at most to facilitate drainage. Prolonged use will cause rhinitis medicamentosa. Oral antihistamines are indicated only if the symptoms are associated with allergy exacerbation. Topical nasal steroids have been recommended recently to help decrease inflammation and to play a prophylactic role following resolution of symptoms in patients with recurrent disease. Nasal saline is useful for thinning secretions, as is guaifenesin (600–1,200 mg twice daily).

Occasionally, maxillary puncture is necessary to obtain material for culture and/or to relieve severe symptoms. This may be done via the inferior meatus or canine fossa. A common indication for this is an immunocompromised patient on multiple recent antibiotics with an occluded sinus.

◆ Outcome and Follow-Up

Acute rhinosinusitis generally resolves with appropriate medical treatment. Subacute rhinosinusitis progresses from 4 to 12 weeks and usually still resolves. Certain patients may relapse, termed recurrent acute rhinosinusitis, with symptoms again lasting less than 4 weeks and recurring four or more times per year. In patients with recurrent disease, CT scanning and more aggressive therapy, including systemic steroids and/or surgery, may be indicated.

Meningitis is the most common intracranial complication from acute rhinosinusitis, often from sphenoid disease. This is managed with IV antibiotics and usually surgical drainage. Orbital and intracranial complications are discussed in detail in prior chapters.

4.2.2   Chronic Rhinosinusitis

◆ Key Features

- Chronic rhinosinusitis is an inflammatory condition of the nose and sinuses.
- By definition of chronic, signs and symptoms last 3 months or longer.
- Several subtypes exist, but their exact definitions remain controversial.

Chronic rhinosinusitis (CRS) is defined as a group of disorders characterized by inflammation of the mucosa of the nose and paranasal sinuses of at least 12 consecutive weeks' duration. Acute rhinosinusitis has been defined as lasting up to 4 weeks. Subacute rhinosinusitis lasts 4 to 12 weeks. CRS occurs secondary to uncontrolled acute or subacute rhinosinusitis and many times requires surgical intervention. Underlying factors such as allergies, cilia motility disorders, and immunodeficiency disorders should be considered in refractory patients.

◆ Epidemiology

Rhinosinusitis (all varieties) is reported to affect 31 million people in United States. CRS results in an estimated 24 million physician visits annually in the United States, 90% of which result in a prescription. U.S. annual expenditure related to the primary diagnosis of sinusitis totals approximately $3.5 billion.

◆ Clinical

Signs and Symptoms

According to updated guidelines, CRS is diagnosed by (1) ≥ 12 weeks of two or more of the following symptoms: mucopurulent drainage, congestion, facial pain/pressure/fullness, decreased olfaction; along with (2) inflammation documented by endoscopic finding of pus, edema or polyps and/or positive computed tomography (CT) scan. Validated quality-of-life (QOL) assessment tools (such as the 20-item Sino-Nasal Outcome Test [SNOT-20] by JF Piccirillo) have indicated that CRS has a large negative impact on patients.

Differential Diagnosis

Intranasal neoplasia, benign or malignant, may present similarly to inflammatory disease. Neoplasms include papillomas (inverting, cylindrical), squamous cell carcinomas or adenocarcinomas, salivary tumors, sarcomas, mucosal melanoma, schwannomas, osteomas, angiofibroma, and olfactory neuroblastoma (esthesioneuroblastoma). Other entities to be considered include nasal manifestations of systemic disease such as limited Wegener's granulomatosis, Churg-Strauss's syndrome, sarcoid, tuberculosis, leprosy, or syphilis. Other causes of localized symptoms include severe periodontal disease or recurrent migraine, which may include throbbing localized headache as well as nasal congestion (primary care providers may label cephalalgia as "sinus headaches," independent of the presence of active sinonasal disease). Temporomandibular joint (TMJ) disorders may cause "sinus" headaches. Rhinitis medicamentosa is common, and patients do not always admit to use of nasal decongestants. In the immunocompromised patient (neutropenia, uncontrolled diabetes mellitus), a high index of suspicion for invasive fungal rhinosinusitis is critical. In certain clinical situations, consider Churg-Strauss's syndrome (vasculitis, asthma, eosinophilia), eosinophilic granuloma spectrum (Langerhans cell histiocytosis), T-cell lymphoma (formerly considered midline lethal granuloma), rhinoscleroma (caused by *Klebsiella rhinoscleromatis*), or rhinosporidiosis (caused by *Rhinosporidium seeberi*; endemic in India and Sri Lanka).

Table 4.7   Exam findings in chronic rhinosinusitis

CT findings	Nasal endoscopy findings
• Mucosal thickening	• Discolored nasal drainage
• Bone changes	• Nasal polyps
• Air-fluid levels	• Edema or erythema, especially at middle meatus or ethmoidal bulla

◆ Evaluation

Controversy exists with regard to definitions and diagnoses of all forms of rhinosinusitis. A diagnosis is generally made on the basis of history in combination with objective exam findings and radiographic assessment, usually CT scanning (**Table 4.7**). As mentioned under Signs and Symptoms, updated 2015 evidence-based guidelines are simplified. Olfactory testing and the SNOT-20 questionnaire are strongly encouraged.

Physical Exam

A full head and neck exam is performed, including a cranial nerve exam. It is important to exclude evidence of complicated sinusitis, such as orbital or intracranial extension of disease. Therefore, note is made of proptosis, periorbital edema, extraocular motility, tenderness, and meningeal signs. Rigid nasal endoscopy should be performed after topical decongestion. Assessment includes position and integrity of the septum; presence of mucosal edema; presence, location, and quality of mucus or purulence; and the presence and quality of polyps or masses. A calcium alginate swab (Calgiswab, Puritan Medical Products, Guilford, ME) or suction trap can be easily used to obtain a sample of any purulence endoscopically from the sinus ostia or middle meatus for culture and sensitivities. The otolaryngologist possesses unique expertise in nasal endoscopy, and this procedure should be part of the exam of all patients presenting with sinonasal complaints.

Consider olfactory testing (especially in patients who note hyposmia/anosmia as a complaint), such as the Smell Identification Test (Sensonics, Inc., Haddon Heights, NJ), formerly called the University of Pennsylvania Smell Identification Test (UPSIT).

Imaging

Thin-section noncontrast coronal and axial CT scanning of the paranasal sinuses is the most useful study. CT staging systems (i.e., Lund-Mackay) have been proposed and may be useful for research or tracking disease over time. CT findings correlate poorly with patients' symptoms. The presence of fluid or soft tissue density opacification of a paranasal sinus is diagnostic. Mucosal thickening without obvious fluid suggests chronic disease. The bony detail of the skull base and orbits should be assessed. Bone erosion or thickening, or the presence of a sinonasal mass, suggests other than acute (chronic) rhinosinusitis and will prompt additional work-up. Fungal disease, presenting as allergic fungal rhinosinusitis, will appear as heterogeneous density. Evidence of expansile disease with bone thinning is seen with allergic fungal rhinosinusitis, mucocele, and low-grade neoplasms. Bony erosion should raise concern for malignancy and is also seen with inflammatory disease such as Wegener's granulomatosis. Bony thickening is seen with long-standing inflammatory disease.

Magnetic resonance imaging (MRI) is helpful for assessing intracranial extension. Fungus may appear as absent signal with both T1 and T2 sequences. However, at present MRI is not recommended as an alternative to CT for routine diagnosis of chronic rhinosinusitis because of its excessively high sensitivity and lack of specificity. The utility of plain X-ray films is very limited.

Labs

Unless the patient is toxic or immunosuppressed, or one suspects complications of rhinosinusitis (orbital or intracranial extension), blood work such as a CBC with differential is not helpful. Bacterial cultures from sinus ostia are useful. The role of fungi is controversial. Fungi are ubiquitous; topical or systemic antifungals are not used unless tissue-invasive fungal infection is present (i.e., in immunosuppressed patients). The role of virus in chronic rhinosinusitis is unclear and is under study.

Microbiology

Inspissated mucus leads to bacterial infection. Importantly, organisms differ from those seen with acute rhinosinusitis. Common microbes include *Staphylococcus aureus*, coagulase-negative *Staphylococcus*, and anaerobic and gram-negative species. Most infections are polymicrobial. Antimicrobial resistance is common.

Pathogenesis and Classification

Etiology is multifactorial, involving environmental, local host, and general host factors. Pathogenic environmental factors include viral infection, air pollution, smoking, and allergy. Smoking is the single most significant factor in recurrent disease; tobacco cessation is strongly encouraged before sinus surgery is performed. Host factors include atopy, immune deficiency, mucociliary clearance problems such as ciliary dyskinesia or cystic fibrosis (probably even subclinical forms of chloride transporter dysfunction), airway hyperactivity, and reactivity to fungus.

Subtypes of chronic rhinosinusitis have been proposed based on inflammatory infiltrate (eosinophilic, neutrophilic, or other) or on various pathophysiologic mechanisms (extrinsic factors, intrinsic factors). The clinical utility of classification has been hampered to some degree by overlap in signs and symptoms. However, categories include chronic rhinosinusitis with or without polyps, chronic rhinosinusitis with eosinophilic mucin, allergic fungal rhinosinusitis (based on the presence of eosinophils and atopy to fungus), and Samter triad (ASA triad) of allergy to aspirin, with asthma, and nasal polyps. CRS is extremely common in patients with acquired immunodeficiency syndrome (AIDS). Finally, the microbiome is an area of active study, although standard measure techniques or treatment recommendations based on microbiome measures are not yet available.

Table 4.8   Treatment strategies in chronic rhinosinusitis

Oral steroids (consider obtaining consent)	Methylprednisolone 32 mg daily × 7 days, then taper
Oral antibiotics	Culture-directed whenever possible
Topical nasal steroid sprays	Mometasone, fluticasone, other
Topical nasal steroid irrigation (off-label use)	Budesonide (one Respule contents added to 240 mL nasal saline) twice daily
Topical nasal antibiotic irrigation, useful for methicillin-resistant *S. aureus* (MRSA; off-label use)	2% mupirocin ointment 22 g in 1 L of normal saline using 50 mL per nostril daily twice daily for 10 days
Surgery	Endoscopic (forceps, microdébrider, balloon catheter dilation)
	Open (trephination, frontal obliteration, other)

◆ Treatment Options

Medical

Uncomplicated chronic rhinosinusitis should be treated medically prior to considering surgery (**Table 4.8**). There is debate regarding what constitutes "maximal medical therapy." Treatment is aimed at infection, inflammation, and underlying factors. A course of systemic steroid tapered over 1 month combined with oral antibiotic therapy has been found useful, especially if polyps are present. Note that oral steroids have risk of serious side effects, and for off-label use it is highly recommended that consent be documented. Methylprednisolone (Medrol, Pfizer, New York, NY) 32 mg orally every day for 1 week, then tapered to 32 mg every other day for 1 week, 24 mg every other day for 1 week, 16 mg every other day for 1 week is a typical regimen. Whenever possible, antibiotic therapy should be culture-directed. Empiric choices include cefuroxime 250 to 500 mg orally twice a day; clarithromycin and doxycycline are alternatives. Antibiotic treatment for CRS may be prolonged. At the end of this treatment, a CT scan is repeated (with image-guidance protocol, if surgery is likely). If symptoms and/or exam and CT findings are not significantly improved, surgery is considered.

Nasal saline irrigations and topical nasal steroids are recommended in updated guidelines. Additional useful medical therapy may include guai-fenesin 600-1200 mg orally twice a day (< 1 week) and saline nasal rinses. Methicillin-resistant *S. aureus* (MRSA) cultured from nasal endoscopy specimens has been seen at initial otolaryngology visit. Nasal irrigation with mupirocin ointment 22 g in 1 L of normal saline using 50 mL per nostril daily for 10 days appears beneficial (this is off-label use). Topical deconges-tants such as oxymetazoline 0.05% (two sprays each nostril twice daily) can be used for 3 to 5 days at most to facilitate drainage. Prolonged use will cause rhinitis medicamentosa. Oral antihistamines are indicated only if the symptoms are associated with allergy exacerbation. Budesonide (Pulmicort

Respules, AstraZeneca, Cambridge, UK; one Respule contents added to 240 mL nasal saline, twice daily for topical nasal irrigation) has been used in some patients with CRS with polyps as a systemic steroid sparing approach (this is off-label use).

Surgical

Endoscopic sinus surgery has become the standard technique for addressing nonneoplastic sinonasal disease. It is also being used for selective neoplastic cases. Open techniques may be necessary in certain cases; for example, open drainage of orbital subperiosteal abscess, or frontal sinus trephination in combination with endoscopic surgery. Preoperative review of the coronal CT scan is critical (**Table 4.9**). Pre- and postoperative care is important for success. Many surgeons employ pretreatment, especially in polyp cases, with methylprednisolone 32 mg orally daily for 5 days prior to surgery, tapered slowly postoperatively, depending on endoscopic exam. Tobacco cessation is mandatory to long-term success. The role and extent of office postoperative débridement is debated.

Endoscopic surgical instrumentation may include through-cutting forceps or powered microdébriders. Tissue-sparing instruments for balloon sinus dilation over a guidewire are widely used.

◆ Outcome and Follow-Up

Chronic rhinosinusitis patients require long-term ongoing care, often including the allergist, rhinologist, and primary physician. Cumulative systemic steroid exposure must be carefully followed to prevent side effects. There is a high rate of revision surgery in CRS patients, especially those with extensive nasal polyposis. It is important for patients to understand that they have a chronic disease condition involving the upper airway and that curing this chronic condition may not be achievable. However, effectively managing symptoms, minimizing disease morbidity, and improving quality of life are reasonable goals. Serial SNOT-20 QOL assessments are useful. Orbital and intracranial complications are discussed in detail elsewhere in this book.

Table 4.9 Preoperative review of coronal CT scan

Shape and integrity of skull base	Height of ethmoidal air cells (in relation to top of maxillary sinus posteriorly—number of cells before skull base)
Shape and integrity of orbit	Sphenoidal sinus anatomy: septations, carotids, optic nerves
Position of uncinate	Anatomic variations: Onodi cell (overriding posterior ethmoidal air cell) Concha bullosa Infraorbital ethmoidal air cell
Location of anterior ethmoidal artery	Hypoplastic maxillary sinus

4.3 Rhinitis

4.3.1 Nonallergic Rhinitis

◆ Key Features

- Many physicians fail to recognize nonallergic rhinitis (NAR), instead treating all rhinitis as allergic.
- Even when allergy has been ruled out, these patients may be diagnosed with "vasomotor rhinitis" (VMR), often a wastebasket diagnosis. Further work-up is often not performed.
- Because NAR encompasses a variety of etiologic factors, careful diagnosis and directed therapy are key to satisfactory treatment.

Rhinitis is defined as inflammation of the nasal lining. It is characterized by symptoms of nasal congestion, rhinorrhea, sneezing, and/or nasal itching. Rhinitis is broadly classified into allergic (AR) and nonallergic (NAR) categories, based on skin testing or in vitro tests for allergen-specific immunoglobulin E (IgE). The term "mixed rhinitis" refers to the presence of both allergic and nonallergic components, and treatment should address both components.

◆ Epidemiology

In the United States, NAR affects 19 million people, and an additional 26 million experience mixed rhinitis. NAR disproportionately affects females, suggesting hormonal influences. It more commonly affects people older than 60 years of age.

◆ Clinical

Signs and Symptoms

Often, VMR is associated with nasal obstruction and thickened postnasal drip. In addition, it can present with copious, watery anterior rhinorrhea, often triggered by changes in temperature, alcohol use, or exposure to odors and aromas. Other common symptoms of NAR include sneezing, congestion, and itching, which can be triggered by inhaled agents, cigarette smoke, foods, chemicals, and medications. All can have an irritant effect on the nasal mucosa.

Differential Diagnosis

NAR is diagnosed after AR has been excluded. Stimulation of the nasal mucosa by endogenous and exogenous agents causes symptoms that characterize rhinitis. In addition, NAR can be exacerbated by hormonal influences such as those experienced during pregnancy, endocrine disturbances such as hypothyroidism, and autonomic dysfunction.

✦ Classification

NAR can be classified into the following subtypes: occupational (irrita-tive-toxic), hormonal, drug-induced, gustatory, inflammatory (eosinophilic), and vasomotor. Rhinitis due to vasculitides and granulomatous diseases (Wegener, sarcoidosis, etc.) is a separate category.

Occupational Rhinitis

Occupational (irritative-toxic) rhinitis is caused by inhalant irritants or toxic agents including chemicals, solvents, and cigarette smoke. Cigarette smoking is the most common cause, and occupational exposure the next leading cause, of this subtype. Cessation and adequate protection from these stimuli result in control of symptoms.

Hormonal Rhinitis

The most commonly reported hormonal rhinitis is rhinitis of pregnancy, seen in 22% of nonsmoking women and in 69% of smokers. Rhinitis of pregnancy is most common during the later stages of pregnancy. Rhinitis of pregnancy resolves within 2 to 4 weeks of delivery.

Drug-Induced Rhinitis

Many common medications have physiologic side effects on the nose, result-ing in nasal congestion. These medications include angiotensin-converting enzyme (ACE) inhibitors, β-blockers, oral contraceptives, antipsychotics, and recently, phosphodiesterase type-5 inhibitors. Some patients may have a non-IgE-mediated sensitivity to nonsteroidal anti-inflammatory drugs (NSAIDs) and aspirin.

Rhinitis medicamentosa is most commonly associated with prolonged use of topical vasoconstrictive nasal sprays such as oxymetazoline. Prolonged use of these medications results in tachyphylaxis, and cessation of use is associated with rebound nasal congestion, which can be severe and refractory to treatment.

Gustatory Rhinitis

Gustatory rhinitis is characterized by watery, often profuse rhinorrhea that develops with ingestion of food. Anticipation of eating or even the smell of food may precipitate clear nasal drainage. The response is mediated by aberrant parasympathetic stimulation of nasal secretomotor fibers on stimulation of salivary secretomotor activity.

Nonallergic Rhinitis with Eosinophilia

Nonallergic rhinitis with eosinophilia (NARES) was originally described as a constellation of perennial sneezing attacks, profuse watery rhinorrhea, and nasal pruritus, as well as nasal congestion in patients who showed a lack of evidence for allergy on skin testing or in vitro testing for specific IgE and who had greater than 20% eosinophils on nasal smears.

Vasomotor Rhinitis

VMR is the most common form of chronic NAR. VMR is a diagnosis of exclusion. VMR is widespread, especially in the elderly, and may be frustrating to treat.

Chemical Sensitivity

A particularly severe form of sensitivity to certain chemical substances is seen on occasion. History generally describes an exposure to a strong or caustic substance with onset of severe or disabling rhinitis symptoms on repeat exposure to even mild or normal chemicals, such as perfumes or cleaning agents. This is poorly understood and has been considered a "multiple chemical sensitivity syndrome." Strict avoidance, if possible, may be effective, although better treatment options remain to be determined.

◆ Evaluation

History

Family and personal history of atopy or allergies, medications, abnormal hormonal status, pregnancy, smoking, and occupational exposure are noted.

Physical Exam

The diagnosis of rhinitis involves a complete head and neck examination, as well as a nasal endoscopy. The size of the nasal conchae and the degree of nasal airway impairment are noted. The reversibility of this hypertrophy is gauged after spraying with topical decongestants. The appearance of the nasal mucosa and secretions is evaluated. Allergic mucosa is classically blue-gray and boggy, whereas erythematous, inflamed mucosa is seen in rhinitis medicamentosa, irritative rhinitis, and granulomatous rhinitis.

Labs

AR should be ruled out by skin allergy testing or by in vitro tests quantifying specific IgE levels. NAR eosinophilic sinusitis can be ruled out by nasal wash cytology or by nasal brushings for eosinophils.

Other Tests

Anterior rhinomanometry, acoustic rhinometry, and nasal peak flows are supplementary tests more commonly used as research tools and not routinely used for diagnosis. Other available tests include serum mediator levels, tests for complement activation, and nasal lavage studies. Nasal lavage studies of the total protein and albumin concentration show significantly higher levels in AR patients as compared with NAR patients and healthy control subjects, likely due to increased vascular permeability.

◆ Treatment Options

Medical

Conservative management should be attempted first. This includes avoidance of irritating substances, cold weather, offending foods, and wine. Regular physical exercise also increases sympathetic input to the nose, correcting for the underlying loss of sympathetic tone. Underlying diseases and medications should be evaluated. Topical anticholinergics, antihistamines, and steroids are commonly used to treat NAR.

Azelastine is approved for use in both AR and NAR. Azelastine is an H1-receptor antagonist. It also inhibits synthesis of leukotrienes, kinins, and cytokines. It also suppresses intercellular adhesion molecules expression and superoxide free radical generation. This anti-inflammatory effect provides relief in NARES and VMR. The antihistaminic effect decreases mucosal edema, prostaglandin production, and stimulation of irritant receptors.

Anticholinergic medications provide relief from rhinorrhea in NAR. Ipratropium bromide is a topical anticholinergic with uncommon systemic side effects. Nasal steroid sprays can also control nasal congestion and rhinorrhea effectively.

Vasculitides and autoimmune granulomatous rhinitis (Wegener's granulomatosis, sarcoidosis, Churg-Strauss's disease) are treated with immunosuppressive drugs.

Surgical

The inferior conchae are lined with vascular mucosa with mucous and serous glands and also contain venous sinusoids surrounded by smooth muscle fibers under autonomic control. Inferior conchal hypertrophy unresponsive to medical therapy can be treated surgically with conchal reduction by a variety of techniques.

Vidian neurectomy and sphenopalatine ganglion block have also been used for intractable VMR. Botulinum toxin (Botox, Pfizer, New York, NY) injection to the sphenopalatine ganglion has also been recently described.

◆ Outcome and Follow-Up

If left untreated, patients continue to suffer from detrimental effects on quality of life. Lifestyle modifications and pharmacologic interventions can be useful, but some forms of NAR, especially in the elderly, are particularly challenging to manage. Once symptoms are adequately controlled, patients can be managed with semiannual or annual follow-up.

4.3.2 Allergy

◆ Key Features

- An allergy is an immune response with deleterious effects.
- Emergencies include anaphylactic shock and angioedema.
- Signs and symptoms often involve otorhinolaryngologic manifestations.

The immune system functions to protect a host from foreign antigens. An allergic reaction is an immune response that causes undesirable effects.

Examples of allergic disease of importance to the otolaryngologist are allergic rhinitis, angioedema, latex allergy, and anaphylaxis.

◆ Epidemiology

An estimated 17% of the population is affected by allergic disease.

◆ Clinical

Important to the clinical management of allergic disease is an understanding of the four types of allergic reactions, as described by Gell and Coombs (**Table 4.10**). Type I is an immediate immunoglobulin E (IgE)-mediated reaction (e.g., urticaria or anaphylaxis); type II is an IgG- or IgM-mediated cytotoxic reaction (e.g., transfusion reaction); type III is a response due to immune complexes, usually IgG (e.g., glomerulonephritis); type IV is a delayed hypersensitivity reaction mediated by T cells (e.g., poison ivy rash, granuloma formation). Inflammatory mediators such as histamine, leukotrienes, and cytokines mediate the effects of an allergic reaction.

Signs and Symptoms

Signs and symptoms may vary widely depending on the allergen and exposure. Nasal effects include sneezing, rhinorrhea, itching, obstructive edema, and supratip crease with so-called allergic salute. Ophthalmologic effects include conjunctival injection, itching, elongated lashes, and allergic shiners. Other airway effects may include chronic mouth breathing, globus sensation with frequent throat clearing, cobblestone appearance to the posterior pharynx, coughing, and wheezing.

Acute allergic emergencies include anaphylaxis and angioedema. Anaphylaxis may present with rapid onset of bronchospasm, laryngeal edema, cough, stridor, itching, urticaria, tachycardia, nausea, and initial hypertension followed by hypotension and cardiovascular collapse. Death may occur rapidly due to airway obstruction or cardiovascular collapse (shock). Angioedema may present with swelling of the lips, oral cavity, tongue, and/or larynx. Progression may be unpredictable and rapid, causing death secondary to airway obstruction.

Table 4.10   Gell and Coombs classification of allergic reactions

Type	Reaction
I: Immediate IgE response, mast cell degranulation	Response within minutes; may include wheezing, urticaria, rhinorrhea, angioedema, anaphylaxis
II: Cytotoxic IgG/IgM reaction	Examples: transfusion reaction with hemolysis; hyperacute graft rejection
III: Immune complex reaction, IgG	Often delayed; may affect various tissues Example: glomerulonephritis, arthritis
IV: Cell-mediated, T-cell response	Example: poison ivy, granuloma formation

Abbreviation: Ig, immunoglobulin.

Differential Diagnosis

Patients presenting with complaints or findings related to possible allergic etiologies may be complex. Considerations include inhalant allergy, food allergy, side effects of medications such as ACE inhibitors, immune disorders such as C1 esterase inhibitor deficiency, various immune deficiencies, or infection.

◆ Evaluation

Work-up must be tailored to the urgency of the situation. In an emergency, evaluation may be limited to a primary assessment, vital signs, and an assessment of the upper airway followed by immediate treatment directed at angioedema or anaphylactic shock. The elective setting enables one to perform a thorough history and physical examination along with appropriate ancillary testing.

Physical Exam

A full head and neck exam is standard. Auscultation of the lungs for wheezing is performed. Note evidence of chronic allergy, such as allergic shiners, supratip nasal crease, as well as nasal conchal edema, nasal mucus, postnasal drainage, and posterior pharyngeal cobblestoning. As for laboratory testing, a scraping of the inferior conchal mucosa for cytology may suggest allergic disease—presence of eosinophils, or nasal mastocytosis. Consider C1 esterase inhibitor levels in cases of recurrent angioedema.

Other Tests

Specific allergy testing may be performed either via blood sample for radioallergosorbent test (RAST) or via skin testing. RAST is useful as a screening for allergen-specific IgE but is insufficient to begin immunotherapy. Skin testing, to elicit a wheal and flare response to specific allergens, can be performed either via the prick test or the serial dilution end point titration (SDET) method, endorsed by the American Academy of Otolaryngic Allergy. SDET provides quantitative data useful for safely beginning immunotherapy. Some allergists use the results of RAST to prescribe immunotherapy. Details of skin testing are beyond the scope of this book; instead see Marple BF, Mabry RL. *Quantitative Skin Testing for Allergy: IDT and MQT*. New York, NY: Thieme; 2006.

◆ Treatment Options

Anaphylaxis

Immediate treatment for anaphylaxis includes airway and circulatory support. Airway support with supplemental oxygen, intubation, or a surgical airway may be indicated. Epinephrine 0.3 mg intramuscularly (IM) or subcutaneously (SC) repeated every 10 minutes up to 1 mg is given (adult dose). Two large-bore intravenous (IV) cannulas should be placed. IV crystalloid bolus, IV diphenhydramine 50 mg, IV H_2 blocker, and IV dexamethasone 8 mg are administered. ICU observation is planned, with further circulatory management with dopamine drip as indicated.

Angioedema

Airway obstruction must be anticipated. IV access and continuous airway monitoring are mandatory. IV diphenhydramine 50 mg, IV H_2 blocker, and IV dexamethasone 8 mg are administered. If airway obstruction is significant, if swelling persists, or if swelling worsens despite medical treatment, elective intubation is performed via awake fiberoptic nasotracheal technique, with a tracheotomy tray available. Direct laryngoscopy is contraindicated, as sedation and paralysis may lead to an inability to mask ventilate, and tongue edema will interfere with visualization of the glottis.

Chronic Allergy Management

Pharmacotherapy includes H_1 blockers, topical nasal steroids, oral steroid tapers used sparingly, topical nasal cromolyn, leukotriene inhibitors, oral decongestants, and topical decongestants used for a maximum of 3 consecutive days to avoid rhinitis medicamentosa. Immunotherapy injections for desensitization may be indicated, based on results of skin testing. Sublingual immunotherapy is an option that has been gaining acceptance, although at present insurance coverage has been less than satisfactory because it has been considered "off-label use." Environmental measures are critical, in terms of avoidance of exposure to allergens such as dust mites, molds, or pets.

◆ Outcome and Follow-Up

Routine follow-up for response to pharmacotherapy and for immunotherapy is indicated. Consultation with a pulmonologist for management of lower airway disease may be helpful.

4.4 Inverted Papillomas

◆ Key Features

- An inverted papilloma is a soft tissue neoplasm often arising from the lateral nasal wall.
- It is benign but can be locally aggressive.
- Malignant degeneration can occur.

An inverted papilloma is considered a benign neoplasm. However, reports suggest that as many as 10 to 20% of cases can contain, or degenerate to, in situ or invasive squamous cell carcinoma. Thus, complete surgical removal is the treatment of choice.

◆ Epidemiology

Males are affected three times more frequently than females. The tumor is more common in older adults.

◆ Clinical

Signs

The patient presents with a polypoid unilateral intranasal mass. Any patient presenting with a unilateral nasal mass should raise suspicion for neoplasm. Allergic fungal sinusitis may present unilaterally as well.

Symptoms

The patient has a unilateral nasal obstruction, with or without sinusitis. Rhinorrhea and/or epistaxis may occur. Histologically, an inverted papilloma consists of in-folded epithelium that may be squamous, transitional, or respiratory.

Differential Diagnosis

The differential diagnosis includes an inverted papilloma, fungiform papilloma (often arises from anterior nasal septum), cylindrical papilloma (often arises from lateral wall; rare tumor), minor salivary gland benign or malignant tumors, lacrimal sac tumors, olfactory neuroblastoma, carcinoma such as squamous cell carcinoma or sinonasal undifferentiated carcinoma, mucosal melanoma, chondrosarcoma, angiofibroma, inflammatory nasal polyp, allergic fungal rhinosinusitis. Other tumors include schwannomas, hamartomas, giant cell granulomas, neurofibromas, and chondromyxoid fibromas.

◆ Evaluation

History

A standard history is taken.

Physical Exam

A full head and neck exam is done, with attention paid to the cranial nerves. Nasal endoscopy with a rigid 0° or 30° endoscope will be useful to assess the intranasal extent and location of soft tissue mass. After imaging excludes possible encephalocele, a biopsy may be obtained in the office or operating room.

Imaging

Computed tomography (CT) provides bony detail and is reviewed with attention to erosive changes at the orbit and skull base. Magnetic resonance imaging (MRI) is helpful in assessing soft tissue tumor extent and can distinguish between inspissated secretion and tumor. CT will often overestimate tumor extent. Images should be reviewed in axial, coronal, and sagittal planes.

◆ Treatment Options

Medical

Definitive treatment requires surgery. Radiotherapy is ineffective and may in fact induce carcinoma.

Surgical

Complete tumor excision is required. Inadequate removal can lead to recurrence, and malignant transformation can occur. Therefore, as summarized by Myers et al, the surgical approach for the management of this tumor must allow (1) adequate exposure for complete removal, (2) an adequate view of the cavity for postoperative examination, and (3) acceptable cosmetic and functional results. Two approaches are commonly employed at present: the open approach via lateral rhinotomy for medial maxillectomy, and the endoscopic approach. Although there has been ongoing debate, most surgeons agree that the procedure utilized should be individualized to the size and location of the tumor and that endoscopic removal can be done in a manner that fulfills these criteria, with a recurrence rate no higher than that for an open approach, in appropriate cases. A midface degloving approach can also be used, especially for tumors located inferiorly (i.e., the area of the premaxilla, nasal septum, or inferior nasal concha).

Regardless of approach, intraoperative frozen pathology should be used to ensure that margins are negative for evidence of residual tumor. Orbital or intracranial extension may require assistance of ophthalmologic or neurosurgical colleagues.

Preoperative Planning

Imaging is reviewed. CT provides bony detail and is reviewed with attention to erosive changes at the orbit and skull base. MRI is helpful for assessing soft tissue tumor extent and can distinguish between inspissated secretion and tumor. CT will often overestimate tumor extent.

A biopsy is required prior to surgery, after imaging is reviewed. Do not biopsy a possible encephalocele; review the MRI. Many surgeons perform biopsy in the operating room combined with endoscopic assessment of the tumor, given concerns for possible hemorrhage following thorough biopsy. If the biopsy indicates malignancy, an open approach to wide resection is often employed if surgery is to be done; radiation or chemoradiation may be options, depending on histology. Endoscopic skull base cancer resection may be performed if appropriate expertise is available.

Open Medial Maxillectomy

A temporary tarsorrhaphy stitch with 5–0 nylon is used to protect the eye. A lateral rhinotomy incision is performed, from just above the medial canthus, along the nasal facial groove, and around the ala, and, if needed, the lip may be split. The periosteum is elevated, as is the periorbita. The anterior and posterior ethmoidal arteries are left as skull base landmarks, indicating the superior extent of dissection. Anterior antrostomy is performed, avoiding injury to the infraorbital nerve. Osteotomies are made along the nasal bone, along the floor of the nose, below the frontoethmoid suture, and at the junction of the lamina papyracea and orbital floor. Posterior attachments are divided with heavy scissors, removing the lateral nasal wall tissue block. Internal maxillary artery branches may require control for hemostasis. Mucosa is stripped from the maxillary, ethmoidal, and sphenoidal sinuses, which are opened. The lacrimal sac is opened and sutured to surrounding tissue. The cavity is packed with Gelfoam (Pfizer, Inc., New York, NY) and antibiotic gauze, and the wound is closed.

Endoscopic Tumor Removal

The following conditions are necessary for endoscopic tumor removal: known histology, adequate imaging studies, surgeon training/experience, and adequate instrumentation. The informed consent must discuss possible conversion to external and/or transoral open procedure. The use of intraoperative computer-assisted surgical navigation (image guidance) is often helpful for endoscopic tumor resection. The techniques used in standard endoscopic sinus surgery are employed, with the goal of complete tumor removal along with a margin of healthy tissue. The nose is topically decongested; an initial rigid endoscopic exam is done for tumor assessment. Local injections are performed using 1% lidocaine with 1:100,000 epinephrine into the sphenopalatine region, middle conchal insertion, and into tumor. Resection is performed with through-cutting instruments; the powered microdébrider is often helpful. It is possible (and typical) to remove the tumor in numerous pieces without compromising the surgery. Often, a tumor stalk can be followed to a precise site of attachment. The bone underlying this attachment site should be abraded with a diamond drill if possible. If the attachment involves a concha, a portion of the concha can be resected. Similarly, the medial wall of the maxillary sinus can be widely removed. If needed, an endoscopic medial maxillectomy may be performed. Bone cannot be examined by frozen section, although mucosa can be sent. If lateral maxillary sinus tumor extension cannot be reached endoscopically, a Caldwell-Luc anterior antrostomy can be used. Steps are taken to ensure that adequate sinus drainage pathways are present. Standard packing, antibiotics, and routine endoscopic sinus surgery postoperative care are used.

An advantage of endoscopic removal is that the exact tumor attachment site is identified and can be followed endoscopically in the office for surveillance for tumor recurrence.

◆ Complications

Major surgical complications can include orbital injury, optic nerve injury, skull base injury with cerebrospinal fluid (CSF) leak, and hemorrhage.

◆ Outcome and Follow-Up

An antibiotic such as cefuroxime axetil 250 mg orally twice a day or clinda-mycin 300 mg orally three times a day is used until any packing is removed, usually at postoperative day 3 or 4. Narcotic analgesic such as oxycodone–acetaminophen 5 mg/325 mg, 1 to 2 tabs orally every 6 hours as needed, is prescribed. Patients are seen in 1 week and then 3 weeks for gentle cavity débridement. Nasal saline irrigation (i.e., NeilMed Sinus Rinse) is done twice daily. Patients are typically seen every 3 to 6 months for tumor recurrence surveillance. Overall recurrence rates up to 20% have been reported, although recurrence should not be expected with adequate margins.

4.5 Anosmia and Other Olfactory Disorders

✦ Key Features

- Olfactory sensory neurons situated in the nasal cavity constitute the first cranial nerve (CN I) and relay olfactory stimuli to the olfactory bulbs of the brain.
- Anosmia, or olfactory loss, can be considered to be conductive (secondary to a process causing nasal obstruction), sensorineural (secondary to a process affecting olfactory neurons or central pathways), or mixed.

The most common causes of olfactory sensory loss are rhinosinusitis, head trauma, or postviral anosmia. Presbyosmia, or age-related decline in olfactory function, is well documented in patients over age 65. Less commonly, effects of drugs or systemic illness have been reported to impact olfactory function adversely.

Anosmia is an absence of olfactory function. Hyposmia (or microsmia) is a decrease in olfactory function. Parosmia is an altered olfactory perception in the presence of stimulus, usually considered foul. Phantosmia is an olfactory perception in the absence of stimulus.

✦ Epidemiology

Approximately 2 to 3 million Americans suffer from chemosensory dysfunction. Olfactory loss is present in 1% of those under age 60 but in > 50% of those over 60 years of age. Presbyosmia is present in most of those > 80 years of age.

✦ Clinical

Signs

In cases of conductive anosmia, nasal endoscopy will usually reveal evidence of obstructive disease, such as mucosal edema, inflammation, mucopus, nasal polyps, or other intranasal mass. In sensorineural anosmia, there may be no obvious exam findings. However, intracranial lesions often cause additional neurologic defects such as altered mental status, urinary incontinence, or seizures. Neoplasms such as an olfactory groove meningioma may cause Foster-Kennedy's syndrome (ipsilateral anosmia, optic atrophy and central scotoma, contralateral papilledema). Objective olfactory testing will reveal the sensory loss.

Symptoms

Many patients are unaware of significant olfactory loss. Those who rely on olfaction, such as cooks, perfumers, firefighters, or chemical workers, are very bothered by hyposmia or anosmia. Acute loss may follow coup/contrecoup injury from even minor head trauma. Fluctuating loss is common with chronic rhinosinusitis. Many anosmics mistakenly complain of loss of taste.

Differential Diagnosis

Obstructive intranasal lesions include polyps, infectious or inflammatory disease, and neoplasia, including Schneiderian papilloma, carcinoma, olfactory neuroblastoma, mucosal melanoma, and metastases. In the absence of obstruction, a sensorineural loss is most often posttraumatic or postviral; thus the history should be corroborative. One should also consider intracranial lesions such as meningioma, neurologic disease such as Parkinson's or Alzheimer's disease, medication side effects, or toxic exposure. Iatrogenic causes such as previous nasal or sinus surgery or prior radiation therapy should be considered. Congenital causes of anosmia include Kallmann's syndrome (hypogonadotropic hypogonadism with anosmia); if suspected, these patients should have an endocrinology consultation. Smoking has also been associated with decreased olfaction, as has the use of over-the-counter intranasal zinc-containing preparations. Other genetic causes are seen rarely, such as ciliopathies.

◆ Evaluation

Objective Olfactory Testing

Validated and easily administered tests of olfactory discrimination are readily available, such as the Smell Identification Test (Sensonics, Inc., Haddon Heights, NJ). This is a "scratch-and-sniff" multiple choice 40-item test that detects anosmia, hyposmia, and malingering and provides scores with age-adjusted norms. More sophisticated tests of olfactory threshold for specific odorants are less commonly employed outside of research centers.

Imaging

In patients without an obvious conductive etiology or history for postviral or posttraumatic anosmia, a head computed tomography (CT) or magnetic resonance imaging (MRI) scan is recommended to rule out an occult skull base or intracranial neoplasm. Thin-section coronal CT with bone algorithms provides excellent detail of the frontoethmoidal and cribriform plate region. Bone dehiscence or soft tissue mass suggests a lesion (e.g., encephalocele, olfactory neuroblastoma). MRI is the test of choice for intracranial lesions.

◆ Treatment Options

Conductive Anosmia

Medical

Medical management for infectious or inflammatory sinonasal disease includes topical nasal steroids, systemic steroid tapers, and oral antibiotics. Oral steroids in combination with culture-directed antibiotics for 4 weeks are considered by many to constitute maximal medical therapy.

Surgical

Endoscopic sinus surgery, with or without septoplasty, can be effective for relieving obstructing disease such as polyposis. Endoscopic or craniofacial approaches to sinonasal or anterior skull base tumors may be indicated.

Sensorineural Anosmia

At present, there is an absence of effective treatment options for postviral anosmia, posttraumatic anosmia, or presbyosmia. Many cases of postviral anosmia or posttraumatic anosmia may recover over 1 to 2 years, but this is difficult to predict. Many patients report parosmias early during recovery. Empiric trial of steroids is employed by many clinicians, and steroid-responsive anosmia is well documented. However, this must be weighed against the risks of steroid use. Oral zinc therapy is often recommended, but the available evidence does not support its use. Olfactory training therapy is safe and has been found to be helpful is some studies: patients are instructed to sniff three different odors (such as citrus, floral perfume, and coffee grounds) for 10 minutes twice daily for several weeks. Appropriate referral for suspected neurologic or systemic disease is imperative.

◆ Outcome and Follow-Up

It is critically important to educate the anosmic patient regarding the importance of working smoke detectors, natural gas detectors, and the labeling and dating of foods to avoid serious injury or death.

4.6 Taste Disorders

◆ Key Features

- The sense of taste is mediated by cranial nerves (CNs) VII, IX, and X.
- Most complaints of taste dysfunction are in fact olfactory disorders.
- Medication effects are the most commonly identifiable cause of taste dysfunction.

Taste or gustation is a proximal chemical sense. Unlike in olfaction (see **Chapter 4.5**), for taste the primary source of stimulus must be in physical contact with the patient. The qualitative descriptors elicited by stimulation of taste receptors include sweet, sour, salty, bitter, and umami (loanword from Japanese that roughly equates to "savory," with its own specific receptors stimulated by glutamates).

◆ Anatomy

Epithelial taste receptor cells are located on the anterior and posterior tongue, the soft palate, and in the larynx. Taste receptor cells are arrayed in sensory end organs, the taste buds, and synapse on primary sensory neurons of the facial nerve (CN VII), the glossopharyngeal nerve (CN IX), or the vagus nerve (CN X). Taste innervation is therefore redundant; that is, a lesion of a single cranial nerve would not abolish all taste input. Taste receptor cells in taste buds turn over and are replaced by proliferative basal cells. This indicates that certain clinical conditions that damage or destroy taste receptors may cause only temporary dysfunction since the system has a capacity for repair.

◆ Epidemiology

Taste loss, whether total (ageusia) or partial (hypogeusia), is much less common than olfactory loss. In a study of a large series of patients with chemosensory complaints, only 4% were found by objective testing to have a true taste deficit; the remainder exhibited olfactory deficits. This reflects the fact that the experience of flavor is mediated by the synergistic stimulation of the olfactory system, the oropharyngeal somatosensory system, and the actual taste receptors of the gustatory system.

◆ Clinical

Taste dysfunction may be a loss or a phantom or altered perception (dysgeusia). Partial loss is most common, and losses are usually quality or compound specific, rather than involving all taste sensation. Causes of taste dysfunction can be categorized as either drug/toxin effects or, less commonly, disease effects such as via periodontal disorders, neurologic disorders, nutritional disorders, infections, or endocrine disorders. Hedgehog inhibitor drugs, used to treat basal cell carcinoma, result in taste loss that can recover upon cessation of the drug. Radiation therapy for head and neck cancer can be another cause of taste dysfunction. Dysgeusia may (rarely) be a seizure manifestation. Iatrogenic injury to the chorda tympani during middle ear surgery can lead to gustatory complaints, such as a persistent metallic taste in the mouth, which gradually subside in most cases. Taste sensation has been shown to decline with age.

Burning mouth syndrome is a challenging problem. Patients complain of a burning oral sensation, often recurrent, with no apparent cause. Evaluation is aimed at eliminating any identifiable cause such as lesion, infection, or drug side effect. Management may include treating identifiable causes, removing offending medications, avoiding harsh toothpastes or mouthwashes, treating reflux, treating thrush, replacing ill-fitting dentures, general oral care and hydration, and trials of medications such as gabapentin for neuropathic pain. Also, modification of diet may be helpful.

◆ Evaluation

History and physical exam should be directed at determining whether the complaint truly relates to a taste disorder or (as is much more common) to an olfactory disorder. Objective testing for olfactory function such as the Smell Identification Test (Sensonics, Inc., Haddon Heights, NJ) can be helpful in this regard. Standardized objective testing for taste receptor function is not widely used. It is important to note that dysgeusia is usually described as one of the taste sensations (sweet, sour, etc.) or as metallic. If described as foul or rotten, this should alert the clinician to the possibility of an olfactory disorder.

✦ Treatment Options

If a taste disorder is identified, management is generally directed at removing or treating underlying causative factors and at supportive measures. Treating local infections such as oral thrush or periodontal disease may be helpful. Stopping possible offending systemic medications, if feasible, may be beneficial.

✦ Outcome and Follow-Up

Good oral care, hydration, nutrition, and xerostomia management with sialogogues are generally supportive measures. Radiation-induced taste dysfunction can recover gradually over many months but may be permanent.

4.7 Rhinologic Manifestations of Systemic Diseases

✦ Key Features

- Nonspecific sinonasal symptoms may be associated with a systemic disease.
- The symptoms are often managed medically to treat underlying disease.
- Radiographic and laboratory evaluation is helpful.

A broad spectrum of infectious, autoimmune, and neoplastic diseases may cause nasal obstruction as well as cosmetic deformity (**Table 4.11**).

✦ Epidemiology

Certain conditions are common in specific geographic areas and should be considered if appropriate. Examples include rhinosporidiosis in Sri Lanka or India and rhinoscleroma in Central America.

✦ Clinical

Signs and Symptoms

Findings with systemic disease processes involving the sinonasal region may be nonspecific and include nasal obstruction, pain, epistaxis, facial numbness, or rhinorrhea. Signs and symptoms of an underlying systemic condition, if active, may be elucidated by a thorough review of systems (e.g., fevers, chills, weight loss, dyspnea, and hematuria).

Differential Diagnosis

Systemic diseases that can involve the nose or sinuses include granulomatous disease such as sarcoidosis or Wegener's granulomatosis and histiocytosis

Table 4.11 Systemic diseases with sinonasal manifestations

Condition	Diagnostic findings	Treatment
Wegener's disease	Septal crusting, perforation, chronic sinusitis, "saddle deformity" (+) c-ANCA Biopsy: granuloma, vasculitis CXR; urinalysis important	Rheumatology consult Systemic steroids, cyclophosphamide, methotrexate, or trimethoprim–sulfamethoxazole
Sarcoidosis	Elevated ACE level Hilar adenopathy on CXR Nasal edema, crusting, pain, obstruction	Systemic steroids
Syphilis	(+) VDRL or RPR, FTA-ABS Nasal erosion at mucocutaneous junction, mucus, scabbing, obstruction, rarely septal smooth mass or perforation	Benzathine penicillin parenteral, or tetracycline
Rhinoscleroma	Africa, Central and South America travel Catarrhal, atrophic, granulomatous, fibrotic stages Biopsy: Mikulicz cells with intracellular Gram (–) organism	Débridement
Rhinosporidiosis	Sri Lanka, southern India Nasal obstruction, rhinorrhea, epistaxis, tumor-like nasal lesions Light microscopy demonstrates organism, *Rhinosporidium seeberi*	Surgical débridement Cauterization of margins Steroid injections for recurrence
Churg-Strauss's disease	Asthma, sinusitis, eosinophilia > 10%, histologically proven vasculitis, mononeuritis multiplex	Systemic steroids Cyclophosphamide Consider sinus surgery for persistent disease
Relapsing polychondritis	Three or more of the following: bilateral auricular chondritis, seronegative arthritis, nasal chondritis, ocular inflammation, audiovestibular injury May involve larynx Elevated ESR, (+) immune complex deposition on biopsy	Systemic steroids Cyclophosphamide, azathioprine, methotrexate, dapsone considered
Lethal midline granuloma	Now considered to be angiocentric T-cell lymphoma Destructive midline nasal lesion	Radiotherapy

Abbreviations: ACE, angiotensin-converting enzyme; c-ANCA, antineutrophil cytoplasmic antibody; CXR, chest X-ray; ESR, erythrocyte sedimentation rate; FTA-ABS, fluorescent treponemal antibody absorbed; RPR, rapid plasma reagin; VDRL, Venereal Disease Research Laboratory test.

X; infectious disease such as syphilis or mycobacteria (both tuberculosis and leprosy). Rhinoscleroma is seen in Central America; rhinosporidiosis is seen in India and Sri Lanka. Neoplastic disease such as T-cell lymphoma (formerly called midline lethal granuloma) affects the nasal cavity. Inflammatory/ immune system disorders affecting the lower respiratory tract and sinuses, such as Churg-Strauss's disease, should be considered in severe asthmatics with severe sinusitis. HIV disease can predispose to sinonasal infections; adenoid hypertrophy in adults should raise suspicion for HIV. Inflammation of nasal cartilage can be seen with relapsing polychondritis.

◆ Evaluation

Physical Exam

A full head and neck examination and a cranial nerve exam are performed. It is important to exclude evidence of complicated sinusitis, such as orbital or intracranial extension of disease. Therefore, note is made of proptosis, peri-orbital edema, extraocular motility, tenderness, and meningeal signs. Nasal endoscopy should be performed after topical decongestion. Assessment includes position of the septum and presence of perforation; presence of mucosal edema; presence, location, and quality of mucus or purulence; and presence and quality of masses. A calcium alginate swab (Calgiswab, Puritan Medical Products, Guilford, ME) or suction trap can be easily used to obtain a sample of any purulence endoscopically from the sinus ostia or middle meatus for culture and sensitivities. Assess for adenoid (pharyngeal tonsil) hypertrophy or nasopharyngeal masses.

Imaging

Thin-section noncontrast coronal and axial computed tomography (CT) scanning of the paranasal sinuses is the most useful study. Staging systems have been proposed and may be useful for research or tracking disease over time. Mucosal thickening or fluid levels are seen easily. The bony detail of the skull base and orbits should be assessed. Bone erosion, thickening, or the presence of a sinonasal mass suggests other than acute rhinosinusitis and will prompt additional work-up. Fungal disease will appear as heterogeneous density. Evidence of expansile disease with bone thinning is seen with allergic fungal rhinosinusitis, mucocele, and low-grade neoplasms. Bony erosion should raise concern for malignancy, and is also seen with inflammatory disease such as Wegener's disease. Bony thickening is seen with long-standing inflammatory disease. Magnetic resonance imaging (MRI) is helpful for assessing intracranial extension. Fungus may appear as an absent signal with both a T1 and T2 MRI sequence. The utility of plain films is very limited.

Labs

Laboratory studies are an important component of the work-up. The angiotensin-converting enzyme (ACE) level may be elevated with sarcoidosis; the anti–neutrophil cytoplasmic antibody (c-ANCA) is elevated with active Wegener's disease; a purified protein derivative test may indicate mycobacterial disease; a Venereal Disease Research Laboratory (VDRL) test can exclude syphilis; erythrocyte sedimentation rate and antinuclear antibody test may indicate rheumatic inflammatory disease. A chest X-ray and urinalysis may be informative for Wegener's disease. Consider human immunodeficiency virus (HIV) testing.

Pathology

A biopsy of an intranasal mass may be helpful. However, one must first exclude the possibility of an encephalocele or a highly vascular lesion such as an angiofibroma; thus, imaging before biopsy is prudent. A biopsy of the margin of a septal perforation may reveal granuloma, vasculitis, or neoplasm but frequently reveals only necrotic tissue or inflammation.

◆ Treatment Options

Medical

Medical therapy directed at the underlying systemic condition is, in general, the treatment of choice. Specific therapy depends upon the diagnosis. Wegener's disease is treated in consultation with a rheumatologist with systemic steroids, cyclophosphamide, methotrexate, or trimethoprim–sulfamethoxazole. Sarcoidosis is treated with systemic steroids. Infectious processes are managed with appropriate antibiotic therapy, ideally based upon cultures and sensitivities. Rhinoscleroma is due to *Klebsiella rhinoscleromatis* and may require aminoglycoside treatment.

Surgical

Surgical treatment of chronic rhinosinusitis due to inflammatory conditions such as Wegener's disease is best performed following systemic anti-inflammatory therapy, once disease is relatively quiescent, if possible. The same principle applies to surgical correction of destructive septal lesions or "saddle nose" deformity. Rhinosporidiosis may require surgical débridement.

◆ Outcome and Follow-Up

Outcome and follow-up depend upon specific diagnosis.

5 Laryngology and the Upper Aerodigestive Tract

Section Editor

Johnathan D. McGinn

Contributors

David Goldenberg

Bradley J. Goldstein

Melissa M. Krempasky

Johnathan D. McGinn

5.0 Anatomy and Physiology of the Upper Aerodigestive Tract

The upper aerodigestive tract is composed of the nasal cavity, nasopharynx, oral cavity, oropharynx, hypopharynx, larynx, trachea, and esophagus. The complex anatomy and physiology supports basic functions in respiration, phonation, deglutition, and the special sense apparatus for the olfactory and gustatory systems. Important aspects of anatomy and physiology are reviewed here. Nasal and paranasal sinus anatomy and physiology are covered in **Chapter 4.0**.

◆ Oral Cavity

General

The vestibule includes the mucosal surface of the lips, buccal mucosa, and buccal/lateral surfaces of the alveolar ridges. The remainder of the oral cavity includes the more medial structures, including the hard and soft palate, mobile tongue (anterior two-thirds), and the oral floor. The oral floor contains the sublingual salivary glands, and the openings of the submandibular ducts (Wharton's ducts), draining the submandibular glands, are found throughout on either side of the midline. The frenulum attaches the anterior tongue to the midline oral floor. Minor salivary glands coat the oral cavity and pharynx.

Musculature

The vestibule includes the orbicularis oris, various levators and depressors, as well as the buccinator, all muscles of facial expression. Tongue musculature involves both intrinsic muscles and extrinsic muscles, including the genioglossus, hyoglossus, and styloglossus, all of which are innervated by the hypoglossal nerve.

Blood Supply

The lingual artery is the primary blood supply to the tongue. The facial artery, a branch of the external carotid, supplies the vestibule via the superior and inferior labial arteries. The greater and lesser palatine foramina in the lateral hard palate house the greater and lesser palatine arteries, branches of the maxillary artery.

Lymphatic Drainage

Facial lymphatics drain primarily to submental, submandibular, and facial nodes of level 1, while the anterior tongue lymphatics drain to upper jugular nodes of level 2, often bilaterally.

Nerve Supply

The hypoglossal nerve, cranial nerve (CN) XII, is the motor supply to the tongue. The lingual nerve (a branch of the mandibular nerve, CN V_3) provides sensation, and taste fibers of the chorda tympani, to the anterior two-thirds of the tongue; CNs IX and X innervate taste buds of the posterior tongue and the base of the epiglottis, respectively. The facial nerve (CN VII) is the motor supply to the orbicularis oris. General sensation to the buccal mucosa is via the second division of the trigeminal nerve (maxillary nerve, CN V$_2$).

Physiology

On average, 1,500 mL of saliva is produced daily from the parotid, sublingual, submandibular, and minor salivary glands.

Detailed swallowing physiology is beyond the scope of this handbook. Briefly, swallowing is divided into active and passive phases. The active phases include a preparatory phase that involves salivation and mastication, and a second oral phase that involves bolus propulsion posteriorly. In the passive phase, CNs IX and X control involuntary laryngeal protective mechanisms and peristalsis.

◆ Pharynx

General

The pharynx extends from the skull base to the sixth cervical vertebra (C6) and is divided into the nasopharynx, superior to the palate; the oropharynx, extending from the palate to the hyoid and from the circumvallate papillae anteriorly; and the hypopharynx, inferior to the hyoid, including the piriform recesses, posterior wall, and postcricoid region (**Fig. 5.1**).

The cervical esophagus extends inferiorly, and the laryngotracheal complex sits anteromedially. Waldeyer's ring of lymphoid tissue includes the adenoids (pharyngeal tonsil) of the nasopharynx, the palatine tonsils of the oropharynx, and the lingual tonsil lining the base of the tongue. Taste buds and minor salivary glands exist in this region as well. The auditory tubes (eustachian tubes) open in the lateral nasopharynx.

Musculature

The superior, middle, and inferior pharyngeal constrictors surround the pharynx, enveloped by the visceral layer of cervical fascia. The palatopharyngeus and stylopharyngeus are supportive. The palatoglossus and palatopharyngeus form the tonsillar pillars.

Blood Supply

The lingual artery supplies the tongue. The palatine tonsils are supplied by external carotid branches via the facial artery, lingual artery, lesser palatine artery, descending palatine artery, and ascending pharyngeal artery.

Lymphatic Drainage

Rich bilateral drainage supplies the base of the tongue and piriform recesses and drains to levels 2 through 4. The tonsils drain primarily to the jugulodigastric region.

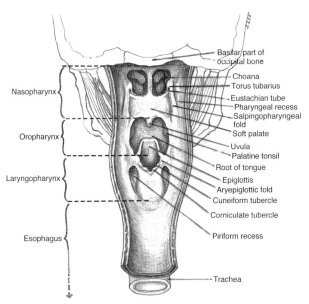

Fig. 5.1 Opened posterior view of the pharynx, demonstrating the boundaries of the nasopharynx, oropharynx, and hypopharynx. (Used with permission from Van de Water TR, Staecker H. *Otolaryngology: Basic Science and Clinical Review*. New York: Thieme; 2006:553.)

Nerve Supply

The palatine tonsils have sensory supply from the glossopharyngeal nerve (CN IX) and the lesser palatine nerve (branch of the maxillary nerve, CN V_2). Referred otalgia is common. CNs IX and X supply motor and sensory innervation to the hypopharynx.

Physiology

Swallowing is discussed with the physiology of the oral cavity, above.

◆ Larynx

General

The larynx can be considered to be a complex valve that regulates airflow. It is a dynamic organ that is involved with both the respiratory/vocal system and the digestive tract because of its position in the pharynx. Its lumen continues superiorly with the pharynx and inferiorly with the trachea; posteroinferiorly it is separated from the pharyngoesophageal lumen. The larynx is divided into the supraglottis, which includes the epiglottis, arytenoids, aryepiglottic fold, false vocal fold, and ventricle; the glottis, which is 1 cm inferior to the laryngeal inlet and includes the true vocal folds; and the subglottis, which extends inferiorly to the inferior border of the cricoid cartilage ring (**Fig. 5.2**).

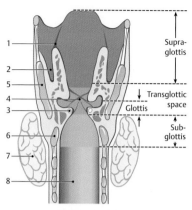

Fig. 5.2 Compartments and individual structures in the larynx. 1. The aryepiglottic fold, forming the boundary between the larynx and hypopharynx. 2. The piriform recess, which belongs to the hypopharynx. 3. Vocal ligament. 4. Anterior commissure. 5. Thyroid cartilage. 6. Cricoid cartilage. 7. Thyroid gland. 8. Trachea. (Used with permission from Behrbohm H et al. *Ear, Nose, and Throat Diseases: With Head and Neck Surgery*, 3rd ed. New York: Thieme; 2009:293.)

Skeleton

Three unpaired cartilages form the main laryngeal structure (**Fig. 5.3**). These are the epiglottis, the thyroid cartilage (from the Greek *thyreos*, meaning oblong shield), and the cricoid (from the Greek *krikos*, meaning ring). Three paired cartilages constitute the remainder of the laryngeal skeleton: the arytenoids, the corniculates, and the cuneiforms. Anterosuperiorly, the larynx is connected to the hyoid bone by the thyrohyoid membrane and muscle, and inferiorly it joins the trachea. Posteriorly, the larynx meets the muscular wall of the pharynx, with the cervical vertebrae posterior to this layer. The thyroid and cricoid cartilages are hyaline cartilage, which may ossify with age. The inferior horns of the thyroid cartilage articulate with the cricoid cartilage; the paired arytenoids articulate with the cranial border of the cricoid lamina. Both of these articulations are synovial joints.

Soft Tissue

Externally, the important membranes include the thyrohyoid membrane, the cricothyroid membrane, and the cricotracheal ligament. Internally, the membranous lining of the larynx is the quadrangular membrane superiorly, extending to the vestibular fold or false vocal fold, and the cricovocal membrane or conus elasticus, extending from the true vocal fold inferiorly. Paired aryepiglottic folds define the opening into the laryngeal lumen superiorly. Lateral and inferior are the piriform recesses, which funnel food and liquid into the esophagus. The paired vocal folds extend from the vocal process of the arytenoids dorsally to the thyroid cartilage ventrally at the anterior commissure. The structure of the vocal folds includes the vocal ligament, lateral cricothyroid ligament, median cricothyroid ligament, the vocalis muscle (thyroarytenoid), and the mucosal covering.

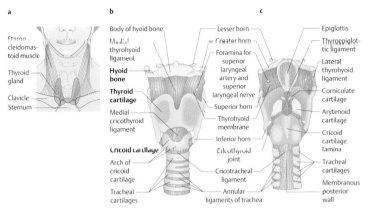

Fig. 5.3 Anatomy of the laryngeal bones and cartilage. (Used with permission from Probst R, Grevers G, Iro H. *Basic Otorhinolaryngology: A Step-by-Step Learning Guide*. New York: Thieme; 2006:338.)

Musculature

The posterior cricoarytenoid exclusively opens (abducts) the vocal folds. The lateral cricoarytenoid and transverse arytenoid (interarytenoid) closes the vocal folds, along with the thyroarytenoid. The thyroarytenoid and the cricothyroid place the vocal folds under tension.

Blood Supply

Arterial supply to the supraglottis arises from the external carotid via the superior laryngeal artery. The inferior laryngeal artery, arising from the subclavian artery via the thyrocervical trunk, supplies the subglottis. Venous drainage is to the internal jugular and brachiocephalic veins.

Lymphatic Drainage

The supraglottis has rich bilateral lymphatic drainage, with connections via the preepiglottic space. The glottis has few lymphatics. The subglottis also has rich bilateral drainage via paratracheal and pretracheal channels. The lymphatic drainage influences the frequency of metastatic spread of laryngeal carcinomas based on the sites of involvement of the primary tumor.

Nerve Supply

The vagus nerve (CN X) supplies the larynx. The superior laryngeal nerve has an external branch, providing motor function to the cricothyroid muscle, and an internal branch, providing sensation to the supraglottis and glottis. The recurrent laryngeal nerve provides motor supply to all other internal laryngeal muscles. On the left, the recurrent nerve passes around the aortic arch; on the right, it passes around the subclavian artery. Both recurrent nerves then ascend along the tracheoesophageal groove to enter the larynx at the inferior cornu of the thyroid cartilage. Importantly, the recurrent laryngeal nerve may branch in the neck prior to entering the larynx. (A nonrecurrent right laryngeal nerve may occur if an aberrant subclavian artery is present.)

Physiology

Briefly, the basic functions of the larynx include airway protection, speech, and respiration. The larynx acts as a sphincter, in concert with pharyngeal structures, to prevent airway aspiration. This is facilitated via epiglottic tilt and contraction of the aryepiglottic folds, false vocal folds, true vocal folds, and adductors. Detailed discussion of the physiology of phonation is beyond the scope of this book.

◆ Esophagus

General

The esophagus lies posterior to the trachea. The esophageal opening is ~15 cm from the upper incisors at the lower border of the cricoid (C6), and the gastroesophageal junction is ~40 cm in adults. The upper esophageal sphincter is formed by the cricopharyngeus muscle at the esophageal opening. A middle physiologic sphincter exists at ~25 cm due to the aortic arch and left bronchus. The lower esophageal sphincter is at the gastroesophageal junction. The esophageal wall has a mucosa, submucosa, muscle layer, and outer fibrous adventitia. There are external longitudinal muscle fibers and internal circular fibers. The superior third is striated muscle, the middle third is mixed, and the inferior third is smooth muscle. The mucosa is stratified squamous, with a transition to columnar epithelium at the junction with the stomach.

Blood Supply

Superiorly, supply is via branches from the inferior thyroid artery originating from the thyrocervical trunk. In the thorax, supply is segmental via branches of the thoracic aorta or via intercostal vessels. Inferiorly, there are branches from the left gastric artery. There is a venous plexus, and drainage parallels supply generally.

Lymphatic Drainage

The cervical lymphatic system includes the deep cervical and paratracheal nodes; the thoracic lymphatics are composed of the posterior mediastinal and tracheobronchial nodes. The abdominal lymphatic system incorporates the left gastric and celiac nodes.

Nerve Supply

The esophagus is served by the glossopharyngeal and vagus nerves and the sympathetics. The myenteric plexus of Auerbach lies between the longitudinal and circular muscle layers.

Physiology

The esophageal phase of swallowing occurs as the bolus passes the upper esophageal sphincter. Primary peristalsis has an initial rapid inhibitory phase followed by a longer wave of contraction. The lower esophageal sphincter relaxes to open for 6 to 8 seconds. There is also a secondary peristaltic wave in a rostral to caudal progression.

5.1 Laryngeal and Esophageal Emergencies

5.1.1 Stridor

◆ Key Features

- Stridor is an indication of airway compromise and should be considered an emergency.
- The priorities are to identify the site of obstruction, restore adequate ventilation, and address the underlying cause.

Stridor is an exam finding defined broadly as noisy breathing due to partial upper airway obstruction, and it is usually high-pitched and harsh. This is to be distinguished from wheezing, which is noise due to reversible collapse of bronchioles of the lower pulmonary airway, and from stertor, a sonorous noise that is due to collapse or obstruction at the upper pharynx, such as snoring.

◆ Clinical

The stridulous patient must be evaluated without delay, as loss of airway may progress rapidly.

Signs and Symptoms

In the adult, development of stridor may be acute or chronic. Symptoms are often nonspecific and variable. Associated symptoms will vary depending on etiology and may include dyspnea, pharyngodynia, dysphagia, odynophagia, and anxiety. Signs include audible noise with breathing and may include fever, cough, hemoptysis, and retractions. Depending on severity and acuity, the patient may be in distress, may be hypoxic, and may also display dysphonia.

Differential Diagnosis

The causes of stridor are numerous. It is useful to categorize based on the anatomic level of obstruction. As a generalization, inspiratory stridor correlates with supraglottic obstruction, expiratory stridor correlates with intrathoracic obstruction (trachea), and biphasic stridor suggests glottic or subglottic obstruction (**Table 5.1**). Differential diagnosis includes an obstructing neoplasm, infection with edema (e.g., supraglottitis), allergy/

Table 5.1   Stridor localization by anatomic site

	Retractions	Stridor*	Voice	Feeding
Naso/oropharynx	Minimal	Stertor[†]	Normal	Normal[†]
Supraglottis	Marked and severe	Inspiratory and high-pitched	Muffled	Abnormal
Glottis/subglottis	Mild to severe	Biphasic and intermediate-pitched	Normal to very abnormal (barking cough)	Normal
Intrathoracic trachea	Mild to severe	Expiratory and low-pitched	Normal (seal-like cough)	Normal

*The quality of the airway noise.
[†]Unless associated with complete nasal obstruction in a neonate.
(Adapted with permission from Van de Water TR, Staecker H. *Otolaryngology: Basic Science and Clinical Review*. New York: Thieme; 2006:214.)

angioedema, foreign body, traumatic injury to the airway (e.g., thyroid cartilage fracture, large hematoma), and bilateral vocal fold immobility (e.g., postoperative iatrogenic injury). Other causes include subglottic stenosis, tracheal stenosis, and tracheomalacia.

◆ Evaluation

One must consider an acutely stridulous patient as a potential airway emergency; prompt evaluation is warranted.

Physical Exam

In critical care algorithms, the ABCs are followed: airway, breathing, circulation. Stridor is a reflection of airway narrowing and is therefore a priority. If the stridulous patient is not ventilating adequately (hypoxic or retaining CO_2), rapid intervention is critical. Establishment of the airway is discussed subsequently under Treatment Options.

History is important in guiding the exam: the timing of onset; known diagnoses, such as history of angioedema or head and neck cancers; previous head and neck surgeries (thyroid surgery, previous tracheotomy); trauma; possible foreign body aspiration; current upper respiratory infection; history of intubations; and any other relevant facts.

On exam, vital signs; pulse oximetry; possibly arterial blood gases; phonation; an oral and pharyngeal exam; and a neck exam for masses, edema, crepitus, or tenderness are important. Unless the adult patient is unstable or not adequately ventilating, a flexible fiberoptic nasopharyngolaryngoscopy is usually safe and extremely helpful. This exam will reveal an estimation of glottic airway diameter, vocal fold mobility, any sites of edema or mass, or the presence of an obstructing laryngeal foreign body. Pediatric patients may selectively undergo flexible fiberoptic examination. Caution must be used, as the examination can precipitate further airway compromise.

Imaging

Plain films of the neck—posteroanterior (PA) and lateral views—may be informative but are being replaced by computed tomography (CT) or magnetic resonance imaging (MRI). In general, one should not send a patient with airway compromise for CT or MRI unless the airway has been secured; loss of the airway during imaging can be disastrous.

Labs

An arterial blood gas (ABG) test may be helpful in determining adequacy of ventilation. Less acutely, a complete blood count (CBC) with differential may be useful in a patient with infection, such as supraglottitis.

◆ Treatment Options

The goals of treatment are (1) to determine the site(s) and degree of obstruction; (2) to stabilize the airway by forced ventilation, intubation, or surgical bypass of the site of obstruction; and (3) to treat the underlying cause.

In an unstable, poorly ventilating patient, the airway must be secured. If possible, the operating room is the safest place to do this. One should approach the airway problem algorithmically, thinking ahead about possible problems (with a plan B and plan C). The algorithm will differ depending on the etiology and the patient. There are useful generalizations, however. (1) It is absolutely critical that the otolaryngologist clearly and authoritatively take control of the airway management. (2) An upright, awake, spontaneously breathing patient is usually the safest situation. (3) One must be prepared for the possibility that sedating and paralyzing a stridulous patient for intubation may result in an inability to mask ventilate, precipitating an emergency. (4) With angioedema, tongue swelling usually precludes the ability to perform direct laryngoscopy.

If intubation is deemed to be impractical (e.g., fiberoptic laryngoscopy indicates that an endotracheal tube will not pass through a narrowed airway), awake tracheotomy is performed. In an emergency where the surgical airway must be most rapidly established, cricothyroidotomy is indicated.

Unless the fiberoptic laryngoscopy suggests otherwise, an awake fiberoptic nasotracheal intubation is often the procedure of choice (if the patient requires intubation). As a backup plan, one should have a Holinger laryngoscope, velvet-eye laryngeal suction, and Eschmann stylet assembled and ready to use. Often, the otolaryngologist can easily intubate a patient with these instruments. A ventilating rigid bronchoscope is also very helpful, if available. In these cases, the patient should be maintained with spontaneous ventilation; if the patient has airway masses or stenosis, then ventilating bronchoscopy can be diagnostic and therapeutic. In addition, a tracheotomy tray should be open and ready to use. Injecting the soft tissue over the cricothyroid membrane with 1% lidocaine and 1:100,000 epinephrine ahead of time will result in vasoconstriction and a much drier operative field if emergency cricothyroidotomy or tracheotomy becomes necessary.

Other strategies for difficult intubation include retrograde intubation by placing a needle and guidewire (from a central line kit) into the cricothyroid membrane or trachea and passing the guidewire up and out of the mouth.

An orotracheal tube may then be blindly passed over the guidewire and into the trachea. There are other techniques, such as fiberoptic intubation through a laryngeal mask airway, video direct laryngoscopy, intubating endoscopes (e.g., Shikani optical stylet), or the use of a lighted stylet to be blindly introduced into the trachea.

Medically, there are helpful strategies to "buy time" or assess response to medical therapy if a patient can maintain ventilation. The patient is maintained in an intensive care unit with continuous pulse oximetry monitoring. Humidified oxygen (e.g., via face tent) will help minimize secretions. Heliox (typically 79% helium/21% oxygen mixture) has been advocated as a short-term intervention to help maximize ventilation while definitive intervention is planned. The gas functions by reducing the viscosity of the inspired air, thus reducing the mechanical work of breathing in the narrowed airway. It can be used while medical intervention is taking effect; this is an excellent means of avoiding intubation. Intravenous (IV) steroids (i.e., dexamethasone 8 mg IV every 8 hours) may reduce airway edema. In some situations, appropriate medical treatment of the underlying problem, such as infection or angioedema, can obviate the need for intubation or surgical airway.

◆ Outcome and Follow-Up

After securing the airway, appropriate management directed at the underlying problem is undertaken. This may include biopsy, treatment of infection, and laboratory or radiographic work-up.

5.1.2   Laryngeal Fractures

◆ Key Features

- Airway obstruction can develop rapidly.
- Evaluate for concurrent injuries such as pneumothorax or esophageal or vascular injury.
- The treatment goals are to ensure an adequate airway, to maintain voice quality, and prevent aspiration.

Laryngeal fractures can be mild, nondisplaced, and isolated. They may also be severe and displaced, with airway compromise and concomitant injuries to other structures of the head, neck, and chest. A fiberoptic laryngeal exam and a computed tomography (CT) scan will usually direct care appropriately.

◆ Epidemiology

Five to ten percent of traumatic injuries involve the neck. Penetrating neck injuries are more common than blunt trauma (see also **Chapter 6.1.4**).

◆ Clinical

Patients usually present with a history of blunt trauma to the anterior neck. Common mechanisms include assault, a strangling or hanging attempt, and vehicular accidents including automobiles, snowmobiles, motorcycles, all-terrain vehicles, and bicycles. A gunshot wound to the neck can result in a cricoid or thyroid fracture alone or in combination with other injury.

Signs and Symptoms

Signs and symptoms may include dysphonia, aphonia, stridor, cough, hemoptysis, dysphagia, and pain. A hallmark of severe injury is subcutaneous emphysema, as well as loss of the normal prominence of the thyroid cartilage.

Differential Diagnosis

Differential diagnosis is based on severity. The injury may be confined to soft tissue or may include cartilage fracture, mucosal disruption, or additional injuries to the pharynx, esophagus, or major vessels.

◆ Evaluation

Physical Exam

A fiberoptic exam and CT are diagnostic. The injury may be occult. A delay in diagnosis contributes to mortality. Trauma algorithms are followed, including ABCs (airway, breathing, circulation). In the presence of laryngotracheal cartilage disruption, intubation is generally contraindicated. An emergency airway is established via a tracheotomy. Transtracheal jet ventilation can be extremely useful while the definitive airway is being established. The remainder of the head and neck exam is directed at determining additional injuries. With a questionable laryngeal fracture, flexible fiberoptic laryngoscopy is performed. The presence of obvious endolaryngeal mucosal disruption, bleeding, or cartilage derangement suggests the injury.

Labs

Laboratory tests are not routinely indicated. When following an inpatient after a laryngeal fracture, a complete blood count (CBC) with differential may be useful to monitor for infection and the development of mediastinitis or sepsis.

Other Tests

Once the airway is deemed stable or stabilized, imaging should be obtained. A CT scan of the neck, viewed with bone windows, provides excellent detail of the laryngeal framework. A chest X-ray is mandatory to evaluate for pneumothorax. A cervical esophagogram is recommended to evaluate for occult esophageal injury.

◆ Treatment Options

The acute treatment goal is maintaining or establishing the airway, as just discussed. The long-term treatment goals include maintaining an adequate airway, a satisfactory voice, and the ability to swallow without aspiration.

Larynx trauma can be categorized as mild or severe. Mild injuries include laryngeal edema, simple endolaryngeal lacerations with minimal cartilage exposure, and nondisplaced fractures. If severity is unclear, an examination under anesthesia with direct laryngoscopy and esophagoscopy is recommended. Patients with mild injuries can usually be managed nonoperatively. Treatment must include observation in a monitored bed (i.e., continuous pulse oximetry), along with intravenous (IV) steroids (Decadron [Merck & Co., Inc., Whitehouse Station, NJ] 8 mg IV every 8 hours × 3 doses), humidified air/O_2, and a soft diet.

Patients with severe mucosal injuries and/or displaced or comminuted cartilage fractures are managed surgically with low tracheotomy followed by exploration and repair. Fractures should be repaired early—ideally, within 24 hours. The basic goals include closure of tracheal defects, coverage of exposed cartilage, removal of devitalized cartilage, and reduction of cartilage fractures. After tracheotomy, direct laryngoscopy and esophagoscopy are performed. If the vocal folds are significantly displaced, laryngofissure is performed with repair of mucosa. Fractures are reduced and reapproximated with Prolene (Ethicon, Somerville, NJ) suture, wire, mesh, or plating. If possible, external perichondrium should be closed. Stenting may be necessary to prevent stenosis or anterior webbing. Indications for stenting are an area of controversy.

◆ Outcome and Follow-Up

Posttreatment follow-up includes ongoing assessment of the airway and swallowing. A barium swallow study with speech-language pathology for evidence of aspiration is important. Consideration of tracheotomy decannulation is based on standard criteria. Further surgical management of webbing or stenosis may be required, as well as long-term use of a T-tube. Patients may require voice therapy.

5.1.3   Caustic Ingestion

◆ Key Features

- Perform an airway assessment and intubation if there is any compromise.
- Identify the ingested substance.
- Do an early endoscopy.

◆ Epidemiology

The incidence of caustic ingestion is estimated at 5,000 to 15,000 cases annually in the United States; 53% of cases occur in children 6 years of age or less. However, only ~3% of deaths secondary to caustic ingestion occur in young children.

◆ Clinical

The patient with caustic ingestion presents with varying findings depending on the type of substance ingested and the quantity.

Signs and Symptoms

With moderate to severe injury, symptoms include oral, neck, and chest pain and dysphagia. Young patients may drool, and older patients may spit secretions or refuse to swallow. Respiratory problems range from coughing and wheezing to stridor and respiratory distress.

Differential Diagnosis

The injury may range from mild to severe as a result of acid versus alkaline ingestion.

◆ Evaluation

It is important to obtain information about the substance ingested. Alkaline substances (lye, ammonia, soaps) cause liquefaction necrosis and deep penetrating injuries to the pharyngeal and esophageal wall. Ingestion of lye (sodium hydroxide, drain cleaner) accounts for ~60% of cases. Acids cause a mucosal surface coagulative necrosis, and deep tissue injury is uncommon. Household bleach is usually less than 5.25% sodium hypochlorite and, therefore, usually causes only mild mucosal irritation.

Physical Exam

Assessment of the airway is the first priority. If there is evidence of airway compromise, the airway should be secured by intubation before edema worsens. This is especially important in children. A head and neck exam and skin survey for caustic burns from the spilled substance are indicated, followed by assessment of the oral and pharyngeal mucosa for injury. Blind nasogastric tube placement is avoided; emesis is not induced; charcoal gastric lavage is not indicated. In the past, the timing of endoscopy was controversial. Currently, esophagoscopy within 24 to 48 hours is recommended. Damage, in terms of an estimate of the depth of injury, is assessed at the proximal extent of injury. Additional advancement of the rigid endoscope is not performed, to avoid further injury.

Labs

Routine preoperative labs are obtained if surgery is planned. A complete blood count (CBC) is followed if there is suspicion of mediastinitis.

Table 5.2   Grading of esophageal caustic burns by endoscopic findings

1st degree	Erythema and punctuate hemorrhages Superficial mucosal injury
2nd degree	Ulceration, exudates, pseudomembranes Partial-thickness injury
3rd degree	Eschar, perforation into or through muscular layer Full-thickness injury

Other Tests

Acutely, a contrast swallow study is not routinely indicated. However, contrast swallow studies are often used to assess the progression of stricture formation during recovery.

◆ Treatment Options

Nonoperative therapy includes hydration, acid-blocking medications, and observation. Steroids do not seem to reduce the incidence of stricture formation; some authors have suggested that they may mask the signs or symptoms of perforation. Antibiotics are often given empirically until perforation has been ruled out. An endoscopy is performed to grade the injury (**Table 5.2**). In general, the scope should not be passed beyond any segments of necrosis or concern for transmural injury. A thoracic surgery consultation is obtained for management of perforation or high-grade injuries. There has been a trend toward early surgical intervention by thoracic surgeons (within 36 hours) to treat deep esophageal injuries. When there is evidence of a high-grade injury on endoscopy, a feeding tube should be placed under direct vision.

◆ Outcome and Follow-Up

Mortality ranges from 0 to 8% overall. Complications including mediastinitis, perforation, and stricture formation range from 10 to 20%. Stricture development generally begins at week 3 or 4; a contrast swallow study or a follow-up endoscopy is helpful at this time.

5.1.4   Laryngeal Infections

◆ Key Features

- Infections of the larynx may be acute or chronic in nature.
- Symptoms and signs include hoarseness, pain, dysphagia, cough, dyspnea, stridor, and signs of systemic illness.
- Therapy is directed at the causative organism and is supportive of any airway issues present.
- Laryngoscopy with biopsy and/or culture may be necessary, as some infections may mimic neoplasms, or required for a definitive diagnosis.

"Laryngitis" is a term used to describe any inflammatory condition of the larynx. Infectious laryngitis may be caused by viral, bacterial, mycobacterial, fungal, and even protozoan organisms. History and physical examination, including laryngoscopy, are instrumental in establishing the diagnosis. The immunologic state of the patient, travel history, and exposure to illness are important factors to address in the history.

◆ Epidemiology

Viral laryngitis is the most common type of laryngitis. Incidence is difficult to establish, as most patients do not seek out care for acute laryngitis issues. Secondary to airway size, laryngitis may present in children with airway symptoms; adults more commonly present with hoarseness and pain complaints.

◆ Clinical

Signs and Symptoms

Viral Laryngitis

Viral laryngitis usually accompanies a viral upper respiratory infection (URI) with systemic viral syndrome. Symptoms include hoarseness, with pitch breaks, and decreased pitch; cough; and pain. Examination shows erythema and edema of the vocal folds. Agents include those causing URIs, with rhinovirus being most common. Treatment is symptomatic, as this should be a self-limited disease. Therapy includes voice rest, hydration, humidification, cough suppressants, and expectorants.

Croup

Croup (laryngotracheitis) is a viral infection seen in children characterized by stridor, a "barky" cough, and fever. This illness is seen primarily in winter but may occur year-round. The severity of the illness varies widely and is based on the degree of subglottic edema. Parainfluenza viruses 1 and 2 and influenza A are the most common etiologic agents. The most important assessment of these patients is evaluating the respiratory status for impending airway intervention and support. Initial home management involves humidification or steam shower, although this is not evidence-based. Racemic epinephrine may be useful to those children with respiratory distress, serving to decrease airway edema rapidly. Admission is no longer thought to be absolutely necessary after this treatment, as the "rebound" concern is rare. Corticosteroids have a clear role in treatment of this condition. Airway intervention including intubation or tracheotomy may be necessary if respiratory decompensation occurs, with respiratory fatigue, hypercarbia, inadequate oxygenation, or worsening neurologic status. For intubated children, an air leak should develop and indicate extubation potential, usually within 2 or 3 days.

Bacterial Laryngitis

Bacterial laryngitis is far less common than viral etiologies. Supraglottitis may involve the entire supraglottis or, more focally, the epiglottis (epiglottitis). The incidence of epiglottitis in children has dramatically fallen since the introduction of the *Haemophilus influenzae* type B vaccine. Adults typically have more diffuse supraglottitis. Patients relate sore throat, fever, odynophagia, muffled voice, and dyspnea. Children may have drooling. Patients may sit in a tripod position, with the torso leaning partially forward, arms positioned at the sides just in front of the torso, and neck extended. Diagnosis is confirmed by the swollen, erythematous epiglottis or supraglottis seen on flexible laryngoscopy. In children, the diagnosis may best be made by lateral neck film and a "thumbprint" sign representing a swollen epiglottis, as manipulation of the airway with flexible endoscopy may precipitate airway compromise. Although historically *H. influenzae* is the most common organism in children, other organisms such as *Streptococcus pneumoniae, Staphylococcus aureus,* β-hemolytic *Streptococcus, Klebsiella pneumoniae,* and parainfluenza virus may be etiologic agents. In severe cases, a secure airway should be established, potentially in an operating room setting. Less emergent airways may be managed with hospital admission and close observation. Adults are less frequently in need of airway interventions than children are. Treatment should include antibiotics that cover β-lactamase-producing *H. influenzae,* such as a second- or third-generation cephalosporin, as well as corticosteroids. Epiglottis abscess is a rare complication of supraglottitis.

Fungal Laryngitis

Although fungal infections occur more commonly in the immunocompromised patient, fungal laryngitis may be seen in many varied patient populations. These infections may present as leukoplakia, either focal or diffuse. Risk factors for fungal laryngitis include those with diminished systemic immune response (e.g., immunocompromised states, diabetes, human immunodeficiency virus [HIV], immunomodulating medications, and severe nutritional deficiencies), or depressed local immune function (e.g., prior local radiation therapy, corticosteroid inhalers, smokers). *Candida* sp. are the most common organisms, but blastomycoses, *Histoplasma, Aspergillus, Cryptococcus,* and coccidiomycosis may be involved. Secondary to the infrequency of these infections and their presentation as leukoplakia, biopsy may be done. Some infections can show pseudoepitheliomatous changes and can even be mistaken for squamous cell carcinoma. Special fungal stains may be necessary. Systemic antifungal agents appropriate for the causative fungal organism are necessary. Topical antifungal medications are not curative, as they require direct contact with the organism, and the larynx is protected from exposure through protective-airway mechanisms.

Tuberculosis

Tuberculosis of the larynx may be seen with pulmonary infection (historically one of the most common laryngeal infections), but may be experienced as an isolated infection in 20 to 40%. Risk factors include exposure in endemic areas, immunocompromised states, and nursing home environments. Patients typically report hoarseness, dysphagia, odynophagia, and cough. The larynx typically is edematous and hyperemic in its posterior third, with some exophytic granular areas. Biopsy, chest radiography, and sputum cultures may be necessary for diagnosis. Treatment is with antimycobacterial drugs, with cultures helpful given the significant drug resistance that may be present.

Actinomycosis

Actinomycosis is an unusual laryngeal infection; it is more commonly known to affect the oral cavity. The fastidious anaerobic gram-positive bacterium has some features resembling fungi. Infections may manifest as edema, abscess, and ulceration. Biopsy may demonstrate the pathognomonic sulfur granules. Treatment typically is with high-dose penicillin given intravenously (IV) or orally depending on the disease severity. Clindamycin is an option for penicillin-allergic patients.

Syphilis

Luetic (syphilitic) infections were once much more common than today. Syphilis may be present in the primary, secondary, or tertiary stage. Laryngeal involvement is rare and may be a component of the secondary or tertiary (gumma) phase. Caused by the *Treponema pallidum* spirochete, these infections may lie dormant for prolonged periods of time. Laryngeal involvement may present as a diffuse hyperemia, ulceration, or maculopapular mucosal rash. Laryngeal syphilis may cause fibrosis, chondritis, and scarring or stenosis. Serologic testing should include Venereal Disease Research Laboratory (VDRL) testing (100% sensitivity in secondary syphilis), with confirmation using fluorescent treponemal antibody absorption (FTA-ABS) and the microhemagglutination assay for *T. pallidum* (MHA-TP). Penicillin G is the primary drug in treatment.

Leprosy

Leprosy, or Hansen's disease, caused by *Mycobacterium leprae*, is very rare in the United States but is seen more often in the Indian subcontinent and Africa. Nasal infection is the primary site of infection in the head and neck, with the larynx being second. Infection favors the supraglottic, with symptoms including hoarseness, muffled voice, odynophagia, and cough. Examination may reveal erythema, nodularity of the mucosa, and ulceration.

However, often the patient has minimal pain, despite the appearance of the tissue. Scarring may develop that leads to stenosis and airway obstruction. Biopsy may reveal "foam cells," with copious *M. leprae* within these cells. Long-term medical therapy is necessary, even 5 to 10 years, with dapsone and rifampin.

Other

The larynx may be involved in other systemic infections, particularly viral infections such as mumps, measles, or varicella (chickenpox).

Differential Diagnosis

There are several causes of symptoms similar to those of laryngeal infection:

- Laryngeal neoplasm
- Airway foreign body
- Autoimmune diseases
- Allergic reaction
- Angioneurotic edema
- Subglottic stenosis
- Laryngopharyngeal reflux

◆ Evaluation

History

The key in evaluation is primarily history, including time course of the condition, exposures, comorbidities, and past medical history.

Physical Exam

A complete, thorough head and neck examination, including flexible naso-laryngoscopy, should be performed. The lungs should also be auscultated to evaluate for concomitant pulmonary issues.

Imaging

The role of imaging is limited. Computed tomography (CT) may be helpful if an abscess is suspected or to aid in evaluating the complication of airway stenosis. If tuberculosis is suspected, chest radiography should be ordered.

Labs

Laboratory testing may include a complete blood count (CBC) or specific serology as appropriate. In some cases (e.g., epiglottitis), laboratory testing would be contraindicated initially. Tissue biopsy and culture may be necessary to confirm a diagnosis for several reasons. First, many of these infections are uncommon; therefore, clinical experience is limited in recognizing the entity definitively. Second, the laryngeal findings may mimic squamous cell carcinoma grossly; the onus is on the clinician to evaluate for this issue. Last, given that the medical therapy may be prolonged and not without side effects and medication interactions, a tissue culture assists in quality care.

◆ Treatment Options

Treatment of laryngeal infections is based on the causative agent. Viral laryngitis is managed with supportive measures. Pharmacologic treatment should be tailored to the organism implicated in the infection.

◆ Outcome and Follow-Up

Follow-up with laryngoscopy should be used to assess resolution of the infection. The frequency of these evaluations is determined by the severity of the infection and the expected time to resolution.

5.2 Neurolaryngology

◆ Key Features

- Neurolaryngeal examination is a key component in the evaluation of any voice disorder.
- Laryngeal dysfunction may be an early sign of systemic neurologic conditions, even before the manifestation of other symptoms.
- In patients with neurologic dysfunction, the other key laryngeal functions beyond phonation should also be assessed (i.e., respiration, airway protection during deglutition).
- Laryngeal electromyography may be helpful in specific clinical scenarios, but controversy exists about its routine use in all neurologic complaints.

Focal and systemic neurologic conditions may affect the laryngeal functions. The laryngeal findings of systemic neurologic conditions may even precede their presentation in other locations. The key in accurately diagnosing these conditions is a careful, detailed history combined with a clinical voice evaluation. Direct visualization of the larynx is important, and may be best done with flexible fiberoptic laryngoscopy. Stroboscopic assessments may also be helpful in assessing the vocal fold mucosal wave and complement the neurolaryngeal exam. The most common neurolaryngeal disorder encountered is vocal fold motion impairment (see **Chapter 5.3.3**). Other common disorders include spasmodic dysphonia, tremor, Parkinson's disease (PD), stroke, and vocal fold dysfunction (VFD).

◆ Clinical

Signs and Symptoms

The laryngeal complaints of patients may concern voice, swallowing, airway, or a combination. Dysphagia is covered in **Chapter 5.4.2**. Airway symptoms may occur with bilateral vocal fold immobility, significant paresis, or paradoxical vocal fold adduction. The features of the vocal concern that should be defined are onset, situational context, perceived quality, pitch, pitch control, fluidity, and stamina.

Differential Diagnosis

Neurologic issues involving the larynx may be either focal or systemic. Therefore, other neurologic features in the remainder of the body should be sought. The systemic diagnosis may have been already determined, or the vocal issue may be the first presenting sign of a new diagnosis. In general, neurolaryngeal illnesses may involve a lack of neuromuscular strength or mobility of the vocal folds or a discoordination of function. The former includes paresis, paralysis, atrophy, and incomplete glottic closure as well as diminished vocal support. These type of conditions may be acute losses (e.g., stroke, surgical injury) or degenerative (e.g., PD, amyotrophic lateral sclerosis [ALS]). The discoordination differential includes tremors, myoclonus, and dystonia.

◆ Evaluation

History

As with many vocal disorders, patients may precisely self-define their vocal concern, but they also may have only a vague description of their problem. A careful history to define their issues includes the timing and situational onset of the symptoms, exacerbating and ameliorating factors, associated symptoms, and vocal quality.

Voice Exam

Evaluation of the voice by the trained listener is essential. This begins even as the patient is relaying their history. Nonlaryngeal factors should be noted, such as articulation issues or hypo- and hypernasality. Laryngeal issues include overall vocal quality (e.g., raspy, breathy, strained, spasmodic), severity of dysfunction, appropriateness of vocal pitch, and presence of voice or pitch breaks. Assistance in this assessment can be provided through the use of certain prepared readings. The most common of these is the "Rainbow Passage," which contains balanced consonants and vowels:

> When the sunlight strikes raindrops in the air, they act like a prism and form a rainbow. The rainbow is a division of white light into many beautiful colors. These take the shape of a long round arch, with its path high above, and its two ends beyond the horizon. There is, according to legend, a boiling pot of gold at one end. People look,

but no one ever finds it. When a man looks for something beyond his reach, his friends say he is looking for the pot of gold at the end of the rainbow.

(Fairbanks G. *Voice and articulation drillbook*. New York, NY: Harper & Row; 1969.) Using predominantly voiced or voiceless phrases may also be of benefit, particularly in spasmodic dysphonia. Appropriate phrases for *ad*ductor spasmodic dysphonia include the following:

- [Counting from 80 to 89]
- "Eeee-eee-eee"
- "We mow our lawn all year."
- "We eat eels every day."
- "We eat eggs every evening."
- "A dog dug a new bone."
- "Where were you one year ago?"
- "We rode along Rhode Island Avenue."

Appropriate phrases for *ab*ductor spasmodic dysphonia include:

- [Counting from 60 to 69]
- "See-see-see"
- "The puppy bit the tape."
- "Peter will keep at the peak."
- "When he comes home, we'll feed him."
- "Harry has a hard head."
- "Tap the tip of the cap, please."
- "Keep Tom at the party."

Some vocal disorders are particular to certain tasks, while others are universal; having a patient sing a well-known tune such as "Happy Birthday" can help determine this fact. The next component, the neurolaryngologic examination, is best done with a flexible endoscope. This allows fluent speech and avoids the distortion and potential inhibitory effects of tongue retraction on direct or indirect laryngoscopy. The larynx should be observed at rest, during normal breathing, and during phonation. Appropriate adduction and abduction with phonation and respiration should be observed. The "/i/--sniff" maneuver should elicit maximal abduction. Asymmetric or paradoxical vocal fold motion may indicate a paresis or dystonia. Rhythmic spontaneous or intention tremor of the larynx should be noted, as well as nonrhythmic myoclonus. Compression of the false folds and supraglottis represents excess use of accessory muscles, suggestive of muscle tension issues or dystonias. Quickly repetitive phonatory tasks (such as /i/–sniff, alternating /i/–/hi/, and /pa/–/ta/–/ka/) may make subtle paresis or discoordination more evident. Glissando (sliding low- to high-pitch /i/) can be used to assess tensioning function.

Imaging

In vocal fold paresis and paralysis, computed tomography (CT) and magnetic resonance imaging (MRI) can confirm that no lesions exist along the course of the vagus and recurrent laryngeal nerves, which could interfere with function. Central nervous system (CNS) imaging may be appropriate if it assists in confirmation of a systemic neurologic condition associated with the neurolaryngeal complaints.

Other Tests

Stroboscopy

Stroboscopic examination allows for the evaluation of not only gross laryngeal mobility and glottic closure but also subtle mucosal wave abnormalities. Assessment of the mucosal wave function may yield additional information regarding the dysphonia; however, not all mucosal wave issues necessarily contribute to vocal complaints.

Laryngeal Electromyography

Laryngeal electromyography (LEMG) can be integrated into the laryngeal functional assessment. Controversy exists as to the extent it should be routinely used in dysphonia. Some agreement exists about its utility in certain circumstances:

1. Needle guidance during botulinum toxin injection to the larynx
2. Diagnosis of vocal fold movement disorders
3. Assessment and prediction of unilateral vocal fold paresis or paralysis after recurrent laryngeal nerve injury
4. Research tool

The validity and interpretation of LEMG in the diagnosis of other neurologic or myopathic disorders is not well defined at this time. Interpretation of LEMG often involves a partnership between the otolaryngologist and a skilled electromyographer, often a neurologist or physical medicine and rehabilitation physician. The factors of fibrillation potentials, fasciculations, recruitment, and action potential characteristics should be noted and can assist in supporting history and examination-generated diagnosis.

◆ Treatment Options

Medical

Medical therapy for neurolaryngeal complaints focuses on attempts to maintain a patent airway, protect the airway from aspiration, and restore normal laryngeal aerodynamics and phonation. Swallowing assessments (e.g., bedside swallow evaluation, fiberoptic endoscopic evaluation of swallowing [FEES], modified barium swallow [MBS]) may be necessary for diagnosis and to determine therapy in some conditions affecting the pharyngeal mobility or protective reflexes of the larynx. After a thorough swallowing evaluation, a speech and language pathology consultation may be beneficial for rehabilitation exercises.

The most common neurolaryngeal disorder, vocal fold paralysis and paresis, is discussed in detail in **Chapter 5.3.3**. Five other common neurolaryngologic issues will be addressed here as examples of treatment: cerebrovascular accident, PD, laryngeal tremor, spasmodic dysphonia, and VFD.

Cerebrovascular accident (stroke) may have multiple effects on laryngeal function. It may alter the ability to protect the airway, swallow, respire, and phonate. Some stroke patients will have language issues (aphasias) rather than laryngeal phonatory issues, and these must be distinguished to design treatment properly. Deficits in stroke may include poor breath support, incomplete glottic closure (even vocal fold paralysis), loss of laryngeal sensation, and discoordination of the laryngoesophageal complex. Specific medication is not recommended but may be instituted for global deficits. Attention should primarily be paid to speech and language pathology therapy to maximize function and minimize aspiration.

PD is caused by progressive degeneration of particular brainstem structures, including the substantia nigra. Seventy to eighty-nine percent of patients experience vocal symptoms, even as the first presenting symptom. Patients with PD can have voices characterized by soft, breathy, monotone speech, occasionally tremor, as well as nonlaryngeal issues such as poor articulation. Specific speech therapy has been designed for PD patients, such as Lee Silverman Voice Treatment (LSVT; LSVT Global, Inc., Tucson, AZ), an intensive therapy involving phonatory effort and glottal closure. Pharmacologic management of PD is beyond the scope of this chapter but primarily involves dopaminergic replacement.

Vocal tremor is rarely restricted to the laryngeal musculature but often involves many muscles involved in phonation. Treatment of vocal tremor may be initiated with medications indicated in essential tremor but has been less well investigated specifically for the larynx. Propranolol (β-adrenergic blocker; reduces tremor amplitude), primidone (neuroleptic; mechanism unknown), and methazolamide (carbonic anhydrase inhibitor) have all been utilized in vocal tremors, but limited studies show efficacy, and dosing is not well defined. Botulinum toxin injections (Botox; Allergan, Dublin, Ireland) can be performed, typically into one or both thyroarytenoid muscles, to reduce tremor amplitude, but they do not eliminate tremor entirely.

Spasmodic dysphonia may be either adductor or abductor, and rarely mixed. Speech therapy has a little role in treating these patients. Botox injection into one or both thyroarytenoid muscles (adductor spasmodic dysphonia) or posterior cricoarytenoid muscle (abductor spasmodic dys-phonia) remains the mainstay of therapy. Unilateral or bilateral injections, as well as dosing, must be titrated to the individual patient through trial and effect. A reasonable starting dose for injection is 1 to 2 U. Some clinicians prefer unilateral injections, as they seem to have the best voice outcome for effect/side effect ratio.

Vocal fold dysfunction (VFD) is likely a spectrum of disorders wherein inappropriate vocal fold adduction occurs during inspiration. Rare organic causes of this occurrence, such as brainstem compression (e.g., Arnold-Chiari malformation) or upper/lower motor neuron injury, should be considered and confirmed if suspected. In classic VFD, this inspiratory adduction creates the characteristic anterior fold adduction with posterior glottic chink. This may occur with laryngeal irritants and psychological stress. The process is often mistaken initially for asthma and can rarely occur synchronously. Therapy directed at vocal fold relaxation and breathing is paramount. Psychological stressors should also be addressed to reduce initiating factors. Any concomitant psychiatric illnesses and symptoms should be managed pharmacologically, if necessary. Acute exacerbations may be managed with the assistance of benzodiazepines and topical laryngeal lidocaine. Some clinicians believe reflux accompanies many patients with VFD and should be treated concurrently.

Surgical

Surgical therapy for laryngeal issues of stroke is limited to palliative measures. Patients with severe impairment of swallowing and airway protection may benefit from tracheotomy for pulmonary hygiene and possible gastrostomy tube placement for enteral nutrition.

PD may involve vocal fold atrophy and has been treated with vocal fold augmentation. Although this therapy aids glottic closure to a degree, issues remain. Overall, PD may be treated surgically through deep brain stimulation, which improves the extremity symptoms, but less so the voice and articulation problems.

Essential tremor has been successfully treated with thalamic deep brain stimulation, but isolated vocal tremor is not an indication for this neurosurgical intervention. Some patients treated with bilateral brain stimulation developed dysarthria, raising concerns over this procedure in vocal tremor.

Spasmodic dysphonia patients do have some surgical options, but currently most patients continue botulinum toxin injections. Recurrent laryngeal nerve section was described by Dedo in 1976. Although it was initially beneficial in half to two-thirds of patients, many had recurrent symptoms years later. The procedure is also complicated by glottic incompetence, strain, and high pitch. Resection of a section of the nerve as described by a group at Vanderbilt University Medical Center (Nashville, TN) improves the rate of recurrence, but 33% needed medialization procedures. Isshiki describes an expansion laryngoplasty for spasmodic dysphonia, but data and follow-up are limited. Berke has modified the recurrent laryngeal nerve section to include only the adductor branch and introduced reinnervation by the ansa cervicalis. Selective nerve section and reinnervation have reported good subjective voice improvements, with 90% having mild or no voice breaks and mild or no dysphonia.

Vocal fold dysfunction has no surgical treatments. Tracheotomy has been used to bypass the larynx but is rarely necessary with nonorganic causes of VFD.

5.3 Voice Disorders

5.3.1 Papillomatosis

◆ Key Features

> - Papillomatosis is the most common benign neoplasm of the larynx.
> - It is a human papillomavirus (HPV)-induced lesion.
> - There is a low chance of malignant conversion.
> - The mainstay of therapy is surgical resection, although adjuvant therapies may be helpful in severe cases.

Papillomatosis may affect any mucosal surface of the head and neck, but it has a predilection for junctions between ciliated respiratory and squamous mucosa. The most common sites are the nasal vestibule, oropharynx, nasopharyngeal surface of the soft palate, upper and lower limits of the laryngeal ventricle, and undersurface of the vocal folds. HPV is the etiologic agent, with some subtypes (HPV-6, HPV-11) predominating. Recurrent respiratory papillomatosis (RRP) typically presents with dysphonia, although some children, and even fewer adults, may present with airway compromise. Treatment is surgical resection, with cold steel dissection, microdébrider, or laser. Adjuvant chemotherapy agents may have some role in recalcitrant cases.

◆ Epidemiology

Laryngeal papilloma can be categorized into two subgroups: juvenile and adult onset. Juvenile usually occurs in children less than 5 years, with 25% presenting in infancy. Incidence of juvenile RRP is 4.3 per 100,000 in the United States. Children are frequently (75%) the firstborn, vaginally delivered offspring of teenage mothers. Males and females are equally affected. Transmission is maternal–neonatal and of higher risk in those with active HPV genital warts (condylomata), although other factors play a role. Adult-onset RRP presents at ages 20 to 40 years, with a 4:1 male/female ratio. Incidence is 1.8 per 100,000. In adults, the disease is likely to be sexually transmitted.

◆ Clinical

Signs and Symptoms

Children may present with airway obstructive symptoms, particularly if they are presenting very young. Children may also have a husky cry or dysphonia. Secondary to the rare nature of the disease and the pediatrician's inability to visualize the larynx, children are frequently misdiagnosed as having other airway problems such as asthma, bronchitis, or croup. Symptoms are present on average 1 year before diagnosis. In some cases, children will present with emergent airway obstruction. Adults typically present with dysphonia, rarely with acute airway compromise. Symptoms are present on average for 6 months before diagnosis.

Differential Diagnosis

Hoarseness in children may be caused by vocal nodules, reflux disease, vocal fold immobility, laryngotracheobronchitis, laryngeal cysts, congenital laryngeal abnormality, or neurologic conditions. Upper airway compromise causes may include congenital laryngeal lesions, laryngeal cysts, vocal fold immobility, subglottic stenosis, a foreign body, and infectious processes, such as epiglottitis or laryngotracheobronchitis.

Hoarseness in adults may be caused by vocal fold nodules, reflux laryngitis, vocal fold cysts or polyps, leukoplakia, vocal fold neoplasms, sulcus vocalis, inflammatory laryngitis (e.g., tobacco abuse, steroid inhalers), vocal fold immobility, hypothyroidism, and systemic illnesses such as sarcoidosis or amyloidosis.

◆ Evaluation

Physical Exam

The physical exam should include a full head and neck examination. Attention should be made to the respiratory status of the patient, to assess whether acute interventions will be necessary to preserve the airway. Vocal quality should be noted. Indirect laryngoscopy can be done on adult patients. Flexible laryngoscopy may be done in adults and nondistressed children to assess location, extent, and functional limitations of the papilloma disease. Videostroboscopy can be useful, when available, to assess the impact of the papilloma on mucosal wave dynamics.

Imaging

Imaging has limited use, except in assessing for other issues causing airway compromise in children or assessing distal pulmonary papillomatosis. High-kilovoltage plain films or airway fluoroscopy may be helpful in this regard but do not specifically assist in the diagnosis of RRP.

Labs

No specific labs are helpful in RRP. Some otolaryngologists recommend HPV typing at the time of resection. This does not alter treatment but can offer some prognostic information, as HPV-11 patients tend to have more aggressive disease, more recurrences, more surgical procedures, and more use of adjuvant therapies.

Pathology

Papillomas contain a pedunculated, vascular, fibrous core with overlying nonkeratinized squamous epithelium. Multiple projections emanate off the central core, giving a frond- or wart-like configuration. Cellular atypia may occur in the epithelium and can be concerning for premalignant changes.

◆ Treatment Options

Medical

Although there are no primary medical therapies for RRP, adjuvant therapy to surgical resections may be necessary. Criteria for adjuvant methods include more than four procedures per year, rapid recurrence with airway compromise, and distant spread of disease. Approximately 10% of juvenile RRP patients require adjuvants.

The most commonly used therapy is recombinant α-interferon. This protein complex is a host defense to viral infection and immunomodulates the host into an antiviral condition. This has been shown to reduce the frequency of operative interventions. It is administered daily for 1 month, then tapered to three times weekly for at least 6 months. Side effects include flu-like symptoms, alopecia, leukopenia, coagulopathy, and neurologic side effects.

Indole-3-carbinol is an herbal supplement derived from cruciferous vegetables. The mechanism is unclear but is believed to be related to alterations in estrogen metabolism. Studies show a majority of patients receive partial to complete response. Dosages for children less than 25 kg are 100 to 200 mg daily and for adults 200 mg twice daily. Side effects include headache and dizziness.

Cidofovir is a cytosine nucleotide analog antiviral agent, designed for herpetic viruses and cytomegalovirus. Intralesional injections have shown good response in some patients. Concern for promoting progression to squamous cell carcinoma has been raised, but such progression is not proven.

Acyclovir has been used systemically, but the benefits are not well defined.

Photodynamic therapy utilizes the uptake of hematoporphyrins by papilloma to sensitize the tissue to red laser light. Disease progression is improved, but remission is not achieved.

Quadrivalent HPV vaccines have recently been released for HPV subtypes 6, 11, 16, and 18, with the indication for treating young girls before sexual activity to reduce the rate of cervical cancers. The hope exists that this use will influence the rate of laryngeal papilloma in future generations, and it may even be applied to males in the future.

Surgical

Surgical resection via microlaryngoscopy remains the mainstay of therapy. Recurrences are typical and multiple procedures are the norm. Juvenile RRP tends to be more aggressive and require more surgeries, likely related to increased growth rate of the RRP and the smaller dimensions of the juvenile larynx prompting earlier intervention for recurrence. Techniques for removal include several modalities and are influenced heavily by surgeon preference. Cold steel dissection of the papilloma may be useful for small isolated lesions, but not diffuse lesions. The CO_2 laser has been the workhorse of RRP for many years. Vaporization of the lesions is a viable treatment option. The laryngeal microdébrider can also be used; it is favored by some surgeons over laser, as it may have less "peripheral damage" given its lack of thermal injury and does not require special intraoperative laser precautions. Several new lasers have been utilized in

RRP, even in the office setting via flexible scopes. These include flexible CO_2 and pulsed dye lasers.

◆ Outcome and Follow-Up

Recommendations regarding postoperative care vary by surgeon (e.g., voice rest). Reflux medications are recommended by many to reduce postoperative scarring exacerbated by any acid exposure, as well as to reduce the potential cofactor of acid exposure in RRP regrowth.

By its very name, RRP is a recurrent problem for patients. The course is variable, with some patients experiencing lifelong recurrences and others manifesting spontaneous remissions. Juvenile-onset RRP does seem to have a higher rate of remission as the children enter adolescence.

Some patients are concerned about spread of RRP to family members or sexual partners. There are no well-documented cases of patient-to-patient transmission of laryngeal RRP. Some theoretical concern exists for caregivers, however, with reported viable virus in laser smoke plumes.

5.3.2   Vocal Fold Cysts, Nodules, and Polyps

◆ Key Features

- Nonneoplastic disorders of the larynx include nodules, cysts, and polyps.
- Dysphonia is a common presenting complaint.
- Large polyps may rarely present with airway obstruction.

Nonneoplastic changes affecting the vocal folds are common causes of chronic hoarseness. An office exam and videostroboscopy can generally lead to an accurate diagnosis. Treatment may involve voice therapy, microscopic voice surgery (microlaryngeal surgery), and behavioral modifications. With accurate diagnosis, appropriate management, and patient compliance, treatment should be highly effective.

◆ Epidemiology

Benign and reactive laryngeal lesions are common disorders; true incidence is difficult to determine.

◆ Clinical

Signs and Symptoms

Patients with various nonneoplastic vocal fold disorders generally complain of hoarseness of variable duration. A history of voice abuse or violent coughing is common. Vocal nodules are almost always seen in young women or young children with a history of voice abuse. Vocal fold polyps are more frequent in men. Stridor is occasionally associated with large vocal polyps. Vocal fold cysts present also with substantial voice changes and usually affect adults. Cysts are thought to be congenital or acquired and seem to arise in the setting of chronic irritation and inflammation after hemorrhage. Reinke's edema, or polypoid chorditis, is a distinct entity from vocal polyps or nodules and usually presents with a pitch disturbance (e.g., females being mistaken for males on the telephone). It is caused by tobacco abuse.

Differential Diagnosis

The major consideration is the possibility of laryngeal squamous cell carcinoma, especially in the setting of tobacco abuse. History and physical examination alone may be insufficient to differentiate early-stage cancer from certain benign conditions. Differential diagnosis includes nodules, cysts, polyps, Reinke's edema, granuloma, papillomatosis, reflux laryngitis, other chronic laryngitis forms, glottic sulcus vocalis, and squamous cell carcinoma.

◆ Evaluation

History

A specific history of severe coughing, anticoagulant use, voice abuse, vocal fatigue, singing, tobacco abuse, or reflux symptoms should be ascertained. Prior intubations, laryngeal trauma, or laryngeal surgeries must not be overlooked. It is important to elicit timing of onset.

Physical Exam

A complete head and neck exam is performed. Office endoscopy and videostroboscopy, if the latter is available, often enable a diagnosis. Vocal nodules are seen as a thickened bilaterally symmetric lesion involving the midmembranous vocal fold contact site, generally found in a young female patient. Vocal fold cysts are usually solitary and visible as a bulge in the affected fold, but when small may be confused with other subepithelial lesions. Characteristic changes in vibration are appreciable on stroboscopic exam. Vocal fold polyps can be variable in size and may be single or multiple. Generally, polyps arise near the vibratory margin of the vocal fold. A feeding vessel or evidence of hemorrhage may be obvious. Large pedunculated polyps are occasionally seen arising from the upper or lower surface of the vocal fold. Reinke's edema appears as symmetric pale thickening of the folds, often with dehydration and thick mucus. Glottic sulcus vocalis may be suggested by stroboscopic findings revealing a segment with reduced vibration, but microlaryngoscopy is often required for definitive diagnosis.

Imaging

Radiologic examination is not indicated in most cases.

◆ Treatment Options

Vocal nodules usually respond to voice therapy alone. Vocal fold cysts may respond to voice therapy; if not, they are removed by microsurgery via cordotomy and microflap. Vocal fold polyps may respond to voice therapy if small but are usually treated with surgery followed by voice therapy and antireflux therapy. Surgery involves excision with microinstruments and the use of short-pulsed CO_2 laser coagulation of a feeding vessel, if present. Reinke's edema may be treated conservatively with voice rest and smoking cessation or treated surgically with submucosal evacuation via a cordotomy, generally placing the incision on the superolateral surface. In all cases, behavioral modification to address tobacco abuse, reflux, voice abuse, and vocal hygiene is important.

◆ Outcome and Follow-Up

In most cases, prognosis should be very good. Prevention of recurrence should involve follow-up monitoring of smoking and other behavioral factors discussed previously.

5.3.3   Vocal Fold Motion Impairment

◆ Key Features

- "Immobility" and "motion impairment" are better terms for this condition than the routine use of "paralysis" given that other etiologies exist for the motion defect.
- Immobility may be due to central or peripheral neural pathology.
- Immobility may also involve fixation of the cricoarytenoid joint or subluxation.
- Unilateral vocal fold immobility creates primarily dysphonia, whereas bilateral vocal fold immobility may create vocal and airway problems.

Vocal fold motion impairment may occur at any age. The impairment may relate to a vocal fold paresis, a vocal fold paralysis, and cricoarytenoid joint fixation or dislocation. A unilateral vocal fold paralysis is more often on the left because the left recurrent laryngeal nerve descends farther into the chest than the right one does. Most patients present with dysphonia, although a bilateral issue may cause airway distress acutely or in a delayed fashion. An evaluation is performed to attempt to rule out etiologies that may require further therapy. Rehabilitation of the voice may be accomplished via medialization of the affected vocal fold to improve glottic closure. Airway impairment secondary to bilateral lesions may be palliated by bypassing the obstruction (tracheotomy) or by increasing the glottic airway area. For bilateral vocal fold paralysis in children, see **Chapter 8.3**.

◆ Clinical

Signs and Symptoms

In pediatric patients, unilateral vocal fold motion problems may be over-looked, particularly if the child has other congenital anomalies or medical issues. A weak cry, with possible feeding or choking problems, may be noted. In some cases aspiration and cyanotic episodes may occur. Rarely, stridor and airway symptoms exist. Bilateral vocal fold motion impairment will typically involve stridor and respiratory insufficiency. A normal cry may be preserved.

In adults, unilateral vocal fold motion impairment presents with dysphonia. The degree of hoarseness varies widely from essentially a normal voice to severe breathy dysphonia. Diplophonia may also be present. If the sensory portion of laryngeal innervation is also involved, then secretion pooling or silent aspiration may occur. This will typically be worse with thin liquids than with thicker liquids or solids. As in children, a bilateral vocal fold may have a relatively preserved voice because of the more medial position of the vocal folds. However, varying degrees of airway obstruction and distress may be noted. Patients may have severe obstruction requiring urgent airway interventions (endotracheal intubation, tracheotomy) or may suffer a more chronic dyspnea with steady or variable symptoms.

Differential Diagnosis

Vocal fold motion impairment may be neurologic (central or peripheral) or mechanical. Vocal fold motion problems may arise from:

- Cervical surgery (thyroidectomy, carotid endarterectomy, anterior cervical fusion)
- Thoracic surgery (pulmonary lobectomy, cardiac bypass or valve surgery, aortic aneurysm repair, esophagectomy)
- Neurologic disease (Guillain-Barré's syndrome, Charcot-Marie-Tooth's disease, Arnold-Chiari malformation, hydrocephalus, cerebrovascular accident, myasthenia gravis, amyotrophic lateral sclerosis [ALS], Lyme disease
- Posterior glottic stenosis
- Endotracheal intubation trauma to cricoarytenoid joint or pressure injury to recurrent laryngeal nerve
- Neck trauma
- Inflammatory diseases (rheumatoid arthritis, Wegener's granulomatosis, sarcoidosis, syphilis, pemphigoid)
- Neoplasms along the course of the recurrent laryngeal nerve (intracranial, cervical, thoracic)
- Laryngeal neoplasm
- Viral neuritis

Vocal fold motion problems may also be idiopathic.

◆ Evaluation

History

The etiology may be evident via the history and timing of the onset of symptoms or may require further evaluation. A careful history for aerodigestive tract symptoms and a history of prior cervical or thoracic surgery, cervical masses, neoplastic disorders, endotracheal intubation, thyroid disease, generalized neurologic symptoms, or viral prodromes should be elicited.

Physical Exam

The physical exam should include a complete head and neck examination, flexible fiberoptic laryngoscopy, and/or videostroboscopy.

Imaging

Imaging involving the course of the recurrent laryngeal nerve is recommended to rule out compressive or infiltrative processes. A computed tomography (CT) scan from the skull base through the aortic arch should be ordered in any patient without an obvious etiology. Some clinicians will use magnetic resonance imaging (MRI) of the brain to evaluate for central nervous system (CNS) lesions or posterior fossa malformations, but this is not routine in the evaluation of vocal fold motion problems.

Labs

Laboratory tests are appropriate if a system illness is suspected as an etiology, but no tests are done routinely. Tests may include rheumatoid factor, antineutrophil cytoplasmic antibody, antinuclear antibody, Venereal Disease Research Laboratory (VDRL) test for syphilis, or Lyme titer. Laryngeal electromyography (LEMG) may be utilized in the immobile fold to assess for denervation and recovery. This may be helpful in differentiating paralysis (fibrillation potentials on LEMG) from fixation (normal action potentials on LEMG). The state of denervation and recovery may be prognosticated by the presence of fibrillation potential (denervation), electrical silence (prolonged denervation with muscle atrophy), or polyphasic action potentials (recovery of some innervation).

◆ Treatment Options

The overall treatment may be guided by the etiology of the vocal fold motion impairment. Treatment of the underlying illness may yield motion recovery in some cases (e.g., immunomodulators for rheumatoid arthritis) or may yield no motion recovery. Rehabilitation of the voice and possibly dysphagia improvement are the goals for most unilateral problems, whereas airway maintenance predominates in bilateral cases.

Medical

No evidence exists for the use of oral steroids in acute-onset vocal fold paralysis. Speech therapy consultation may be beneficial for maximizing vocal function, given the limitations of a nonfunctional fold. Additionally, as some patients may experience dysphagia or aspiration symptoms, the therapist may be able to assess the swallow function clinically and make recommendations about therapeutic maneuvers to improve symptoms.

Surgical

Medialization of the impaired vocal fold is performed to provide better glottic closure and thus more normal phonatory dynamics. Techniques may provide temporary or permanent solutions. Injection augmentation may utilize absorbable or permanent materials. This may be performed transcutaneously, under endoscopic guidance in the office, or during operative microlaryngoscopy. Open approaches (medialization laryngoplasty) involve making a thyroid ala window and placing preformed or surgeon-carved Silastic (Dow Corning Corp., Auburn, MI) implants, or layered polytetrafluoroethylene (Gore-Tex, W.L. Gore and Associates, Flagstaff, AZ). Arytenoid adduction may be beneficial in some patients as an adjuvant to reduce posterior glottic gap. Reinnervation of the thyroarytenoid muscle may assist in vocal fold tone and improved glottic closure. The main purpose of reinnervation is to prevent laryngeal muscular atrophy.

◆ Outcome and Follow-Up

In the case of vocal fold paralysis, clinical recovery may require as long as 12 months. Therefore, serial evaluations may be necessary to document the recovery and to reevaluate for vocal issues benefiting from intervention. A functional voice initially may worsen over time as vocal fold atrophy and final fold position manifest. LEMG may provide some prognostic information regarding recovery.

5.3.4 Voice Rehabilitation

◆ Key Features

- Voice therapy encompasses techniques employed in the management schema for patients with voice disorders.

Vocal rehabilitation often involves a multidisciplinary approach combining the services of both otolaryngologists and speech-language pathologists. Speech-language pathologists offer several therapeutic approaches with consideration of the patient's variables: the etiology of the voice disorder, the vocal demands of the patient, and patient cooperation/compliance. Vocal rehabilitation methods include resonant voice therapy, vocal function exercises, confidential voice therapy, manual circumlaryngeal reposturing, and Lee Silverman Voice Therapy (LSVT; LSVT Global, Inc., Tucson, AZ). Comprehensive vocal rehabilitation often includes a combination of one or more therapeutic approaches.

◆ Epidemiology

Vocal disorders amenable for voice therapy include several possible etiologies, including benign midmembranous vocal fold lesions, functional voice disorders, vocal fold paralysis or paresis, laryngeal movement disorders, and progressive neurogenic disorders such as Parkinson's disease (PD) and amyotrophic lateral sclerosis (ALS).

◆ Clinical

Signs

Signs of vocal disorders include perceptual, acoustic, and physiological variables. These variables are often defined by the patient as one or more of nine common symptoms of voice problems.

Symptoms

The nine most common symptoms of voice problems are:

- Hoarseness
- Vocal fatigue
- Breathiness of voice
- Reduced phonatory range
- Aphonia or total loss of voice
- Pitch breaks or inappropriate pitch level
- Strain
- Tremor
- Pain

Table 5.3 Voice handicap index

Pitch	Evaluation of monopitch, inappropriate pitch, pitch breaks, reduced pitch range
Loudness	Evaluation of monoloudness, loudness variation, reduced loudness range
Quality	Hoarse or rough, breathy, tension, tremor, strain/struggle, sudden voice interruptions, diplophonia
Other behaviors	Stridor, throat clearing, habitual cough

Differential Diagnosis

Differential diagnosis of voice disorders must include evaluation of all perceptual, acoustic, and physiological variables to determine the most appropriate voice therapy approach.

◆ Evaluation

Evaluation of voice disorders should include evaluation of perceptual, acoustic, and physiological components of vocal function.

Perceptual Evaluation

Perceptual evaluation includes evaluation of pitch, loudness, quality, and other related features. Perceptual evaluation is often subjective based on the assessment of the voice by both the speech-language pathologist and the patient. The Voice Handicap Index is a quality of life instrument used by a patient to rank his or her voice in areas of functional, physical, and emotional impact of the voice (**Table 5.3**).

Acoustic Evaluation

Acoustic evaluation includes evaluation of the variables related to movement of the vocal folds and sound production from the vocal tract. This assessment can be completed with the use of computer voice analysis systems such as Visi-Pitch or Computerized Speech Laboratory (both from Pentax Medical, Montvale, NJ). Assessment includes measurement of the following parameters:

- Fundamental frequency
- Amplitude
- Signal-to-noise ratio
- Vocal rise and fall time
- Vocal tremor
- Maximum phonation time
- Frequency breaks
- Habitual pitch

Physiological Evaluation

Physiological evaluation relates to the aerodynamics, vibratory behaviors, and muscle activity of the vocal folds. This evaluation can be completed with videostroboscopic evaluation of the larynx, electroglottography, electromyography, and laryngeal endoscopy. The parameters of videostroboscopy include:

- Evaluation of vocal fold edge and texture
- Degree of glottic closure
- Phase closure
- Vertical level
- Amplitude of vibration

- Mucosal wave
- Vibratory behavior
- Phase symmetry
- Periodicity

◆ Treatment Options

Several voice rehabilitation programs exist including general vocal hygiene, resonant voice therapy, vocal function exercises, confidential voice therapy, manual circumlaryngeal reposturing, and LSVT. Often, comprehensive voice therapy includes a combination of elements from each of these therapy approaches and close interaction with an otolaryngologist's treatment program.

Vocal Hygiene

Vocal hygiene is a vital component of all voice rehabilitation. This includes focus on adequate hydration, reduction and elimination of vocal abusive and misuse behaviors, proper warm-up and cool-down of the voice, adequate voice rest, modification of contributing environmental factors, and voice amplification.

Resonant Voice Therapy

Resonant voice therapy focuses on establishing adequate oral and nasal resonance of the voice. This includes tasks focusing through a hierarchy including lip and tongue trills, nasal humming (/mmmm/), nasal words, rote and structured tasks, and conversation.

Vocal Function Exercises

Vocal function exercises are a series of structured vocal exercises that are used to maintain or establish muscle balance within the larynx, strength, and ease of phonation. These exercises promote complete closure of the true vocal folds and are thought to encourage equal open and closed phases of the vocal folds. Four exercises are used.

1. Sustain vowel /ee/.
2. Produce word "knoll" with a pitch glide starting with a high pitch.
3. Produce word "knoll" with pitch glide starting with low pitch.
4. Sustain vowel /oo/ on designated notes C, D, E, F, and G.

It is important to focus on these exercises as speaking tasks and not singing tasks. These exercises are not used primarily for speech tasks but are best when paired with another therapy approach such as resonant voice therapy.

Confidential Voice Therapy

Confidential voice therapy is used to reduce increased glottal closure by producing a glottal gap during phonation and creating a low-intensity, breathy vocal quality. Although focusing on creating a breathy vocal quality, this approach also accomplishes reduction of loudness, rate, and hyperfunction.

Manual Circumlaryngeal Reposturing

Manual circumlaryngeal reposturing is a hands-on method of vocal rehabilitation focused on relaxation of extraneous muscle tension. This includes
direct physical manipulation and massage of the laryngeal area. This
method usually works quickly to break muscle patterns that interfere with
vocal production. Areas of focus include the base of tongue, the cornu of the
hyoid bone, thyrohyoid space, and the posterior borders of the thyroid cartilage. Voice production is then trained for similar use of the larynx during
phonation without physical manipulation.

Lee Silverman Voice Therapy

LSVT is a voice therapy approach designed specifically for patients with voice
disorders associated with PD. This approach includes specific exercises to promote increased vocal volume. The speech–language pathologist is required to
undergo specialized training prior to instruction. The therapy course is based
on an intensive program of four sessions per week for 1 month.

◆ Outcome and Follow-Up

Follow-up with repeat laryngeal visualization and follow-up with an otolaryngologist is recommended following a completed course of voice therapy,
especially in cases involving vocal pathology such as vocal fold nodules,
polyps, paresis, or paralysis. This ensures resolution of the pathology and
determination of whether continued medical treatment is necessary.

5.4 Swallowing Disorders

5.4.1 Zenker's Diverticulum

◆ Key Features

- Zenker's diverticulum is a posterior pharyngeal pulsion diverticulum.
- It occurs in an area of potential weakness (Killian-Jamieson, Laimer-Hackermann area, Killian's dehiscence) in the inferior posterior part of the pharynx.
- It occurs in men twice as often as in women.
- It is found more often on the left.

Zenker's diverticulum is a pouch that develops in the pharynx just above the
upper esophageal sphincter. Typically, this causes dysphagia, regurgitation,
halitosis, and generalized irritation. It typically manifests in a posterolateral
fashion, with 90% appearing on the left side.

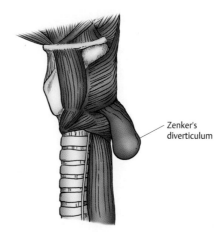

Fig. 5.4 Illustration of laryngopharyngeal anatomy, including Zenker's diverticulum. (Used with permission from Stewart MG, Selesnick SH. *Differential Diagnosis in Otolaryngology—Head and Neck Surgery*. New York: Thieme;2011:287.)

◆ Epidemiology

Zenker's diverticulum is 2.5 times more common in men than women and typically occurs in older patients (eighth or ninth decade). It occurs more frequently in European countries or in patients of European heritage. Persons of African descent are rarely affected.

◆ Clinical

Signs and Symptoms

Patients typically complain of dysphagia, regurgitation of undigested food, a feeling of food sticking in the throat, a globus sensation, and a persistent cough (especially after eating). Signs or symptoms may include aspiration, unintentional weight loss, and halitosis. Occasionally, a soft swelling may be palpable in the neck, typically in the left side.

Differential Diagnosis

The differential diagnosis includes pharyngeal malignancy, esophageal malignancy, and dysphagia due to central nervous system (CNS) etiology.

◆ Evaluation

History

A history is often suggestive of Zenker's diverticulum. Questions should be asked pertaining to weight loss, regurgitation, halitosis, and signs or symptoms associated with aspiration, such as frequent choking and coughing. There is typically no pain except in the presence of carcinoma.

Physical Exam

A full head and neck exam should be performed. On laryngoscopy, signs of laryngitis and pooling of saliva in the hypopharynx secondary to underlying cricopharyngeal hypertrophy may be seen. Less commonly, undigested food particles may be seen.

Imaging

Video fluoroscopy with barium typically demonstrates the pouch, especially near the end of the second stage of swallowing. This test is usually diagnostic, and no further imaging exams are typically necessary. Of note, ensuring the unilaterality of the pouch during this exam is important.

Pathology

Zenker's diverticulum is a herniation or false diverticulum of the esophageal mucosa posteriorly between the cricopharyngeus muscle and the inferior pharyngeal constrictor muscles (**Fig. 5.4**). Although rare, it is important to recognize that a small percentage of patients with Zenker's diverticulum may have a squamous cell carcinoma in the pouch (0.5 to 1%).

◆ Treatment Options

Medical

In a medically infirm patient, botulinum toxin (Botox; Allergan, Dublin, Ireland) injections to the middle pharyngeal constrictor (formerly called oropharyngeus) muscle may be effective.

Surgical

Treatment is typically surgical and reserved for symptomatic patients or patients with aspiration and pneumonia. Surgical management of Zenker's diverticulum entails division of the cricopharyngeus muscle to eliminate the potentially elevated pressure zone and elimination of the diverticular pouch as a reservoir of food and secretions. Surgical treatment may be endoscopic or open. Operative intervention is usually undertaken when the diverticulum is at least 3 cm in length.

Endoscopic treatment includes endoscopic identification of the pouch and stapler transection of the cricopharyngeal bar, or the common wall between the pouch and the cricopharyngeal introitus is divided to make a common lumen.

Open surgical techniques include open diverticulectomy, inversion, cricopharyngeal myotomy, or diverticulopexy in which the diverticulum is inverted and sutured to the prevertebral fascia. Open techniques are typically performed through a left neck incision.

◆ Outcome and Follow-Up

Long-term follow-up care is not routinely required.

5.4.2 Dysphagia

◆ Key Features

- Dysphagia may reflect dysfunction at any level of the swallowing reflex from the oral cavity to the distal esophagus.
- Evaluation requires a detailed history, full head and neck examination, and often endoscopic evaluations and imaging studies.
- Swallowing therapy may be beneficial to those with upper aerodigestive tract dysfunction who have no medically or surgically correctable problem.

"Dysphagia" is a term encompassing a large area of clinical symptoms. Patients complain of "trouble swallowing." A careful, detailed history may be necessary to elicit the exact nature of the patient's problems with swallowing. Dysfunction may be due to physical obstructive phenomena, neuromuscular weakness, or discoordination.

◆ Epidemiology

Dysphagia affects all age groups, dependent on the etiology of the symptom. The elderly are disproportionately affected, however. Some estimate that 50% of nursing home patients suffer with swallowing problems. The percentage of stroke patients who relate dysphagia is 50 to 75%.

◆ Clinical

Signs and Symptoms

Patients may relate very specific aspects of the swallowing reflex that are problematic for them, or they may simply have a generic complaint of trouble swallowing. Dysphagia is associated with symptoms including choking, gagging, globus, odynophagia, difficulty initiating swallow, drooling, aspiration, coughing, nasal reflux, and regurgitation. A history of pneumonia is concerning for chronic aspiration. Weight loss may be a sign of dysphagia significant enough to reduce caloric intake, or potentially a neoplastic process. Children with dysphagia may have similar symptoms but also prolonged feeding times, repeated swallow efforts, or unusual posturing during feeding.

Dysphagia may involve one or more of the phases of the swallowing reflex, including oral preparatory, pharyngeal, or esophageal phases. Specific symptoms may direct the examiner's attention to one of these sites.

Differential Diagnosis

- Neurologic disorder (e.g., myasthenia gravis, Parkinson's disease [PD], amyotrophic lateral sclerosis [ALS], multiple sclerosis, cerebral palsy,

mental retardation or developmental delay, muscular dystrophy, postpolio syndrome, cranial neuropathies)
- Neurologic injury (e.g., cerebrovascular accident, traumatic brain injury, neurosurgical or skull base procedures with cranial neuropathies)
- Obstruction (e.g., upper aerodigestive tract neoplasms, esophageal web, strictures, achalasia, foreign body, cricopharyngeal dysfunction, cervical spine osteophytes)
- Other (e.g., xerostomia, gastroesophageal reflux disease [GERD], presbyphagia or presbyesophagus, neck irradiation, cleft lip/palate, hypopharyngeal diverticulum, tracheotomy)

◆ Evaluation

Physical Exam

The physical exam should include all components of the upper aerodigestive tract. The oral cavity should be examined and note made of labial competence; salivary function; tongue mobility, symmetry, and strength; palatal motion; mucosal lesions or masses; and gag reflex. The pharyngeal examination should include mirror examination and/or flexible nasopharyngoscopy. In addition to examining for symmetry, mass effect, and mucosal lesion, the presence of pooled secretions is a key finding. Saliva and liquid or food residue in the vallecula, piriform recesses, and postcricoid area indicate either an obstruction of material passage somewhere between the cricopharyngeus and the stomach, or a sensory defect of the hypopharynx and larynx.

Laryngeal examination is a component of the pharyngeal evaluation. A "wet voice" may indicate retained secretions in the hypopharynx and laryngeal introitus. The sensation, general mobility, and ability to completely close the vocal folds should be assessed. Neck examination should note symmetry, contour, presence of masses, and presence of laryngeal elevation with swallow. Normal presence of laryngeal crepitus (easy mobility and click encountered on moving the larynx over the cervical spine) should be elicited. Cranial nerves (CNs) should be assessed, particularly those associated with the swallow mechanism: CNs V, VII, IX, X, and XII.

Imaging

Plain film radiography has a limited role in the assessment of dysphagia. Cervical films may demonstrate foreign bodies, cervical osteophytes, and air–fluid levels in the cervical esophagus or diverticulum. Chest radiographs may show pneumonia or evidence of chronic aspiration, as well as esophageal air–fluid levels. The mainstay of evaluation is the modified barium swallow (MBS), or rehabilitation swallow. This test is typically done in conjunction with a speech pathologist. Cinefluoroscopic examination involves having the patient swallow contrast containing a coated material of different consistencies. This allows for an anatomic evaluation of the upper aerodigestive tract but also a functional assessment of bolus preparation, transfer, and transit. Patients may vary in their ability to manage various consistencies of food; the MBS enables identification of this fact, as well as information about therapeutic consistency changes. Retained material may be noted. Additionally, laryngeal penetration and aspiration may be identified. Rehabilitation maneuvers may be tried under fluoroscopy by the speech pathologist and feedback about their effectiveness can be immediately ascertained. Computed tomography (CT) and magnetic resonance imaging (MRI) may be necessary to investigate asymmetry for the pharynx and esophagus or when tumor is suspected.

Other Tests

Fiberoptic endoscopic evaluation of swallowing (with or without sensory testing), or FEES, is another technique available to assess the swallow mechanism. This can be an alternative to an MBS. A flexible endoscopy is passed through the nose and positioned to visualize the oropharynx and hypopharynx and larynx during swallowing trials. Trailed substances are colored with food dye, and the examination is recorded to ease assessment of rapid events and subtle findings. Sensory testing is accomplished via an air pulse delivered through the flexible laryngoscope and identification of the presence and strength of the laryngeal adductor reflex. Formal esophagoscopy is useful if esophageal pathologies are suspected. This technique also allows for biopsy and sometime interventions. Some otolaryngologists have adopted in-office, nonsedated transnasal esophagoscopy for assessing the esophagus. Esophageal manometry and pH probe testing may be adjuvants to assess for esophageal dysmotility and reflux issues.

◆ Treatment Options

Medical

Dysphagia secondary to nonobstructive phenomena is typically managed with therapy techniques. Most of these techniques require voluntary action on the part of the patient, although some require little patient cognition. Techniques may involve head and neck positioning during the swallow, food consistency changes, and sensory enhancement therapy. A speech pathologist with an interest in swallow rehabilitation should be consulted. Many patients perform better with various consistencies of food: dietary modification and thickening agents may help a patient maintain oral intake. Nutritional supplements may be useful in the nutritionally compromised patient. If reflux is a component of the dysphagia or is thought to be the underlying etiology, medical therapy may be tried.

Surgical

Surgery may be directed to obstructive phenomena such as tumors, strictures, webs, cricopharyngeal hypertonicity, or hypopharyngeal diverticulum. Vocal fold immobility that contributes to aspiration issues may benefit from medialization thyroplasty. Procedures for chronic aspiration exist (see **Chapter 5.4.3**). If oral intake is deemed unsafe due to aspiration, feeding gastrostomy may be necessary.

◆ Outcome and Follow-Up

The etiology largely determines the treatment outcome and follow-up

5.4.3   Aspiration

◆ Key Features

- Aspiration involves the passage of secretions or material into the lower airways.
- Aspiration is an important source of morbidity in the neuromuscularly impaired and debilitated.
- The most common cause of aspiration is neuromuscular dysfunction.
- Chronic aspiration may have severe medical consequences, and medical, sometimes surgical, interventions need to be enacted.

In general, the lower airway should not be exposed to upper aerodigestive tract secretions or materials. Aspiration of small amounts of material during sleep (reported in 50% normal patients) may be tolerated if the tracheobronchopulmonary system clearing mechanisms are functional. Large episodes of aspiration or chronic aspiration may yield complications whose severity is determined by the nature and volume of the material aspirated. Aspiration may be primary (swallowed dietary materials or secretions) or secondary (regurgitated diverticulum or gastric contents).

◆ Clinical

Signs and Symptoms

The presence of chronic aspiration may be evident to the patient and healthcare providers or may be "silent," with no cough generated. Dysphagia is intimately associated with aspiration, as most patients with noted aspiration will also complain of "trouble swallowing" (see **Chapter 5.4.2**). Symptoms of chronic aspiration include choking or coughing when swallowing (may be with specific types of dietary intake, all food, or even the patient's own secretions). Some patients may also complain of chronic cough independent of swallowing, related to the bronchopulmonary complications of the chronic aspiration. Productive cough, fevers, and dyspnea in a patient with dysphagia is concerning for this issue. Also, recurrent lower respiratory infections in a patient with predisposing comorbidities should make the clinician suspicious of this issue.

Differential Diagnosis

Some conditions may share respiratory symptoms with the complications of chronic aspiration. The key differential diagnosis is for those diseases that may predispose to chronic aspiration:

- Neuromuscular
  - Degenerative diseases
    - Alzheimer's disease
    - Amyotrophic lateral sclerosis (ALS)
    - Multiple sclerosis
    - Progressive supranuclear palsy
    - Parkinson's disease (PD)
    - Huntington's disease
  - Disorders
    - Myasthenia gravis
    - Myopathy (dermatomyositis, inclusion body myositis)
    - Muscular dystrophy
    - Poliomyelitis and postpolio syndrome
    - Guillain-Barré's syndrome
    - Cranial neuropathies
- Central nervous system (CNS) injury
  - Cerebrovascular accident
  - Head trauma
  - Anoxic brain injury
  - Postsurgical
  - Encephalitis/meningitis
  - Cerebral palsy
- Upper aerodigestive tract disorders
  - Vocal fold immobility
  - Stricture (web, reflux, caustic ingestion, postsurgical)
  - Zenker's diverticulum
  - Cricopharyngeal dysfunction
  - Postirradiation/chemoradiation
  - Postsurgical dysfunction
  - Neoplasms
  - Achalasia
  - Reflux
- Other
  - CNS/skull base neoplasm
  - Severe deconditioning or systemic illness
  - Intoxication
  - Mental retardation or developmental delay
  - Presence of a tracheotomy tube

✦ Evaluation

After a detailed history and physical examination (including nasopharyngoscopy), several options exist for evaluation. A bedside swallow evaluation by a speech pathologist is reasonable for those with mild dysphagia, but secondary to the morbidity that may accompany aspiration; if aspiration is suspected, an objective evaluation is warranted.

Imaging

Modified barium swallow (MBS) has been the traditional imaging study for evaluation of dysphagia and aspiration. This test may demonstrate the passage of contrast material into the trachea and bronchi. Laryngeal penetration or retained contrast within the piriform recesses or vallecula are concerning because of their aspiration potential. Therapeutic maneuvers may be performed under cinefluoroscopy and their impact determined immediately, thus aiding in care planning.

Scintigraphy has been proposed to demonstrate and quantify aspiration. Overall, it offers few advantages beyond MBS and fiberoptic endoscopic evaluation of swallowing (FEES) (see Other Tests). Chest radiography (plain film or computed tomographic [CT] radiography) may be helpful in demonstrating pneumonia and chronic pulmonary disease stemming from aspiration (e.g., bronchiectasis).

Other Tests

FEES involves the transnasal endoscopic monitoring of dyed food and liquid ingestion. Observations are made regarding premature leakage, retained materials, laryngeal penetration, or aspiration. This study is typically video-recorded so that slow motion review may be performed to assess for subtle evidence of swallowing dysfunction.

✦ Treatment Options

Initial management in a patient who has concerns for chronic aspiration is to ensure NPO (nothing by mouth) status, to minimize the volume of potential aspirate until confirmation can be made. Good oral care and speech therapy assessment are appropriate in all patients. Alternative nutrition routes such as nasogastric tubes or percutaneous feeding conduits should be considered, depending on clinical circumstances, for those with prolonged inadequate nutrition.

Medical

A variety of speech therapy techniques are available to assist in safe swallowing. These include consistency changes (e.g., thickening agents, alternating consistencies), as well as positioning maneuvers (e.g., chin tuck, head turn) and swallowing maneuvers (e.g., double swallow, swallow–cough, swallow–cough–swallow, effortful swallow). If a patient is deemed to be inappropriate for any oral intake, alternative feeding conduits should be utilized. If aspiration of secretions is an issue, surgical procedures may be necessary.

Table 5.4 Surgical management of chronic aspiration

Procedure	Description	Advantages	Disadvantages
Irreversible			
Narrow-field laryngectomy	Removal of larynx, preserving hyoid and strap muscles	Definitive separation of respiratory and digestive tracts	Definitively irreversible Negative psychosocial features for patients Transcervical approach Loss of phonation
Glottic closure	Median thyrotomy with suture closure of true and false vocal folds	High success rate Theoretical, but difficult reversal	Transcervical approach Tracheotomy Loss of phonation
Subperichondrial cricoidectomy	Subperichondrial resection of cricoid with closure subglottic mucosa and strap muscle reinforcement	High success rate Possible under local anesthesia	Transcervical approach Tracheotomy Loss of phonation Fistula potential
Reversible			
Laryngotracheal separation	Transection of the trachea with creation of tracheostoma and closure of subglottis	Among the most dependable of reversible procedures	Transcervical approach Tracheotomy Loss of phonation Fistula potential
Laryngotracheal diversion	Transection of the trachea with creation of tracheostoma and anastomosis of proximal trachea to esophagus	Among the most dependable of reversible procedures "Aspirated" secretions into proximal trachea diverted to esophagus	Transcervical approach Tracheotomy Loss of phonation Fistula potential
Epiglottic flap laryngeal closure	Larynx is closed by denuding edges of epiglottis and aryepiglottic folds and suturing epiglottis over the glottis	Potential speech preservation if posterior glottis is kept open	Transcervical approach Tracheotomy Possible dehiscence 50% prevention of aspiration Supraglottic stenosis after reversal

continued

Table 5.4 Surgical management of chronic aspiration *(Continued)*

Double-barrel tracheotomy	Transection of trachea with externalization of both ends of the trachea	Decreased fistulization	Transcervical approach Skin contamination with secretions
Partial cricoidectomy	Submucosal resection of posterior cricoid with cricopharyngeal myotomy and tracheotomy, serves to narrow laryngeal inlet and widen esophageal inlet	Preserves the voice	Transcervical approach Tracheotomy Persistent aspiration
Vertical laryngoplasty	Denuding of lower edge of the epiglottis, aryepiglottic folds, arytenoids with vertical tubing of the epiglottis, leaving superior opening	Preservation of voice Described for total glossectomy patients to reduce need for laryngectomy	Transcervical approach Persistent aspiration
Endolaryngeal stenting	Endolaryngeal stent placed to occlude the larynx	Simple to place	Leakage around the stent and aspiration Endolaryngeal injury Airway compromise if tracheotomy tube displaced Patient discomfort

Medical therapy should also involve treatment for the complications of the aspiration. These may include intubation, ventilator support, bronchoscopy, antibiotics, and pulmonary toilet.

Surgical

If medical management fails to correct the aspiration problem or is deemed inadequate, several surgical techniques are available. Placement of a tracheotomy tube facilitates pulmonary toilet and, with a cuffed tube inflated, may decrease aspiration events. An inflated cuffed tracheotomy tube, however, will not prevent aspiration. The presence of a tracheotomy tube may worsen or even cause aspiration: the laryngeal elevation accompanying a swallow is limited by tracheal tethering by the tube, and laryngeal sensation gradually decreases when airflow through the glottis ceases. A speaking valve may aid in swallowing by improving subglottic pressures necessary to clear secretions, and maintenance of laryngeal sensation. Directed surgical procedures may be helpful in reducing aspiration (e.g., chemical or surgical cricopharyngeal myotomy for cricopharyngeal dysfunction, vocal fold medialization for vocal fold immobility).

Laryngeal surgical management of chronic aspiration may be classified as reversible and irreversible (**Table 5.4**). Each of these techniques has advantages and disadvantages that may influence its use. Reversible procedures all have the potential advantage of being reversible if the underlying aspiration condition improves sufficiently.

◆ Complications

Complications may include chronic lung disease and pulmonary fibrosis.

◆ Outcome and Follow-Up

Outcome depends on the etiology of aspiration.

5.5 Acid Reflux Disorders

◆ Key Features

- Laryngopharyngeal reflux is distinct from classic gastroesophageal reflux disease (GERD).
- The work-up may involve an endoscopy, barium studies, and a pH probe.
- Extraesophageal manifestations relate to the pharynx, larynx, and lungs.

◆ Epidemiology

Twenty-five to forty percent of healthy adult Americans experience symptomatic gastroesophageal reflux disease (GERD) manifested as heartburn. Laryngopharyngeal reflux (LPR) typically does not cause heartburn or esophagitis. Certain foods, medications, hormones, and physical states (e.g., obesity) can decrease the pressure of the lower esophageal sphincter, thus worsening LPR or GERD symptoms.

◆ Clinical

Signs

GERD: esophagitis, Barrett's esophagus
LPR: coughing, throat clearing, laryngeal erythema

Symptoms

GERD symptoms typically include postprandial heartburn and regurgitation. LPR symptoms may be more subtle and include hoarseness, globus sensation, dysphagia, chronic throat clearing, halitosis, sensation of postnasal drainage, chronic cough, laryngospasm, and otalgia.

◆ Evaluation

A suggestive history and exam findings usually prompt a "therapeutic trial" of behavioral changes and twice-daily use of a proton pump inhibitor. Ancillary testing should be employed if this regimen fails or if symptoms are atypical or worsening, due to risk of malignancy.

Physical Exam

Nasolaryngopharyngoscopy may reveal laryngeal erythema and edema of arytenoids and interarytenoid space, laryngeal pachydermia, and vocal fold granulomas.

Imaging

A barium swallow study is useful for initial screening and to identify structural abnormalities.

Labs

Laboratory tests are seldom useful.

Other Tests

A dual-channel 24-hour pH monitoring probe is the gold standard. Esophagogastroduodenoscopy identifies the presence and severity of esophagitis and the possible presence of Barrett's esophagus. The role of screening endoscopy is evolving. With the advent of the transnasal esophagoscope (TNE), the routine screening of reflux patients for occult esophagitis or Barrett's esophagus has become more commonplace.

Pathology

Transient lower esophageal sphincter relaxation is a manometric finding. The Reflux Symptom Index (RSI), a patient-completed survey, is useful for scoring or grading.

◆ Treatment Options

Medical

Behavioral modification: weight loss, smoking cessation, avoid eating before sleep, avoid caffeine, alcohol, peppermint, chocolate, and spicy and acid foods.

H_2 receptor antagonists: ranitidine (e.g., Zantac, Boehringer Ingelheim Pharmaceuticals, Ridgefield, CT) 150 mg orally twice daily. These agents block histamine at the H_2 receptors, particularly those in the gastric parietal cells, to inhibit acid secretion. Tachyphylaxis may develop to H_2 blockers after several weeks of use.

Proton pump inhibitors (PPIs): esomeprazole (e.g., Nexium, Pfizer, New York, NY) 20 to 40 mg orally twice daily. These agents inhibit gastric acid secretion by inhibition of the H^+/K^+-ATPase system in the gastric parietal cells.

Prokinetics: metoclopramide (Reglan, Ani Pharmaceuticals, Baudette, MN) 10 mg orally four times daily. These agents increase lower esophageal sphincter pressure to help reduce reflux and also accelerate gastric emptying.

Surgical

About 20% of patients have a progressive form of reflux disease and may develop severe complications. For these patients, surgical treatment should be considered. The indications for this include Barrett's esophagus; strictures; respiratory manifestations (e.g., cough, wheezing, aspiration); ear, nose, and throat manifestations (e.g., hoarseness, sore throat, otitis media); and dental manifestations (e.g., enamel erosion).

With laparoscopic fundoplication, symptoms resolve in ~92% of patients.

◆ Complications

Complications of untreated or resistant GERD include esophagitis, pneumonia, asthma, and interstitial lung fibrosis. Barrett's esophagus is one of the most serious complications of GERD, because it may progress to cancer.

◆ Outcome and Follow-Up

Patients should understand that there is a need for long-term maintenance therapy. Many physicians advocate mandatory esophagoscopy, if patients continue to experience symptoms, to rule out Barrett's esophagus changes and cancer. Others advocate screen endoscopy in patients with a positive response to PPI treatment.

5.6 Laryngeal Manifestations of Systemic Diseases

◆ Key Features

- Systemic diseases may generate vocal and airway consequences.
- Management of the underlying systemic illness may or may not enable reversal of the laryngeal issues. Systemic diseases may manifest as laryngeal symptoms and findings. A careful clinical history and appropriate testing should yield a diagnosis. Frequently, consultation with colleagues from other services more familiar with the overall systemic illness may be needed.

◆ Rheumatoid Arthritis

Rheumatoid arthritis is a chronic, inflammatory condition affecting synovial joints with progressive arthritis and deformity. All synovial joints are vulnerable, with hands and feet the most commonly affected. Women are three times more likely to develop the disease, usually between the third and seventh decade. A juvenile form of the disease also exists. The cricoarytenoid joint may be involved in this process in 25 to 50% of those with long-standing disease. Symptoms may include hoarseness, globus, and airway compromise. Examination may show inflammatory changes of the arytenoid region, diffuse laryngeal myositis, and rheumatoid nodules within the vocal folds or unilateral or bilateral vocal fold motion impairment. Treatment may include nonsteroidal anti-inflammatory drugs (NSAIDs) or corticosteroids. Local injections of steroids into the cricoarytenoid joint region have shown success in improving joint mobility.

◆ Relapsing Polychondritis

Relapsing polychondritis is a chronic and recurrent autoimmune inflammatory condition affecting all cartilage subtypes. The laryngotracheal complex may be involved in 40 to 50% of patients. Disease may affect the airways focally or diffusely. Symptoms may include hoarseness, dyspnea, stridor, laryngotracheal tenderness, or dysphagia. Airway symptoms may be secondary to acute inflammatory and swelling, laryngotracheal collapse secondary to replacement of cartilage by fibrosis, or subglottic stenosis. Treatment is as necessary for any airway obstruction, but in general, therapy consists of corticosteroids and other immunosuppressive agents.

◆ Wegener's Granulomatosis

Wegener's granulomatosis is an autoimmune disorder characterized by necrotizing granulomas and vasculitis. The upper and lower respiratory tract and renal systems are primarily affected, although vasculitis may occur anywhere. The larynx is involved primarily in the subglottic and upper tracheal region, and pathology is seen in the early phase of ~ 10 to 15% of patients. Biopsy may demonstrate the characteristic granulomas. Antineutrophilic cytoplasmic antibodies are elevated in 90% of cases. Airway management of the subglottic stenosis may be necessary and involve dilations, laser resection, or tracheotomy. Formal laryngotracheoplasty or tracheal resection should be reserved for chronic, nonactive disease.

◆ Sarcoidosis

Sarcoidosis is a systemic granulomatous disease of unknown etiology, with a U.S. predilection for African Americans and those of Scandinavian descent. Women are more often affected than men. Pulmonary and lymphatic systems are most commonly affected. Laryngeal involvement may occur in 1 to 5% of affected individuals. The supraglottic structures are typically most involved, with sparing of the true vocal folds. Airway compromise may occur from enlargement of the supraglottic structures due to the noncaseating, granulomatous infiltration. Treatment may include systemic steroids, but local steroid injection into the involved larynx itself has been described. Serial, conservative laser ablation of excessive tissue may also be needed.

◆ Amyloidosis

Multiple variants of amyloidosis exist, including primary and secondary systemic amyloidosis and amyloidosis associated with multiple myeloma, as well as a localized form. In the aerodigestive tract, submucosal and intramuscular deposits of fibrillar protein–polysaccharides complex occur. The larynx is seldom involved. Presentation varies from mild hoarseness symptoms, secondary to small submucosal vocal fold deposits causing mucosal stiffness, to airway compromise, secondary to large supraglottic, glottic, or subglottic deposits. Biopsy is used for diagnosis, with the classic apple-green birefringence under polarized light microscopy with Congo red stain. Treatment with local resection may be necessary if symptoms warrant.

◆ Epidermolysis Bullosa

This is a rare, hereditary connective tissue disorder based on a defect in the dermal basement membrane. Blisters form secondary to separation of the epidermis and dermis, often after minimal trauma. Milder forms may heal without event unless secondary infections occur, with more severe forms creating mucosal scarring. When the larynx is involved in the process, webbing, stenosis, and synechiae may form. Intubation should be avoided, to avoid any trauma that may precipitate the bulla formation and subsequent scarring.

◆ Pemphigoid

Pemphigoid is an autoimmune disease involving antibodies against components of the basement membrane. Blisters form on both cutaneous and mucosal surfaces. Bullous pemphigoid typically heals without scarring, unless secondary scarring occurs. Cicatricial pemphigoid occurs in older patients and may result in significant mucosal scarring. This scarring may occur in the larynx or esophagus, resulting in vocal, airway, and swallowing symptoms. Clinical features and biopsy can make the diagnosis. Laser resection of symptomatic scarring may be necessary. Systemic immunosuppression may be used in significant cases.

◆ Angioneurotic Edema

Angioedema involves plasma extravasation into tissues, resulting in swelling. Multiple forms exist, but idiopathic, medication-related (angiotensin-converting enzyme [ACE] inhibitors), and hereditary forms are most commonly encountered by the otolaryngologist. Airway edema may form within the lips, tongue, pharynx, and larynx. Hereditary angioneurotic edema typically presents early in life and is characterized by multiple edema events. Hereditary forms are associated with a defect in C1 esterase inhibitor. Levels of this enzyme may be performed to help make the diagnosis. Treatment acutely involves airway management as necessary. Edema may progress, so airway monitoring should be considered, even if acute intervention is not necessary. The hereditary form may be treated acutely with C1-inhibitor concentrate, with androgens being helpful in chronic prevention. ACE inhibitor–related events should be treated acutely with medication cessation and consideration for steroids. Angioneurotic edema may occur any time after initiation of the drug, hours to years later.

◆ Neuromuscular Disease

Numerous systemic neuromuscular disorders may cause laryngeal symptoms. These findings may range from vocal fold paresis to paralysis and discoordination of vocal fold motion during speech, respiration, and swallowing. Diseases include myasthenia gravis, amyotrophic lateral sclerosis (ALS), Parkinson's disease (PD), Guillain-Barré's syndrome, multiple sclerosis, Charcot-Marie-Tooth's disease, and postpolio syndrome.

◆ Other

Many other systemic conditions may cause laryngeal symptoms. Hypothyroidism (myxedema) and allergic disease may both cause vocal fold edema and hoarseness.

6 Head and Neck Surgery

Section Editor

Neerav Goyal

Contributors

Eelam A. Adil

Michele M. Carr

David Goldenberg

Bradley J. Goldstein

Neerav Goyal

Melissa M. Krempasky

Heath B. Mackley

Francis P. Ruggiero

Sohrab Sohrabi

6.0 Anatomy of the Neck

Surgically, it is useful to consider the neck anatomy in terms of compartments or levels and to consider fascial layers. The neck is covered by a layer of superficial fascia, and the deep cervical fascia can be divided into superficial, middle, and deep layers (**Fig. 6.1**). This is relevant in terms of spread of infection and lymphatic spread of cancer. The neck can be grossly divided into the anterior and posterior neck. Posteriorly, of course, are the cervical spine and paraspinal muscles. Anterolaterally, the neck contents are considered in terms of nodal levels I though VI (**Fig. 6.2**).

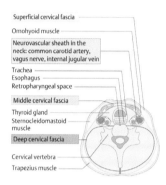

Superficial cervical fascia

Omohyoid muscle

Neurovascular sheath in the neck: common carotid artery, vagus nerve, internal jugular vein

Trachea
Esophagus
Retropharyngeal space

Middle cervical fascia

Thyroid gland
Sternocleidomastoid muscle

Deep cervical fascia

Cervical vertebra

Trapezius muscle

Fig. 6.1 Cervical fascial planes. (Used with permission from Probst R, Grevers G, Iro H. *Basic Otorhinolaryngology: A Step-by-Step Learning Guide.* Stuttgart/New York: Thieme;2006:313.)

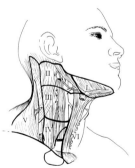

Fig. 6.2 Nodal levels I through VI. (Used with permission from Van de Water TR, Staecker H. *Otolaryngology: Basic Science and Clinical Review.* Stuttgart/New York: Thieme;2006:606.)

327

Each level contains a compartment of fibrofatty lymph node–bearing tissue that is addressed for removal during neck dissection procedures for cancer. Level I consists of the submental region and the submandibular area containing the submandibular gland. Level II is the upper jugular chain lymph node region, level III is the middle jugular chain, and level IV is the inferior jugular chain region. Level V is the posterior triangle from the anterior border of the trapezius to the posterior border of the sternocleidomastoid muscle. Level VI is the node-bearing tissue of the central compartment. The visceral structures of the neck are included in the central compartment and include the laryngotracheal complex, the thyroid and parathyroids, and the cervical esophagus.

◆ Blood Supply

The common carotid artery ascends into the neck and bifurcates into the internal and external carotid artery approximately at the level of the hyoid bone. The internal carotid has no branches in the neck and delivers important blood supply to the brain, along with the vertebral arteries. The external carotid supplies the head and neck structures via multiple branches (in order, starting inferiorly): the superior thyroid, ascending pharyngeal, lingual, facial, occipital, posterior auricular, superficial temporal, and maxillary arteries (**Fig. 6.3**). Venous drainage tends to parallel major arteries, with variable anterior and external jugular branches superficially, and large common facial veins joining into the internal jugular vein, which feeds the subclavian veins. The carotid sheath, formed by all three layers of the deep cervical fascia, contains the carotid artery, jugular vein, and vagus nerve. Important delicate lymphatics from the thoracic duct carry chyle into the jugular vein near its junction with the subclavian in the left neck; however, accessory thoracic ducts commonly occur on the right.

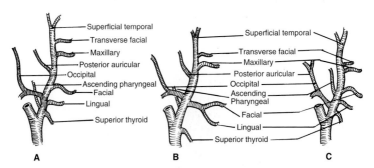

Fig. 6.3 The branching of the arteries originating from the carotid artery can be quite variable. (Used with permission from Van de Water TR, Staecker H. *Otolaryngology: Basic Science and Clinical Review.* Stuttgart/New York: Thieme;2006:603.)

◆ Innervation

The 12 cranial nerves (CNs) supply the head and neck region with motor, sensory, and special sensory fibers. They are, in order, the olfactory, optic, oculomotor, trochlear, trigeminal, abducens, facial, vestibulocochlear, glossopharyngeal, vagus, spinal accessory, and hypoglossal. In the neck there are surgically important aspects of CN anatomy. The hypoglossal (XII) emerges from the skull base at the hypoglossal canal and courses beneath the digastric and submandibular contents as motor supply to the tongue. The pars nervosa of the jugular foramen contains the glossopharyngeal (IX), vagus (X), and accessory nerves (XI). The vagus runs within the carotid sheath, and the recurrent laryngeal branches course in the tracheoesophageal groove to supply the vocal folds; the superior laryngeal nerves arise from the vagus in the upper neck. The accessory nerve courses posteroinferiorly through the neck, entering the anterior border of the sternocleidomastoid, emerging from the posterior border near Erb's point, and continuing into the trapezius.

The facial nerve (VII) exits the skull base at the stylomastoid foramen, and its main motor branches course within the parotid gland to innervate the muscles of facial expression, while the lingual nerve supplies parasympathetics to the submandibular gland and sensation to the anterior tongue and is encountered deep to the submandibular gland. Important cervical nerves are encountered in the neck as well. The great auricular nerve (it is not named great*er*, since there is no *lesser* auricular nerve) transmits sensory fibers of C2–3 to the auricular area (**Fig. 6.4**). This nerve is encountered along the sternocleidomastoid, coursing superiorly from Erb's point. The phrenic nerve (C3–5) is deep to the floor fascia (deep layer of the deep cervical fascia) along the anterior scalene muscle, supplying motor fibers to the diaphragm. Also, the brachial plexus is in the same plane, deep to the fascia on the middle scalene. The cervical sympathetic trunk runs deep to the carotid. CN anatomy is reviewed in **Appendix B** of this book.

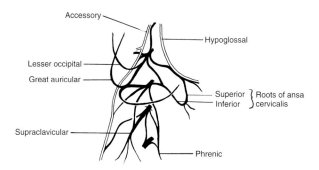

Fig. 6.4 Cervical plexus. (Used with permission from Van de Water TR, Staecker H. *Otolaryngology: Basic Science and Clinical Review.* Stuttgart/New York: Thieme;2006:603.)

6.1 Neck Emergencies

6.1.1 Necrotizing Soft Tissue Infections of the Head and Neck

◆ Key Features

- Necrotizing fasciitis is a soft tissue infection that causes necrosis of fascia and subcutaneous tissue but initially spares skin and muscle.
- It is rare in the head and neck; when it occurs it is usually associated with immunosuppression or odontogenic infection.
- Half of patients develop systemic bacteremia.
- Necrotizing soft tissue infections require aggressive treatment to combat the associated high morbidity and mortality.

Necrotizing soft tissue infections rarely may involve the face and neck, scalp, and eyelids.

◆ Epidemiology

In the head and neck, dental infections are the most common etiology, followed by trauma, peritonsillar and pharyngeal abscesses, and osteoradio-necrosis. Immunocompromised patients are most susceptible. Predisposing conditions include diabetes mellitus, obesity, arteriosclerosis, alcoholism, chronic renal failure, hypothyroidism, malignancy, and poor nutrition. Gas-producing wound infections are usually produced by bacteria of the Clostridia class. Onset of symptoms is usually 2 to 4 days after the insult.

◆ Clinical

Signs

The signs of a necrotizing soft tissue infection include a low-grade fever, and the skin becomes smooth, warm, tense and shiny with no sharp demarcation. The infected skin also develops a dusky discoloration with poorly defined borders. Soft tissue crepitus is common from gas formation (though not necessary for the diagnosis). Later in the disease process, bullae may develop. Systemic symptoms get more severe with typical signs of septicemia. The last stage of the disease is characterized by cyanotic skin discoloration typical of necrosis. Patients may present with a benign clinical picture yet with a leukocytosis not consistent with the clinical picture.

Symptoms

There is sudden severe pain and swelling. There may be anesthesia of the involved skin.

Differential Diagnosis

The differential diagnosis includes other deep neck space infections, pyoderma gangrenosum, radiation necrosis, cellulitis, and erysipelas.

◆ Evaluation

Physical Exam

When clinical hard signs are present (i.e., crepitus, skin necrosis, bullae, hypotension), a physical exam may be helpful. Unfortunately, the signs and symptoms are often very subtle on presentation.

Imaging

Plain soft tissue films of the neck (looking for gas in soft tissue) may be obtained. Computed tomography (CT) is the most useful study to detect gas in areas inaccessible to palpation and to identify areas where the infection has spread. In addition, it can detect vascular thrombosis, erosion of vessels, and mediastinitis. Magnetic resonance imaging (MRI) has also been suggested, as it can demonstrate areas of enhancement or infection that crosses fascial planes.

Labs

Routine blood work is needed to look for metabolic abnormalities such as hyponatremia and hypoproteinemia due to fluid sequestration and hypocalcemia as a result of subcutaneous fat saponification. Additionally, a complete blood count will note a significantly elevated white blood cell count.

Microbiology

Group A hemolytic streptococci and *Staphylococcus aureus,* alone or in synergism, are frequently the initiating infecting bacteria. However, other aerobic and anaerobic pathogens may be present, including *Bacteroides, Clostridium, Peptostreptococcus,* Enterobacteriaceae, coliforms, *Proteus, Pseudomonas,* and *Klebsiella* species.

Pathology

The pathology shows a localized necrosis of skin that is secondary to thrombosis of nutrient vessels as they pass through involved fascia. Tissue hypoxia resulting from small vessel vasculitis and thrombi and impaired host defenses help facilitate anaerobic bacterial growth.

◆ Treatment Options

Prompt measures offer hope for survival of the patient.

Medical

High-dose intravenous (IV) broad-spectrum antibiotics are recommended. Hyperbaric oxygen therapy is sometimes used in addition to surgical and antimicrobial treatment.

Surgical

Aggressive surgical debridement until there are bleeding viable borders is necessary. This may require multiple trips to the operating room for irrigation and debridement and/or bedside dressing changes and debridement. Initially, it is important not to close the wound with larger defects, due to the progressive nature of the disease process. If the necrotizing process involves the neck, avoid tracheotomy through the infected area.

◆ Outcome and Follow-Up

The overall mortality rate has been reported to be as high as 70%.

6.1.2   Ludwig's Angina

◆ Key Features

- Ludwig's angina is a rapidly expanding, diffuse inflammation of the submandibular and sublingual spaces.
- It is most often caused by dental infections.
- The condition is often found in immunocompromised patients, such as those with diabetes or human immunodeficiency virus/acquired immunodeficiency syndrome (HIV/AIDS) or drug abusers.

Ludwig's angina is a rapidly spreading bilateral cellulitis of the sublingual and submaxillary spaces. Before the advent of antibiotics, the mortality associated with Ludwig's angina approached 50%, but today, mortality rates are in the range of 8 to 10%. The most common cause of death is respiratory compromise.

◆ Epidemiology

Ludwig's angina represents up to 13% of all deep neck infections. Typically, young adults present with Ludwig's angina; it is unusual in children. The infection generally spreads from a dental or periodontal infection. Other causes include upper respiratory infections, floor-of-mouth trauma, mandibular fractures, sialadenitis, IV drug abuse, trauma and tonsillitis, and immunocompromised states such as diabetes or HIV/AIDS. Forty percent of Ludwig's angina cases involve oral anaerobes.

◆ Clinical

Signs

The signs of the infection include an inability to close the mouth, trismus, drooling, sitting upright, inability to swallow and dysphonia, dyspnea, stridor, fever, chills, and tachycardia. Note that stridor, dyspnea, decreased air movement, or cyanosis suggest impending respiratory compromise.

Symptoms

The symptoms of Ludwig's angina are severe neck pain and tenderness, submandibular and submental swelling, fever, malaise, and dysphagia.

Differential Diagnosis

The differential diagnosis includes other deep neck space infections, an infected cyst, tumor, and cellulitis.

◆ Evaluation

Physical Exam

On physical examination, the patient will often present with carious molar teeth, neck rigidity, and drooling. There is a "woody" or "brawny" induration of involved spaces with little to no fluctuance. The patient's mouth floor is swollen, and the tongue may be swollen or elevated. The patient may describe difficulty breathing and may have audible breathing.

Imaging

A computed tomography (CT) scan is most useful.

Labs

Blood cultures are usually negative; if the swelling is aspirated or drained, samples should be sent for Gram stain, culture, and sensitivity.

◆ Treatment Options

Airway control is the first priority of treatment, followed by IV antibiotics and timely surgical drainage. Blind oral or nasotracheal intubation or attempts with neuromuscular paralysis are contraindicated in Ludwig's angina, as they may precipitate an airway crisis.

Medical

Aggressive empiric high-dose, IV antibiotics are recommended—cefuroxime plus metronidazole. If the patient is allergic to penicillin, prescribe clindamycin plus a quinolone. Once culture and sensitivity results have been obtained, antibiotic therapy may be changed accordingly.

Surgical

To establish airway control, a tracheotomy may be indicated. Surgical drainage was once universally required but now may be reserved for cases in which antibiotic treatment fails. On external incision and drainage, often straw-colored material, as opposed to frank purulence, is found. Consider placement of a passive drain to allow continued drainage as the infection resolves.

◆ Complications

A spontaneous rupture may lead to asphyxia, aspiration, or pneumonia. The infection may spread to other deep neck compartments.

◆ Outcome and Follow-Up

The offending tooth should also be removed if the infection's origin is odontogenic.

6.1.3   Deep Neck Infections

◆ Key Features

- Deep neck infections are most commonly caused by tonsillar, peritonsillar, or odontogenic infections.
- They may involve surrounding nerves, vessels, bones, and other soft tissue.
- Microbiology typically reveals mixed bacterial flora, including anaerobic species.
- Deep neck spaces have avenues of communication with each other: infection in one space can spread to adjacent spaces.

Deep neck infections hold the potential for severe complications. Complex head and neck anatomy often makes early recognition of deep neck infections challenging, and a high index of suspicion is necessary to avoid delay in treatment. Aggressive monitoring and management of the airway are the most urgent aspects of care, followed by appropriate antibiotic coverage and surgical drainage, as needed. Risk factors for deep neck infection include diabetes mellitus, HIV, steroid therapy, chemotherapy, and other sources of immune compromise.

◆ Clinical

Signs and Symptoms

Pain and swelling of the neck are the most prevalent symptoms. Fever, malaise, and dysphagia may occur. Other common symptoms are deep space–specific and include dysphagia, odynophagia, trismus, dysphonia, otalgia, and dyspnea.

In the pediatric population, fever, neck mass, and stiffness are most prevalent, followed by sore throat, poor oral intake, drooling, and lymphadenopathy. Stridor, dyspnea, decreased air movement, and cyanosis suggest impending respiratory compromise.

Differential Diagnosis

The differential diagnosis includes infected congenital cysts, lymphangitis, tumor, cellulitis, and necrotizing fasciitis.

◆ Evaluation

History, physical examination, laboratory work, and diagnostic imaging each provide important clues for assessing a patient for a deep neck infection.

Physical Exam

Initial evaluation of the airway is always the first priority, and any signs of respiratory distress or impending airway compromise should be immediately and aggressively managed.

Imaging

A contrast-enhanced computed tomography (CT) scan is most useful. Ultrasound may be more accurate than CT in differentiating a drainable abscess from cellulitis. Magnetic resonance imaging (MRI) provides better soft tissue definition than CT. MRI also avoids exposure to radiation and interference from dental fillings.

Labs

Labs should include a complete blood count (CBC) with differential, serum glucose, and electrolytes; coagulation studies; HIV screening in adults; blood cultures; and appropriate cultures of aspirates obtained before antibiotics are instituted, if possible.

Microbiology

Infections are commonly polymicrobial and reflect the oropharyngeal flora. Frequently isolated aerobes include *Streptococcus viridans*, *Klebsiella pneumoniae*, *Staphylococcus aureus*, and, less frequently, *Streptococcus pneumoniae*, *Streptococcus pyogenes*, *Neisseria* species, and *Haemophilus influenzae*. Common anaerobic isolates include *Peptostreptococcus*, *Bacteroides fragilis*, pigmented *Prevotella* and *Porphyromonas* spp., *Fusobacterium* spp., and *Eikenella corrodens*.

◆ Treatment Options

Airway control is the first priority of treatment, followed by IV antibiotics and timely surgical drainage. Airway management, if necessary, should be undertaken under controlled conditions, in the operating room if possible, with either awake fiberoptic intubation or awake tracheotomy. Blind oral or nasotracheal intubation or attempts with neuromuscular paralysis may precipitate an airway crisis.

Medical

Every patient who has a deep neck infection should be given empiric antibiotic therapy until culture and sensitivity results are available. Empiric therapy should be effective against the aerobic and anaerobic bacteria that are commonly involved.

Either penicillin in combination with a β-lactamase inhibitor (e.g., amoxicillin with clavulanic acid) or a β-lactamase-resistant antibiotic (e.g., cefoxitin, cefuroxime, imipenem, or meropenem) in combination with a drug that is highly effective against most anaerobes (e.g., clindamycin or metronidazole) is recommended for optimal empiric coverage. Once available, the results of the culture and sensitivity tests can enable tailoring of adequate antibiotic therapy.

In select cases, an uncomplicated deep neck abscess or cellulitis can be effectively treated with antibiotics and careful monitoring, without surgical drainage. Simultaneous medical treatment for associated comorbidities such as diabetes mellitus can improve the overall immune status of a patient.

Surgical

Indications for surgery include airway compromise, critical condition, septicemia, complications, descending infection, diabetes mellitus, or no clinical improvement within 48 hours of the initiation of parenteral antibiotics. In addition, abscesses > 3 cm in diameter that involve the prevertebral, anterior visceral, or carotid spaces, or that involve more than two neck spaces, should be surgically drained.

Surgical drainage (**Table 6.1**) can be performed in several ways, including simple intraoral or extraoral incision and drainage for superficial abscesses, a more extensive external cervical approach with drain placement for more complicated infections, and minimally invasive techniques such as image-guided needle aspiration and indwelling catheter placement.

Table 6.1   Surgical approaches for drainage of deep neck infections

Infection site	Surgical approaches for drainage
Peritonsillar	Intraoral needle aspiration or incision and drainage
Submandibular space	Supramylohyoid—intraoral drainage Inframylohyoid—extraoral surgical drainage
Parapharyngeal space	External cervical approach along the anterior border of the sternocleidomastoid muscle CT-guided transoral drainage
Masticator space	External incision along inferior border of mandible Intraoral approach via retromolar trigone
Parotid space	External parotidectomy incision
Retropharyngeal space	Transoral External cervical approach
Prevertebral space	External cervical approach
Carotid space	External cervical approach

◆ Complications

Complications include mediastinitis, aspiration pneumonia, lung abscess, empyema, Lemierre's syndrome (suppurative thrombophlebitis of the internal jugular vein), carotid artery aneurysm or rupture, osteomyelitis involving the mandible or cervical vertebral bodies, meningitis, intracranial abscess, and disseminated intravascular coagulation.

◆ Outcome and Follow-Up

The initiating etiology, if recognized (an infected tooth, a tonsillar abscess), and predisposing systemic conditions (diabetes mellitus) should be addressed.

6.1.4 Neck Trauma

◆ Key Features

- Neck trauma can be either penetrating or blunt.
- There is potential injury to the larynx, trachea, esophagus, major vessels, and nerves.
- Airway management is always the priority.
- Cervical spine injury must be excluded.
- The zone of the neck where the trauma occurs will help dictate the management algorithm.

Factors in the mechanism of neck trauma determine the location of injury, the injury characteristics, the tissues and organs involved, and the extent of damage to the tissues and organs.

◆ Epidemiology

Neck trauma accounts for 5 to 10% of all serious traumatic injuries. Blunt trauma to the neck typically results from motor vehicle crashes, but it also occurs with sports-related injuries, clothesline injury, strangulation, or blows from the fists or feet. Blunt trauma has become much less common since routine seatbelt use was established.

For penetrating trauma, > 95% of wounds result from guns and knives, with the remainder resulting from motor vehicle accidents, household injuries, industrial accidents, and sporting events. The male-to-female ratio of penetrating neck trauma is 5:1.

◆ Clinical

Critical organs and structures are at risk from neck trauma; clinical manifestations may vary greatly. The presence or absence of signs and symptoms can sometimes be misleading, serving as a poor predictor of underlying damage.

Signs

Signs of airway injury include:

- Subcutaneous emphysema—tracheal, esophageal, or pulmonary injury
- Air bubbling through the wound
- Stridor or respiratory distress—laryngeal and/or esophageal injury
- Voice changes: hoarseness, diplophonia, breathiness
- Cyanosis

  Signs of vascular injury include:

- Hematoma (expanding)—vascular injury
- Active external hemorrhage from the wound site—arterial vascular injury
- Bruit/thrill—arteriovenous fistula
- Pulselessness/pulse deficit
- Distal ischemia (neurologic deficit in this case)

  Signs of pharyngoesophageal injury include:

- Hematemesis, inability to tolerate secretions
- Neck crepitus
- Development of mediastinitis

Symptoms

- Clinical manifestations may vary greatly depending on involved organs and systems.
- Dysphagia—tracheal and/or esophageal injury
- Hoarseness—tracheal and/or esophageal injury
- Oronasopharyngeal bleeding—vascular, tracheal, or esophageal injury
- Neurologic deficit—vascular and/or spinal cord injury
- Hypotension—nonspecific; may be related to the neck injury or may indicate trauma elsewhere

Differential Diagnosis

Considerations with neck trauma include cervical spine injury, laryngotracheal injury, vascular injury, and pharyngoesophageal injury.

◆ Evaluation

History

History, if available, can provide important details regarding the mechanism of injury.

Physical Exam

Advanced Trauma Life Support (ATLS) protocols are followed. The exam begins with ABCs (airway, breathing, circulation), followed by secondary assessment once a patient has a safe airway and is hemodynamically stable. All patients with neck trauma should be assumed to have a cervical spine injury until this has been ruled out.

With blunt trauma, injury to the larynx or trachea is the most common serious finding and often presents with subcutaneous air, hoarseness, or odynophagia. In a stable patient, flexible fiberoptic laryngoscopy can reveal evidence of injury such as blood, motion impairment, or edema.

With penetrating trauma, determine which vertical zones of the neck are involved (**Fig. 6.5**; **Table 6.2**). Zone I extends from the clavicle to the cricoid cartilage; zone II extends from the cricoid to the mandibular angle; zone III extends from the mandibular angle to the skull base.

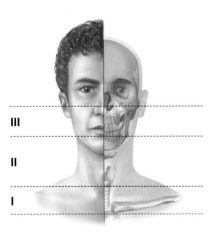

Fig. 6.5 Zones of the neck for evaluation of penetrating trauma. (Used with permission from Schuenke M, Schulte E, Schumacher U. *Head, Neck, and Neuroanatomy.* 2nd ed. Stuttgart/New York: Thieme; 2016. *Thieme Atlas of Anatomy*; vol 3, illustration by Karl Wesker.)

III

II

I

Table 6.2 Zones of the neck and management of penetrating trauma

Zone	Anatomy	Contents	Management
I	Clavicle to cricoid	Common carotid, vertebral, and subclavian arteries and the trachea, esophagus, thoracic duct, and thymus	Angiography, esophagram
II	Cricoid to mandibular angle	Internal and external carotid arteries, jugular veins, pharynx, larynx, esophagus, recurrent laryngeal nerve, spinal cord, trachea, thyroid, and parathyroids	Surgical exploration if symptomatic
III	Mandibular angle to skull base	Distal extracranial carotid and vertebral arteries and the uppermost segments of the jugular veins	Angiography

Imaging

Controversy exists regarding aspects of trauma management, with trends moving away from surgical exploration in stable patients and with expanding use of imaging and observation. There is an inherent delay with any imaging study; accordingly, transport to the operating room should not be delayed by an imaging study when the patient's condition warrants emergent surgery.

Penetrating zone I and III injuries should undergo angiographic evaluation of the carotids. Zone I injuries should also undergo esophageal studies such as Gastrografin (Bracco Diagnostics, Inc., Princeton, NJ) swallow study.

Cervical spine radiography is routine and should be reviewed for emphysema, fractures, displacement of the trachea, and the presence of a foreign body.

Computed tomography (CT) scans prove most useful when bony or soft tissue damage is a consideration. Magnetic resonance imaging (MRI) or MR angiography is used for evaluation of the patient exhibiting neurologic impairment with minimal or absent abnormalities of the cervical spine on plain radiograph.

CT angiography offers advantages over conventional catheter angiography. It is readily accessible, can be rapidly performed, and causes fewer complications than catheter angiography. Additionally, some experts assert that subtle disruptions of the vessel wall may be detected on CT angiography. Artifacts secondary to metal can obscure vascular detail and can limit CT angiography.

Labs

As necessary, a trauma panel, CBC, electrolytes, other warranted blood chemistry levels, and blood type and crossmatching should be obtained.

◆ Treatment Options

Establishment of the airway is the first priority. If there is airway compromise, a surgical airway, rather than endotracheal intubation, is usually preferred. With neck injuries, a patient may have a laryngotracheal separation or near separation that can be worsened by an endotracheal intubation. Either a cricothyroidotomy or tracheotomy is performed if there is respiratory distress. Bleeding is initially managed with direct pressure and establishment of large-bore IV access to permit fluid resuscitation (**Fig. 6.6**).

- Endoscopy
  - Laryngoscopy, bronchoscopy, pharyngoscopy, and esophagoscopy may be useful in the assessment of the aerodigestive tract. Rigid endoscopes are superior to flexible scopes, as insufflation may worsen an injury.

- Angiography
  - Angiography is routinely used to evaluate stable patients sustaining penetrating wounds to zones I and III that pierce the platysma.
  - A four-vessel study is a prerequisite.
  - Drawbacks include cost and the inherent danger of any vascular, particularly arterial, invasive procedure.

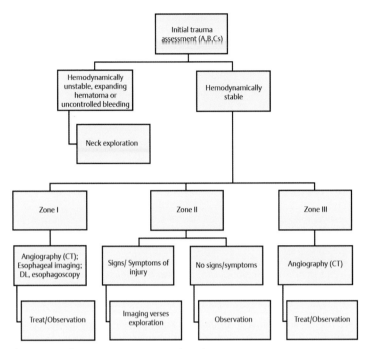

Fig. 6.6 Neck trauma management algorithm.

The unstable patient (hemodynamic instability, severe hemorrhage, expanding hematoma) is taken to the operating room. The stable patient is categorized as symptomatic or asymptomatic. Signs or symptoms of injury to the airway, esophagus, vessels, or nerves (i.e., hemoptysis, hoarseness, dysphagia, crepitus) dictate further work-up/interventions. If the penetrating injury is in zone II, neck exploration is generally done; if the injury is zone I, angiography and esophageal studies are performed. If the injury is in zone III, angiography should be performed. Asymptomatic patients are also typically imaged as above if the injury is zone I or III and observed if the injury is zone II.

In general, vascular injuries are managed with either embolization or surgical control. Surgery involves exploration and management of injuries of the carotid sheath, esophagus, and laryngotracheal complex (**Table 6.3**).

Table 6.3 Specific injuries sought and treated during neck exploration

Carotid artery injuries	Esophageal injuries
Vertebral artery injuries	Nerve injuries
Jugular vein injury	Thoracic duct injuries
Laryngotracheal injuries	Thyroid injuries

There is no role for probing or local exploration of the neck in the trauma bay or emergency room, because this may dislodge a clot and initiate uncontrollable hemorrhage.

◆ Outcome and Follow-Up

Standard postoperative management for neck surgery is followed. Overall mortality is 1 to 2%.

6.2 Approach to Neck Masses

◆ Key Features

- A neck mass may be inflammatory, congenital, or neoplastic.
- It may be anterior (midline), lateral, posterolateral, or supraclavicular.
- The patient's history should include age, duration, progression, pain, infection, smoking, prior cancer, exposure to tuberculosis, and animal exposure.

Neck masses are relatively common and may present at any age group. The differential diagnosis is broad, and both benign and malignant processes should be considered. A systematic approach is crucial to developing a rapid diagnosis and treatment plan.

Age is an important factor in evaluating a neck mass. The age groups include pediatric, young adult, and older adult (> 40 years). Each age group exhibits a certain relative frequency of disease occurrences, which can guide the diagnostician to further differential considerations. In general, neck masses in children are more commonly inflammatory or infectious. This is also true in young adults, although lymphoma is a consideration. In older adults, a neck mass should be considered neoplastic until proven otherwise.

The location of congenital neck masses is important; these lesions are often characterized by their location. The location of malignant neck masses, particularly if metastatic, may help identify the primary tumor (**Fig. 6.7**).

◆ Clinical

Signs and Symptoms

Depending on the cause, the neck mass may be painless (early neoplasm or congenital mass) or painful (infection or trauma). Depending on the etiology, associated symptoms may be those of an upper respiratory infection, toothache (infectious or inflammatory mass), or dysphagia, odynophagia, hoarseness, otalgia, hemoptysis, weight loss, night sweats, and fever (neoplasm).

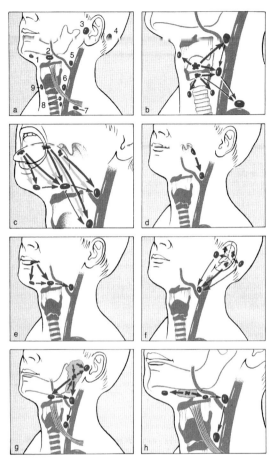

Fig. 6.7 Head and neck masses. **(a)** Typical sites of regional lymph node metastases: 1. submental lymph nodes; 2. submandibular lymph nodes; 3. parotid and preauricular lymph nodes; 4. retroauricular lymph nodes; 5. lymph nodes of the jugulofacial venous angle; 6. deep cervical lymph nodes; 7. lymph nodes in the juguloclavicular venous angle: lower deep cervical lymph nodes and supraclavicular lymph nodes; 8. pre- and peritracheal lymph nodes; 9. prelaryngeal lymph nodes. **(b)** Laryngeal carcinoma. **(c)** Carcinoma of different parts of the tongue. Note the tendency to contralateral metastases. **(d)** Tonsillar carcinoma. **(e)** Lower lip carcinoma. **(f)** Carcinoma of the external ear. Note the segmental lymphatic efferent from the auricle. **(g)** Parotid carcinoma. Note the intraglandular lymph node metastases. **(h)** Submandibular gland carcinoma. (Used with permission from Becker W, Naumann HH, Pfaltz CR. *Ear, Nose and Throat Diseases: A Pocket Reference.* 2nd ed. Stuttgart/New York: Thieme;1994:516.)

Differential Diagnosis

See **Table 6.4**.

Table 6.4   Differential diagnosis of neck masses

Congenital	Neoplastic malignant	Neoplastic benign	Systemic, inflammatory and infectious disease
Branchial cleft cyst	Head and neck metastasis	Hemangioma	Lymphadenitis—bacterial, viral
Dermoid cyst	Thyroid metastasis	Thyroid: neoplasm or goiter	Deep neck abscess
Thyroglossal duct cyst	Lymphoma	Lymphangioma	Cat scratch disease
Laryngocele	Salivary gland tumor	Salivary gland tumor	Tuberculosis or atypical mycobacterium
Ectopic thyroid tissue		Lipoma	Sarcoidosis, Kikuchi-Fujimoto's disease, Kimura's disease, Castleman's disease
		Carotid body tumor or paraganglioma	Sialadenitis

◆ Evaluation

History

A thorough review of the developmental time course of the mass, associated symptoms, personal habits prior to the trauma or infection, irradiation, or surgery is important. Ask about smoking, tobacco chewing, alcohol use, fever, pain, weight loss, night sweats, exposure to tuberculosis, animals, pets, and occupational/sexual history.

Physical Exam

All mucosal surfaces of the nasopharynx, oropharynx, larynx, and nasal cavity should be visualized by direct examination or by indirect mirror or fiberoptic visualization. State of dentition should be noted. The oropharyngeal surfaces should be palpated. Regarding the neck mass, emphasis on location, tenderness, mobility, and consistency of the neck mass can often place the mass within a general etiologic grouping.

Imaging

Computed tomography (CT) is important and can better elucidate the nature of a neck mass and its association with surrounding structures. Criteria such as heterogeneity of the center of the mass, blurred borders, and a round shape are suggestive of malignancy. CT may also be able to identify additional neck masses not clinically palpable and/or the primary tumor. Contrast should be used except in a suspected thyroid lesion, as it may interfere with radioactive iodine imaging studies or therapy.

Magnetic resonance imaging (MRI) is comparable to CT, but it is more expensive and has longer imaging time. With contrast, it is especially good for vascular and neural delineation. Angiography is recommended if a primary vascular neck mass is suspected and synchronous embolization is being considered. Ultrasound is helpful in differentiating solid from cystic masses and congenital cysts from solid lymph nodes and glandular tumors.

Labs

A routine complete blood count test may reveal an infectious process. More specialized laboratory tests may become necessary as the investigation proceeds.

Other Tests

- Fine-needle aspiration biopsy (FNAB): Currently, FNAB is the standard of diagnosis for neck masses and is indicated in any neck mass that is not an abscess and persists despite appropriate antibiotic therapy. FNAB separates inflammatory and reactive processes that usually do not require surgery from neoplastic lesions, either benign or malignant.
- Panendoscopy: If careful examination in the office does not identify the etiology of the neck mass and a tumor is suspected, the upper aerodigestive tract should be examined under anesthesia. Biopsies should be performed on any suspicious mucosal lesions.

◆ Treatment Options

Medical

A tender, mobile mass or one highly suggestive of inflammatory or infectious etiology may warrant a short clinical trial of antibiotics and observation with close follow-up. Use steroids judiciously; steroids may shrink a neck mass caused by lymphoma, lulling the physician and patient into a false sense that the condition is improving.

Surgical

- Open excisional biopsies should be avoided in cases in which a nonlymphoma malignancy (epidermoid, melanoma) is suspected. If FNAB results are negative or equivocal but suspicion for malignancy persists, an open excisional biopsy of the cervical lymph node may be performed. The patient and surgeon should be prepared to proceed immediately with a complete neck dissection depending on the results of frozen sections.
- Open excisional biopsies may be performed for lymphomas or granulomatous disease.
- Inflamed congenital masses are typically treated with antibiotics and then surgically removed after inflammation has subsided.

- Infectious processes causing neck masses are treated medically. Surgery, in the form of incision and drainage, is used in cases that do not respond to appropriate medical therapy.

6.3 Head and Neck Cancer

◆ Key Features

- Head and neck cancer comprises a heterogeneous group of tumors, consisting predominantly of squamous cell carcinoma (SCC) of the upper aerodigestive tract.
- This type of cancer is linked to tobacco smoking and alcohol.
- There is a propensity for second primary tumors (between 4 and 7% per year), especially if the patient is still smoking.
- Multimodality treatment includes surgery, radiation, and chemotherapy.
- Adult with persistent neck mass is SCC until proved otherwise.

Head and neck cancer, predominantly SCC, can affect the oral cavity, pharynx, larynx, hypopharynx, cervical esophagus, nose, and paranasal sinuses. The goal of treatment is cure or palliation with preservation of function. Specific sites and subsites of head and neck cancer are discussed in subsequent chapters.

Table 6.5 Tumor differentiation grading using the Broder classification (tumor grade [G])

G1: Well differentiated
G2: Moderately well differentiated
G3: Poorly differentiated
G4: Undifferentiated

Note: There is no statistically significant correlation between degree of differentiation and the biologic behavior of the cancer; however, vascular invasion is a negative prognostic factor.

◆ Epidemiology

Head and neck SCC accounts for ~ 5% of cancers in the United States. This corresponds to an estimated 17 per 100,000 Americans per year with newly diagnosed SCC of the head and neck. These cancers are more common in men and typically occur in patients over age 50. The etiology includes tobacco use (smoking and smokeless) and alcohol consumption. Eighty-five percent of head and neck SCC are linked to tobacco use. The synergistic effect of alcohol and smoking increases the risk of disease many more times than the simple additive risk of either risk factor alone. In SCC, mutations in the *TP53* gene correlate with drinking and smoking habits. Approximately 15% of patients have a viral etiology. Epstein-Barr virus (EBV) has been implicated in the development of nasopharyngeal carcinoma. Human papillomavirus (HPV) infection is another factor implicated in the carcinogenesis of upper aerodigestive tract tumors. In particular, HPV-16 can be isolated in up to 72% of oropharyngeal cancers. The recent increase in cancers of the tongue and tonsils in developed countries, particularly in younger patients, has been associated with HPV.

During the past 20 years, the overall incidence of head and neck SCC has been declining in the United States, a decline that is attributed to a decrease in the prevalence of smoking. In other parts of the world, head and neck SCC is attributed to habitual and cultural habits such as chewing *paan* (betel leaf with areca nut), smoking *khat* (*Catha edulis*), and drinking *yerba maté*.

◆ Clinical

Signs

Signs may include hoarseness, muffled speech, trismus, and recurrent epistaxis. Many patients present with a neck mass as chief complaint, representing metastatic nodal disease from an occult primary tumor in the upper aerodigestive tract (**Table 6.6**).

Table 6.6   Incidence of cervical lymph node metastases associated with carcinomas of the upper aerodigestive tract

Tumor location	Incidence of cervical lymph node metastases at diagnosis (%)
Oral cavity	30–65
Oropharynx	39–83
Nasopharynx	60–90
Hypopharynx	52–72
Supraglottis	35–54
Glottis	7–9
Nasal cavity and paranasal sinuses	10–20
Salivary glands	25–50
Thyroid gland	18–84*

*Depends on age and histologic subtype. (Adapted with permission from Probst R, Grevers G, Iro H. *Basic Otorhinolaryngology: A Step-by-Step Learning Guide*. Stuttgart/New York: Thieme; 2006:333.)

Symptoms

Symptoms of head and neck SCC are variable and depend on the site and stage of the primary tumor (see "Staging of Head and Neck Cancer"). Early symptoms may be vague and mimic benign disease and are therefore discovered only at advanced stages of disease. Symptoms may include dysphagia, odynophagia, a globus sensation, changes in voice (this includes both hoarseness and velopharyngeal insufficiency), referred otalgia, CN hypoesthesia, nasal obstruction, epiphora, and hyposmia.

Differential Diagnosis

- Upper respiratory infections such as pharyngitis, laryngitis, deep neck infections or abscesses
- Congenital masses and cysts
- Upper airway manifestations of rheumatologic and autoimmune diseases
- Hematologic malignancies (lymphoma)
- Tuberculosis
- Fungal infections

◆ Evaluation

History

History should include questions about risk factors, breathy voice or prolonged hoarseness, dysphagia, hemoptysis, difficulty breathing, shortness of breath, otalgia, and unintentional weight loss, fevers, or chills ("B symptoms").

Physical Exam

Physical exam should include careful inspection of the oral and oropharyngeal mucosa for lesions and palpation of the tonsillar region and tongue base for firm nodules or masses.

An indirect mirror or flexible fiberoptic laryngoscopy should be performed. During this examination, the patient should be asked to perform several maneuvers such as tongue protrusion, puffing out the cheeks, lightly coughing, and speaking to better visualize and access the larynx and the hypopharynx. Specifically, these assessments are done to assess for asymmetry or the presence of any visible masses or ulcerations. It is also important that laryngeal motility be assessed, as this is critical in tumor staging. The neck should be examined in a systematic fashion. Any palpable lymph nodes should be assessed with regard to size, location, texture, and mobility.

Imaging

A contrast-enhanced computed tomography (CT) or magnetic resonance imaging (MRI) scan of head and neck should be obtained to assess local and regional extent of disease and involvement of adjacent structures, such as the great vessels of the neck and the prevertebral fascia. Specific characteristics of regional lymphadenopathy, if present, should be noted, such as extracapsular spread, central necrosis, and size of involved lymph nodes. Criteria for pathologic lymph nodes include nodes that have a round shape with loss of a hilum, presence of central necrosis, and/or lymph nodes larger than 10 mm (15 mm in level 1).

A metastatic work-up may consist of a chest radiograph with liver function tests, CT scan of the chest and abdomen, or, alternatively, a fluorodeoxyglucose–positron emission tomography (FDG-PET) scan.

Labs

Blood count, electrolyte, and liver function tests should be performed to assess nutritional status.

Other Tests

Fine-needle aspiration biopsy (FNAB) is a highly accurate technique for the investigation of cervical lymph node metastases in head and neck SCC and is the first-line test in a patient with lymphadenopathy. Sensitivity of this test is improved when performed with ultrasound guidance. It is best to avoid open biopsy of a neck mass, because of the problems of tumor spillage and violation of fascial planes.

Patients in whom a suspicion of head and neck SCC exists should undergo biopsy of suspicious primary site lesions. Because of the propensity for second primary tumors that accompany head and neck SCC, these patients should undergo a panendoscopy (triple endoscopy), consisting of laryngoscopy, esophagoscopy, and bronchoscopy together, to search for simultaneous lesions. This may also lend insight into the extent of the primary lesion, particularly important in the smoking patient. This is a point of controversy, and PET scanning may play a greater role in the future. Mention should be made that in the current literature, the sensitivity of PET scanning is not adequate to replace panendoscopy: for instance, the larynx has baseline activity on PET due to patient breathing and/or talking during the scan.

Pathology

Ninety percent of head and neck cancers are SCCs.

◆ Treatment Options

Treatment of head and neck SCC consists of surgery, radiotherapy, chemotherapy, or a combination of these. Surgical resection remains the gold standard for treatment of head and neck cancer. Surgery may address the primary tumor as well as cervical metastasis.

Radiation therapy for SCC of the head and neck involves the delivery of high-energy ionizing radiation to targeted tissues. Radiation doses can be delivered by different methods, including fractionation, hyperfractionation, accelerated fractionation, and intensity-modulated radiotherapy (IMRT).

Chemotherapy for SCC of the head and neck involves the systemic administration of cytotoxic drugs that target rapidly dividing cells. Individual chemotherapeutic agents effective in the therapy of head and neck cancer include cisplatin, methotrexate, 5-fluorouracil, taxanes, ifosfamide, and bleomycin. Currently, chemotherapy is not a primary therapy for the treatment of head and neck cancer, but either it can be used as an induction agent followed by surgery and/or radiation, or it can be given concurrently with radiation treatment.

Of the molecularly targeted agents, cetuximab is an IgG1 chimeric antibody directed against the epidermal growth factor receptor (EGFR).

Other therapy methods for head and neck cancer include photosensitizers and interstitial laser therapy, photodynamic therapy, immune therapy, gene therapy, and targeted therapy against HPV.

✦ Cancer of Unknown Primary

Patients with head and neck cancer can initially present with a painless neck mass. In 2 to 8% of these patients, the tumor origin is not known. This is classified as a cancer of unknown primary (CUP), carcinoma of unknown primary origin, or occult primary malignancy. A primary tumor is considered unknown only *after* a thorough investigation (including physical exam, imaging, and biopsies) has been completed.

Treatment of CUP is controversial. Surgical excision in the form of a neck dissection followed by radiation therapy allows a lower total dose of radiation to be used. Primary radiation therapy provides treatment to both the upper aerodigestive tract and its locoregional metastasis but forces the radiation oncologist to treat a wider field, as the primary site is unknown. Chapter 6.3.8 discusses the management of this diagnosis in more detail.

✦ Outcome and Follow-Up

The treatment of head and neck SCC, whether surgical or chemoradiation, often leaves the patient with significant speech and swallowing deficits. Therefore, is it paramount for a multidisciplinary team to treat head and neck SCC. This team can include the surgical oncologist, medical and radiation oncologist, oral surgeon, prosthodontist, speech language and swallowing pathologist, nurse, and social worker.

Patients with regional neck disease prior to treatment should have a CT scan or an integrated FDG-PET/CT. There is controversy about the need for a planned neck dissection following radiotherapy in patients with high-risk disease. Most recurrences of SCC occur within 3 years of the initial treatment. The National Comprehensive Cancer Network (NCCN) guidelines suggest routine follow up after treatment. This includes follow up every 1 to 2 months the first year, every 2 to 6 months the second year, every 4 to 8 months the third through fifth years and annual follow up afterwards.

Patients should be told of the risk of a second primary tumor and encouraged to report any new symptoms. The risk of a second primary carcinoma is highest in those who continue to smoke. Patients should be counseled for tobacco cessation.

✦ Staging of Head and Neck Cancer

• With the publication and the 2018 implementation of the American Joint Committee on Cancer (AJCC) 8th edition, the classification of the regional lymph node metastases and their effect on stage grouping are fairly consistent throughout all anatomic sites of head and neck cancer (except nasopharynx and HPV-associated oropharynx cancer). Additionally, extranodal extension (ENE) has been included in the staging criteria. This can be determined clinically (fixation of the node to the skin or muscles, or nerve dysfunction) or pathologically and can be supported (but not determined) radiologically. HPV associated oropharyngeal cancers have separate nodal classification. For non-HPV associated cancers, the clinical and pathologic nodal (N) categories are as follows:

Regional Lymph Nodes (N)*

NX: Regional lymph nodes cannot be assessed

N0: No regional lymph node metastasis

N1: Metastasis to a single ipsilateral lymph node measuring ≤ 3 cm in greatest diameter and ENE negative

N2: Further divided into three categories:

    N2a: Single ipsilateral lymph node > 3 and ≤ 6 cm and ENE negative (pathologic staging also includes a single ipsilateral or contra-lateral lymph node ≤ 3 cm and ENE positive)

    N2b: Multiple ipsilateral lymph nodes ≤ 6 cm and ENE negative

    N2c: Bilateral or contralateral lymph nodes ≤ 6 cm in greatest dimension and ENE negative

N3: Now further divided into two categories:

    N3a: Metastasis to a lymph node > 6 cm, ENE negative

    N3b: Metastasis to a single lymph node that is ENE positive (pathologic staging includes single lymph nodes that are ENE positive >3cm), or metastasis to multiple lymph nodes with any ENE positive

A designation of "U" or "L" can be attached to the N category to indicate nodes above ("U") or below ("L") the lower border of the cricoid. Similarly, clinical and pathologic ENE should be recorded as ENE (−) or ENE (+). Clinical and pathologic staging are similar with the differences noted in parenthesis.

*Superior mediastinal lymph nodes are considered regional lymph nodes (level VII). Midline nodes are considered ipsilateral nodes.

- Distant metastatic disease is divided into two categories:

    M0: Absence of distant disease

    M1: Presence of distant metastatic disease

- The T category of a tumor indicates the extent of the primary tumor and varies by anatomic subsite. This can be measured by size, as in the oral cavity, oropharynx, and salivary glands; by involvement of varying subsites, as in the nasopharynx, hypopharynx, and larynx; or by extent of invasion and destruction, as in the maxillary sinus. With the new edition, it is also effected by HPV status in the oropharynx. The specific T stage criteria are discussed in each subsite section.

- Across all anatomic sites of the head and neck (except the nasopharynx), the following classifications apply for HPV negative (p16 negative) cancers (**Table 6.7**):

Stage I disease: Includes only T1 N0 M0 tumors

Stage II disease: Includes only T2 N0 M0 tumors

Stage III disease: Includes T3 N0 M0 and T1–3 disease that is N1 M0

Stage IV disease: Includes T4 tumors with or without nodal disease, as well as any tumor with N2 or N3 disease or evidence of distant metastatic disease

Table 6.7 Cancer stage groupings

	N0	N1	N2	N3
T1	Stage I	Stage III	Stage IVA	Stage IVB
T2	Stage II	Stage III	Stage IVA	Stage IVB
T3	Stage III	Stage III	Stage IVA	Stage IVB
T4a	Stage IVA	Stage IVA	Stage IVA	Stage IVB
T4b	Stage IVB	Stage IVB	Stage IVB	Stage IVB
M1	Stage IVC	Stage IVC	Stage IVC	Stage IVC

Please refer to the site-specific sections for TNM categories and staging for nasopharynx and HPV-associated oropharynx cancers.

Table 6.8 Tumor differentiation grading using the Broder classification (tumor grade [G])

G1: Well differentiated
G2: Moderately well differentiated
G3: Poorly differentiated
G4: Undifferentiated

Note: There is no statistically significant correlation between degree of differentiation and the biologic behavior of the cancer; however, vascular invasion is a negative prognostic factor.

6.3.1 Chemotherapy for Head and Neck Cancer

◆ Key Features

- Concurrent chemotherapy with definitive radiotherapy is a safe and effective means to treat locally advanced squamous cell carcinoma (SCC) of the head and neck.
- Concurrent chemotherapy with postoperative radiotherapy (i.e., chemoradiotherapy) improves survival in select high-risk patients.
- Palliative chemotherapy can reduce symptoms and modestly extend survival in an incurable setting.
- Newer biologic and cytotoxic agents continue to cause the treatment of head and neck cancer to evolve.

The role of chemotherapy in head and neck cancer is expanding, and its utility varies with the stage of the disease. For patients with metastatic or incurable locoregional disease, chemotherapy is palliative. For patients with potentially curable locoregional head and neck cancer, chemotherapy is an integral component of the multimodality approach. Chemotherapy in the definitive treatment of head and neck cancer is an adjuvant therapy. Strictly defined, an adjuvant therapy is an addition to the potentially curative modality (primary surgery or definitive radiation) that improves outcomes. Broadly speaking, adjuvant therapies can be preoperative (or preradiotherapy), concurrent with radiation, or postoperative (or postradiotherapy). Most early adjuvant chemotherapy trials in cancer were postoperative in nature, so "adjuvant therapy" has also been used to describe only postoperative (or postradiotherapy) chemotherapy. This has given rise to the term "neoadjuvant" chemotherapy to describe preoperative (or preradiotherapy) chemotherapy. "Induction chemotherapy" and "neoadjuvant chemotherapy" are synonymous.

◆ Neoadjuvant Chemotherapy

Advantages of neoadjuvant chemotherapy (i.e., induction chemotherapy) include an intact vascular bed for better drug delivery, reduced tumor bulk to improve the ease of resection, and early eradication of regional and distant micrometastases. Disadvantages include delaying surgery in potentially curable patients with chemoresistant disease, relying on clinical staging to make treatment decisions, the morbidity of "overtherapy," and patient nonadherence after chemotherapy. Neoadjuvant cisplatin and 5-fluorouracil (5-FU) followed by radiotherapy in responders was an organ preservation strategy described in the frequently cited Veterans' Administration (VA) Laryngeal Cancer Study Group. Subsequent results have shown this approach to be inferior to concurrent cisplatin with radiation, but newer induction regimens including docetaxel have reintroduced neoadjuvant chemotherapy followed by radiotherapy as a viable option. Neoadjuvant chemotherapy before surgery has not been found to be helpful in randomized trials.

◆ Concomitant Chemoradiotherapy

The simultaneous use of chemotherapy and radiation continues to be the standard for locally advanced SCC (stages III to IVb). The primary benefit has been in decreasing locoregional failure, which has translated into roughly a 10% overall survival benefit. The effect on decreasing metastatic disease has been inconsistent. It is believed that chemotherapy may have some benefit against radioresistant hypoxic tumor cells. However, the simultaneous use of chemotherapy and radiotherapy has significantly increased grade 3 and 4 toxicities, which can be potentially lethal or lead to treatment breaks that decrease the radiation's efficacy. In patients who are receiving surgery and are found to have high-risk features (positive margins, N2 disease, nodal extracapsular extension), postoperative cisplatin with radiation has proven superior to radiation alone. Cisplatin, 5-FU, taxanes, and mitomycin C all act as radiosensitizing agents.

◆ Adjuvant Therapy

The use of postoperative or postradiation chemotherapy has not been found to be helpful in randomized trials, although it is commonly done for three cycles in nasopharyngeal cancer based on the Intergroup Trial showing that concurrent cisplatin with radiation, followed by three cycles of cisplatin plus 5-FU, improved survival over radiation alone. It is controversial whether the cycles given after radiation add any independent benefit. Newer agents have recently been approved for second-line therapy in treating head and neck SCC (recurrent or metastatic). These agents, pembrolizumab and nivolumab, are immune checkpoint inhibitors targeting the PD-1 protein on immune cells.

◆ Types of Chemotherapeutic Agents Used for Head and Neck Cancer

Platinum-Based Alkylating Agents

The cytotoxic effects of alkylating agents (e.g., cisplatin) are based on their interaction with DNA. These agents cause substitution reactions, cross-linking reactions, or strand-breaking reactions. These agents alter the information coded in the DNA molecule, resulting in inhibition of or inaccurate DNA replication with resultant mutation or cell death.

Antimetabolites

The cytotoxic effect of antimetabolites (e.g., methotrexate) is due to their structural similarity to naturally occurring metabolites involved in nucleic acid synthesis. They inhibit critical enzymes involved in nucleic acid synthesis and become incorporated into the nucleic acid and produce incorrect codes. Both of these mechanisms result in an inhibition of DNA synthesis and ultimate cell death.

Antitumor Antibiotics

Antitumor antibiotics (e.g., mitomycin, bleomycin) are antimicrobial compounds produced by *Streptomyces* species in culture. They are cytotoxic in that they affect the structure and function of nucleic acids by intercalation between DNA base pairs (doxorubicin), DNA strand fragmentation, or cross-linking of DNA.

Alkaloids

Alkaloids (e.g., vincristine, vinblastine) bind to free tubulin dimers and disrupt the balance between microtubule polymerization and depolymerization, resulting in the net dissolution of microtubules, destruction of the mitotic spindle, and arrest of cells in metaphase.

Taxanes

Taxanes (e.g., paclitaxel, docetaxel) are compounds that disrupt equilibrium between free tubulin and microtubules, causing stabilization of ordinary cytoplasmic microtubules and the formation of abnormal bundles of microtubules.

EGFR Inhibitors

Epidermal growth factor receptor (EGFR) is a protein found on the surface of some cells, to which epidermal growth factor binds, causing the cells to divide. It is found at abnormally high levels on the surface of many types of cancer cells, so these cells may divide excessively in the presence of epidermal growth factor (EGFR, ErbB1, and HER1). Cetuximab (Erbitux, Eli Lilly and Company, Indianapolis, IN) specifically targets EGFR and binds to EGFR with higher affinity than its natural ligands. Binding results in the internalization of the antibody-receptor complex without activation of the intrinsic tyrosine kinase. Consequently, signal transduction through this cell pathway is blocked, which inhibits tumor growth and leads to apoptosis.

During a recent multinational, randomized study to compare radiotherapy alone with radiotherapy plus cetuximab in patients with locoregionally advanced head and neck cancer, cetuximab was found to improve locoregional control and reduce mortality.

PD-1 Inhibitors

Programmed cell death protein 1 (PD-1) is a protein found on the surface of lymphocytes and generally prevents the immune system from attacking its host. Many neoplasms have proteins that bind PD-1 preventing the immune response to the tumor. Drugs that inhibit the activation of PD-1 (immune checkpoint inhibitors) allow for the immune system to be active against cancer cells. Two drugs currently on the market have recently been FDA approved for the treatment of head and neck cancer as second-line therapy, pembrolizumab (Keytruda, Merk and Company, Kenilworth, NJ) and nivolumab (Opdivo, Bristol-Meyer-Squibb, New York City, NY). Of note, by inhibiting this checkpoint, both drugs also allow the immune system to affect the host body, resulting in side effects including mucositis, hypophysitis, thyroiditis, pneumonitis, and other inflammatory conditions.

In recent trials, each drug individually has shown increased survival over current chemotherapy regimens in recurrent or metastatic head and neck cancer.

◆ Complications

Each drug or combination of chemotoxic drugs can cause specific side effects, and some can be permanent. These side effects may be so severe that chemotherapy must be ceased. In general, chemotherapy may cause the following side effects: fatigue, nausea, vomiting, hair loss, xerostomia, anorexia, immunocompromise, diarrhea, mucositis, and death. Please refer to **Table 6.9** for specific toxicities related to the chemotherapeutic agents.

Table 6.9 Chemotherapy agents

Class	Examples	Mechanism	Toxicities
Platinum-based alkylating agents	Cisplatin, carboplatin	Cause DNA substitution reactions, cross-linking reactions, or strand-breaking reactions	Nephrotoxicity, neurotoxicity, ototoxicity, hemolytic anemia, myelosuppression
Antimetabolites	Methotrexate	Inhibit critical enzymes involved in nucleic acid synthesis	Hepatotoxicity, neutropenia

(continued)

Table 6.9 Chemotherapy agents *(Continued)*

Antitumor antibiotics	Mitomycin, bleomycin, doxorubicin	DNA fragmentation, cross-linking, or intercalation	Pulmonary fibrosis (bleomycin), cardiomyopathy (doxorubicin)
Alkaloids	Vincristine, vinblastine	Bind to free tubulin dimers; arrest cells in metaphase	Peripheral neuropathy, hyponatremia, alopecia, neutropenia
Taxanes	Paclitaxel, docetaxel	Disrupt equilibrium between free tubulin and microtubules	Neutropenia, hair loss
EGFR inhibitors	Cetuximab	Bind to EGFR preventing tyrosine kinase pathway	Rash, pruritus
PD-1 inhibitors	Pembrolizumab, Nivolumab	Binds to PD-1, prevents T-cell apoptosis	Rash, pneumonitis, hypophysitis, thyroiditis, mucositis

6.3.2 Radiotherapy for Head and Neck Cancer

◆ Key Features

- Definitive radiotherapy is a safe and effective means to treat various cancers of the head and neck, either in inoperable patients or as an alternative to surgery for organ preservation.
- Postoperative radiotherapy decreases local failure in select high-risk patients.
- Palliative radiotherapy can reduce local symptoms in an incurable setting.
- Radiation can be improved by sensitizing tumor cells preferentially or by decreasing radiation damage to normal tissues.

Ionizing radiation is a locoregional therapy whereby photons (gamma rays or X-rays), electrons, neutrons, protons, or heavier particles (e.g., mesons, alpha particles, carbon ions) cause cells to undergo death during either mitosis or apoptosis, primarily through the creation of DNA double-strand breaks. The therapeutic ratio of radiation depends on the difference in sublethal repair between normal tissues and tumor cells, the use of radio-protectors and/or radiosensitizers, and the use of advanced methods to limit the irradiation of normal tissues.

◆ Fundamental Concepts of Radiation

Radiation dose is defined as the amount of energy (joules) imparted per unit mass (kg). The SI metric unit of dose is the gray (Gy), defined as 1 J/kg. Historically, the unit used was the rad, which is equivalent to 0.01 Gy, or 1 cGy.

Each radiation treatment is called a fraction because for most situations the total radiation dose is given over multiple sessions. A standard fraction is 1.8 to 2 Gy per fraction, and a standard course is five fractions per week, with one fraction given per day. Fractionation is biologically advantageous because of the processes of tumor reoxygenation and reassortment into more radiosensitive parts of the cell cycle. Increasing the number of fractions preferentially spares normal tissues by giving them more time to repair sublethal damage. The number of fractions cannot be increased indefinitely because of tumor repopulation, which significantly reduces radiation's efficacy if the total treatment time exceeds 7 weeks.

Various alternative fractionation strategies have been used to try to enhance radiation's effectiveness. Accelerated radiation delivers treatment faster than standard fractionation (> 10 Gy per week). Hyperfractionated radiation is the use of fraction sizes smaller than 1.8 Gy. Hypofractionated radiation is the use of fraction sizes larger than 2.0 Gy. These strategies can be combined, as in accelerated hyperfractionation.

◆ Methods of Radiation Delivery

Radiation is broadly divided into brachytherapy and teletherapy. Brachytherapy is the placement of radioisotopes near or inside the target. In squamous cell carcinoma (SCC) of the head and neck, this is most commonly done by placing catheters in a tumor or operative bed and using an afterloading device to push the source into the catheters for predetermined periods of time to deliver a prescribed dose to the entire target volume. The exposure time ranges from over 2 to 3 days in low-dose rate applications, most commonly with cesium-137, to 10 to 30 minutes in high-dose rate applications, most commonly with iridium-192. With differentiated thyroid cancer, orally administered iodine-131 (^{131}I) preferentially binds to tumor cells, with ablative doses of 100 to 150 mCi delivering 250 to 300 Gy.

Teletherapy, or external beam radiation, is the delivery of radiation by pointing an external source of radiation at the target. The most common source in modern radiotherapy is the linear accelerator, which can generate high-energy (4 to 25 MeV) photons and electrons. Gamma Knife radiosurgery units (Elekta, Stockholm, Sweden) use cobalt-60 sources that emit 1.25-MeV photon beams. Intraoperative radiation can be focally delivered to internal structures with a linear accelerator or portable X-ray generator in the operating room. External beam radiation is further subdivided by the technology used.

Conventional radiation planning uses X-ray films to define the target volume. Plans are generally limited to a small number of angles, and radiation beams are shaped by fabricating Wood's metal (Bolton 158, Bolton Metal Product Co., Bellefonte, PA) blocks. Three-dimensional (3D) conformal radiation uses computed technology (CT)-based treatment planning systems to improve target identification and evaluate dose distribution more accurately. This increases dose conformality to the target by making it easier to use more fields from virtually any beam angle. Intensity-modulated radiation therapy (IMRT) improves dose conformality further by delivering different doses to different sections within the same beam, and it optimizes the choice and intensity of beams by using a software algorithm to simultaneously test more plans than a human could within a reasonable period of time. Image-guided radiotherapy (IGRT) further improves dose conformality by using real-time imaging to confirm that the patient is in the appropriate position on the couch before delivering radiation, thereby decreasing setup error and allowing tighter margins. Stereotactic radiosurgery (SRS) is the use of a highly conformal large single fraction of external beam radiotherapy, using either a Gamma Knife or a linear accelerator. A Gamma Knife uses cobalt-60 with up to 201 sources aimed at the same point in space to produce a small area with a high dose and sharp dose dropoff. A common trait of all modern systems is that increased dose conformality to the target requires a high level of patient setup consistency, and this is achieved using custom masks or external frames that connect to the patient couch.

◆ Rationale for Definitive (Curative) Radiotherapy

Primary radiotherapy in the treatment of SCC of the nasopharynx, oropharynx, oral cavity, and glottis has long been considered an option even in resectable disease. The primary justification for this is not increased efficacy over surgery but organ and functional preservation without compromising long-term efficacy. This is an option in both early (stage I or II) and advanced (stage III or IV) disease. For patients with advanced disease, definitive radiation with chemotherapy with or without planned neck dissection, with surgery to the primary reserved for salvage, had an equivalent rate of survival compared with surgery followed by radiation in randomized trials of cancers of the larynx, hypopharynx, and other areas of the pharynx. For patients with early-stage lesions of the larynx, no randomized trials of laryngectomy versus other modalities exist, but a large amount of mature data exist regarding the long-term efficacy of definitive radiation. The results of these trials cannot be extrapolated to all cases, and it is likely that surgery should be the primary modality in some patient subsets. Tumor control, functional outcome, and quality of life should be considered by a multimodality treatment team before choosing an individual patient's treatment plan.

Definitive radiation, with or without chemotherapy depending upon the histology, is also used in mucosal melanoma, skin cancer, salivary gland cancer, lymphoma, and plasmacytoma. In select cases, conformal radiation using IMRT, SRS, or brachytherapy can be used in previously irradiated sites to salvage locally recurrent cases.

◆ Rationale for Adjuvant Radiotherapy

Postoperative radiotherapy is used if there is residual disease or a significant risk of occult residual disease. Randomized evidence supports the use of postoperative radiation for SCC that is stage III or IV or that has close or positive margins. The addition of current chemotherapy to adjuvant radiation has proven to be better than radiation alone in large randomized trials. Randomized data for other tissue types do not exist, but postoperative radiation is commonly given in high-risk cases of Merkel cell carcinoma, salivary gland carcinoma, skin cancer, and thyroid cancer. Preoperative radiation is generally reserved for marginally unresectable disease, but it is more standard in olfactory neuroblastomas to make the definitive surgery smaller and less morbid.

◆ Rationale for Palliative Radiotherapy

In the noncurative setting, radiotherapy is used to treat areas that are causing or at a high risk to cause local symptoms. Common indications in head and neck cancer to treat the primary lesion include uncontrolled bleeding, pain, dysphagia, and a compromised airway. Metastatic disease to the bone, brain, and lung can also be palliated effectively using radiation.

◆ Complications

Radiation side effects can be characterized as acute or late. Acute effects occur during or within the first few weeks after radiotherapy and tend to be transient. Late effects occur months to years after treatment and tend to be permanent. Common acute side effects include dermatitis, mucositis, taste changes, xerostomia, fatigue, facial hair loss, decreased sweating, anorexia, and weight loss. Less common acute effects include cough, hoarseness, nausea, and sialadenitis. Common late effects include xerostomia, trismus, hypothyroidism, soft tissue fibrosis, dysphagia, and taste changes. Less common late effects include soft tissue necrosis, osteoradionecrosis, laryngeal edema, spinal cord myelopathy, carotid stenosis, and second malignancy. Acute effects are generally managed supportively because of their transient nature. Aggressive dental support, stretching exercises, and proper skin care can minimize some late effects. Routine evaluation for hypothyroidism and xerostomia should also be performed, as pharmacologic interventions can improve these conditions.

◆ Improving the Therapeutic Ratio of Radiation

Radiation can be improved by sensitizing tumor cells preferentially or by decreasing radiation damage to normal tissues. Hyperfractionation and accelerated radiation regimes have improved outcomes in stage III or IV SCC compared with standard fractionation, whereas hypofractionation has improved local control in early-stage glottic lesions. Radiation sensitizers with proven efficacy in randomized trials include concurrent platinum agents, mitomycin C, and cetuximab. Normal tissues can be spared using IMRT, submandibular gland transfer, and amifostine. Future improvements are expected as imaging, radiation delivery, and new agents continue to be further developed.

6.3.3   Sinonasal Cancer

◆ Key Features

> • Sinonasal cancer initially may mimic benign sinus disease.
> • Tumors of the paranasal sinuses often present with advanced disease.
> • Cure rates are generally ≤ 50%.
> • Most patients die of direct extension into vital areas.

Malignant tumors of the sinonasal tract are extremely rare, accounting for 0.2% of all invasive cancers and 3% of head and neck cancers. Cancers of the maxillary sinus are the most common. Tumors of the ethmoid sinuses are less common (20%), and cancers of the sphenoid and frontal sinuses are rare (< 1%). Local extension often makes it difficult to access the sinus of origin.

◆ Epidemiology

Chemical carcinogens such as chromium, nickel, thorium dioxide, and tanning chemicals have been implicated in the development of carcinoma of the paranasal sinuses. Exposure to wood dust has been implicated specifically in adenocarcinoma of the ethmoid. Interestingly, tobacco use was previously thought not to play a role in sinonasal carcinogenesis. However, up to a fivefold increased risk of sinonasal carcinoma has been observed with heavy smoking. Rarely, sinonasal cancers may present as a second primary tumor in tobacco users with other head and neck cancers.

◆ Clinical

Signs and Symptoms

The clinical presentation of sinus malignancies is nonspecific and often mimics benign disease; thus, diagnosis is often delayed for months. Key indicators of malignancy are cranial neuropathies, proptosis, and pain of maxillary dentition; trismus; palatal and alveolar ridge fullness; or frank erosion into the oral cavity. Symptoms include nasal obstruction, discharge, stuffiness, congestion, recurrent epistaxis, unilateral tearing, diplopia, exophthalmos, infraorbital nerve hypoesthesia, cheek swelling, facial asymmetry, hearing loss, and serous otitis media due to nasopharyngeal extension.

Differential Diagnosis

The differential diagnosis includes benign sinus disease, benign sinus tumors, and metastatic tumors to the sinus.

✦ Evaluation

History

The patient history should include known carcinogen exposure, tobacco usage, and prolonged benign sinus symptoms and signs.

Physical Exam

A complete head and neck examination, including nasal endoscopy, should be performed. The sinonasal, ocular, and neurologic systems should be studied in detail. Evidence of nerve hypesthesia, diplopia, proptosis, and loose dentition should be carefully evaluated. Suspicious lesions should be biopsied.

Imaging

Imaging should include either a contrast-enhanced computed tomography (CT) scan or magnetic resonance imaging (MRI). There may be a role for integrated ^{18}F fludeoxyglucose (FDG) positron emission tomography (PET)/CT.

Other Tests

A definitive diagnosis requires a biopsy. Special attention should be paid to cranial nerve (CN) function because malignant paranasal tumors are associated with a high incidence of cranial neuropathies compared with inflammatory or benign sinus disease. Be cautious about in-office biopsy, as these tumors can have high vascularity.

Pathology

Squamous cell carcinoma (SCC) is the most frequent type of malignant tumor in the paranasal sinuses (70–80%). Minor salivary gland tumors constitute 10 to 15% of these neoplasms. Some 5% of cases are lymphomas. Other tumors include sinonasal undifferentiated carcinoma (SNUC), chondrosarcoma, osteosarcoma and malignant melanoma, and olfactory neuroblastoma (**Fig. 6.8**).

Inverted papilloma, a benign tumor with a tendency to recur (see **Chapter 4.4**), may transform into a malignant SCC of the paranasal sinuses in a small percentage of cases.

✦ Treatment Options

Most stage T1 or T2 maxillary sinus carcinomas are treated by surgery alone, provided adequate resection margins are obtained. This may be en bloc surgical resection or endoscopic sinus surgery, depending on the extent of disease and experience of the surgeon. The specific approach is determined by the location of disease and histology (**Fig. 6.9**).

T3 and T4 lesions are treated by combination therapy with surgery and radiation. The issue of whether radiation is more effective before or after surgery remains controversial. Chemotherapy alone is generally used as a palliative measure.

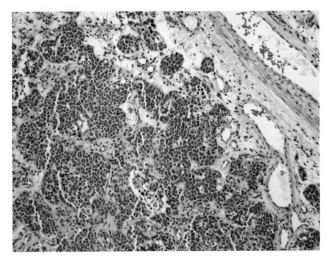

Fig. 6.8 Low-grade forms of olfactory neuroblastoma tumor have a distinct lobular array of small blue cells set in a neurofibrillary or vascular stroma. As the grade increases, the tumor becomes more solid, with increased nuclear pleomorphism and mitotic activity. (Used with permission from Har-El G, Day T, Nathan C-A, Nguyen SA. *A Multidisciplinary Approach to Head and Neck Neoplasms.* New York: Thieme; 2013. *Otorhinolaryngology—Head and Neck Surgery Series.*)

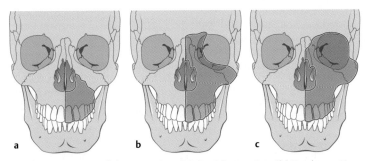

Fig. 6.9 Resection of the upper jaw. **(a)** Partial resection. **(b)** Total resection. **(c)** Total resection with exenteration of the orbit. (Used with permission from Behrbohm H, Kaschke O, Nawka T, Swift A. *Ear, Nose, and Throat Diseases: With Head and Neck Surgery.* 3rd ed. Stuttgart/New York: Thieme; 2009:227.)

◆ Outcome and Follow-Up

For maxillary tumors, malignancy behind Öhngren's plane is regarded to carry a much poorer prognosis because of the rapid spread to the orbit and middle cranial fossa (**Fig. 6.10**). Despite improvements in surgical ablative and reconstructive techniques, radiation delivery modalities, and imaging technologies, disease-free survival at 5 years remains < 50%, independent of stage. Five-year disease-free survival for patients with advanced-stage cancer drops to 25%.

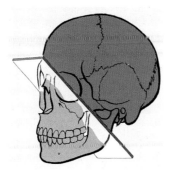

Fig. 6.10 Öhngren's plane passing through the medial canthus and the mandibular angle. It divides the maxillary sinus into a superoposterior part and an inferoanterior part. Cancer limited to the latter part typically carries a better prognosis. (Used with permission from Becker W, Naumann HH, Pfaltz CR. *Ear, Nose, and Throat Diseases: A Pocket Reference.* 2nd ed. Stuttgart/New York: Thieme; 1994:293.)

◆ Staging of Nose and Paranasal Sinus Cancer: For All Carcinomas Excluding Mucosal Malignant Melanoma

Primary Tumor (T): Maxillary Sinus

TX: Cannot be assessed

Tis: Carcinoma in situ

T1: Tumor limited to the maxillary sinus mucosa with no erosion or destruction of bone

T2: Tumor causing bone erosion or destruction, including extension into the hard palate and/or middle nasal meatus, except extension to posterior wall of maxillary sinus and pterygoid plates

T3: Tumor invades any of the following: bone of the posterior wall of maxillary sinus, subcutaneous tissues, floor or medial wall of orbit, pterygoid fossa, or ethmoid sinuses

T4a: Tumor invades anterior orbital contents, skin of cheek, pterygoid plates, infratemporal fossa, cribriform plate, or sphenoid or frontal sinuses

T4b: Tumor invades any of the following: orbital apex, dura, brain, middle cranial fossa, cranial nerves other than maxillary division of trigeminal nerve (V_2), nasopharynx, or clivus

Primary Tumor (T): Nasal Cavity and Ethmoid Sinus

TX: Cannot be assessed

Tis: Carcinoma in situ

T1: Tumor restricted to any one subsite, with or without bone invasion

T2: Tumor invading two subsites in a single region or extending to involve an adjacent region within the nasoethmoidal complex, with or without bone invasion

T3:   Tumor extends to invade the medial wall or floor of the orbit, maxillary sinus, palate, or cribriform plate

T4a: Tumor invades any of the following: anterior orbital contents, skin of nose or cheek, minimal extension to anterior cranial fossa, pterygoid plates, or sphenoid or frontal sinuses

T4b: Tumor invades any of the following: orbital apex, dura, brain, middle cranial fossa, cranial nerves other than maxillary division of trigeminal nerve (V_2), nasopharynx, or clivus

Regional Lymph Nodes (N)*

NX: Regional lymph nodes cannot be assessed

N0:   No regional lymph node metastasis

N1:   Metastasis to a single ipsilateral lymph node measuring ≤ 3 cm in greatest diameter and ENE negative

N2:   Further divided into three categories:

N2a: Single ipsilateral lymph node > 3 and ≤ 6 cm and ENE negative (pathologic staging also includes a single ipsilateral or contralateral lymph node ≤ 3 cm and ENE positive)

N2b: Multiple ipsilateral lymph nodes ≤ 6 cm and ENE negative

N2c: Bilateral or contralateral lymph nodes ≤ 6 cm in greatest dimension and ENE negative

N3:   Now further divided into two categories:

N3a: Metastasis to a lymph node > 6 cm, ENE negative

N3b: Metastasis to a single lymph node that is ENE positive (pathologic staging includes single lymph nodes that are ENE positive >3cm), or metastasis to multiple lymph nodes with any ENE positive

A designation of "U" or "L" can be attached to the N category to indicate nodes above ("U") or below ("L") the lower border of the cricoid. Similarly, clinical and pathologic ENE should be recorded as ENE (−) or ENE (+). Clinical and pathologic staging are similar with the differences noted in parenthesis.

*Superior mediastinal lymph nodes are considered regional lymph nodes (level VII). Midline nodes are considered ipsilateral nodes.

Distant Metastasis (M)

M0:   No distant metastasis

M1:   Distant metastasis

American Joint Committee on Cancer Stage Groupings of Sinonasal Cancers Except Mucosal Malignant Melanoma (8th edition)

Stage 0 disease: Carcinoma in situ (TisN0M0)

Stage I disease: Includes only T1 N0 M0 tumors

Stage II disease: Includes only T2 N0 M0 tumors

Stage III disease: Includes T3 N0 M0 and T1 -3 disease that is N1 M0

Stage IVA disease: Includes T4a disease with N0-N2 M0 disease and T1-T3 disease that is N2 M0

Stage IVB disease: Includes T4b disease with any nodal disease or T1-T4a disease with N3 disease without distant metastases (M0)

Stage IVC disease: Any disease with distant metastases (M1)

See **Table 6.7** in Chapter 6.3.3.

6.3.4   Nasopharyngeal Cancer

◆ Key Features

- There is a high frequency of nasopharyngeal cancer (NPC) among patients of Chinese ethnicity and descent.
- It is associated with Epstein-Barr virus (EBV) exposure.
- The diagnosis must be excluded in patients with asymptomatic cervical lymphadenopathy and unilateral serous otitis media.

Nasopharyngeal cancer (NPC) is a distinct type of head and neck cancer that differs from other malignancies of the upper aerodigestive tract with respect to epidemiology, pathology, clinical presentation, and responses to treatment. NPC is an uncommon neoplasm in most parts of the world but is endemic in East Asia. Seventy percent of patients with newly diagnosed NPC present with locally advanced disease. Latent EBV infection seems to be crucial in the pathogenesis of NPC. Studies have established that NPC cells express two distinct EBV latent membrane proteins: LMP-1 and LMP-2. These proteins are attractive targets for adaptive immunotherapy.

◆ Anatomy

The nasopharynx is bounded superiorly by the basi-occiput and basi-sphenoid, posteriorly by the C1 and C2 cervical bodies, anteriorly by the choanae, and inferiorly by the soft palate. The lateral walls are occupied primarily by the eustachian tube orifice. Immediately posterior to the eustachian tube orifice is the Rosenmüller fossa (pharyngeal recess), where most nasopharyngeal carcinomas originate.

◆ Epidemiology

NPC occurs most often in China, where it is the third most common malignancy among men, with an incidence rate of 15 to 50 per 100,000.

NPC rates are also high in Vietnamese and Filipino men. There is an intermediate incidence in Inuit (Eskimos) and in the populations of the Mediterranean basin. Emigration from high- to low-incidence areas reduces the incidence of NPC in first-generation Chinese, but incidence still remains at seven times the rate seen in Caucasians. NPC occurs in younger patients, including children, but the peak incidence is seen in people aged 55 to 64 years. Males are affected three times more often than females.

◆ Clinical

Signs and Symptoms

Early signs and symptoms are subtle and variable and are often initially ignored by both patient and physician. Cervical lymphadenopathy is the most common sign (50–90% of patients), followed by blood-stained nasal discharge or epistaxis, unilateral serous otitis media, and cranial neuropathies (most often CN VI, followed by CN V). Five to seven percent of all patients have systemic metastases at presentation, most often to bone.

Symptoms include unilateral nasal obstruction, unilateral hearing loss and otalgia, diplopia, facial or neck pain, and paresthesia.

Differential Diagnosis

- Minor salivary gland tumors
- Juvenile nasopharyngeal angiofibroma
- Adenoid hypertrophy
- Tornwaldt cysts
- Fibromyxomatous polyps
- Choanal polyps, fibromas
- Papillomas
- Osseous/fibroosseous tumors
- Craniopharyngiomas
- Extracranial meningiomas
- Chordomas

◆ Evaluation

History

History should include questions about epistaxis, nasal obstruction and discharge, hearing loss or clogged ear, headache, diplopia, facial pain, and numbness.

Physical Exam

The physical exam should include a fiberoptic nasopharyngoscopy. The neck should be examined in a systematic fashion. Any lymph nodes should be assessed with regard to size, location, and mobility.

Imaging

Imaging is required for staging and treatment planning for NPC. Computed tomography (CT) and magnetic resonance imaging (MRI) are recommended for the diagnostic process and evaluation of tumoral extent and bone erosion and to delineate tumor extension into the parapharyngeal and retropharyngeal spaces, the oropharynx, the orbit, and the intracranial compartment.

A chest X-ray, liver ultrasound, and a bone scan are recommended for all patients with nodal disease. The role of positron emission tomography (PET) in the staging of nasopharyngeal carcinoma has not been well established.

Labs

The quantitative analysis of cell-free EBV DNA in plasma of patients has been studied, and data suggest a possible value of this tool in screening and monitoring treatment. High IgA antibody levels to EBV capsid antigen and early antigen (EA) provide a valuable screening tool for early cases in high-incidence populations.

Other Tests

A dental examination is required before instituting radiotherapy to reduce the development of postradiotherapy complications. Patients should continue with meticulous dental care and fluoride prophylaxis.

Pathology

Classic nasopharyngeal carcinoma has been classified into three types by the World Health Organization (WHO):

Type 1: Keratinizing squamous cell carcinoma (SCC)

Type 2 (2a): Nonkeratinizing or poorly differentiated carcinoma

Type 3 (2b): Undifferentiated carcinoma (lymphepithelioma)

WHO types II and III exhibit between 82 and 100% positivity with respect to EBV antibody titers. Type 1 may have an association with cigarette and alcohol consumption and accounts for up to 30% of cases in nonendemic areas and < 5% in endemic areas. Several genetic markers of the human leukocyte antigen (HLA) system have been investigated in patients with NPC in China and other parts of Asia. HLA-A2 and HLA-BS-in-2 were associated with an increased incidence, whereas HLA-A11 was associated with a decreased risk. See the histology slides in **Fig. 6.11**.

◆ Treatment Options

Medical

Radiotherapy is the cornerstone of the definitive treatment for NPC. This is because NPCs are particularly radiosensitive, whereas the tumor is in a relatively inaccessible location, making surgical excision difficult and highly morbid. External beam is most commonly delivered by opposed lateral fields to encompass the primary tumor and upper neck. Radiation doses of 70 to 76 Gy in fractions of 1.8 to 2.0 Gy per day to the primary and anatomic structures at risk within the vicinity of the nasopharynx. Because there is a high incidence of subclinical neck disease, radiation doses between 50 and 60 Gy are used to electively treat the neck.

Recent data shows a clear role for concomitant chemoradiotherapy followed by adjuvant chemotherapy, which provides statistically significant improvement in overall survival and disease-free survival.

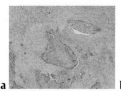 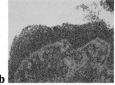 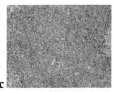

a   b   c

Fig. 6.11   (a) Histology slide showing type I squamous cell nasopharyngeal carcinoma (hematoxylin and eosin, ×200). **(b)** Histology slide showing type II nonkeratinizing squamous cell nasopharyngeal carcinoma (hematoxylin and eosin, ×200). **(c)** Histology slide showing type III undifferentiated nasopharyngeal carcinoma (hematoxylin and eosin, ×200). (Used with permission from Lund VJ, Howard DJ, Wei WI. *Tumors of the Nose, Sinuses, and Nasopharynx.* Stuttgart/New York; Thieme; 2014:539.)

EBV DNA titers seem to be an important index for prognostication. EBV DNA titers correlate with stage, treatment response, relapse, and survival.

Adoptive immunotherapy with EBV-specific CTL (cytotoxic T cell lymphocytes) awaits further exploration.

Surgical

The role of surgery in NPC is largely confined to the treatment of residual or recurrent disease either in the nasopharynx or in the neck, though there is literature from China discussing the use of surgery as a primary-modality treatment. Neck dissection for postradiation residual or recurrent nodal disease is the most common indication for surgery.

◆ Outcome and Follow-Up

Overall survival with the use of conventional radiotherapy alone in the treatment of NPC is in the range of 50 to 76%. Patients with stage I and II disease have a high rate of cure with radiotherapy alone. Seventy percent of patients with NPC present with locally advanced stage III or IV disease. For these patients, radiotherapy delivered in combination with chemotherapy has become the standard of care. The prognosis for those with distant metastatic spread remains poor.

◆ Staging of Nasopharyngeal Cancer

Primary Tumor (T)

TX: Primary tumor cannot be assessed

T0:   No tumor identified, but EBV-positive cervical node(s) involvement

Tis: Carcinoma in situ

T1:   Tumor confined to nasopharynx, or extension to oropharynx and/or nasal cavity without parapharyngeal involvement

T2:   Tumor with extension to parapharyngeal space, and/or adjacent soft tissue involvement (medial pterygoid, lateral pterygoid, prevertebral muscles)

T3: Tumor with infiltration of bony structures at skull base, cervical vertebra, pterygoid structures, and/or paranasal sinuses

T4: Tumor with intracranial extension, involvement of cranial nerves, hypopharynx, orbit, parotid gland, and/or soft tissue infiltration beyond the lateral surface of the pterygoid muscle

Regional Lymph Node (N)

NX: Regional lymph nodes cannot be assessed

N0: No regional lymph node metastasis

N1: Unilateral metastasis in cervical lymph node(s) and/or unilateral or bilateral metastasis in retropharyngeal lymph node(s), ≤ 6 cm in greatest dimension, above the caudal border of cricoid cartilage

N2: Bilateral metastasis in cervical lymph node(s), ≤ 6 cm in greatest dimension, above the caudal border of cricoid cartilage

N3: Unilateral or bilateral metastasis in cervical lymph node(s), > 6 cm in greatest dimension, and/or extension below the caudal border of cricoid cartilage

Distant Metastasis (M)

M0: No distant metastasis

M1: Distant metastasis

American Joint Committee on Cancer Stage Groupings of Nasopharynx Cancers (8th Edition)

Stage 0 disease: Carcinoma in situ (TisN0M0)

Stage I disease: Includes only T1 N0 M0 tumors

Stage II disease: Includes T0–N1M0 and T2 N0–N1 M0 tumors

Stage III disease: Includes T3 N0 M0 and T0–3 disease that is N2 M0

Stage IVA disease: Includes T4 disease with N0-N2 M0 disease and T0-T4 disease that is N3 M0

Stage IVB disease: Any disease with distant metastases (M1) (**Table 6.10**)

Table 6.10 Cancer Stage Groupings for Nasopharynx Cancer

	N0	N1	N2	N3
T0	N/A	Stage II	Stage III	Stage IVA
T1	Stage I	Stage II	Stage III	Stage IVA
T2	Stage II	Stage II	Stage III	Stage IVA
T3	Stage III	Stage III	Stage III	Stage IVA
T4	Stage IVA	Stage IVA	Stage IVA	Stage IVA
M1	Stage IVB	Stage IVB	Stage IVB	Stage IVB

6.3.5   Oral Cavity Cancer

◆ Key Features

- A nonhealing or bleeding sore in the mouth or on the lip is the most common presentation.
- A persistent white or red patch on oral mucosa needs to be investigated.
- History of tobacco smoking or chewing occurs in most cases.
- Lip cancer may be caused by sun exposure.

The oral cavity extends from the vermilion borders of the lips anteriorly to the junction of the hard and soft palates superiorly and to the line of circumvallate papillae posteriorly. Oral cancer should be identified early, and screening is useful. It is frequently preceded by an identifiable premalignant lesion. The progression from dysplasia may occur over a period of years.

◆ Epidemiology

Thirty thousand people are diagnosed yearly with oral cancer in the United States, and it causes > 8,000 deaths. It constitutes < 5% of US cancers, but in India, the incidence is far greater. For all stages combined, the 5-year relative survival rate is 59%, and the 10-year survival rate is 44%. It typically occurs in those over the age of 45 and occurs in men twice as often as in women. The number of new cases of this disease has been decreasing during the past 20 years. Tobacco smoking and alcohol are the primary risk factors. Smokeless tobacco in the Western world and paan (betel leaf with areca nut) in Asia are also risk factors for oral cancer. Other suspected risk factors include viral infection (human papillomavirus [HPV]), a diet low in fruits and vegetables, vitamin A deficiency, genetic susceptibility, and immunosuppressive drugs or immunocompromised conditions. Recently there has been a growing number of young patients with oral cancers, particularly involving the tongue.

◆ Clinical

Signs

Signs may include uncomfortable or poorly fitting dentures, loosening of the teeth, changes in articulation, a mass in the neck, weight loss, and persistent halitosis.

Symptoms

Symptoms depend on site and stage of the primary tumor and its effect on function of that area. They include a nonhealing white or red (leukoplakia, erythroplakia) patch or sore in the mouth (most common symptom), persistent pain in the mouth, and a thickening in the cheek or the floor of the mouth. More advanced disease may cause a sore throat, difficulty chewing, dysphagia, trismus or tongue tethering, numbness of the tongue or mouth, and pain around the teeth or jaw.

Differential Diagnosis

- Oral and pharyngeal infections such as pharyngitis or stomatitis
- Chancre
- Benign oral or odontogenic lesions
- Denture sores
- Aphthous ulcers or herpetic sores
- Lesion due to cheek biting
- Oral manifestations of systemic diseases
- Necrotizing sialometaplasia

◆ Evaluation

History

Evaluation begins with a detailed history inquiring about tobacco and alcohol usage, oral pain, referred otalgia, dysphagia, articulation changes, and weight loss.

Physical Exam

A physical exam should include a complete head and neck exam. Specific attention should be directed at the site of the lesion. The lesion size should be noted, as should its infiltration and spread to adjacent oral cavity or oropharyngeal subsites such as the floor of the mouth, alveolus, and tongue base. A bimanual examination of the lesion, the surrounding floor of the mouth, and the submandibular triangle should be performed.

Careful palpation of the neck may reveal adenopathy. The main routes of lymph node drainage from the oral cavity are into the first-echelon nodes (i.e., buccinator, jugulodigastric, submandibular, and submental). Tumor sites close to the midline commonly drain bilaterally.

Imaging

Contrast-enhanced computed tomography (CT) of the head and neck is a necessary component of initial evaluation. Tumor size and spread may be evaluated as well as discrete nodal disease, bony destruction, and vascular involvement. Magnetic resonance imaging (MRI) may be helpful in the evaluation of oral cancer because it provides a higher contrast between normal tissue and tumor on T2-weighted images, has no beam artifact from dental material, and provides multiplanar imaging.

The combination of positron emission tomography (PET) and CT is a useful diagnostic and staging modality in the evaluation of the patient with head and neck cancer.

A chest CT may be used to rule out pulmonary metastasis. Periapical dental radiographs provide fine detail and may show minimal invasion. Panoramic dental radiographs may show gross bony destruction.

Labs

Routine preoperative laboratory studies are employed.

Other Tests

Patients with suspected oral cancer must undergo a biopsy for pathologic diagnosis. The first test for the evaluation of a neck mass presenting with an oral cavity lesion is fine-needle aspiration biopsy (FNAB).

The routine use of panendoscopy, which includes bronchoscopy, esophagoscopy, and laryngoscopy, is recommended. It allows for the complete evaluation of the upper aerodigestive tract and helps rule out the presence of a synchronous tumor. The mucous membranes of the upper aerodigestive tract are carefully evaluated, and biopsy samples of any abnormal-looking areas are taken. This is particularly important in the patient who smokes.

Toluidine blue staining and photodynamic agents such as 5-aminolevulinic acid (ALA) may be used to enhance detection of oral lesions. Oral brush biopsy (OralCDx; CDx Diagnostics, Suffern, NY) can be used in the screening of oral precancer and cancer.

A dental evaluation should be performed, with attention to dental hygiene, dentition status, and integrity of the mandible.

Pathology

Ninety percent of oral cancers are squamous cell carcinomas (SCCs), and they may be preceded by various precancerous lesions. Non-SCC oral cancers may also include minor salivary gland tumors. Other rarer cancers may be of odontogenic apparatus origin, lymphomas, soft tissue sarcomas, or melanomas.

There is no significant correlation between degree of squamous differentiation (see **Table 6.5**) and the biologic behavior of oral cancer. Vascular and perineural invasion thickness and depth of invasion are all negative prognostic factors.

Verrucous carcinoma (VC) is a locally aggressive, clinically exophytic, low-grade, well-differentiated SCC with minimal metastatic potential. It is also known as Ackerman's tumor. An HPV infection is thought to facilitate or cause verrucous carcinoma. Associations with verrucous carcinoma have been found in patients who chew tobacco and betel nut. Fully developed lesions are white cauliflowerlike papillomas with a pebbly surface that may extend and coalesce over large areas of the oral mucosa. Overall, patients with verrucous carcinoma have a favorable prognosis; the course of verrucous carcinoma lesions is characterized by slow, continuous local growth.

Proliferative verrucous leukoplakia (PVL) is a particularly aggressive form of oral leukoplakia that commences with a hyperkeratosis, spreads to become multifocal and verruciform in appearance, and later becomes malignant. It is significant because it has a high recurrence rate and the potential to develop into verrucous carcinoma or SCC in 60 to 70% of the affected patients. PVL is more commonly found in elderly females and is associated with tobacco use or alcohol abuse in 30 to 50% of patients. The etiology of PVL is unknown. An association with HPV infection, particularly strains 16 and 18, has been implicated in some cases. The most common locations are the gingiva or alveolar ridge, the tongue, and the buccal mucosa. The gingiva is the most likely site for the malignant transformation of PVL. PVL often begins as a focal lesion spreading laterally over time and can be multifocal. Early in its course, it is a flat hyperkeratotic lesion that becomes progressively verrucous and histologically often exhibits varying degrees of epithelial dysplasia.

◆ Treatment Options

Surgical resection and radiotherapy are the current treatments of choice. Surgery is considered the primary and preferred modality of treating cancers of the oral cavity.

Lip Cancer

Most lip SCCs present on the lower lip (88–95%), 2 to 7% present on the upper lip, and 1% on the oral commissure. Basal cell carcinoma is more common on the upper lip.

Treatment of Lip Cancer

- For T1 and T2 lesions, radiotherapy and surgery produce similar cure rates; the method of treatment is determined by functional and cosmetic factors.
- Advanced lesions of the lip generally require a combination of surgery and radiotherapy.
- Patients with upper lip and oral commissure SCC have a worse overall prognosis.
- The 5-year survival for stage I and II lesions is 90%.

Oral Tongue Cancer

Seventy-five percent of tongue cancers occur on the posterior lateral aspect, 20% on the anterior lateral aspect, and 3 to 5% on the lingual dorsum. At the time of diagnosis, 75% oral tongue cancers are T2 or smaller. Forty percent of patients with oral tongue cancer demonstrate clinical evidence of neck metastasis at presentation.

Treatment of Oral Tongue Lesions

- Early tongue cancer: Wide local excision is often used for T1 lesions that can be resected transorally.
- For larger T1 and T2 lesions, either surgery or radiotherapy is an acceptable treatment.
- Deeply infiltrative lesions (> 4 mm depth) can be treated with surgery with postoperative radiotherapy and a selective neck dissection.
- Selected patients with T4 tongue cancer can be treated with combined surgery (i.e., total glossectomy, sometimes requiring laryngectomy due to the high risk of postoperative aspiration) and postoperative radiotherapy.
- For T1 and T2 lesions, 20 to 30% of patients harbor metastatic disease in cervical lymph nodes. Thus, therapy (surgery or radiotherapy) aimed at the neck should be considered as part of definitive treatment.

- The 5-year survival is 75% for stage I and II oral tongue cancers and < 40% for stage III and IV oral tongue cancers.

Buccal Mucosa Cancer

Carcinomas of the buccal mucosa represent 5 to 10% of oral cancers. The most common area is in the region of the third mandibular molar. Lesions < 1 cm in diameter can be treated by surgery alone if the oral commissure is not involved. If involved, radiotherapy should be considered. Premalignant conditions include submucosal fibrosis and lichen planus. The latter has a reported transformation rate of 0.5 to 3%, whereas the former has a malignant transformation rate of 0.5%.

Treatment of Buccal Mucosa Cancers

- Lesions smaller than 1 cm in diameter can be managed by surgery alone if the commissure is not involved. If the commissure is involved, radiotherapy (including brachytherapy) should be considered.
- Advanced lesions of the buccal mucosa can be treated with surgical resection alone, radiotherapy alone, or surgical resection plus postoperative radiation.
- The 5-year survival for buccal mucosa cancer is 75% for stage I, 65% for stage II, 30 to 65% for stage III, and 20 to 50% for stage IV buccal cancer.

Floor of Mouth Cancer

Cancers of the floor of the mouth represent 28 to 35% of oral cancers. Thirty-five percent of patients with floor of mouth cancer present with T3 or T4 disease. The most common presentation of cancer of the floor of the mouth is a painless inflamed superficial ulcer with poorly defined margins. Preexistent or coincident leukoplakia can be observed in adjacent tissues in ~ 20% of cases.

Treatment of Floor of Mouth Cancer

Note that a cancer involving the gingiva adjacent to recent dental extraction is at high risk for bony extension via the tooth socket.

- For T1 lesions, either transoral surgery or radiotherapy is an acceptable treatment.
- For small T2 lesions (≤ 3 cm), surgery may be used if the lesion is attached to the periosteum, whereas radiotherapy may be used if the lesion encroaches on the tongue.
- For large T2 lesions (> 3 cm), surgery and radiotherapy are alternative methods of treatment, the choice of which depends primarily on the expected extent of disability from surgery.
- External-beam radiotherapy with or without interstitial radiotherapy should be considered postoperatively for larger lesions.
- For more advanced lesions, surgery should incorporate rim resection plus neck dissection or partial mandibulectomy with neck dissection as appropriate.

- The 5-year survival for floor of mouth cancer is 90% for stage I, 80% for stage II, 65% for stage III, and 30% for stage IV.

Retromolar Trigone Cancer

Retromolar trigone cancers account for ~ 10% of all oral cancers. These cancers typically present with advanced disease, and 50% of patients have regional metastasis at the time of diagnosis.

Treatment of Retromolar Trigone Cancer

For small lesions without detectable bone invasion, limited resection of the mandible may be performed. Radiotherapy may be used initially, with surgery reserved for radiation failure. Selective neck treatment should be performed—for advanced stages, multimodality therapy with surgery and postoperative radiation is most often used.

Hard Palate Cancer

Cancer of the hard palate accounts for 5% of all oral cavity malignancies. Ten to 25% of patients with head and neck SCC of the hard palate present with regional metastasis. (Only 53% of hard palate cancers are SCC; minor salivary gland malignancies make up the rest.)

Treatment of Cancer of the Hard Palate

For both early and advanced disease, surgery (inferior maxillectomy with surgical obturator) is used for primary therapy. Radiotherapy has a role depending on factors such as close or positive surgical margins, evidence of perineural involvement, or the presence of lymph node metastases. The prosthodontist is important in the care of these patients for oral rehabilitation. The 5-year survival for hard palate cancer ranges from 40 to 60%.

Advanced Oral Cavity Cancer

Clinical trials for advanced oral tumors evaluating the use of chemotherapy preoperatively, before radiotherapy, as adjuvant therapy after surgery, or as part of combined-modality therapy are appropriate.

◆ Outcome and Follow-Up

The National Comprehensive Cancer Network (NCCN) guidelines suggest routine follow up after treatment. This includes follow up every 1 to 2 months the first year, every 2 to 6 months the second year, every 4 to 8 months the third through fifth years and annual follow up afterwards. Patients with regional neck disease prior to treatment should undergo CT scan or integrated ^{18}F fludeoxyglucose (FDG)-PET/CT 12 weeks after the completion of radiotherapy to assess for residual disease that may necessitate postradiotherapy neck dissection. The risk of a second primary carcinoma is highest in those who continue to smoke, and patients should be strongly urged to quit.

See **Fig. 6.12**.

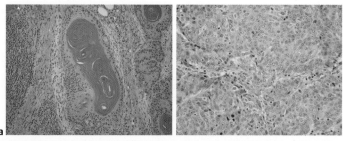

Fig. 6.12 Squamous cell carcinoma. **(a)** Well-differentiated squamous cell carcinomas are often extensively keratinized (a keratin pearl is seen in the center of a nest), with mild cytologic atypia and mitotic activity limited to the parabasal zones. **(b)** In contrast, poorly differentiated squamous cell carcinomas grow as cords or sheets of highly pleomorphic cells with frequent mitoses. There is little evidence of maturation within the tumor nests. (Used with permission from Har-El G, Day T, Nathan C-A, Nguyen SA. *A Multidisciplinary Approach to Head and Neck Neoplasms.* New York: Thieme;2013. *Otorhinolaryngology—Head and Neck Surgery Series.*)

◆ Staging of Oral Cavity Cancer

Primary Tumor (T) (now includes Depth of Invasion [DOI])

TX: Primary tumor cannot be assessed

Tis: Carcinoma in situ

T1:   Tumor ≤ 2 cm in greatest dimension, and ≤ 5 mm DOI

T2:   Tumor ≤ 2 cm and DOI >5 mm and ≤ 10 mm or tumor > 2 cm and ≤ 4 cm, and ≤ 10 mm DOI

T3:   Tumor > 4 cm in greatest dimension or any tumor >10 mm DOI

T4a: Moderately advanced local disease

    Lip: Tumor invades through the cortical bone, the inferior alveolar nerve, the floor of the mouth, or the skin of the face (i.e., the chin or nose).

    Oral cavity: Tumor invades the adjacent structures, such as the cortical bone [mandible, maxilla], the maxillary sinus, or the skin of the face.

T4b: Very advanced local disease. Tumor invades the masticator space, pterygoid plates, or skull base and/or encases the internal carotid artery.

Regional Lymph Nodes (N)*

NX: Regional lymph nodes cannot be assessed

N0:   No regional lymph node metastasis

N1:   Metastasis to a single ipsilateral lymph node measuring ≤ 3 cm in greatest diameter and ENE negative

N2:   Further divided into three categories:

    N2a: Single ipsilateral lymph node > 3 and ≤ 6 cm and ENE negative (pathologic staging also includes a single ipsilateral or contralateral lymph node ≤ 3 cm and ENE positive)

N2b: Multiple ipsilateral lymph nodes ≤ 6 cm and ENE negative

N2c: Bilateral or contralateral lymph nodes ≤ 6 cm in greatest dimension and ENE negative

N3: Now further divided into two categories:

N3a: Metastasis to a lymph node > 6 cm, ENE negative

N3b: Metastasis to a single lymph node that is ENE positive (pathologic staging includes single lymph nodes that are ENE positive >3cm), or metastasis to multiple lymph nodes with any ENE positive

A designation of "U" or "L" can be attached to the N category to indicate nodes above ("U") or below ("L") the lower border of the cricoid. Similarly, clinical and pathologic ENE should be recorded as ENE (–) or ENE (+). Clinical and pathologic staging are similar with the differences noted in parenthesis.

*Superior mediastinal lymph nodes are considered regional lymph nodes (level VII). Midline nodes are considered ipsilateral nodes.

Distant Metastasis

M0: No distant metastasis

M1: Distant metastasis

American Joint Committee on Cancer Stage Groupings for Oral Cavity Cancers (8th edition)

Stage 0 disease: Carcinoma in situ (TisN0M0)

Stage I disease: Includes only T1 N0 M0 tumors

Stage II disease: Includes only T2 N0 M0 tumors

Stage III disease: Includes T3 N0 M0 and T1 -3 disease that is N1 M0

Stage IVA disease: Includes T4a disease with N0-N2 M0 disease and T1-T3 disease that is N2 M0

Stage IVB disease: Includes T4b disease with any nodal disease or T1-T4a disease with N3 disease without distant metastases (M0)

Stage IVC disease: Any disease with distant metastases (M1) (**Table 6.11**)

Table 6.11 Cancer stage groupings

	N0	N1	N2	N3
T1	Stage I	Stage III	Stage IVA	Stage IVB
T2	Stage II	Stage III	Stage IVA	Stage IVB
T3	Stage III	Stage III	Stage IVA	Stage IVB
T4a	Stage IVA	Stage IVA	Stage IVA	Stage IVB
T4b	Stage IVB	Stage IVB	Stage IVB	Stage IVB
M1	Stage IVC	Stage IVC	Stage IVC	Stage IVC

6.3.6   Oropharyngeal Cancer

✦ Key Features

- Oropharyngeal cancer includes cancer of the palatine tonsil, tongue base, soft palate, and oropharyngeal wall.
- Oropharyngeal cancer is primarily linked to tobacco and alcohol use.
- Human papillomavirus (HPV) is a risk factor for cancer of the tonsil.
- Neck metastasis may be cystic.

The oropharynx is located between the soft palate superiorly and the hyoid bone inferiorly; it communicates with the oral cavity anteriorly, the nasopharynx superiorly, and the supraglottic larynx and hypopharynx inferiorly. Oropharyngeal cancers are typically detected at a more advanced stage than oral cancer. The oropharynx is an important component in swallowing; therefore, treating these tumors is challenging and often requires a multidisciplinary approach and posttreatment rehabilitation.

✦ Epidemiology

In the United States, an estimated 8,300 new cases of pharyngeal cancer (including cancers of the oropharynx and hypopharynx) are diagnosed yearly, with an estimated mortality of 2,000. It affects men three times more than women. Seventy-five percent of oropharynx cancers occur in the palatine tonsil. Tobacco (including smokeless tobacco) and alcohol abuse represent the most significant risk factors for the development of oropharynx cancer. Viral infection with HPV is an important risk factor for squamous cell carcinoma (SCC) of the oropharynx and may be a positive prognostic factor.

✦ Clinical

Signs

Signs include changes in articulation, muffled speech, a mass in the neck, unintentional weight loss, hemoptysis, and persistent halitosis.

Symptoms

Symptoms may include pain, dysphagia, globus sensation, referred otalgia, trismus, and fixation of the tongue. Cancers of the base of the tongue and tonsil are typically insidious.

Differential Diagnosis

- Oropharyngeal infections such as pharyngitis or stomatitis
- Chancre
- Benign oropharyngeal or odontogenic lesions
- Aphthous ulcers or herpetic sores
- Oral manifestations of systemic diseases

◆ Evaluation

History

Evaluation begins with a detailed history inquiring about tobacco and alcohol usage, sexual history, oral pain, odynophagia, referred otalgia, dysphagia, hemoptysis, articulation or speech changes, and unintentional weight loss.

Physical Exam

The physical exam should include a complete head and neck exam, with specific attention directed at the site of the lesion. The lesion size should be noted, as should its apparent infiltration and spread to adjacent pharyngeal or oral cavity subsites such as oral tongue, hypopharynx, nasopharynx, and vallecula. Palpation of the lesion should be performed if possible in an awake patient. In advanced cases, the primary origin of the lesion, such as the tongue base or tonsil, is not always discernible. Fiberoptic laryngoscopy should be performed. Inspection and palpation of the neck often reveal adenopathy.

Imaging

Clinical staging may understage oropharynx tumors, especially the tongue base extension. Both contrast-enhanced computed tomography (CT) and magnetic resonance imaging (MRI) are able to assess oropharynx tumor extent as well as regional spread. Neck metastasis from oropharynx cancer may be cystic in morphology; this finding by itself should raise suspicion of a cancer in the tonsil or tongue base.

At minimum, a chest CT should be used to rule out pulmonary metastasis or second primary. Alternatively, an integrated ^{18}F fludeoxyglucose (FDG)–positron emission tomography (PET)/CT may be used in a combined staging and metastatic work-up.

Labs

Standard preoperative laboratories, as indicated, should be obtained.

Other Tests

Patients with suspected cancer of oropharynx must undergo a biopsy and a sample of the lesion taken for pathologic examination. This may be done in an office setting in cases of tonsil cancer and soft palate cancer, but it is not usually possible in cases of tongue base lesions. If neck metastases are evident, they should be sampled by fine-needle aspiration biopsy (FNAB).

Because of the propensity for second primary tumors, panendoscopy (triple endoscopy—laryngoscopy, esophagoscopy, and bronchoscopy together) has been advocated. This is particularly important in patients who smoke or in patients with large, bulky tumors to establish the true extent of these lesions.

Pathology

Histologically, 90% of oropharynx cancers are SCCs. Basaloid SCC is an uncommon but aggressive SCC variant. Other cancers of the oropharynx include minor salivary gland carcinomas, lymphomas, and "lymphoepithelial-like" carcinomas.

◆ Treatment Options

For stage I oropharynx cancer, surgery or radiotherapy may be used depending on the expected functional deficit. Radiation clinical trials evaluating hyperfractionation schedules should be considered.

For stage II oropharynx cancer, surgery and radiation therapies are equally successful in controlling disease. Radiotherapy may be the preferred modality when the functional deficit is expected to be great.

The management of stage III oropharynx cancer is complex and requires a multidisciplinary approach to establish the optimal treatment. A combination of surgery with postoperative radiotherapy and/or chemotherapy is most often used. An alternative is chemoradiation therapy alone, based on the patient's initial nodal involvement.

In stage III tonsil cancer, hyperfractionated radiotherapy yields a higher control rate than standard fractionated radiotherapy.

In advanced unresectable oropharyngeal cancer, radiotherapy or chemoradiation is used.

Treatments currently under investigation include chemotherapy with radiation clinical trials as well as with radiosensitizers, radiation clinical trials evaluating hyperfractionation schedules and/or brachytherapy, particle-beam radiotherapy, and hyperthermia combined with radiotherapy.

Recently, transoral robotic-assisted surgery (TORS) for resection of select oropharyngeal tumors has gained momentum. Clinical trials are currently underway to evaluate the outcomes of TORS versus radiation therapy.

◆ Outcome and Follow-Up

The overall 5-year disease-specific survival for patients with all stages of disease is ~ 50%. Patients with HPV-positive tumors who are nonsmokers have a better prognosis. The National Comprehensive Cancer Network (NCCN) guidelines suggest routine follow up after treatment. This includes follow up every 1 to 2 months the first year, every 2 to 6 months the second year, every 4 to 8 months the third through fifth years and annual follow up afterwards.

◆ Staging of Oropharyngeal Cancer (HPV Negative)

Primary Tumor (T)

TX: Primary tumor cannot be assessed

Tis: Carcinoma in situ

T1: Tumor ≤ 2 cm in greatest dimension

T2: Tumor > 2 cm but ≤ 4 cm in greatest dimension

T3: Tumor > 4 cm in greatest dimension or extension to lingual surface of epiglottis

T4: Moderately advanced or very advanced local disease

    T4a: Moderately advanced local disease. Tumor invades the larynx, extrinsic muscle of tongue, medial pterygoid, hard palate, or mandible.*

    T4b: Very advanced local disease. Tumor invades lateral pterygoid muscle, pterygoid plates, lateral nasopharynx or skull base or encases carotid artery.

*Note: Mucosal extension to the lingual surface of the epiglottis from primary tumors of the base of the tongue and vallecula does not constitute invasion of the larynx.

Regional Lymph Nodes (N)*

NX: Regional lymph nodes cannot be assessed

N0: No regional lymph node metastasis

N1: Metastasis to a single ipsilateral lymph node measuring ≤ 3 cm in greatest diameter and ENE negative

N2: Further divided into three categories:

    N2a: Single ipsilateral lymph node > 3 and ≤ 6 cm and ENE negative (pathologic staging also includes a single ipsilateral or contralateral lymph node ≤ 3 cm and ENE positive)

    N2b: Multiple ipsilateral lymph nodes ≤ 6 cm and ENE negative

    N2c: Bilateral or contralateral lymph nodes ≤ 6 cm in greatest dimension and ENE negative

N3: Now further divided into two categories:

    N3a: Metastasis to a lymph node > 6 cm, ENE negative

    N3b: Metastasis to a single lymph node that is ENE positive (pathologic staging includes single lymph nodes that are ENE positive >3cm), or metastasis to multiple lymph nodes with any ENE positive

A designation of "U" or "L" can be attached to the N category to indicate nodes above ("U") or below ("L") the lower border of the cricoid. Similarly, clinical and pathologic ENE should be recorded as ENE (−) or ENE (+). Clinical and pathologic staging are similar with the differences noted in parenthesis.

*Superior mediastinal lymph nodes are considered regional lymph nodes (level VII). Midline nodes are considered ipsilateral nodes.

Please refer to the next chapter for staging of HPV positive oropharyngeal cancer.

6.3.7 Human Papillomavirus and Head and Neck Cancer

◆ Key Features

- HPV-related oropharyngeal cancer is increasing in incidence.
- Between 70 and 90% of newly diagnosed oropharyngeal cancers in the United States are HPV-positive.
- Patients with HPV-related head and neck cancers tend to be younger and healthier and have an improved prognosis compared to those with HPV-negative tumors.
- Neck metastasis may be cystic.

Human papillomavirus (HPV) is the most common sexually transmitted infection. Infections can occur in the oral cavity (as well as in the cervix or anorectal or urogenital tract). Persistent high-risk HPV infection (primarily HPV16) is associated with development of malignancy. Most HPV infections clear within one year spontaneously and do not require treatment. Some infections may become persistent, especially in immunocompromised patients or active smokers. Routine HPV testing of oropharyngeal squamous cell carcinoma and head and neck squamous cell cancers of unknown primary are recommended. Testing should include high-risk HPV in situ hybridization (ISH) and/or p16 immunohistochemistry (IHC).

Discussing HPV may be unfamiliar territory in otolaryngology—head and neck surgery practice, and it can be a potentially sensitive topic that can be challenging to navigate with patients. Patients and partners have questions and concerns regarding acquisition and transmission of HPV infection, but partners of patients with HPV-related oropharyngeal cancer do not have a higher rate of oral HPV infection.

◆ Epidemiology

HPV is the most common sexually transmitted infection in the United States, and it is estimated that a majority of the sexually active population will have at least one HPV infection during their lifetimes. HPV is a double-stranded DNA virus that can infect human skin and mucosa, including the oropharynx, genitals, and anus. More than 150 types of HPV infections have been identified, and these can be divided into low-risk and high-risk types. Low-risk infections, most commonly HPV6 and 11, are associated with development of benign lesions such as genital warts or respiratory papillomatosis. High-risk infections, most commonly HPV16 and 18, are associated with development of malignancies including cervical, anorectal, urogenital, and oropharyngeal cancer.

In a patient with a cancer of unknown primary, the tumors frequently are found to be HPV-positive.

Pathophysiology

The mechanism of viral oncogenesis is through HPV viral proteins E6 and E7, which disrupt cell cycle pathways. The E6 protein binds and degrades p53, allowing cell cycle escape, and E7 inhibits another tumor suppressor, retinoblastoma (Rb) protein.

◆ Clinical

HPV-positive tumors often present with small primary oropharyngeal tumors (**Fig. 6.13**). Nodal disease may be large and cystic in nature.

◆ Treatment Options

Current guidelines do not differentiate treatment recommendations based on HPV tumor status. Patients are treated with chemotherapy, radiation, transoral robotic surgery (TORS), open surgery, or a combination of these. HPV-positive tumor status may serve as eligibility for certain clinical trials investigating de-escalation of treatment.

◆ Outcomes and Follow-Up

Despite late stage at diagnosis HPV-positive patients have significantly improved prognosis compared to HPV-negative patients. Three-year overall survival is 82% for HPV-positive patients.

◆ Staging of HPV+ Oropharyngeal Cancer

Primary Tumor (T)

T0: No primary identified

T1: Tumor ≤ 2 cm in greatest dimension

T2: Tumor > 2 cm but ≤ 4 cm in greatest dimension

T3: Tumor > 4 cm in greatest dimension or extension to lingual surface of epiglottis

T4: Moderately advanced local disease; tumor invades the larynx, extrinsic muscle of tongue, medial pterygoid, hard palate, or mandible or beyond*

*Mucosal extension to lingual surface of epiglottis from primary tumors of the base of the tongue and vallecula does not constitute invasion of the larynx.

Regional Lymph Node (N)

Clinical N (cN)

NX: Regional lymph nodes cannot be assessed

N0: No regional lymph node metastasis

N1: One or more ipsilateral lymph nodes, ≤ 6 cm

N2: Contralateral or bilateral lymph nodes, ≤ 6 cm

N3: Lymph node(s) > 6 cm

Pathologic N (pN)

NX: Regional lymph nodes cannot be assessed

pN0: No regional lymph node metastasis

pN1: Metastasis in ≤ 4 lymph nodes

pN2: Metastasis in > 4 lymph nodes

Distant Metastasis (M)

M0: No distant metastasis

M1: Distant metastasis

American Joint Committee on Cancer Stage Groupings for HPV positive Oropharyngeal Cancers (8th Edition)

Clinical staging is as follows:

Stage I disease: T0-T2, N0-N1 disease that is M0

Stage II disease: T3N0-N1 M0 and T0-T3 disease that is N2 M0

Stage III disease: T4 tumors with or without nodal disease as well as any tumor with N3 disease without metastases

Stage IV disease: any tumor with metastatic disease

Please refer to **Table 6.12**.

Table 6.12   Clinical staging of HPV + oropharynx cancer

	N0	N1	N2	N3
T0	N/A	Stage I	Stage II	Stage III
T1	Stage I	Stage I	Stage II	Stage III
T2	Stage I	Stage I	Stage II	Stage III
T3	Stage II	Stage II	Stage II	Stage III
T4	Stage III	Stage III	Stage III	Stage III
M1	Stage IV	Stage IV	Stage IV	Stage IV

Staging based on pathologic criteria for HPV associated (p16-positive) oropharyngeal cancer is different and is as follows:

Stage I disease: T0-T2, N0-N1 disease that is M0

Stage II disease: T3-T4N0-N1 M0 and T0-T2 disease that is N2 M0

Stage III disease: T3-T4 with N2M0 disease

Stage IV disease: any tumor with metastatic disease

Please refer to **Table 6.13**.

Table 6.13   Pathologic staging of HPV + oropharynx cancer

	N0	N1	N2
T0	N/A	Stage I	Stage II
T1	Stage I	Stage I	Stage II
T2	Stage I	Stage I	Stage II
T3	Stage II	Stage II	Stage III
T4	Stage II	Stage II	Stage III
M1	Stage IV	Stage IV	Stage IV

Histologic Grade (G)

No grading system exists for HPV-mediated oropharyngeal tumors.

Histopathologic Type

The histopathology of HPV-mediated p16+ oropharyngeal cancers is characteristic and easily recognizable (**Fig. 6.13**).

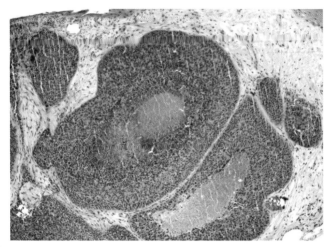

Fig. 6.13 Basaloid squamous cell carcinomas are aggressive tumors, often arranged as nests of small dark cells with central necrosis. Tumor cells at the periphery of the nests frequently align with elongated nuclei at right angles to the stroma, giving a palisaded appearance. When located in the oropharynx, these tumors often harbor human papillomavirus. (Used with permission from Har-El G, Day T, Nathan C-A, Nguyen SA. *A Multidisciplinary Approach to Head and Neck Neoplasms.* New York: Thieme;2013. *Otorhinolaryngology—Head and Neck Surgery Series.*)

6.3.8 Cancer of Unknown Primary

◆ Key Features

- When clinicians are unable to determine the origin of a metastatic cervical lymphadenopathy, after thorough investigation, the cancer is said to originate from an unknown primary site.
- The typical presentation of an unknown-primary cancer of the head and neck is a painless neck mass.
- When the primary is ultimately found, it is most often in the oropharynx.
- When the primary is ultimately found, it may be very small.
- Risk factors include human papillomavirus (HPV), smoking, and alcohol.

Patients with head and neck cancer typically present with a painless neck mass. This is known as cancer of unknown primary (CUP), carcinoma of unknown primary origin, or occult-primary malignancy. Unknown-primary carcinoma presenting as cervical lymph node metastasis accounts for approximately 2 to 9% of all head and neck malignancies. A primary tumor is considered unknown only *after* a thorough investigation (including physical exam, imaging, and biopsies) has been completed.

Evaluation of possible CUP begins with a thorough history and physical examination, including flexible fiberoptic laryngoscopy. Fine-needle aspiration biopsy (FNAB) of the neck mass provides a histologic diagnosis, which may assist with finding the primary tumor, but 90% are attributable to squamous cell carcinoma (SCC). Without an identified primary tumor, this biopsy should also be tested for HPV and EBV positivity to assist with localizing the primary. As p16 can be expressed at other sites besides the oropharynx, HPV In Situ Hybridization (ISH) is also recommended to help confirm a likely oropharyngeal primary.

Once a diagnosis of cancer has been established, imaging studies can assist with localization of the primary site. Computed tomography (CT) is faster and more cost-effective, but magnetic resonance imaging (MRI) has a higher sensitivity for small tumors given its better soft tissue delineation. Positron emission tomography (PET)-CT may be considered and may help rule out primary sites below the diaphragm. It has recently been recommended that imaging evaluation begin with a CT and chest X-ray, followed by MRI or PET-CT if the primary site is still not found.

The next step is to perform panendoscopy with biopsies whether or not the primary site was located on imaging. Panendoscopy typically includes bronchoscopy, esophagoscopy, and direct laryngoscopy. If no obvious tumor is visualized, palatine tonsillectomy and guided biopsies are performed. Most advocate a unilateral tonsillectomy limited to the side of the neck mass, but others advocate bilateral tonsillectomies in this circumstance. The most common sites of CUP include the palatine tonsil and base of the tongue, followed by the nasopharynx and piriform recess. Each of these sites should at least be inspected, with consideration of guided biopsies.

◆ Transoral Robotic Surgery and CUP

Recently, transoral robotic surgery (TORS) was found to be an effective approach in identification of CUP origin. Visual examination of the oropharynx under 3D magnification helps to identify malignant, vascular, and mucosal changes. Transoral tonsillectomy and lingual tonsillectomy with frozen analysis are valuable diagnostic procedures in cases with no identifiable mucosal abnormality.

◆ HPV and CUP

Squamous cell carcinoma of unknown primary site (SCCUPS) of the head and neck typically has a favorable prognosis. It is suspected that the historical good outcome is a reflection of a high percentage of previously unrecognized HPV association. It is unknown whether the incidence of unknown-primary carcinoma of the head and neck is rising at a rate similar to that of HPV-associated oropharyngeal cancer.

HPV-associated oropharyngeal cancer has been present for many years, but an increasing incidence has been observed in the last decades. An increased incidence of HPV-related CUP would therefore be expected. This is particularly relevant to consider because it has been observed that

HPV-positive cancers are prone to early metastasis and so are diagnosed at an advanced N-stage with a very small T-site.

Treatment of CUP is controversial. Surgical excision in the form of a neck dissection followed by radiation therapy allows use of a lower total dose of radiation. Primary radiation provides treatment to both the upper aerodigestive tract and its locoregional metastasis but forces the radiation oncologist to treat a wider field, as the primary site is unknown.

With improved visualization and freedom of motion, TORS is becoming an innovative surgical modality that allows detection and complete resection of oropharyngeal subsites with minimal morbidity.

◆ Staging for Cancer of Unknown Primary

- If EBV positive, use nasopharyngeal staging (**Chapter 6.3.4**)
- If HPV positive, use p16 positive oropharyngeal staging (**Chapter 6.3.7**)
- If EBV and HPV negative use the following:

Regional Lymph Nodes (N) *

NX: Regional lymph nodes cannot be assessed

N0: No regional lymph node metastasis

N1: Metastasis to a single ipsilateral lymph node measuring ≤ 3 cm in greatest diameter and ENE negative

N2: Further divided into three categories:

  N2a: Single ipsilateral lymph node > 3 and ≤ 6 cm and ENE negative (pathologic staging also includes a single ipsilateral or contra- lateral lymph node ≤ 3 cm and ENE positive)

  N2b: Multiple ipsilateral lymph nodes ≤ 6 cm and ENE negative

  N2c: Bilateral or contralateral lymph nodes ≤ 6 cm in greatest dimension and ENE negative

N3: Now further divided into two categories:

  N3a: Metastasis to a lymph node > 6 cm, ENE negative

  N3b: Metastasis to a single lymph node that is ENE positive (pathologic staging includes single lymph nodes that are ENE positive >3cm), or metastasis to multiple lymph nodes with any ENE positive

A designation of "U" or "L" can be attached to the N category to indicate nodes above ("U") or below ("L") the lower border of the cricoid. Similarly, clinical and pathologic ENE should be recorded as ENE (−) or ENE (+). Clinical and pathologic staging are similar with the differences noted in parenthesis.

*Superior mediastinal lymph nodes are considered regional lymph nodes (level VII). Midline nodes are considered ipsilateral nodes.

American Joint Committee on Cancer Stage Groupings for Cancer of Unknown Primary (8th Edition)

Stage III disease: Includes N1 M0 disease
Stage IVA disease: Includes N2 M0 disease
Stage IVB disease: Includes N3 M0 disease
Stage IVC disease: Any disease with distant metastases (M1)

6.3.9   Hypopharyngeal Cancer

◆ Key Features

- Hypopharyngeal cancer occurs in the piriform recesses, the posterior hypopharyngeal, or postcricoid region.
- Patients present with dysphagia, globus sensation, hoarseness, and referred otalgia.
- It usually presents in advanced stages of disease.
- It has a high propensity for regional metastasis at presentation.

The hypopharynx is the part of the pharynx that lies behind the larynx and connects the oropharynx and the esophagus. It is subdivided into three subsites: the paired piriform recesses, the posterior hypopharyngeal wall, and the postcricoid region. Sixty-five to 85% of cancers of the hypopharynx involve the piriform recesses, 10 to 20% involve the posterior pharyngeal wall, and 5 to 15% involve the postcricoid area.

◆ Epidemiology

Cancer of the hypopharynx is uncommon, with ~ 2,500 new cases diagnosed in the United States each year. Cancer of the hypopharynx typically presents in advanced stages, and the incidences of regional metastases and distant metastases are also among the highest of all head and neck cancers. Cancer of the hypopharynx is typically seen in men over 55 years old with a history of tobacco product use and/or alcohol ingestion.

An exception is an increased incidence of postcricoid cancer in women aged 30 to 50 years with Plummer-Vinson's syndrome. Asbestos may pose an independent risk for the development of cancer of the hypopharynx.

◆ Clinical

Signs and Symptoms

Signs include muffled speech, hoarseness, a mass in the neck, hemoptysis, unintentional weight loss, airway obstruction, and persistent halitosis. The incidence of regional metastases is 50 to 70% at presentation. Symptoms include dysphagia, chronic sore throat, hoarseness, globus sensation, and referred otalgia.

Differential Diagnosis

Differential diagnosis may include pharyngeal infections such as pharyngitis or candidal infection, benign hypopharynx or upper esophageal lesions, and pharyngeal manifestations of systemic diseases.

◆ Evaluation

History

A detailed history should include questions about smoking and alcohol usage, prolonged hoarseness, dysphagia, odynophagia, hemoptysis, otalgia, and unintentional weight loss.

Physical Exam

The physical exam should include a complete head and neck exam. Specific attention should be directed to the site of the lesion. A fiberoptic laryngoscopy should be performed. The lesion size should be noted, as should its infiltration of and spread to adjacent laryngeal and hypopharyngeal subsites. During this examination, the patient should be taken through maneuvers such as protrusion of the tongue, puffing out the cheeks, lightly coughing, and speaking, the better to visualize and access the pharynx and larynx. It is important that laryngeal motility be assessed, as this is critical in tumor staging. Inspection and palpation of the neck often reveals adenopathy. On neck examination, loss of the grating sensation (laryngeal crepitus) of the laryngeal cartilages over the prevertebral tissues may indicate deep pharyngeal wall involvement with fixation of the larynx. Impeding airway obstruction should be recognized and addressed.

Imaging

Chest imaging with a chest radiograph or computed tomography (CT) scan should be performed to rule out pulmonary metastasis or a pulmonary second primary.

Superficial mucosal lesions in the piriform recess may be seen on barium swallow studies, although this is not the imaging modality of choice. Negative findings on swallow study despite progressive or continuous symptoms should not preclude an endoscopic examination. CT and magnetic resonance imaging (MRI) are used to image the primary tumor and regional lymph nodes prior to definitive treatment. They provide information about the location and extent of tumor involvement and demonstrate the interface of tumor with cartilage, muscles, soft tissues, and blood vessels. Alternatively, an integrated ^{18}F fludeoxyglucose (FDG)–positron emission tomography (PET)/CT may be used in a combined staging and metastatic work-up.

Labs

Blood count, electrolyte, and liver function tests should be performed to assess nutritional status.

Other Tests

Patients with suspected cancer of the hypopharynx must undergo a biopsy and a sample of the lesion taken for pathologic examination. This biopsy may be coupled with a triple endoscopy (panendoscopy) to evaluate the patient for the presence of synchronous second primary tumors. The direct laryngoscopic exam under anesthesia is a critical part of staging and treatment planning.

Pathology

Ninety-five percent of cancers of the hypopharynx are squamous cell carcinomas (SCCs).

◆ Treatment Options

The treatment of cancer of the hypopharynx is controversial, in part because of its low incidence and the inherent difficulty in conducting adequately powered, prospective, randomized clinical studies. In general, both surgery and radiotherapy are the mainstays of most curative efforts aimed at this cancer.

Stage I Tumors

Laryngopharyngectomy with neck dissection has been the most frequently used therapy for surgical hypopharyngeal cancers. In very select cases, a partial laryngopharyngectomy may be successfully used. Radiotherapy may be used as a primary treatment modality and should include the neck.

Stage II Tumors

Laryngopharyngectomy with neck dissection has been the most frequently used therapy. Neoadjuvant chemotherapy has been used to reduce tumors and render them more definitively treatable with either surgery or radiation.

Stage III and IV Tumors

Most often, a combination of surgery and radiation is given postoperatively. Patients with stage III or IV cancer of the hypopharynx should be considered for treatment with combined postoperative adjuvant radiotherapy and chemotherapy.

◆ Outcome and Follow-Up

The prognosis of cancer of the hypopharynx is poor, with most series reporting a < 25% 5-year survival rate. Presentation at a late stage, multisite involvement within the hypopharynx, unrestricted soft tissue tumor growth, an extensive regional lymphatic network enabling development of metastases, and restricted surgical options for complete resection contribute to an overall poor prognosis. The National Comprehensive Cancer Network (NCCN) guidelines suggest routine follow up after treatment. This includes follow up every 1 to 2 months the first year, every 2 to 6 months the second year, every 4 to 8 months the third through fifth years and annual follow up afterwards.

◆ Staging of Hypopharyngeal Cancer

Primary tumor (T)

TX: Primary tumor cannot be assessed

Tis: Carcinoma in situ

T1: Tumor limited to one subsite of hypopharynx and/or ≤ 2 cm in greatest dimension

T2:   Tumor invades more than one subsite of hypopharynx or an adjacent site, or measures > 2 cm but ≤ 4 cm in greatest dimension without fixation of hemilarynx

T3:   Tumor > 4 cm in greatest dimension or with fixation of the hemilarynx or extension into the esophagus

T4:   Moderately advanced and very advanced local disease

   T4a: Moderately advanced local disease: tumor invades the thyroid/cricoid cartilage, hyoid bone, thyroid gland, or central compartment soft tissue*

   T4b: Very advanced local disease: tumor invades prevertebral fascia, encases carotid artery, or involves mediastinal structures

*Note: Central compartment soft tissue includes prelaryngeal strap muscles and subcutaneous fat.

Regional Lymph Nodes (N)*

NX: Regional lymph nodes cannot be assessed

N0:   No regional lymph node metastasis

N1:   Metastasis to a single ipsilateral lymph node measuring ≤ 3 cm in greatest diameter and ENE negative

N2:   Further divided into three categories:

   N2a: Single ipsilateral lymph node > 3 and ≤ 6 cm and ENE negative (pathologic staging also includes a single ipsilateral or contralateral lymph node ≤ 3 cm and ENE positive)

   N2b: Multiple ipsilateral lymph nodes ≤ 6 cm and ENE negative

   N2c: Bilateral or contralateral lymph nodes ≤ 6 cm in greatest dimension and ENE negative

N3:   Now further divided into two categories:

   N3a: Metastasis to a lymph node > 6 cm, ENE negative

   N3b: Metastasis to a single lymph node that is ENE positive (pathologic staging includes single lymph nodes that are ENE positive >3cm), or metastasis to multiple lymph nodes with any ENE positive

A designation of "U" or "L" can be attached to the N category to indicate nodes above ("U") or below ("L") the lower border of the cricoid. Similarly, clinical and pathologic ENE should be recorded as ENE (–) or ENE (+). Clinical and pathologic staging are similar with the differences noted in parenthesis.

*Superior mediastinal lymph nodes are considered regional lymph nodes (level VII). Midline nodes are considered ipsilateral nodes.

American Joint Committee on Cancer Stage Groupings for Hypopharyngeal Cancer (8th Edition):

Stage 0 disease: Carcinoma in situ (TisN0M0)

Stage I disease: Includes only T1 N0 M0 tumors

Stage II disease: Includes only T2 N0 M0 tumors

Stage III disease: Includes T3 N0 M0 and T1 -3 disease that is N1 M0

Stage IVA disease: Includes T4a disease with N0-N2 M0 disease and T1-T3 disease that is N2 M0

Stage IVB disease: Includes T4b disease with any nodal disease or T1-T4a disease with N3 disease without distant metastases (M0)

Stage IVC disease: Any disease with distant metastases (M1) (**Table 6.14**)

Table 6.14 Cancer stage groupings

	N0	N1	N2	N3
T1	Stage I	Stage III	Stage IVA	Stage IVB
T2	Stage II	Stage III	Stage IVA	Stage IVB
T3	Stage III	Stage III	Stage IVA	Stage IVB
T4a	Stage IVA	Stage IVA	Stage IVA	Stage IVB
T4b	Stage IVB	Stage IVB	Stage IVB	Stage IVB
M1	Stage IVC	Stage IVC	Stage IVC	Stage IVC

6.3.10 Laryngeal Cancer

◆ Key Features

- Laryngeal cancer is the second most common head and neck cancer.
- The most common site is the glottis.
- It may present early with hoarseness.
- Treatment options are based on site and extent of disease.

Cancer arising from the squamous epithelium of the larynx is a common head and neck cancer, with well-known risk factors. Proper staging is complex but crucial for treatment formulation. The larynx plays a unique role in respiration, speech, and swallowing. The complex anatomy of the larynx explains the unique patterns of spread of laryngeal cancer:

- The preepiglottic fat is located in the anterior and lateral aspects of the larynx and is often invaded by advanced cancers.
- The recurrent laryngeal nerve innervates the intrinsic laryngeal muscles. Invasion of this nerve causes hoarseness clinically and fixation of the vocal folds.
- The anterior commissure invasion may be a conduit for tumor spread.

The larynx is divided into three anatomic regions: the supraglottic larynx, the glottis, and the subglottic region. The supraglottic larynx includes the epiglottis, the preepiglottic space, the laryngeal aspects of the aryepiglottic folds, the false vocal folds, the arytenoids, and the ventricles. The inferior boundary is a horizontal plane drawn through the apex of the ventricle. This corresponds to the area of transition from squamous to respiratory epithelium. The glottis extends from the true vocal folds inferiorly to roughly 1 cm below the true folds, including the paraglottic space and the anterior and posterior commissures extending inferiorly ~ 1 cm. The sub-glottic larynx has its superior border at the inferior border of the glottis, ~ 1 cm below the true vocal folds, and extends inferiorly to the trachea.

Laryngeal cancer can also be classified by anatomic location. Signs, symptoms, and tumor behavior vary depending on the site and the extent of disease.

◆ Epidemiology

For 2016, the Surveillance, Epidemiology, and End Results (SEER) program of the National Cancer Institute, US National Institutes of Health, estimated that 13,340 men and women would be diagnosed with cancer of the larynx in the United States, with 3,620 patient deaths. Risk factors include smoking and drinking alcohol, which act synergistically; laryngeal papillomatosis; radiation exposure; immunosuppression; and occupational exposure to metals, plastics, and asbestos. Laryngeal carcinoma is more common in African Americans than in European Americans, with a ratio of 3.5:1.

◆ Clinical

Signs and Symptoms

The common symptoms of *supraglottic cancers* include mild odynophagia, mild dysphagia, and mass sensation. Later symptoms include severe dysphagia and aspiration and referred ear pain (otalgia). The mechanism of the referred ear pain is through the activation of the internal branch of the superior laryngeal branch of cranial nerve (CN) X with referral to Arnold's nerve (auricular branch of CN X). Twenty-five to 50% have nodal metastasis to the cervical lymph nodes. Supraglottic tumors often spread to nodes on both sides of the neck.

Glottic cancers account for over half of all laryngeal cancers and present typically with hoarseness. Voice change often happens early and can help diagnose early-stage cancer, improving prognosis. Additionally, the vocal folds' sparse lymphatics leads to a relatively low incidence of nodal metastasis. Advancing glottic cancer can spread posteriorly to the arytenoid complex, causing vocal fold fixation, or anteriorly to the commissure, where it can invade the thyroid cartilage.

Subglottic cancer is uncommon. It may produce biphasic stridor or airway obstruction. Patients may be asymptomatic until advanced stages of disease, and thus the prognosis is worse. Lymphatics drain through the cricothyroid and cricotracheal membranes to the pretracheal, paratracheal, and inferior jugular nodes, and occasionally to mediastinal nodes.

Differential Diagnosis

- Hyperkeratosis
- Papillomas
- Polyps
- Fibromas
- Granulomas
- Laryngoceles
- Laryngeal manifestations of systemic, infectious, or autoimmune disease

◆ Evaluation

The most important adverse prognostic factors for laryngeal cancers include increasing T stage and N stage (see the "Staging of Laryngeal Cancer" section). Other prognostic factors may include sex, age, performance status, and a variety of pathologic features of the tumor, including grade and depth of invasion.

History

History should focus on timing and duration of symptoms and assessment of risk factors. A full understanding of the patient's general medical health, nutritional and cardiopulmonary status, social support, and compliance are crucial for planning of therapy.

Physical Examination

A thorough physical examination of the head and neck should be performed, including inspection of the oral mucosa, laryngoscopy, bimanual palpation of the floor of the mouth and the base of the tongue, and a careful assessment of the cervical lymph nodes and thyroid cartilage contour.

Imaging

Contrast-enhanced computed tomography (CT) scans obtained with appropriate section thickness aid in the evaluation of laryngeal cancer and neck masses. Positron emission tomography (PET)-CT can assist in identifying metastasis and set a baseline of future follow-up for recurrence. At the very least, a chest CT should be performed to rule out a secondary pulmonary malignancy or metastatic disease.

Other Tests

Suspension direct laryngoscopy provides an opportunity for examination under general anesthesia, palpation, and biopsy. Extent of the tumor and the overall condition of the airway mucosa can be evaluated. Panendoscopy (i.e., laryngoscopy, esophagoscopy, and bronchoscopy together) can be performed to rule out synchronous malignancies.

Fine-needle aspiration biopsy (FNAB) of a neck mass may yield a positive result when the certainty of an enlarged lymph node is in question.

Pathology

Ninety to 95% of laryngeal cancers are squamous cell carcinomas (SCCs). Other less common types of laryngeal malignancies include adenoid cystic carcinoma, with a characteristic indolent course of growth and perineural invasion. Rarely, cancer can be of neuroendocrine, stromal, or mesenchymal origin.

◆ Treatment Options

Stage I Laryngeal Cancer

Supraglottis

Standard treatment options include:

- External-beam radiotherapy alone
- Supraglottic laryngectomy

Glottis

Standard treatment options include:

- Radiotherapy
- Cordectomy for very carefully selected patients with limited and superficial T1 lesions
- Partial or hemilaryngectomy or total laryngectomy, depending on anatomic considerations
- Laser excision (endoscopic laryngectomy)

Subglottis

- Radiotherapy alone

Stage II Laryngeal Cancer

Supraglottis

Standard treatment options include:

- External-beam radiotherapy, supraglottic laryngectomy, or total laryngectomy, depending on location of the lesion, clinical status of the patient, and expertise of the treatment team
- Postoperative radiotherapy, indicated for positive or close surgical margins

Glottis

Standard treatment options include:

- Radiotherapy
- Partial or hemilaryngectomy or total laryngectomy, depending on anatomic considerations; under certain circumstances, laser microsurgery may be appropriate.

Subglottis

- Lesions can be treated successfully by radiotherapy alone with preservation of normal voice.

Stage III Laryngeal Cancer

Supraglottis

Standard treatment options include:

- Surgery with or without postoperative radiotherapy
- Definitive radiotherapy with surgery for salvage of radiation failures
- Chemotherapy administered concomitantly with radiotherapy; can be considered for patients who would require total laryngectomy for control of disease

Glottis

Standard treatment options include:

- Surgery with or without postoperative radiotherapy
- Definitive radiotherapy with surgery for the salvage of radiation failures

- Chemotherapy administered concomitantly with radiotherapy; can be considered for patients who would require total laryngectomy for control of disease

Subglottis

Standard treatment options include:

- Laryngectomy plus isolated thyroidectomy and tracheoesophageal node dissection, usually followed by postoperative radiotherapy
- Treatment by radiotherapy alone, indicated for patients who are not candidates for surgery

Stage IV Laryngeal Cancer

Supraglottis

Standard treatment options include:

- Total laryngectomy with postoperative radiotherapy
- Definitive radiotherapy with surgery for salvage of radiation failures
- Chemotherapy administered concomitantly with radiotherapy; can be considered for patients who would require total laryngectomy for control of disease

Glottis

Standard treatment options include:

- Total laryngectomy with postoperative radiotherapy
- Definitive radiotherapy with surgery for salvage of radiation failures
- Chemotherapy administered concomitantly with radiotherapy; can be considered for patients who would require total laryngectomy for control of disease

Subglottis

Standard treatment options include:

- Laryngectomy plus total thyroidectomy and bilateral tracheoesophageal node dissection, usually followed by postoperative radiotherapy
- Treatment by radiotherapy alone, indicated for patients who are not candidates for surgery

Treatment Types

Radiation

Radiation is sometimes preferred because of the good oncologic results, preservation of the voice, and the possibility of surgical salvage in patients whose disease recurs locally.

Surgery

Surgical treatment options should be reviewed carefully to ensure adequate pulmonary and swallowing function postoperatively.

- *Transoral laser microsurgery:* Transoral laser microsurgery is ideal for the treatment of early to intermediate glottic and supraglottic cancer. It may be performed under suspension microlaryngoscopy with a laser. The tumor may be transected and removed piecemeal. This treatment has the same indications and contraindications as open partial laryngectomies. A functional cricoarytenoid unit must be preserved. Survival and laryngeal preservation are comparable to other conventional treatments.

- *Transoral robotic surgery (TORS):* Transoral robotic-assisted supraglottic laryngectomy may be appropriate for certain supraglottic cancers.

- *Partial laryngectomy:* Several procedures constitute partial laryngectomies:

  o *Vertical hemilaryngectomy:* When disease is small and involves only one vocal fold and arytenoid cartilage, a vertical hemilaryngectomy can be performed. This procedure removes, unilaterally, the true vocal fold from anterior to commissure to vocal process of arytenoid, as well as the false vocal fold, the ventricle paraglottic space, and the overlying thyroid cartilage. Resection can be extended to include the whole arytenoid. A frontolateral hemilaryngectomy additionally removes the anterior commissures, part of the contralateral vocal fold, and the overlying thyroid cartilage.

  o *Supraglottic laryngectomy:* Supraglottic laryngectomy can be performed in tumors limited to the supraglottic region with normal vocal fold mobility, with 2-mm margin at the anterior commissure. It is contraindicated if disease extends anteriorly into the thyroid cartilage or the anterior neck or posteriorly to postcricoid or intra-arytenoid areas or prevertebral fascia, and in patients with poor pulmonary function. This procedure may remove the entire epiglottis and aryepiglottic folds, false vocal folds, preepiglottic space, and part of the thyroid cartilage, and it can be extended to include the vallecula, wall of the piriform recess, and the base of the tongue up to the circumvallate papillae. Supraglottic laryngectomy may be performed open or transorally utilizing a robotic platform.

  o *Supracricoid laryngectomy:* Supracricoid laryngectomy can be performed for removal of large tumors, even certain T4 tumors of the glottis and supraglottis. However, it is contraindicated in subglottic extension, 10 mm anteriorly or 5 mm posteriorly, and with involvement of both arytenoid cartilages, the hyoid bone, the base of the tongue, or the cricoid cartilage. Supracricoid laryngectomy resects both true and both false vocal folds, the paraglottic space, and the entire thyroid cartilage, as well as the epiglottis and one arytenoid if necessary. Reconstruction involves cricohyoidoepiglottopexy or cricohyoidopexy if the epiglottis is removed.

- *Total laryngectomy:* A total laryngectomy may be performed in the event of radiation failure with unclear extent of recurrence, in the event of chondroradionecrosis, or when other conservation techniques are not feasible. A total laryngectomy removes the entire larynx, including the thyroid and cricoid cartilages, part of the thyroid gland, and the paratracheal lymph nodes, and it may involve removal of the overlying strap muscles.

✦ Complications

- Psychosocial trauma from surgery and/or radiotherapy
- Vocal fold–powered voice loss in some procedures
- Aspiration pneumonia, in some procedures
- Osteoradionecrosis
- Chondroradionecrosis
- Chronic pain
- Breathing difficulties
- Stoma infections
- Potential stoma malignancies

✦ Outcome and Follow-Up

Consideration should be given to airway protection, nutritional support, and voice rehabilitation. Establishing a stable airway via tracheotomy should be considered preoperatively for tumors threatening the airway or obscuring intubation. Preemptive gastrostomy tube placement can ensure maximized preoperative and postoperative nutritional status. If voice preservation is not possible in the treatment plan, a noninvasive option for voice rehabilitation is an electrolarynx. Alternately, patients can learn techniques for producing esophageal voice, using expulsion of air through the esophagus to generate the base vibration for speech. With tracheoesophageal puncture, a fistula can be created between the cervical trachea and the esophagus to allow efficient swallowing of air for esophageal voicing.

Close oncologic follow-up care is necessary because second primary cancers, recurrences, and late metastases are all strong possibilities, especially if the patient continues to smoke.

✦ Staging of Laryngeal Cancer

Primary Tumor: Supraglottis (T)

TX: Primary tumor cannot be assessed

Tis: Carcinoma in situ

T1:   Tumor limited to one subsite of supraglottis *with normal vocal fold mobility*

T2:   Tumor invading mucosa of more than one adjacent subsite of supraglottis or glottis or region outside the supraglottis (e.g., the mucosa of the base of the tongue, vallecula, or medial wall of piriform recess) *without fixation of the larynx*

T3:   Tumor limited to larynx *with vocal fold fixation* and/or invading any of the following: the postcricoid area, preepiglottic tissues, paraglottic space, and/or minor thyroid cartilage erosion (e.g., inner cortex)

T4:   Moderately advanced to advanced disease

   T4a: Moderately advanced local disease; tumor invading through the thyroid cartilage and/or invading tissues beyond the larynx (e.g., the trachea, the soft tissues of the neck including the deep extrinsic muscles of the tongue, the strap muscles, the thyroid, or the esophagus)

T4b1 Very advanced local disease; tumor invading the prevertebral space, encasing the carotid artery, or invading the mediastinal structures

Primary Tumor: Glottis (T)

TX: Primary tumor cannot be assessed

Tis: Carcinoma in situ

T1:   Tumor limited to the vocal fold(s) (may involve anterior or posterior commissure) *with normal mobility*

T1a: Tumor limited to one vocal fold

T1b: Tumor involves both vocal folds

T2:   Tumor extending to the supraglottis and/or the subglottis *and/or with impaired vocal fold mobility*

T3:   Tumor limited to the larynx *with vocal fold fixation* and/or invasion of the paraglottic space, and/or the inner cortex of thyroid cartilage

T4:   Moderately advanced to advanced disease

T4a: Tumor invading through the outer cortex of the thyroid cartilage and/or invading tissues beyond the larynx (e.g., the trachea, the soft tissues of the neck including the deep extrinsic muscles of the tongue, strap muscles, the thyroid, or the esophagus)

T4b: Tumor invading the prevertebral space, encasing the carotid artery, or invading mediastinal structures

Primary Tumor: Subglottis (T)

TX: Primary tumor cannot be assessed

Tis: Carcinoma in situ

T1:   Tumor limited to the subglottis

T2:   Tumor extending to the vocal fold(s) *with normal or impaired mobility*

T3:   Tumor limited to the larynx *with vocal fold fixation*

T4:   Moderately advanced to advanced disease

T4a: Tumor invading the cricoid or thyroid cartilage and/or invades the tissues beyond the larynx (e.g., the trachea, the soft tissues of the neck including the deep extrinsic muscles of the tongue, the strap muscles, the thyroid, or the esophagus)

T4b: Tumor invading the prevertebral space, encasing the carotid artery, or invading the mediastinal structures

T Category Considerations

- Supraglottis: Normal vocal fold mobility (T1), fixation of the larynx (T2), and vocal fold fixation (T3) may be determined only clinically.
- Glottis: Normal vocal fold mobility (T1), impaired vocal fold mobility (T2), and vocal fold fixation (T3) may be determined only clinically.

- Subglottis: Normal or impaired vocal fold mobility (T2) and vocal fold fixation (T3) may be determined only clinically.

Regional Lymph Nodes (N)*

NX: Regional lymph nodes cannot be assessed

N0:   No regional lymph node metastasis

N1:   Metastasis to a single ipsilateral lymph node measuring ≤ 3 cm in greatest diameter and ENE negative

N2:   Further divided into three categories:

> N2a: Single ipsilateral lymph node > 3 and ≤ 6 cm and ENE negative (pathologic staging also includes a single ipsilateral or contralateral lymph node ≤ 3 cm and ENE positive)
>
> N2b: Multiple ipsilateral lymph nodes ≤ 6 cm and ENE negative
>
> N2c: Bilateral or contralateral lymph nodes ≤ 6 cm in greatest dimension and ENE negative

N3:   Now further divided into two categories:

> N3a: Metastasis to a lymph node > 6 cm, ENE negative
>
> N3b: Metastasis to a single lymph node that is ENE positive (pathologic staging includes single lymph nodes that are ENE positive >3cm), or metastasis to multiple lymph nodes with any ENE positive

A designation of "U" or "L" can be attached to the N category to indicate nodes above ("U") or below ("L") the lower border of the cricoid. Similarly, clinical and pathologic ENE should be recorded as ENE (−) or ENE (+). Clinical and pathologic staging are similar with the differences noted in parenthesis.

*Superior mediastinal lymph nodes are considered regional lymph nodes (level VII). Midline nodes are considered ipsilateral nodes.

Distant Metastasis (M)

MX: Distant metastasis cannot be assessed

M0:   No distant metastasis

M1:   Distant metastasis

American Joint Committee on Cancer Stage Groupings of Supraglottis, Glottis, and Subglottis (8th edition)

Stage 0 disease: Carcinoma in situ (TisN0M0)

Stage I disease: Includes only T1 N0 M0 tumors

Stage II disease: Includes only T2 N0 M0 tumors

Stage III disease: Includes T3 N0 M0 and T1 -3 disease that is N1 M0

Stage IVA disease: Includes T4a disease with N0-N2 M0 disease and T1-T3 disease that is N2 M0

Stage IVB disease: Includes T4b disease with any nodal disease or T1-T4a disease with N3 disease without distant metastases (M0)

Stage IVC disease: Any disease with distant metastases (M1)

See **Table 6.7** in Chapter 6.3.3.

6.3.11 Speech Options after Laryngectomy

◆ Key Features

- Partial laryngectomy may make phonation difficult, resulting in dysphonia.
- Total laryngectomy, associated with removal of the larynx and modification of the respiratory tract, results in a total loss of phonatory ability (aphonia).
- Evaluation for appropriate post–total laryngectomy communication is multifactorial.
- The three primary options for communication are the electrolarynx, tracheoesophageal puncture, and esophageal speech.

Surgery to the larynx, whether in the form of total or partial laryngectomy, has the potential to impact the vocal communication system greatly. Partial laryngeal surgery often requires intensive vocal rehabilitation, and full functionality may never be regained. Total laryngectomy results in aphonia, and there are several communication options to replace this function.

◆ Epidemiology

The annual incidence of diagnosed head and neck cancer in the United States is ~ 45,660 cases. Of these, cancer of the larynx accounts for 25% of cases (see **Chapter 6.3.10**). Cancers diagnosed in the first or second stage are more likely to be treated with local surgical excision or chemoradiation therapy; cancers of the larynx in the third or fourth stage are more likely to result in a total removal of the larynx in combination with chemotherapy and radiotherapy. Of the three communication options for postlaryngectomy, 55% of individuals use an electrolarynx as a primary communication method, 31% use a tracheoesophageal puncture prosthesis, and 6% use the esophageal speech method (8% remain nonvocal).

◆ Clinical

Signs and Symptoms

Following partial laryngeal surgery, patients often present with dysphonia characterized by a weak, strained, or breathy vocal quality. Patients who have had a total laryngectomy have a total inability to phonate postoperatively secondary to removal of the larynx, including the vocal folds.

Differential Diagnosis

In patients with partial laryngeal surgery, it is important to determine whether the current vocal qualities are a result of surgical treatment versus an advancement or recurrence of the carcinoma. Any change in previous alaryngeal communication abilities of individuals following a total laryngectomy can indicate recurrence of cancer and should be carefully evaluated.

◆ Evaluation

Evaluation for communication methods following total laryngectomy include an evaluation of physical changes from surgery and chemoradiation therapy to assess for the ability for electronic larynx placement either transcervically (neck-type) or intraorally (mouth-type), stoma size and placement for stomal occlusion with tracheoesophageal puncture voicing. Additionally, manual dexterity, motivation level, and financial/insurance resources should be considered.

◆ Treatment Options

After Partial Laryngeal Surgery

Voice rehabilitation following partial laryngeal surgery should include treatment with a speech-language pathologist and should focus on appropriate vocal hygiene, adequate breath support, decreased muscle tension, and oral resonance (see **Chapter 5.3.4**).

After Total Laryngectomy

Electrolarynx

A battery-powered electronic device called an electrolarynx is used. Depending on anatomic changes following surgery, an electrolarynx can be placed either transcervically (neck-type) or intraorally (mouth-type). The electrolarynx produces a vibration that is transmitted intraorally through a straw attached to the device or through the tissues of the neck or cheek.

The electrolarynx offers a communication option immediately after surgery, is relatively easy to use, and has a lower one-time cost (when compared with the tracheoesophageal puncture voice prosthesis). Disadvantages include a mechanical sound quality, requirement for one free hand during communication, and unfamiliarity of the sound to most listeners.

Tracheoesophageal Puncture Voice Prosthesis

For the tracheoesophageal puncture voice prosthesis, a small fistula is surgically placed in the tracheoesophageal wall, ~ 1 cm below the upper lip of the stoma. This fistula is kept patent by the insertion of a one-way valved prosthesis. Voicing is then achieved by passing air from the trachea to the esophagus via stomal occlusion with either manual finger occlusion or a hands-free stomal attachment.

The voice prosthesis allows for an esophageal sound production, which is then shaped by the oral cavity for speech production. Individuals with a laryngectomy often feel this method allows speech to be most comparable to preoperative speech in terms of quality, fluency, and ease of production. Disadvantages include anatomic variations and mechanical problems. Anatomic variations include hypertonicity or flaccidity of the pharyngoesophageal muscle segment, stomal stenosis, and stoma irregularity. Mechanical problems include size, fit, prosthesis breakdown (secondary to *Candida* infection or gastroesophageal reflux disease), or dislodgement. Other disadvantages include the cost of the prosthesis (which must be replaced every few months), accessibility to a speech-language pathologist or otolaryngologist trained to change and maintain indwelling valves, and manual dexterity for cleaning and management.

Esophageal Speech

Speech is produced from a learned method of vibrating the pharyngoesophageal muscle segment. Air is introduced into the esophagus through the oral cavity and is then passed back out of the esophagus past the pharyngoesophageal segment. This can be done using either a glossopharyngeal press method or an inhalation method.

Esophageal speech enables communication without the use of mechanical or prosthetic devices and allows more natural sound production. Disadvantages include an increased time period for learning this method (estimated 4 to 6 months of regular speech therapy and daily practice), limited success rates, and decreased ability to control volume. Use of esophageal speech is becoming rarer, with fewer speech therapists trained in teaching patients this modality of postlaryngectomy speech and improvements with tracheoesophageal speech.

◆ Outcome and Follow-Up

Any patient with laryngeal carcinoma must follow up with an otolaryngologist for at least 5 years postoperatively. A patient with an indwelling tracheoesophageal puncture voice prosthesis must follow up with a speech-language pathologist or otolaryngologist trained in prosthesis management for all changes, approximately every 3 months. A patient with a nonindwelling tracheoesophageal puncture voice prosthesis (i.e., one that is removed, cleaned, and reinserted by the patient on a frequent basis) should follow up with a speech-language pathologist or an otolaryngologist yearly for tract evaluation and fitting. Additionally, follow-up should occur immediately for prosthesis dislodgement or significant change in sound quality, as this can indicate a more significant problem, recurrence, or aspiration or may allow tract stenosis or closure.

6.3.12 Referred Otalgia in Head and Neck Disease

◆ Key Features

- Referred otalgia is the sensation of ear pain originating from a source outside the ear.
- If no otic source for otalgia can be identified, then malignancy must be investigated and excluded.

By definition, referred otalgia is the sensation of ear pain originating from a source outside the ear. Many remote anatomic sites share innervations with the ear, and noxious stimuli to these areas may be perceived as otalgia

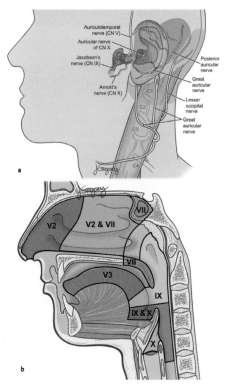

Fig. 6.14 Sources of referred otalgia. **(a)** The sensory innervation of the ear and periauricular area is from multiple nerves, including branches from cranial nerves (CN) V, VII, IX, and X as well as spinal nerve C2 and C3 rootlets. **(b)** Multiple areas in the head and neck share sensory innervation with the ear. (Used with permission from Sclafani AP, ed. *Total Otolaryngology—Head and Neck Surgery*. New York, NY: Thieme;2015:117.)

(**Fig. 6.14**). In adult patients, especially those at risk, if no otic source for otalgia can be identified, malignancy must be investigated and excluded, especially for adult patients with known risk factors.

The sensory innervation of the ear is provided by the auriculotemporal branch of the fifth cranial nerve (CN) (mandibular nerve [CN V$_3$]), contributions from C2 and C3 through the cervical plexus via the great auricular nerve, the tympanic nerve [branch of CN IX], the auricular nerve [branch of CN X], and the sensory branch of CN VII [Ramsay-Hunt branch], which innervates a portion of the external auditory canal and surrounding concha.

The explanation for complex sensory innervation of the ear ultimately lies in the ear's embryologic development. The otic vesicle comes to rest central to branchial arches 1, 2, 3, and 4. The sensory and motor nerves of these arches are CN V, CN VII, CN IX, and CN X, respectively.

✦ Etiology

Etiology for referred otalgia includes:

- Dental disorders
- Ill-fitting dentures
- Bruxism
- Cervical osteoarthritis
- Cervicofacial myofascial pain syndrome
- Posttraumatic neuralgia (greater auricular neuroma)
- Chronic pharyngitis
- Eagle's syndrome
- Postviral neuralgia (Ramsay-Hunt's syndrome, postherpetic neuralgia)
- Temporal arteritis
- Parotid neoplasia
- Gastroesophageal reflux

Lesions of the anterior two-thirds of the tongue and inferior oral cavity tend to refer pain to the ear via CN V_3. Lesions of the lateral base of the tongue, the tonsillar region, and the inferior two-thirds of the nasopharynx cause deep, intense otalgia via sensory impulses through CN IX. Lesions of the supraglottic larynx communicate sensory afferents via the internal laryngeal branch of the superior laryngeal nerve of CN X. Lesions of the posterior oropharynx, the inferior nasopharynx, the medial aspect of the base of the tongue, and the hypopharynx tend to refer pain to the ear owing to the overlapping innervations of both CN IX and X (via the pharyngeal plexus).

✦ Evaluation

The evaluation of a patient with otalgia begins with a detailed history and a thorough head and neck examination. Questions addressed include the character and timing of the otalgia, exacerbating and alleviating factors of the otalgia, the patient's past otologic history, the symptoms associated with the otalgia (tinnitus, hearing loss, vertigo), the presence of constitutional symptoms (to detect malignancies), and sinus and dental questions.

A head and neck examination is fundamental in evaluating otalgia. A thorough otologic examination, with a tuning fork test at two frequencies (256 and 512 Hz), is important. The CNs are examined and compared bilaterally. The nose, sinuses, oral cavity, oral pharynx, and neck are inspected and palpated to look for sources of referred otalgia. In assessing otalgia in the setting of a normal otologic examination, a fiberoptic nasopharyngolaryngoscopy is mandated to look for lesions that can be potentially noxious to the trigeminal (CN V), facial (CN VII), glossopharyngeal (CN IX), or vagus (CN X) nerves. Attention should be directed to the endolarynx to examine the mucosa for signs of malignancy and gastroesophageal reflux.

◆ Treatment Options

Treatment consists of appropriate treatment of the source of otalgia in combination with pain management.

6.3.13 Neck Dissection

◆ Key Features

- The presence of cervical lymph node metastasis reduces survival of patients with head and neck squamous cell carcinoma (SCC) by up to 50%.
- Neck dissection or lymphadenectomy is a surgical procedure in which the fibro-fatty contents of the neck are removed for the prevention or treatment of cervical metastasis.
- Neck dissection is most commonly used in the treatment of cancers of the upper aero-digestive tract, skin of the head and neck, thyroid, and salivary glands.

Cancers of the head and neck tend to metastasize to cervical lymph nodes. The term "neck dissection" refers to the systematic removal of lymph nodes in the neck. To eradicate cancer in the cervical lymph nodes and to help determine the need for additional therapy (staging) when no lymph nodes are clinically identified, neck dissection may be performed. Although used most commonly for the management of cancers of the upper aerodigestive tract, neck dissection is also used for malignancies of the skin of the head and neck, the thyroid, and the salivary glands.

The original surgical procedure described for the treatment of metastatic neck cancer was a radical neck dissection (RND), first described by Crile in 1906; until several decades ago, this was considered to be the standard procedure for the management of clinically positive neck disease in the setting of head and neck cancer. More recently, a shift toward more conservative surgical procedures has been adopted. This shift aims at removing lymphatic tissue but preserving adjacent nonlymphatic structures. In addition, specific nodal groups at risk for metastatic disease, as predicted by the size, location, and other features of the primary tumor, are addressed in a selective fashion in certain cases.

◆ Classification of Neck Levels

The evaluation of the drainage pattern of the primary tumor site in the upper aerodigestive tract has led to the understanding and identification of nodal groups at risk for cervical metastases. The neck has been divided into six such groups, called neck levels.

Level 1: The Submandibular and Submental Triangles

Level 1 consists of the submandibular and submental triangles. The submandibular triangle is bordered by the mandible superiorly, the posterior belly of the digastric muscle posteroinferiorly, and the anterior belly of the digastric muscle anteroinferiorly. Its floor is the hyoglossus muscle. The submental triangle is the region between the bilateral anterior bellies of the digastric muscle and the hyoid bone. Level 1 can be divided into Levels 1A and 1B by the anterior belly of the digastric muscle.

Level 2: The Jugular-Digastric Region

Level 2 is known as the jugular digastric region. Its boundaries are the skull base superiorly, the carotid bifurcation inferiorly, the posterior border of the sternocleidomastoid muscle, and the lateral border of the sternohyoid and sternothyroid muscles medially. Level 2 can be divided into 2A and 2B by the course of the accessory nerve (CN XI).

Level 3: The Middle Jugular Region

Level 3 is the middle jugular region. It is bordered by the carotid bifurcation superiorly, the junction of the omohyoid and sternocleidomastoid muscle at the jugular vein inferiorly, the posterior border of the sternocleidomastoid muscle laterally, and the lateral border of the sternohyoid muscle medially.

Level 4: The Lower Jugular Region

Level 4 is the lower jugular region and extends from the omohyoid superiorly to the clavicle inferiorly. It extends to the posterior border of the sternocleidomastoid muscle and the lateral border of the sternohyoid muscle medially. The fascia overlying the phrenic nerve and the brachial plexus is the deep boundary.

Level 5: The Posterior Triangle

Level 5 is also known as the posterior triangle. It includes the lymph nodes between the posterior border of the sternocleidomastoid muscle and the anterior border of the trapezius muscle. It also extends to the clavicle inferiorly. The course of the accessory nerve is encompassed in this triangle. The "supraclavicular region" is also found in level 5. Level 5 can be divided into level 5A and 5B by the horizontal line at the level of the cricoid cartilage.

Level 6: The Anterior Compartment

Level 6 is the anterior compartment and includes the midline lymph nodes adjacent to the trachea and thyroid gland. The borders of this region are the hyoid bone superiorly, the sternal notch inferiorly, and the carotid sheath laterally.

♦ Classification of Neck Dissections

The current classification of neck dissection has been developed by the Committee of Head and Neck Surgery & Oncology of the American Academy of Otolaryngology—Head and Neck Surgery and is based on the following principles:

1. An RND is the standard basic procedure for removal of lymph nodes from the neck, and all other procedures represent a modification of this procedure. It is defined as the en bloc removal of the nodal groups between the mandible and the clavicle. An RND includes the removal of the internal jugular vein, the accessory nerve, and the sternocleidomastoid muscle.

2. When modification of the RND involves preservation of a nonlymphatic structure, the procedure is termed a modified neck dissection.

3. When modification involves preservation of one or more lymph groups that are routinely removed in an RND, the procedure is termed a selective neck dissection (SND). The procedure is usually performed if there is no palpable neck disease (clinically N0 neck) but the risk of occult metastasis to the cervical lymph nodes is likely > 20%. For example, a T1 N0 SCC of the oral tongue extending deeper than 4 mm is an indication to perform an SND involving levels 1 to 3, possibly level 4. SNDs include a supraomohyoid neck dissection, a lateral compartment neck dissection, a posterior lateral neck dissection, and anterior compartment neck dissection.

   - Supraomohyoid neck dissection involves removal of levels 1 through 3 and is usually performed in the setting of oral cavity tumors and N0 neck disease.

   - Lateral compartment neck dissection includes levels 2 through 4 and is used in conjunction with the surgical resection of tumors of the larynx, hypopharynx, oropharynx, and thyroid.

   - Posterior lateral neck dissection includes levels 2 through 5. It may include the retroauricular and suboccipital nodal regions as well. Posterior lateral neck dissection is typically performed for cutaneous malignancies of the scalp and face.

   - Anterior compartment or central compartment neck dissection includes level 6 and is used for tumors found in the larynx, the hypopharynx, the subglottis, the cervical esophagus, and the thyroid. Anterior neck dissection is commonly performed for papillary thyroid cancer with metastases to the lymph nodes.

4. When modification involves removal of addition lymph node groups or nonlymphatic structures relative to the RND, the procedure is termed an extended RND. An extended RND involves the additional removal of muscles, nerves, vessels, and lymph nodes as dictated by primary disease or the presence of metastases found in surgery. An extended neck dissection may involve the retropharyngeal lymph nodes, the hypoglossal nerve, portions of the prevertebral musculature and the carotid artery. Also, certain parotid gland malignancies may require total parotidectomy combined with neck dissection.

◆ Complications of Neck Dissection

Complications may be divided into intraoperative or postoperative. It is important to remember that certain medical conditions, such as postradiation treatment, poor nutritional status, hypothyroidism, alcoholism, and diabetes, may increase the risk of intraoperative and postoperative complications.

Intraoperative complications of neck dissections include hemorrhage and damage to adjacent CNs. During a submandibular submental dissection, the marginal mandibular branch of the facial nerve, the hypoglossal nerve, and the lingual nerve are all at risk. Injury to the phrenic nerve may cause hemidiaphragm paresis but is typically symptomatic only in patients with significant pulmonary disease. Injury to the vagus may cause vocal fold paralysis. Injury to the brachial plexus is rare but can occur, causing upper extremity weakness. Injury to the sympathetic trunk may cause Horner's syndrome. Postoperative complications include hematoma, shoulder dysfunction, wound infection, salivary or chylus fistula, and carotid artery blowout.

6.3.14 Robotic-Assisted Head and Neck Surgery

◆ Key Features

- Robotic systems allow excellent visualization, stability, and increased range of motion for head and neck surgery.
- The technology enables minimally invasive techniques in the head and neck region.
- Current clinical applications in otolaryngology include transoral resection of oral, oropharyngeal, and supraglottic tumors.
- Other applications include transaxillary and facelift incision thyroidectomies.
- Further applications are expected to follow in the near future.

Robotic-assisted surgery is an emerging technology whose application to otolaryngology—head and neck surgery has been challenging because of the spatial and technical limitations of the head and neck region. Yet the value of robots for head and neck surgery has recently been demonstrated and is growing. The word "robot," from the Czech word *robota*, meaning forced labor, was coined for Karel Čapek's 1921 science fiction play *R.U.R. (Rossum's Universal Robots)*. The development of electronic and digital data processing and control systems made real robots possible, and the era of robots in surgery commenced in 1994 when the first AESOP (Automated Endoscopic System for Optical Positioning, a voice-controlled camera holder) prototype robot was used clinically.

◆ The Robots

The robotic da Vinci Surgical System, or dVSS (Intuitive Surgical Inc., Sunnyvale, CA), is in use in fields such as general surgery, urology, gynecology, cardiothoracic surgery, and recently otolaryngology—head and neck surgery. The dVSS provides several advantages over conventional laparoscopy, such as three-dimensional (3D) vision, motion scaling, intuitive movements, visual immersion, and tremor filtration.

In 2015 the Medrobotics Flex Robotic System (Medrobotics, Raynham, MA) received FDA clearance for use in head and neck surgery, representing a newer generation of robotic technology for transoral surgery. It combines a highly flexible robotic scope with a variety of flexible instruments to work in the oral cavity, oropharynx, hypopharynx and larynx.

◆ Transoral Robotic-Assisted Surgery

A surgical camera and instrumentation are passed through the patient's open mouth and controlled by the surgeon sitting at the adjacent console. The surgeon directs the graspers and cautery or laser to the tumor location and resects under direct visualization. Transoral robotic-assisted surgery (TORS) may preclude the need for mandibulotomy and tracheotomy and allow thorough resection of tumors under direct visualization.

The dVSS is composed of the following:

- Four robotic hands: Named EndoWrist instruments, they function like hands. They can grasp objects, twist, and turn. The robotic hands are relatively small and allow the surgeon to make very precise movements.
- 3D camera: This is a high-definition camera that gives the surgeon a 3D image of the surgical field. The camera includes significant magnification, enabling the surgeon to zoom in on the operative field as needed.
- Console: The surgeon sits at the console, where he or she controls the four robotic hands and sees images from the 3D camera.

The four robotic hands and the 3D camera are inserted through incision(s) or a natural orifice, depending on the specific procedure. The two access points most used to date for the dVSS are transoral access for tongue base, tonsil, supraglottic, parapharyngeal, and skull base tumors as well as obstructive sleep apnea surgery; and transaxillary access for scarless thyroidectomy. Further options—facelift, transcervical, and transoral access for neck tumors—are currently under investigation.

The Medrobotics Flex Robotic System is specifically designed and FDA-cleared for TORS. Unlike previous robotic-surgical instruments, which were linear and dependent on different angled cameras (0° and 30°) in order to change viewing direction, the Flex Robotic System is based on a flexible robotic scope and flexible instrumentation.

The Flex Robotic System consists of four primary components:

- The Flex Console, which houses the physician control handle, a touch screen visual display, and the touch screen monitor

- The Flex Base, a reusable assembly that transfers electronic signals from the console into mechanical motions
- The Flex Scope, a sterile, single-use component that mounts on the Flex Base and houses the flexible portion of the robot and components to move it
- The Flex Cart and Stand as support for the Flex Base and Flex Scope; part of the operating table must be positioned appropriately to reach the oral cavity.

Setup time for the entire system is reported at less than 10 minutes. In preparation for surgery, the Flex Base is placed midline on the patient and the Flex Scope is positioned directly at the opening of the oral cavity. In this system, there are no external arms. The instrument arms are coaxial to the scope, allowing for a smaller initial opening and more movement within a limited-size surgical cavity. The instruments can be exchanged without the need for assistance. The Flex Robotic System has a smaller footprint, allowing more room within the operating theater and for greater unit portability.

◆ Transaxillary Thyroidectomy

The goals of minimally invasive thyroid surgery are to maintain an acceptable level of safety while improving cosmesis. The patient is placed in the supine position under general anesthesia. The lesion-side arm is raised and fixed for the shortest distance from the axilla to the anterior neck. A skin incision is made in the anterior axillary fold. A subplatysmal plane is developed immediately superficial to the pectoralis major and clavicle. Once the subplatysmal plane is sufficiently large, retractors are placed and the dVSS robotic arms are docked.

A second skin incision is made on the medial side of the anterior chest wall for insertion of the fourth robot arm. The operation then proceeds in similar fashion to an open thyroidectomy. The application of the remote access robotic axillary thyroidectomy in the United States yielded a number of significant complications not previously encountered in thyroid surgery, including brachial plexus injury, esophageal perforation, and high-volume blood loss from damage to the great vessels. The rate of conversion to an anterior cervical approach is reported to be up to 2%.

◆ Robotic Facelift Thyroidectomy

Robotic facelift thyroidectomy was developed to overcome some of the limitations associated with the robotic axillary thyroidectomy. Robotic facelift thyroidectomy incorporates a single postauricular modified facelift incision as the access site, a fixed retractor system, and utilization of the surgical robot. This technique, while not "minimally invasive," reduces the extent of dissection by approximately 38% as compared to transaxillary thyroidectomy, shortening the recovery time, reducing postoperative discomfort, and permitting drainless outpatient surgery.

◆ Advantages of Robotic-Assisted Surgery

- Robotic-assisted surgery allows for minimally invasive techniques with small incisions, less blood loss, and reduced recovery time.
- It allows access to areas typically inaccessible with conventional laparoscopic techniques.
- It increases the surgeon's dexterity while minimizing tremor.
- It provides excellent optics and improved visualization (3D view with depth perception).

◆ Disadvantages of Robotic-Assisted Surgery

- The cost is high.
- The size of the system may be awkward: older systems especially have relatively large footprints and cumbersome robotic arms.
- There is a lack of compatible instruments and equipment.
- The surgeon has no tactile feedback ("feel of tissue")— this is somewhat resolved in the Medrobotics system.
- No billing codes have yet been established for TORS.

6.3.15   Skin Cancer of the Head, Face, and Neck

6.3.15.1   Basal Cell Carcinoma

◆ Key Features

- Basal cell carcinoma is the most common skin cancer (80%).
- It is derived from basilar keratinocytes.
- Basal cell carcinoma is slow-growing, rarely metastasizing.
- It has a high cure rate from excision with minimal margins.

Basal cell carcinoma (BCC) is the most common cancer in humans. As sun exposure is the heaviest risk for developing BCC, 90% of these cancers are found in the head and neck region. Although prevention is best (by reducing sun exposure), BCC is rarely aggressive with very low rates of metastasis (< 1%) and can usually be treated with complete surgical excision.

◆ Epidemiology

No great epidemiologic source exists for BCC, as it is usually included under the "non-melanoma" skin cancer data. The National Cancer Institute estimates > 1,000,000 new cases of BCC and squamous cell carcinoma (SCC) combined, with mortality figures of < 2,000 individuals. In the United States, BCC is more common in the Sunbelt states. Farmers, construction workers, and other workers who spend many hours in the sun have a skin cancer risk. Risk factors also include light-pigmented skin and blue/green eyes. Persons of African descent rarely develop BCC, but there is higher incidence in albino Africans, pointing to the central protective role of melanin. Genetic conditions with high BCC incidence include xeroderma pigmentosum (autosomal recessive defect in DNA repair protein) and nevoid BCC syndrome (i.e., Gorlin's syndrome, which is an autosomal dominant condition involving jaw cysts, bifid ribs, scoliosis, palmar pits, and multifocal BCC in situ in childhood). Other risk factors include damage to skin via ultraviolet (UV) B radiation (sun, tanning beds), ionizing radiation exposure, arsenic exposure, prior trauma or chronic irritation, and immunosuppression.

◆ Clinical

Signs and Symptoms

Basal cell carcinoma usually presents as an indolent growth or discolored patch on the skin, rarely with itching, bleeding, and ulceration. The appearance of the lesion varies with the type (see Pathology).

Differential Diagnosis

- Actinic keratosis
- Seborrheic keratosis
- Keratoacanthoma
- Nevi
- Bowen's disease
- SCC
- Melanoma

◆ Evaluation

Physical Exam

A routine physical exam should be performed with an emphasis on the scalp, folds around the nose, lips, canthi, and ears, as these areas carry higher risk of recurrence.

Other Tests

No imaging or laboratory tests are necessary, but suspicious lesions should be biopsied.

Pathology

There are four histopathologic types of BCC:

Nodular

This the most common form of BCC (60–80%). It most often appears on the head, neck, and upper back. The lesions appear as waxy papules with central depression or rolled edges and a pearly translucency. Often, telangiectasias appear over the surface, which can lead to bleeding and crusting, especially with ulceration.

Morpheaform

This form constitutes 10 to 20% of BCC. This is the most aggressive variety, with the worst prognosis. It appears commonly on the face as a sclerotic, sometimes depressed, plaque with yellowish color and irregular borders. Bleeding and ulceration are rare, and this lesion may be mistaken for a scar. These tumor cells express collagenases, which allow them to travel along peripheral nerves and embryonic fusion planes.

Pigmented

This type is very similar to the nodular type, but with the additional characteristic of pigmentation, which may resemble a benign nevus or melanoma. These lesions are more commonly found on darker-skinned individuals.

Superficial

This type appears commonly on the trunk (rarely on the head and neck) as a scaly, indurated patch with an irregular border, often mimicking psoriasis or eczema or resembling actinic keratosis. Growth is slow with low rates of erosion and invasion. Multiple superficial BCCs have been associated with arsenic exposure.

◆ Treatment Options

Medical

The application of 5-fluorouracil (5-FU) has some success with BCC. Imiquimod is an agonist for the toll-like receptor (TLR) 7 and/or 8, inducing a helper T cell cytokine cascade and interferon production. It purportedly acts as an immunomodulator. It is available as a 5% cream and is used in schedules ranging from twice weekly to twice daily over 5 to 15 weeks.

External beam radiation can be used effectively and has gained favor over superficial X-rays by many radiation oncologists. Ionizing radiation is a good treatment option for patients who are not surgical candidates, especially those patients who have facial tumors.

Treatment for Metastatic or Locally Advanced Basal Cell Carcinoma

BCCs frequently exhibit constitutive activation of the Hedgehog/PTCH1-signaling pathway. Two inhibitors of Smoothened (SMO), a transmembrane protein involved in the Hedgehog pathway, are approved for the treatment of adults with metastatic BCC, patients with locally advanced BCC that has recurred after surgery, and patients who are not candidates for surgery or radiation therapy.

Surgical

Most commonly, BCC is removed in the ambulatory setting by curettage with electrodesiccation, using a looped blade to scrape away the lesion from

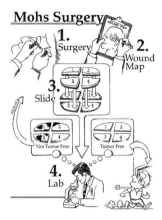

Fig. 6.15 Steps in Mohs micrographic excision. (Used with permission from Papel ID, ed. *Facial Plastic and Reconstructive Surgery*. 3rd ed. New York: Thieme; 2009:683.)

normal skin, vigorously and in multiple directions. This is best used for small nodular or superficial BCCs, with a 90% success rate, but should not be used with aggressive types of BCC or in cosmetically or functionally sensitive areas. Surgical excision with 4-mm margins has a 95% cure rate and can be performed for any BCC variant. Primary closure has better cosmetic outcome than healing by secondary intention. The most effective procedure (96–99% cure rate) is Mohs micrographic excision (**Fig. 6.15**). In this technique, the tumor is removed and the margin mapped, color-coded, and then examined thoroughly for remaining cancer while the patient is still in the operating room. If there is remnant cancer, the surgeon returns to that specifically mapped area and removes tissues, repeating this process until all margins are clear. This procedure is best used for cosmetically or functionally sensitive areas in which wide margins cannot be easily removed or for aggressive, recurring, or large tumors.

Cryosurgery can also reliably treat small, nonaggressive BCC.

◆ Outcome and Follow-Up

Patients who are diagnosed with BCC have a 35 to 40% chance of developing another tumor within 3 years and a 50% chance of developing another (not recurrent) basal cell carcinoma within 5 years. Therefore, regular skin screenings are recommended. Wearing hats (to protect the head and neck from sun exposure) and sunblock usage should be encouraged.

◆ Staging of Cutaneous Basal Cell Carcinoma

Primary Tumor (T)

TX: Primary tumor cannot be assessed

Tis: Carcinoma in situ

T1:   Tumor < 2 cm in greatest dimension

T2:   Tumor ≥ 2 cm and < 4 cm in greatest dimension

T3:   Tumor > 4 cm in maximum dimension or minor bone erosion or perineural invasion or deep invasion

T4:   Tumor with gross cortical bone/marrow, skull base invasion, and/or skull base foramen invasion

   T4a: Tumor with gross cortical bone/marrow invasion

   T4b: Tumor with skull base invasion and/or skull base foramen involvement

*Perineural invasion for T3 classification is defined as tumor cells within the nerve sheath of a nerve lying deeper than the dermis or measuring 0.1 mm or larger in caliber, or presenting with clinical or radiographic involvement of named nerves without skull base invasion or transgression; Deep invasion is defined as invasion beyond the subcutaneous fat or > 6 mm (as measured from the granular layer of adjacent normal epidermis to the base of the tumor).

Regional Lymph Nodes (N)*

NX: Regional lymph nodes cannot be assessed

N0:   No regional lymph node metastasis

N1:   Metastasis to a single ipsilateral lymph node measuring ≤ 3 cm in greatest diameter and ENE negative

N2:   Further divided into three categories:

   N2a: Single ipsilateral lymph node > 3 and ≤ 6 cm and ENE negative (pathologic staging also includes a single ipsilateral or contralateral lymph node ≤ 3 cm and ENE positive)

   N2b: Multiple ipsilateral lymph nodes ≤ 6 cm and ENE negative

   N2c: Bilateral or contralateral lymph nodes ≤ 6 cm in greatest dimension and ENE negative

N3:   Now further divided into two categories:

   N3a: Metastasis to a lymph node > 6 cm, ENE negative

   N3b: Metastasis to a single lymph node that is ENE positive (pathologic staging includes single lymph nodes that are ENE positive >3cm), or metastasis to multiple lymph nodes with any ENE positive

A designation of "U" or "L" can be attached to the N category to indicate nodes above ("U") or below ("L") the lower border of the cricoid. Similarly, clinical and pathologic ENE should be recorded as ENE (−) or ENE (+). Clinical and pathologic staging are similar with the differences noted in parenthesis.

*Superior mediastinal lymph nodes are considered regional lymph nodes (level VII). Midline nodes are considered ipsilateral nodes.

Distant Metastasis (M)

MX: Distant metastasis cannot be assessed

M0:   No distant metastasis

M1:   Distant metastasis

American Joint Committee on Cancer Stage Groupings of Non Melanoma Cutaneous Malignancy of the Head and Neck (8th Edition)

Stage 0 disease: Carcinoma in situ (TisN0M0)

Stage I disease: Includes only T1 N0 M0 tumors

Stage II disease: Includes only T2 N0 M0 tumors

Stage III disease: Includes T3 N0 M0 and T1 -3 disease that is N1 M0

Stage IVA disease: Includes T4a disease with N0-N2 M0 disease and T1-T3 disease that is N2 M0

Stage IVB disease: Includes T4b disease with any nodal disease or T1-T4a disease with N3 disease without distant metastases (M0)

Stage IVC disease: Any disease with distant metastases (M1)

Table 6.15   Cancer stage groupings

	N0	N1	N2	N3
T1	Stage I	Stage III	Stage IVA	Stage IVB
T2	Stage II	Stage III	Stage IVA	Stage IVB
T3	Stage III	Stage III	Stage IVA	Stage IVB
T4a	Stage IVA	Stage IVA	Stage IVA	Stage IVB
T4b	Stage IVB	Stage IVB	Stage IVB	Stage IVB
M1	Stage IVC	Stage IVC	Stage IVC	Stage IVC

6.3.15.2   Cutaneous Squamous Cell Carcinoma

◆ Key Features

- Squamous cell carcinoma (SCC) is the second most common skin cancer.
- Its aggressiveness is related to size and lymphatic spread.
- Surgical excision is the mainstay of treatment.

Squamous cell carcinoma is the second most common skin cancer in humans after basal cell carcinoma (BCC), covered in the previous chapter. SCC is more aggressive than BCC, as it frequently grows vertically, leading to lymphatic penetration and metastasis. In addition to sun exposure, chronic damage to skin and immunosuppressive states are risk factors. SCCs arising from previously damaged skin (scar, burn, or chronic injury, such as Marjolin ulcer) and large primary lesions (> 2 cm) are more aggressive, with higher rates of recurrence and metastasis. Lesions < 2 cm have 5% recurrence and 7% metastasis rates. Lesions > 2 cm have double the recurrence rate and three times the rate of lymphatic metastatic spread. As in the case of BCC, prevention is best, by reducing sun exposure and repeated injury; however, SCC can usually be treated successfully with surgical excision of the primary lesion along with affected lymphatic tissue.

◆ Epidemiology

The National Cancer Institute estimates over 1,000,000 new cases of BCC and SCC combined per year in the United States, with mortality figures of < 2,000 individuals. The epidemiologic factors of SCC are UV-B light exposure, related genetic sensitivity to the sun, chemical carcinogen exposure, previous radiation exposure, and chronic inflammation, immunosuppression, and human papillomavirus (HPV) infection.

◆ Clinical

Signs and Symptoms

The skin appearance of SCC is diverse: SCC may appear as a scaly, rough patch on an erythematous base on sun-exposed skin. The lesion may look like a scar but does not heal and often bleeds and ulcerates. Similarly, a nonhealing ulcer or wound may house SCC. SCC may also arise from erythroplakic lesions. The appearance of the lesion varies with the type.

Differential Diagnosis

- Bowen's disease
- Cutaneous horn
- Actinic keratosis
- Keratoacanthoma
- Wart
- Blastomycosis
- BCC
- Melanoma

◆ Evaluation

History

An appropriate history should include a special emphasis on previous and current cutaneous lesions or discolorations.

Physical Exam

A routine physical exam should be performed. Lymph nodes in the parotid gland and the neck should be assessed, especially with lesions involving the nose, ear, and temple.

Imaging

No imaging or laboratory tests are necessary for isolated cutaneous lesions (if adenopathy suspected, imaging is needed to assist with staging), but computed tomography (CT), magnetic resonance imaging (MRI), and positron emission tomography (PET) are useful for determining the extension of tumor if advanced.

Other Tests

Suspicious lesions require either a one-punch biopsy or two shave biopsies, which include the level of the middermis.

Pathology

Histologically, SCC can be graded as well, moderately, and poorly differentiated. Grossly, it can be ulcerative, infiltrative, or exophytic.

Variants

Variants of SCC include the following:

- Spindle cell, a biologically aggressive variant of SCC, may resemble soft tissue sarcoma, but it can be differentiated with a positive vitronectin antibody test. The spindle cells are elongated nuclei in a whorled pattern. Although it is a rare variant, it is more commonly seen at sites of previous scars or chronic injury.

- Adenoid (acantholytic) displays pseudoglandular differentiation with a separation of keratinocytes from each other. Histologically, it may resemble adenocarcinoma, but clinically it appears as typical SCC, usually in the elderly, in the periauricular region. This variant is also considered biologically aggressive.

- Indolent variants include Bowen's disease (SCC in situ), which is characterized histologically by hyperkeratosis, parakeratosis, and acanthosis with thickened and elongated rete ridges.

- Keratoacanthoma is a relatively common low-grade malignancy that originates in the pilosebaceous glands and closely and pathologically resembles SCC (rapid growth around hair follicle, spontaneous resolution in 4 to 6 months).

- Verrucous carcinoma is a low-grade variant of SCC with little potential for distant metastases. However, it has the potential to cause local destruction and has a higher rate of local recurrence.

◆ Treatment Options

The treatment of SCC is surgical excision. Small, well-differentiated tumors can be removed safely with 4-mm margins, while lesions > 2 cm, moderately undifferentiated with subcutaneous fat involvement, require at least 6-mm margins, including a portion of subcutaneous fat. If parotid or cervical lymph nodes are clinically involved, superficial parotidectomy and modified radical neck dissection is recommended. Mohs micrographic excision can be employed, especially in cosmetically sensitive areas (**Table 6.16**).

Radiotherapy is effective as the primary therapy for poor surgical candidates and cosmetically sensitive areas or as adjunct therapy to minimize recurrence, treat positive or narrow margins, treat lymphatic spread, or debulk large lesions prior to excision.

Table 6.16 Treatment options for SCC and BCC

Mohs micrographic excision

If one or more of these factors are present:

- Recurrent tumor
- Tumor size larger than 2 cm in diameter
- Tumors with an aggressive histology (such as morpheaform, infiltrative, micronodular BCC, or poorly differentiated SCC)
- Tumors with ill-defined margins
- Tumors that are incompletely excised
- Tumors with perineural invasion
- Tumor location where maximal conservation of normal tissue is important (such as eyelid, nose, ear, lip, digit, genitalia)

Otherwise consider

Standard excision

Use at least

- 4- to 6-mm margins to a depth of mid to deep subcutaneous tissue if small (< 2 cm) primary BCC > SCC with clinically well-defined borders and nonaggressive histology

or

- 7-mm margins to a depth that includes all of the subcutaneous tissue if factor(s) are present for consideration of Mohs but Mohs is unavailable or patient refuses Mohs.

Radiation therapy

- If patient is a poor surgical candidate
- Refuses surgery
- As postoperative treatment, if Mohs or standard excision shows perineural invasion or positive margins

Consider therapies other than radiation therapy if the patient has connective tissue disease (i.e., lupus, scleroderma) or is < 50 years old.

Less commonly used modalities

These modalities are primarily used for superficial BCC and SCC on the trunk and extremities:

- Cryosurgery
- Curettage and electrodesiccation
- Laser
- Photodynamic therapy

Adapted from Papel ID, ed. *Facial Plastic and Reconstructive Surgery*, 4th ed. New York: Thieme;2016:583.

◆ Outcome and Follow-Up

After treatment of early disease, patients should be followed every 6 months for 2 years, and then yearly. More advanced disease should be followed more frequently (3 to 6 months) for 2 years, with increased intervals subsequently. Previous SCC greatly increases chance of secondary tumors; patients should receive full skin exams yearly. Protection against sun exposure (wide-brim hats, sunblock) should be stressed.

◆ Staging of Cutaneous SCC

Primary Tumor (T)

TX: Primary tumor cannot be identified

Tis: Carcinoma in situ

T1:   Tumor < 2 cm in greatest dimension

T2:   Tumor ≥ 2 cm, and < 4 cm in greatest dimension

T3:   Tumor ≥ 4 cm in maximum dimension, or minor bone erosion or perineural invasion or deep invasion*

T4:   Tumor with gross cortical bone/marrow, skull base invasion, and/or skull base foramen invasion

   T4a: Tumor with gross cortical bone/marrow invasion

   T4b: Tumor with skull base invasion and/or skull base foramen involvement

*Perineural invasion for T3 classification is defined as tumor cells within the nerve sheath of a nerve lying deeper than the dermis or measuring 0.1 mm or larger in caliber, or presenting with clinical or radiographic involvement of named nerves without skull base invasion or transgression. Deep invasion is defined as invasion beyond the subcutaneous fat or > 6 mm (as measured from the granular layer of adjacent normal epidermis to the base of the tumor.

Regional Lymph Nodes (N)*

NX: Regional lymph nodes cannot be assessed

N0:   No regional lymph node metastasis

N1:   Metastasis to a single ipsilateral lymph node measuring ≤ 3 cm in greatest diameter and ENE negative

N2:   Further divided into three categories:

   N2a: Single ipsilateral lymph node > 3 and ≤ 6 cm and ENE negative (pathologic staging also includes a single ipsilateral or contra-lateral lymph node ≤ 3 cm and ENE positive)

   N2b: Multiple ipsilateral lymph nodes ≤ 6 cm and ENE negative

   N2c: Bilateral or contralateral lymph nodes ≤ 6 cm in greatest dimension and ENE negative

N3:   Now further divided into two categories:

   N3a: Metastasis to a lymph node > 6 cm, ENE negative

N3b: Metastasis to a single lymph node that is ENE positive (pathologic staging includes single lymph nodes that are ENE positive >3cm), or metastasis to multiple lymph nodes with any ENE positive

A designation of "U" or "L" can be attached to the N category to indicate nodes above ("U") or below ("L") the lower border of the cricoid. Similarly, clinical and pathologic ENE should be recorded as ENE (–) or ENE (+). Clinical and pathologic staging are similar with the differences noted in parenthesis.

*Superior mediastinal lymph nodes are considered regional lymph nodes (level VII). Midline nodes are considered ipsilateral nodes.

Distant Metastasis (M)

M0: No distant metastasis

M1: Distant metastasis

American Joint Committee on Cancer Stage Groupings of Cutaneous Squamous Cell Carcinoma (8th Edition)

Stage 0 disease: Carcinoma in situ (TisN0M0)

Stage I disease: Includes only T1 N0 M0 tumors

Stage II disease: Includes only T2 N0 M0 tumors

Stage III disease: Includes T3 N0 M0 and T1 -3 disease that is N1 M0

Stage IVA disease: Includes T4a disease with N0-N2 M0 disease and T1-T3 disease that is N2 M0

Stage IVB disease: Includes T4b disease with any nodal disease or T1-T4a disease with N3 disease without distant metastases (M0)

Stage IVC disease: Any disease with distant metastases (M1)

Table 6.17 Cancer stage groupings

	N0	N1	N2	N3
T1	Stage I	Stage III	Stage IVA	Stage IVB
T2	Stage II	Stage III	Stage IVA	Stage IVB
T3	Stage III	Stage III	Stage IVA	Stage IVB
T4a	Stage IVA	Stage IVA	Stage IVA	Stage IVB
T4b	Stage IVB	Stage IVB	Stage IVB	Stage IVB
M1	Stage IVC	Stage IVC	Stage IVC	Stage IVC

Histopathologic Type

The classification applies only to carcinomas of the skin, primarily cutaneous SCC (CSCC) and other carcinomas. It also applies to the adenocarcinomas that develop from eccrine or sebaceous glands and to the spindle cell variant of CSCC. Microscopic verification is necessary to group by histologic type. One form of *in situ* CSCC or intraepidermal CSCC is often referred to as Bowen's disease. This lesion should be assigned Tis.

6.3.15.3 Melanomas of the Head, Face, and Neck

✦ Key Features

- Melanomas of the head, face, and neck arise from neuroendocrine cells and stain strongly with HMB-45 and S-100.
- Melanomas are aggressive: locally invasive, distant metastasis, and poorest prognosis of skin cancers.
- Depth of invasion is the key for treatment and prognosis.
- Treat with wide local excision and chemotherapy.

Approximately 20% of melanomas occur in the head and neck region; 80% of these arise from the skin (most commonly the cheek, scalp, ear, and neck); the rest are mucosal (most commonly the anterior septum, middle and inferior conchae, hard palate, and gingiva). In cases of melanoma, the depth of invasion is the key to staging and prognosis. Suspicious lesions should be excised completely with a margin dictated by the depth of the lesion. Risk factors include UV-B light exposure, severe sunburns (more than three before age 20), large congenital nevi, familial dysplastic syndrome, fair skin, and blue or green eyes.

Mucosal melanoma of the head and neck is relatively rare. Mucosal melanomas show far more aggressive behavior than skin melanomas do and are more inclined to metastasize into regional and distant sites or recur locally, regionally, or in distant locations, resulting in a high rate of cause-specific death. The prognosis is grim, with most published reports documenting a 5-year survival rate of 10 to 15%.

The presence of a pigmented lesion in the oral or nasal cavities should raise suspicion of mucosal melanoma; a biopsy of the lesion should be promptly obtained. Diagnosis of pathologic disease is dependent on the identification of intracellular melanin.

✦ Epidemiology

The National Cancer Institute estimates 76,380 new cases of and 10,130 deaths from melanoma occurred in the United States in 2016. There has been a clear upward trend in incidence over time. Melanoma has the highest rate of increase in incidence and the third highest increase in mortality among cancers in the United States. The highest prevalence of melanoma is in white males. Late-stage presentations (metastases) are more common in persons of African descent.

◆ Clinical

Signs and Symptoms

Melanomas usually present as macular or nodular areas of discoloration on the skin, sometimes aggravated by itching, ulceration, and bleeding. The ABCDEs point to melanoma:

1. **A**symmetric shape
2. **B**order irregularity
3. **C**olor variation (within parts of lesion, or over time)
4. **D**iameter (6 mm, or increase in size)
5. **E**volution (changes in time)

Mucosal melanomas usually present as macular, nodular, or ulcerated lesions on mucosa, causing epistaxis, nasal obstruction, or mass in the oral cavity.

Differential Diagnosis

- Seborrheic keratosis
- Pigmented basal cell cancer
- Solar lentigines
- Atypical nevi
- Hemangioma
- Melanoacanthoma
- Focal argyrosis
- Olfactory neuroblastoma
- Other neuroendocrine carcinomas

◆ Evaluation

Physical Exam

A routine physical exam, focusing on sun damage and commonly affected areas (cheek, scalp, neck, etc.), on the ABCDEs of lesions as above, and palpation for lymphadenopathy. Mucosal melanomas can present as pigmented, friable lesions on mucosal surface, though they can also present as amelanotic masses.

Imaging

Imaging is not often used in early disease, but in more advanced disease and for metastatic work-up positron emission tomography (PET)–computed tomography (CT) and magnetic resonance imaging (MRI) are useful.

Labs

Lactate dehydrogenase (LDH) in distant metastatic work-up.

Other Tests

Immunohistochemical staining; HMB-45 (homatropine methylbromide) and S-100.

Pathology

Superficial Spreading (60–70%)

Most common type; common in younger people; multicolored with notched border; usually from preexisting nevi at dermal–epidermal junction; radial growth (diameter increase) precedes vertical growth (ulceration); can invade all levels of dermis

Nodular (15–30%)

Most aggressive; worst prognosis; appears as dark (blue/black/red) pigmented nodule; 5% amelanotic; can arise de novo (unrelated to sun exposure); no radial growth, but rapid vertical growth with frequent bleeding and ulceration; regional and distant lymphadenopathy

Acral Lentiginous (10%)

High incidence in Asians and Africans; large, dark, with irregular border on soles, palms, and subungual lateral growth

Lentigo Maligna (5%)

Best prognosis; common in elderly over sun-damaged skin; large, flat, tan or brown; grows slowly; stays in dermal–epidermal junction and spreads radially; bleeding or sudden change in size signal vertical growth and invasion

◆ Treatment Options

Treatment should be based on staging: there are three commonly used staging systems (see Staging of Melanomas of the Head, Face, and Neck). Breslow, Clark, and the American Joint Committee on Cancer (AJCC) are similar staging systems in that they are all based on depth of invasion. The microstage of malignant melanoma is determined by histologic examination by the vertical thickness of the lesion in millimeters (Breslow classification) and/or the anatomic level of local invasion (Clark classification). Currently, the most widely used system is the AJCC. AJCC melanoma staging guidelines have incorporated serum LDH for the classification of stage IV disease.

Medical

Interferon is usually given after surgical excision as an adjuvant therapy. High-dose treatment with interferon α2b increases disease-free survival and overall survival over observation; low-dose treatment is less effective (ECOG 1694 trial). Side effects of treatment include immunosuppression, anorexia, nausea/vomiting, liver toxicity (increased aspartate aminotransferase [AST]), and neurologic/neuropsychiatric problems.

Surgical

Complete surgical excision provides the best prognosis. The local treatment for melanomas is surgical excision with margins based on Breslow thickness and anatomic location: for in situ lesions, 0.5- to 1-cm margins. For most melanomas 2 to 4 mm in thickness, this means 2- to 3-cm radial excision margins. Clinically enlarged or matted lymph node beds require lymphadenectomy.

Melanoma that has spread to distant sites is rarely curable with standard therapy, though high-dose interleukin-2 (IL-2) has been reported to produce durable responses in a small number of patients.

Sentinel Lymph Node Biopsy

Fifteen to 35% of clinically negative nodes are sentinel lymph node positive. Biopsy is indicated for lesions > 1 mm deep. Preoperative lymphoscintigraphy can map the first echelon of draining nodes. Intraoperatively, inject isosulfan blue (Lymphazurin; Medtronic, Minneapolis, MN) dye at the primary site, locate the sentinel node with a radioactive probe, and send for a frozen section. A positive sentinel node requires neck dissection and possibly adjuvant therapy.

◆ Outcome and Follow-Up

Even with 1-mm lesions with negative margins of resection, the recurrence rate is high. Ulceration and thickness of the primary lesion make recurrence much more likely. Mucosal melanomas have a high rate of recurrence. A history of melanoma itself is a risk factor for new primaries. Also, nodal disease can appear after primary excision. Therefore, patients should be monitored closely with routine history and physical exams, and possible chest X-ray and serum LDH for metastases.

For skin melanoma, prognosis is multifactorial and primarily depends on tumor thickness, the presence or absence of histologic ulceration, and lymph node involvement (most important). Despite advances in the treatment of metastatic disease, the detection and treatment of cutaneous melanoma in its thin, early phase remains the best chance for cure.

Melanoma of the Mucosal Membrane

Lesions of the oral cavity have a higher prevalence of lymph node metastasis than those occurring in either the nasal or the pharyngeal cavities. Overall, 18% of patients with mucosal melanoma have lymphatic metastases at presentation. The average distant metastatic rate at presentation is 10%.

Primary site recurrence occurs in ~ 40% of nasal cavity lesions, 25% of oral cavity lesions, and 32% of pharyngeal tumors. Overall primary site recurrence ranges from 55 to 66% and from 16 to 35% for nodal recurrence. Most recurrences occur within the first 3 years.

◆ Staging of Melanomas of the Head, Face, and Neck

Skin Melanoma

Clark's Levels: Invasion Through

Level I: Lesions involving only the epidermis (in situ melanoma); not an invasive lesion

Level II: Invasion of the papillary dermis that does not reach the papillary–reticular dermal interface

Level III: Invasion fills and expands the papillary dermis but does not penetrate the reticular dermis

Level IV: Invasion into the reticular dermis but not into the subcutaneous tissue

Level V: Invasion through the reticular dermis into the subcutaneous tissue

Breslow's Levels

Level I: Lesions < 0.76 mm

Level II: Lesions 0.76 to 1.49 mm

Level III: Lesions 1.5 to 3.99 mm

Level IV: Lesions > 3.99 mm

Primary Tumor (T)

TX: Primary tumor thickness cannot be assessed (e.g., shave biopsy/ curettage)

T0:   No evidence of primary tumor (e.g., unknown primary or completely regressed melanoma)

Tis: Melanoma in situ (i.e., not an invasive tumor: anatomic level I)

T1:   Melanoma ≤ 1.0 mm in thickness, with or without ulceration

   T1a: Melanoma < 0.8 mm without ulceration

   T1b: Melanoma ≥ 0.8 mm and ≤ 1.0 mm in thickness with or without ulceration, or < 0.8 mm with ulceration

T2:   Melanoma 1.1 to 2 mm in thickness, with or without ulceration

   T2a: Melanoma 1.1 to 2.0 mm in thickness, no ulceration

   T2b: Melanoma 1.1 to 2.0 mm in thickness, with ulceration

T3:   Melanoma 2.1 to 4.0 mm in thickness, with or without ulceration

   T3a: Melanoma 2.1 to 4.0 mm in thickness, no ulceration

   T3b: Melanoma 2.1 to 4.0 mm in thickness, with ulceration

T4:   Melanoma > 4.0 mm in thickness, with or without ulceration

   T4a: Melanoma > 4.0 mm in thickness, no ulceration

   T4b: Melanoma > 4.0 mm in thickness, with ulceration

Regional Lymph Nodes (N)

NX: Regional lymph nodes cannot be assessed

N0:   No regional lymph node metastasis

N1:   Metastasis in 1 regional lymph node or in-transit, satellite and or microsatellite metastases without involved lymph nodes

   N1a: Clinically occult (microscopic) metastasis

   N1b: Clinically apparent (macroscopic) metastasis

   N1c: No regional lymph node disease but present in-transit, satellite, and/or microsatellite metastases

N2:   Metastasis in 2 or 3 regional nodes or in-transit, satellite and/or microsatellite metastases with one involved lymph node

  N2a: Clinically occult (microscopic) metastasis

  N2b: Clinically apparent (macroscopic) metastasis

  N2c: In-transit, satellite and/or microsatellite metastases with one involved lymph node

N3:   Metastasis in four or more regional lymph nodes, or matted metastatic nodes, or in-transit metastasis or satellites(s) with metastasis in two or more regional node(s)

  N3a: Clinically occult (microscopic) metastasis

  N3b: Clinically apparent (macroscopic) metastasis or matted nodes

  N3c: In-transit, satellite and or microsatellite metastases with two or more involved lymph nodes or any matted nodes

Distant Metastasis (M)

M0:   No evidence of distant metastasis

M1:   Distant metastasis (documented in this specimen)

  M1a: Metastasis in skin, subcutaneous tissues, or distant lymph nodes

   M1a(0): LDH normal

   M1a(1): LDH elevated

  M1b: Metastasis to lung

   M2a(0): LDH normal

   M2a(1): LDH elevated

  M1c: Metastasis to all other non-CNS visceral sites

   M1c(0): LDH normal

   M1c(1): LDH elevated

  M1d: Distant metastasis to CNS

   M1d(0): LDH normal

   M1d(1): LDH elevated

Specify site, if known. The (0) or (1) suffices are not used if LDH is not recorded or is unspecified.

American Joint Committee on Cancer Stage Groupings of Cutaneous Melanoma (8th Edition)

Clinical Staging

  Stage 0 disease: Carcinoma in situ (TisN0M0)

  Stage IA disease: Includes only T1a N0 M0 tumors

  Stage IB disease: Includes T1b-T2a N0 M0 tumors

  Stage IIA disease: Includes T2b-T3a N0 M0 tumors

  Stage IIB disease: Includes T3b-T4a N0 M0 tumors

Stage IIC disease: Includes only T4b N0 M0 tumors

Stage III disease: Any tumor with nodal disease without metastases

Stage IV disease: Any tumor with metastases

Pathologic Staging

Stage 0 disease: Carcinoma in situ (TisN0M0)

Stage IA disease: Includes T1a-T1b N0 M0 tumors (note that pT1bN0M0 is stage IA, while above cT1bN0M0 is stage IB)

Stage IB disease: Includes only T2a N0 M0 tumors

Stage IIA disease: Includes T2b T3a N0 M0 tumors

Stage IIB disease: Includes T3b-T4a N0 M0 tumors

Stage IIC disease: Includes only T4b N0 M0 tumors

Stage IIIA disease: Includes T1a-T2a N1a or N2a M0 disease

Stage IIIB disease: Includes T0 N1b-N1c M0 disease or T1a-T2a N1b/c or N2a M0 disease, T2b/T3a N1a-N2b M0 disease or

Stage IIIC disease: Includes T0 N2-N3 M0 disease, T1a-T3a N2c or N3 disease, T3b/T4a tumors with nodal disease and M0, T4b N1a-N2c M0 disease

Stage IIID disease: Includes T4b N3 M0 disease

Stage IV disease: Any tumor with metastases

◆ Staging of Mucosal Melanoma

Primary Tumor

T3:   Tumors limited to mucosal disease

T4:   Moderately advanced or very advanced disease

  T4a: Moderately advanced disease: tumor involving deep soft tissue, cartilage, bone, or overlying skin

  T4b: Very advanced disease: tumor involving brain, dura, skull base, lower cranial nerves (CNs IX, X, XI, XII), masticator space, carotid artery, prevertebral space, or mediastinal structures

Regional Lymph Nodes

NX: Regional lymph nodes cannot be assessed

N0:   No regional lymph node metastases

N1:   Regional lymph node metastases present

Distant Metastasis

M0:   No distant metastasis

M1:   Distant metastasis

No prognostic stage grouping currently proposed.

6.3.16   Malignant Neoplasms of the Ear and Temporal Bone

◆ Key Features

- Squamous cell carcinoma (SCC) is the most common malignancy of the middle ear and temporal bone, accounting for 60 to 80% of these lesions.
- Basal cell carcinoma (BCC) may be slightly more prevalent than SCC on the auricle but accounts for ~ 20% of neoplasms of the middle ear and temporal bone.
- A host of other malignant neoplasms can affect the ear and temporal bone, including melanoma, sarcomas, hematologic malignancies, and metastatic lesions.

Squamous cell carcinoma (SCC) is the most common malignancy affecting the external auditory canal (EAC). Patients may present with painless bloody otorrhea. Physical examination may reveal the appearance of granulation tissue, and a biopsy is necessary to differentiate from chronic otitis.

◆ Epidemiology

For cutaneous malignancies of the auricle, controversy exists regarding whether SCC or BCC is more common. The main causative factor is sun exposure; median age is ~ 70 years. Melanoma is less common.

The incidence of temporal bone cancer is ~ 6 per million, with no clear sex predilection. Chronic suppurative otitis media (CSOM) may be a precursor, but no definitive correlation has ever been proved.

◆ Clinical

Signs

Swelling of the ear canal with or without aural polyps may be a sign of a malignant neoplasm of the ear. Facial nerve weakness or other cranial nerve (CN) palsies may be identified. Hearing loss will most likely be conductive, but an aggressive lesion with otic capsule invasion can present with sensorineural hearing loss and vertigo.

Symptoms

Tumors of the ear canal mimic otitis externa with drainage and discomfort. Tumors of the temporal bone or middle ear mimic otitis media with painless drainage but may be bloody. Patients may present with hearing loss (conductive or sensorineural) and facial palsy.

Differential Diagnosis

Neoplasms must be differentiated from an infectious lesion by a biopsy. Although this chapter deals primarily with SCC, there is a long list of other malignancies that can affect the temporal bone, including BCC, adenocarcinoma, sarcoma, melanoma, lymphoma, and metastatic tumors. Benign lesions such as ear canal osteomas, paragangliomas, schwannomas, meningiomas, hemangiomas, endolymphatic sac tumors, and eosinophilic granulomas also need to be ruled out.

◆ Evaluation

Physical Exam

A full head and neck exam is necessary. Begin with a thorough skin and scalp evaluation looking for other skin lesions. Any skin abnormality on the auricle or in the canal requires a biopsy. The parotid gland and neck are carefully palpated. Complete CN exam is documented as well. Evaluation of temporomandibular joint function is important to exclude gross involvement or tumor invasion.

Imaging

Computed tomography (CT) of the temporal bones without contrast is the study of choice for temporal bone involvement. Degree of erosion of the ear canal is noted, as is involvement of the middle ear or any deeper structures. A neck CT with contrast evaluates the parotid gland and the cervical lymph nodes. The parotid gland may be involved by both direct extension and intraparotid nodal metastasis. Magnetic resonance imaging (MRI) of the brain is helpful in evaluating possible dural extension or intracranial metastatic lesions. Arteriography with balloon occlusion may be needed to evaluate suspected intrapetrous carotid artery invasion. Positron emission tomography (PET) scanning may be helpful in evaluating nodal disease or distant metastases.

Labs

Biopsy is necessary. An audiogram will be helpful in counseling patients regarding hearing rehabilitation after treatment.

Pathology

Pathology of SCC is the same as SCC elsewhere (see **Chapter 6.3.15.2**). There are many different subtypes: well differentiated, moderately differentiated, poorly differentiated, clear cell, spindle cell, and verrucous.

◆ Malignant Neoplasms of the Ear and Temporal Bone Other Than SCC

Melanoma

Melanoma of the auricle accounts for almost 1% of all melanomas. T stage is based on Breslow level. Surgical excision with 1- to 2-cm margin and neck dissection or sentinel node assessment for tumors 1 mm or thicker, or greater than Clark's level IV, is indicated.

Malignant Glandular Tumors

Adenoid cystic carcinoma and ceruminous adenocarcinoma present as painful obstructing ear canal masses. They are treated surgically like SCC with postoperative radiation. Lateral parotidectomy is also indicated, along with postoperative radiation.

Chondrosarcoma

Chondrosarcomas occur at the skull base, off midline at the petroclival junction. There are five subtypes and three grades; conventional is the most common subtype, and most tumors are grade I or II. Chondrosarcomas most commonly present with headache, diplopia, or hearing loss plus CN deficits, and most arise during the fourth or fifth decade of life. CT shows bony destruction and calcification; MRI reveals bright T2 and enhancement with contrast. Surgical excision by any number of approaches is necessary.

Chordoma

Chordoma is a locally aggressive disease process with a low rate of metastasis. It originates from notochord remnant. There are three subtypes. It is usually found midline at the clivus. Patients most commonly present with headache or diplopia and usually are 40 to 50 years of age. Over 90% of patients die of disease, but < 10% have metastasis. CT shows a midline erosive mass that may enhance with contrast, and MRI images are bright on T2 and enhance with contrast. Multiple midline and lateral approaches are available.

Sarcoma

Sarcoma is the most common malignancy of the temporal bone in children, especially rhabdomyosarcoma. There are multiple types, and it usually presents with otitis media, drainage, polyps, and bleeding. Most cases respond to either chemotherapy or radiotherapy, so surgery is limited to diagnostic biopsy, with aggressive resection reserved for treatment failures.

Metastasis

Metastasis is most commonly hematogenous from breast, lung, and kidney. It may also spread via cerebrospinal fluid or leptomeningeal spread. Patients present with hearing loss, facial paralysis, and headache. Survival is usually less than one year.

◆ Treatment Options

Treatment is based the T stage according to the modified University of Pittsburgh staging system:

- T1: Tumor limited to EAC without bony erosion
- T2: Tumor limited to EAC with bony erosion less than full thickness, and < 5 mm of soft tissue involvement
- T3: Tumor with full-thickness erosion of the EAC with < 5 mm of soft tissue involvement or middle ear or mastoid involvement or facial palsy
- T4: Tumor eroding the cochlea, petrous apex, carotid canal, jugular foramen, dura, medial wall of middle ear, or > 5 mm of soft tissue involvement

Medical

Chemotherapy may have some role in treatment as an adjunct to surgery, usually given postoperatively and in palliative management. Radiotherapy is recommended postoperatively for all lesions T2 or greater.

Surgical

The surgical approach depends on site and stage of lesion. There are many common surgical approaches (**Fig. 6.16a,b**), beginning with sleeve resection of the ear canal with some form of mastoidectomy for T1 lesions isolated to the ear canal. Lesions within the canal, but not extending into the middle ear, are approached with a lateral temporal bone resection that removes the ear canal en bloc. The medial margin of resection is the middle ear and the facial nerve canal.

Lesions that extend into the middle ear can be resected with subtotal temporal bone resection, which is a lateral temporal bone resection and piecemeal removal of any residual deeper tumor remnants. Total temporal bone resection is reserved for deeply invasive T4 lesions, and its utility is controversial.

Neck dissection and parotidectomy are often part of the resection, certainly if there is clinically evident nodal spread. Pedicled flap or free flap may be required for reconstruction.

Melanoma is discussed in **Chapter 6.3.15.3**; it requires wider margins and sentinel node assessment except for early-stage lesions.

◆ Outcome and Follow-Up

Accurate outcomes and survival rates are difficult to find in the literature. T1 tumors treated with surgery probably have a 5-year survival rate > 90%. T2 tumors treated with surgery and radiation have 5-year survivals of ~ 90%. T3 and T4 tumors treated with surgery and radiation have 5-year survival rates < 50%.

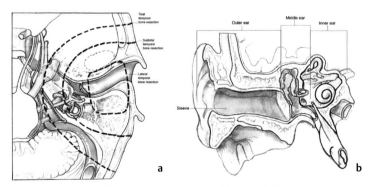

Fig. 6.16   Anatomic illustrations of **(a)** temporal bone and **(b)** sleeve resections.

6.3.17   Lymphomas of the Head and Neck

◆ Key Features

- The basic categories are Hodgkin's lymphoma (HL) and non-Hodgkin's lymphoma (NHL).
- NHL occurs more than five times as frequently as HL.
- NHL is the second most common malignancy in human immunodeficiency virus (HIV)-positive patients.
- Lymphomas are the most common nonepithelial tumors of the head and neck.
- The extranodal sites in the head and neck are the thyroid, orbit, salivary glands, and sinonasal passages.

The otolaryngologist—head and neck surgeon usually serves a well-defined, important role in the management of lymphomas. A high index of suspicion for lymphoma as a cause of common complaints in the head and neck region can lead to early diagnosis and improved outcome. Beyond the role of diagnostician, the head and neck surgeon will often be the one who obtains tissue for diagnosis. NHL usually originates in lymphoid tissues and can spread to other organs; it is much less predictable than HL and has a far greater predilection to disseminate to extranodal sites. The prognosis depends on the histologic type, stage, and treatment. For staging of HL and NHL, see **Table 6.18**.

Table 6.18   American Joint Committee on Cancer/Ann Arbor Staging System for Hodgkin's and non-Hodgkin's lymphoma

Stage I	Involvement of a single lymph node region (I); or localized involvement of a single extralymphatic organ or site in the absence of any lymph node involvement (IE) (rare in Hodgkin's lymphoma)
Stage II	Involvement of two or more lymph node regions on the same side of the diaphragm (II); or localized involvement of a single extralymphatic organ or site in association with regional lymph node involvement with or without involvement of other lymph node regions on the same side of the diaphragm (IIE); the number of regions involved may be indicated by a subscript; for example, II_3
Stage III	Involvement of lymph node regions on both sides of the diaphragm (III), which also may be accompanied by extralymphatic extension in association with adjacent lymph node involvement (IIIE), by involvement of the spleen (IIIS), or both (IIIE,S)

(continued)

Table 6.18   American Joint Committee on Cancer/Ann Arbor Staging System for Hodgkin's and non-Hodgkin's lymphoma *(Continued)*

Stage IV	Diffuse or disseminated involvement of one or more extralymphatic organs, with or without associated lymph node involvement; or isolated extralymphatic organ involvement in the absence of adjacent regional lymph node involvement, but in conjunction with disease in distant site(s); any involvement of the liver or bone marrow, or nodular involvement of the lung(s)
A and B classification (symptoms). Each stage should be classified as either A or B according to the absence or presence of defined constitutional symptoms.	1. *Fevers:* Unexplained fever with temperature above 38°C 2. *Night sweats:* Drenching sweats that require change of bedclothes 3. *Weight loss:* Unexplained weight loss > 10% of the usual body weight in the 6 months before diagnosis

Used with permission from American Joint Committee on Cancer: *AJCC Cancer Staging Handbook*. 8th ed. New York: Springer; 2017.

◆ Epidemiology

Non-Hodgkin's Lymphoma

In 2016, there were 72,580 estimated new cases of NHL and 20,150 deaths from NHL in the United States.

Hodgkin's Lymphoma

In 2016, there were 8,500 estimated new cases of HL and 1,120 deaths from HL in the United States. Over 75% of all newly diagnosed patients with adult HL can be cured with combination chemotherapy and/or radiotherapy. The median patient age is in the low to mid-20s, with half of the patients between 15 and 30 years of age; HL is rare in patients younger than age 10 and after age 60. The age distribution is bimodal, with a peak in the low 20s and a second peak in the low 40s.

◆ Clinical

HL often presents as an asymptomatic neck mass. It arises almost exclusively in nodal tissue; it manifests as enlarged rubbery painless nodes in the low neck and/or supraclavicular fossa, or above the hyoid in the submental, submandibular, periauricular, or periparotid nodes. Disease spreads in an orderly fashion to contiguous nodal regions. For diagnostic criteria of NHL, see **Table 6.19**.

◆ Evaluation

History

A detailed history, with special attention to the constitutional (B) symptoms of temperature higher than 38°C (100°F), night sweats, and weight loss of > 10% of total body weight over 6 months. Pruritus as a systemic symptom

Table 6.19   Diagnostic criteria for common lymphomas of the head and neck

Histologic subtype	Cell type	Additional CD markers	Associated oncogene	Translocation (incidence in subtype)	Cellular activity	Typical head and neck site	Typical behavior
Small lymphocytic lymphoma	B	CD5⁺, CD10⁻, CD23⁺	ND	ND	ND	Anterior orbit, nodes	Indolent
Follicular	B	CD5⁻, CD43⁻, CD10⁺, CD23±	BCL2	t(14;18) (q32;q11)90%	Suppression of apoptosis	Nodes, pharyngeal lymphoid ring, salivary glands	Indolent
Diffuse large cell	B	CD5⁻, CD10⁺, CD23±, CD43⁻, CD30±	BCL2	t(14;18) (q32;q11) 20%	Suppression of apoptosis	Pharyngeal lymphoid ring, nodes, salivary glands, thyroid, orbit, sinonasal tract	Aggressive
			BCL6	3q27 40%	Zinc finger transcription factor		
			BCL8	t(14;15) (q32;q11–13) 3–4%	Transcription factor		
Mucosa-associated lymphoid tissue (MALT)	B	CD5⁻, CD10⁻, CD23	ND	t(11;18) (q21;q21) 35%	ND	Salivary glands, orbit, thyroid, pharyngeal lymphoid ring	Indolent
Marginal zone (monocytoid)	B		ND	ND	ND	Nodes, neurotropic presentation	Indolent

(continued)

Table 6.19 Diagnostic criteria for common lymphomas of the head and neck (*Continued*)

		BCL1 (cyclin-D)	t(11;14) (q13;q32) 70%	C1/S progression	Pharyngeal lymphoid ring, nodes	Aggressive
Mantle	B	CD5+, CD10±, CD23−, CD43+				
Burkitt	B	CMYC	8q24 100%	Transcription activation; cell cycle control	Pharyngeal lymphoid ring, parapharyngeal site	Aggressive
Primary system C or primary cutaneous anaplastic large cell	T	CD30+ / ALK/NPM	t(2;5) (p23;q35) ND	Tyrosine kinase	Skin	Variable
Angiocentric lymphoma (AKA), lethal midline granuloma, nasal T-cell lymphoma, nasal (T-NK cell) lymphoma	T	CD56+, CD4+ / ND	ND	ND	Sinonasal tract	Aggressive

Abbreviation: ND, no data.

Data from Tsang RW, Gospodarowicz MK. Non-Hodgkin's lymphoma. In: Gunderson LL, Tepper JE, eds. *Clinical Radiation Oncology.* Philadelphia, PA: Churchill Livingstone; 2000:1158–1188.

remains controversial and is not considered a B symptom. A history relating to lymphadenopathy or extranodal disease involvement, such as unilateral tonsillar hypertrophy or nasal obstruction, is a concern.

Physical Exam

A complete head and neck physical examination should be performed, focusing on identifying and documenting the extent of lymphadenopathy, the pharyngeal lymphoid (Waldeyer) ring, or skin involvement.

Imaging

Knowledge of the anatomic extent of disease is required for treatment planning. Clinical staging for patients with HL includes a history, physical examination, laboratory studies (including erythrocyte sedimentation rate [ESR]), and thoracic and abdominal/pelvic computed tomography (CT) scans. Positron emission tomography (PET) scans, sometimes combined with CT scans, have replaced gallium scans and lymphangiography for clinical staging.

Labs

A complete blood cell count with differential, ESR, serum protein electrophoresis, chemistries, and liver function tests should be obtained.

Other Tests

Fine-needle aspiration biopsy (FNAB) can be sufficient to confirm recurrence in an already well-characterized lymphoma and will occasionally be sufficient to secure initial diagnosis, but excisional biopsy is generally preferred to afford assessment of nodal or extranodal tissue architecture. Core needle biopsy is an alternative if excisional biopsy is not possible.

Bone marrow involvement occurs in 5% of patients; biopsy is indicated in the presence of constitutional B symptoms or anemia, leukopenia, or thrombocytopenia.

Pathology

Pathologists currently use the World Health Organization (WHO) modification of the Revised European-American Lymphoma (REAL) classification for the histologic classification for adult HL; see **Table 6.20**.

Table 6.20   World Health Organization/Revised European-American Lymphoma (WHO/REAL) classification for adult Hodgkin's lymphoma

Classical Hodgkin's lymphoma
Nodular sclerosis Hodgkin's lymphoma
Mixed-cellularity Hodgkin's lymphoma
Lymphocyte depletion Hodgkin's lymphoma
Lymphocyte-rich classical Hodgkin's lymphoma
Nodular lymphocyte–predominant Hodgkin's lymphoma

◆ Treatment Options

Medical

Hodgkin's Lymphoma

Patients with nonbulky stage IA or IIA disease are considered to have clinical early-stage disease. These patients are candidates for chemotherapy, combined-modality therapy, or radiotherapy alone. Patients with stage III or IV disease, bulky disease, or the presence of B symptoms will require combination chemotherapy with or without additional radiotherapy.

Radiotherapy can be helpful. In adult HL, the appropriate dose of radiation alone is 25 to 30 Gy to clinically uninvolved sites and 35 to 44 Gy to regions of initial nodal involvement.

Non-Hodgkin's Lymphoma

For indolent lymphomas, no initial therapy is recommended while asymptomatic. At the onset of symptoms or complications, a single-agent oral alkylator therapy may induce and maintain clinical remission. Relapses are common.

Aggressive lymphomas are treated with a goal of cure. Localized stage I disease may be treated with radiation alone. For bulkier or clinically staged localized disease, chemotherapy is the mainstay of treatment. An intensive but abbreviated chemotherapy course followed by consolidation radiotherapy has, until recently, been the treatment of choice. Emerging experience suggests that CHOP (cyclophosphamide, doxorubicin [hydroxydaunorubicin], vincristine [Oncovin; Eli Lilly, Indianapolis, IN], and prednisone) plus rituximab (anti-CD20 monoclonal antibody) may be the most efficacious protocol in elderly patients. Disseminated aggressive disease is best treated with full-intensity, full-course chemotherapy.

Surgical

In both NHL and HL, surgery is typically performed to establish diagnosis. It consists of an excisional biopsy of enlarged or suspicious lymph nodes. Occasionally, palatine, lingual or nasopharyngeal tonsil tissue is excised and submitted. The specimen should be adequately sampled, handled, and fixed. When possible, care should be taken to provide intact samples large enough to provide meaningful nodal architecture information on which to base pathologic diagnosis. All permanent specimens should be submitted dry or in saline, but not in formalin, to allow immunohistochemical and flow cytometric studies to complement traditional pathology.

◆ Outcome and Follow-Up

The most important prognostic factors in HL are subtype and stage. Lymphocyte-predominant disease has an excellent prognosis; the prognosis of the nodular sclerosis variant is also very good. Lymphocyte-depleted classic HL has the worst prognosis. Other poor prognostic factors include constitutional symptoms, age > 45 years, bulky mediastinal disease, extranodal disease, elevation of LDH or ESR, and more than five disease foci in the spleen in pathologically staged patients.

Because HL is often curable and frequently occurs in younger populations, consideration of immediate and delayed complications of therapy is important. The most worrisome of these complications are secondary malignancies, which occur with an overall incidence of 5%. Complications of radiotherapy include those specific to head and neck irradiation, such as xerostomia and mucositis, as well as generalized fatigue and weight loss.

6.3.18   Idiopathic Midline Destructive Disease

♦ **Key Features**

- Idiopathic midline destructive disease (IMDD) is a progressive destructive lesion of the midface and upper airway region.
- Sinonasal natural killer cell or T cell (NK/T cell) lymphomas are associated with the disease.
- Non-Hodgkin's lymphoma of the midface region is one of the rarest forms of extranodal lymphoma, representing < 0.5% of cases.
- The incidence of these tumors is substantially higher among Asian and South and Central American populations.

IMDD, also known as lethal midline granuloma or extranodal NK/T cell lymphoma: nasal type, is a rare disorder characterized by ulceration and necrosis of the midline facial tissues and obstruction of the upper airway region.

♦ **Epidemiology**

IMDD affects a wide age range, peaking in the sixth decade. Males are predominantly affected, and the disease is much more common in persons resident in East Asia (e.g., Japan, Taiwan, China, Korea, Thailand). In Asian groups, > 90% of cases have T cell markers, and Epstein-Barr virus (EBV) has been consistently demonstrated in the cell genome.

♦ **Clinical**

Signs and Symptoms

Initial symptoms are usually those of a nonspecific rhinitis or sinusitis with nasal obstruction and nasal discharge. Epistaxis and facial swelling may occur. As the disease progresses, ulcerations spread, destroying the soft tissues, cartilage, and bone. Subsequently, facial pain and facial deformities develop. Signs may include cranial nerve (CN) palsies, diplopia, and proptosis due to intraorbital or skull base extension. Death after a long duration may be the result of cachexia, hemorrhage, meningitis, or intercurrent infection.

Differential Diagnosis

- Wegener's granulomatosis
- Malignant lymphoma
- Churg-Strauss's syndrome
- Polyangiitis
- Drug abuse

◆ Evaluation

Physical Exam

A complete head and neck exam including a nasal endoscopy should be performed. The most common finding is the presence of a nasal septal perforation.

Imaging

No specific imaging findings are present. The main role of imaging is to evaluate the extent of the disease, monitor its progression over time, and ascertain the effect of treatment. Computed tomography (CT) with high-resolution bone algorithms is the best method to evaluate bone changes, whereas magnetic resonance imaging (MRI) should be used to determine the extent of soft tissue, orbital, and intracranial involvement.

Pathology

Because the abnormal tissue is largely necrotic, multiple biopsy specimens are often required before a diagnosis is made. IMDD seems to be closely associated with EBV. This is unusual, as typically this virus is associated with B cell lymphomas.

◆ Treatment Options

Left untreated, IMDD is uniformly fatal.

Medical

Treatment for sinonasal NK/T-cell lymphomas consists of the combination of an anthracycline-based chemotherapy regimen (e.g., CHOP—cyclophosphamide, doxorubicin hydrochloride [hydroxydaunorubicin], vincristine sulfate [Oncovin], and prednisone) along with locoregional radiotherapy. Generally, the initial response to radiotherapy is so rapid and dramatic that the use of involved-field radiotherapy has been accepted as the preferred treatment option for localized disease. Overall, ~ 20 to 30% of patients treated with radiotherapy alone experience systemic failure in extranodal sites, and local recurrence rates range from 31 to 67%.

Surgical

Biopsy for diagnosis and debridement of necrotic tissue are the only surgical interventions.

◆ Outcome and Follow-Up

Patients with IMDD have poor survival outcomes, with the cumulative probability of survival at 5 years ranging from 37.9 to 45.3%.

6.3.19 Paragangliomas of the Head and Neck

◆ Key Features

- Paragangliomas of the head and neck are highly vascular tumors.
- Other terms used for tumors of the same histology are carotid body tumor, chemodectoma, and glomus tumor.

Paragangliomas are neuroendocrine tumors that develop from paraganglia, small organs of the autonomic nervous system. Paragangliomas may develop at four sites within the head and neck: the carotid body (carotid body [glomus caroticum] tumors), the ganglia of the vagus nerve (glomus vagale tumors), the jugular bulb (glomus jugulare tumors), and the middle ear (glomus tympanicum tumors). Treatment of head and neck paragangliomas is primarily surgical, although radiation and observation may be appropriate under certain circumstances.

◆ Epidemiology

Paragangliomas are rare tumors, accounting for < 1% of all head and neck tumors. In most cases, these are solitary lesions; bilateral or multicentric lesions occur in 3% of cases. Ten to 15% of patients have familial paragangliomas; patients with the familial tumors have much higher rates of bilaterality and multicentricity. The carotid body and jugular bulb are the most common sites of head and neck paragangliomas. Rare sites of involvement are the larynx, nasal cavity, paranasal sinuses, and thyroid gland.

◆ Clinical

Signs and Symptoms

Presentation of paragangliomas relates to the location at which the tumor arises. Carotid body and vagal paragangliomas present as slow-growing, nontender neck masses. A typical lateral neck mass may be seen, accompanied in some cases by the oropharyngeal bulge suggestive of parapharyngeal space involvement. More advanced or neglected lesions may have associated ipsilateral cranial neuropathies.

Differential Diagnosis

Initially, all etiologies of a lateral neck mass should be considered. Radiographic or clinical localization to the parapharyngeal space focuses the investigation; the most common parapharyngeal space lesions are salivary gland tumors (most common), paragangliomas, and nerve sheath tumors (schwannomas and neurofibromas).

◆ Evaluation

Physical Exam

A complete head and neck exam with attention to cranial nerve (CN) function is appropriate. The neck mass associated with a paraganglioma is frequently pulsatile, owing to its intimate relationship to the carotid vessels. Additional neck masses, suggesting lymph node metastasis or multifocality, should also be sought.

Imaging

Computed tomography (CT) scanning with contrast is useful, demonstrating the hypervascular tumor and its relationship with the neck vessels. Magnetic resonance imaging (MRI) provides similar information with the added benefits of no radiation exposure, greater soft tissue differentiation, and three planes of view. Formal angiography has been replaced by MRI, magnetic resonance angiography (MRA), or CT in the diagnostic realm, but it is still required when embolization is needed preoperatively. Octreotide scan is also a helpful nuclear medicine scan that can help confirm a paraganglioma and also identify other potential paragangliomas in the body.

Labs

A history of signs and symptoms of excess catecholamines should be explicitly sought. If symptoms such as flushing, labile or difficult-to-control hypertension, or excessive perspiration are described, preoperative testing for serum and urine catecholamines (and their metabolites) should be ordered. Although "functional" (catecholamine-secreting) paragangliomas of the head and neck are unusual (1–3%), pheochromocytomas of the adrenal medulla, which may constitute a portion of a syndrome of which the head and neck paraganglioma is the presenting feature, are much more frequently metabolically active.

Pathology

Grossly, paragangliomas are polypoid, well circumscribed, and firm to rubbery in consistency. Paragangliomas have a characteristic histologic appearance, with tumor cells arranged in clusters called "Zellballen," which are separated by a fibrovascular stroma (**Fig. 6.17**). Roughly 10% of paragangliomas are malignant. Malignancy is determined solely on the basis of metastasis rather than on any histologic features of the primary tumor.

◆ Treatment Options

The major goal of treatment is prevention of morbidity due to progressive cranial neuropathies. In most cases, this goal is best achieved by surgical extirpation via a cervical incision. Many surgeons employ preoperative embolization to decrease blood loss and improve visualization with larger

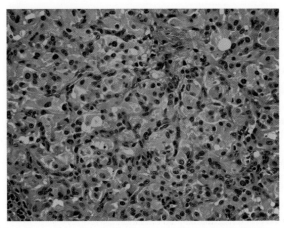

Fig. 6.17 Paraganglioma: a "Zellballen" or compact nested pattern is evident, with plump eosinophilic tumor cells surrounded by spindled S100-positive sustentacular cells. (Used with permission from Har-El G, Day T, Nathan C-A, Nguyen SA. *A Multidisciplinary Approach to Head and Neck Neoplasms*. New York: Thieme;2013. *Otorhinolaryngology—Head and Neck Surgery Series*.)

tumors. The need for internal carotid artery sacrifice and revascularization with saphenous vein grafting should always be considered, especially in larger tumors and tumors that radiographically encapsulate the internal carotid artery. The Shamblin criteria can be used to evaluate the patient, and type III tumors have a higher association with both cranial neuropathies and the need for carotid reconstruction.

On the other hand, surgery itself may result in new cranial neuropathies and significant associated morbidity. This merits consideration of other management strategies in selected cases. Other options include close observation with serial imaging and external beam radiation. Notably, external beam radiation appears to be tumoristatic rather than tumoricidal with paragangliomas.

In the very elderly or infirm patient, and in those with multiple (especially bilateral) tumors, all options are considered carefully. In the fragile patient, surgery may be postponed unless significant growth is noted radiographically or worsening of cranial neuropathies is identified clinically. In patients with bilateral disease, treatment, which may include any combination of surgery, observation, and external beam radiation, is tailored to achieve a goal of CN preservation on at least one side, as intractable swallowing dysfunction and/or tracheotomy dependence are the inevitable consequence of bilateral CN X or XII impairment.

◆ Outcome and Follow-Up

Patients should be closely observed for any local recurrence, although these are usually rare. Contralateral tumors should be sought and resected.

6.3.20 Peripheral Nerve Sheath Tumors

◆ Key Features

- Peripheral nerve sheath tumors (PNSTs) include schwannomas and neurofibromas.
- Schwannomas account for 6 to 8% of intracranial neoplasms.
- PNSTs are the most common tumors of the poststyloid parapharyngeal space.
- Vestibular schwannomas (see **Chapter 3.8**) are the most common cranial nerve schwannomas, followed by trigeminal and facial schwannomas and then those of the glossopharyngeal, vagus, and spinal accessory nerves.
- Benign PNSTs include neurilemoma (schwannoma), neurofibroma, and ganglioneuroma.
- Malignant PNSTs include malignant neurofibrosarcoma, schwannosarcoma, and sympathicoblastoma.

PNSTs are divided into two major groups: schwannomas (neurilemomas) and neurofibromas. Schwannomas are slow-growing, usually benign tumors that may arise from any nerve that is ensheathed in Schwann cells. In the parapharyngeal space, this includes cranial nerves (CNs) V_3, IX, X, XI, and XII; the sympathetic trunk; and the upper cervical nerves. In the parapharyngeal space, schwannomas often present as neck masses.

Neurofibromas, in contrast, are unencapsulated and intimately involved with the nerve of origin. Neurofibromas are often multiple.

◆ Epidemiology

About 30% of all schwannomas arise in the head and neck. They are the most common benign neurogenic neoplasm of the parapharyngeal space. In this setting, most arise from the vagus nerve or the sympathetic trunk. Neurofibromas may occur as a manifestation of neurofibromatosis type 1 (NF-1; formerly known as von Recklinghausen's disease); in these patients, the incidence of malignant transformation is increased. Malignant PNSTs constitute ~ 10% of all soft tissue sarcomas and are more often found in the setting of neurofibromatosis. The most common head and neck area of involvement of malignant PNSTs is the neck, though it may arise from the tongue or soft palate.

◆ Clinical

Signs and Symptoms

Benign schwannomas of the parapharyngeal space most frequently present as neck masses. Other features of PNSTs at presentation may include an oropharyngeal bulge and ipsilateral cranial neuropathies.

Differential Diagnosis

- Paraganglioma
- Deep lobe parotid tumor
- Parapharyngeal space salivary gland
- Lymphoma
- Metastatic disease

◆ Evaluation

History

A history should include a family history of neurofibromatosis and other syndromes.

Physical Exam

A complete head and neck examination, including examination of CN function, is appropriate. Cranial neuropathies may or may not correlate with the nerve of origin of the tumor; that is, in some cases, adjacent nerves may develop palsies due to compression while the nerve of origin continues to function normally. Other than the mass, many patients will be asymptomatic.

Imaging

MRI is the imaging modality of choice for schwannomas and is frequently diagnostic. Schwannomas have low signal intensity on T1-weighted images and high signal intensity on T2-weighted images. Administration of gadolinium causes intense enhancement of schwannomas.

Pathology

Benign schwannomas arise from the nerve sheath and consist of Schwann cells in a collagenous matrix. Histologically, schwannomas are characterized by regions of tightly packed spindle cells. The terms *Antoni type A neurilemoma* and *type B neurilemoma* are used to describe varying growth patterns in schwannomas. Type A tissue has elongated spindle cells arranged in irregular streams and is compact in nature. Type B tissue has a looser organization, often with cystic spaces intermixed within the tissue.

Malignant PNSTs may be classified into three major categories, with epithelioid, mesenchymal, or glandular characteristics.

◆ Treatment Options

The surgical approach chosen depends on the location and extent of the lesion within the parapharyngeal space, the presence or absence of involvement of adjacent spaces, and the preferences of the surgeon. Options include cervical, cervical–parotid, cervical–parotid with mandibulotomy, and submandibular approaches. Differentiation of schwannomas from neurofibromas is of relevance to surgeons because schwannomas can be easily shelled out while preserving nerve contiguity. In most neurofibromas, however, the nerve is incorporated within the mass, and the required surgery includes resection and subsequent nerve grafting to preserve and restore function. In the case of schwannomas, this type of relationship between tumor and nerve presents the possibility of enucleation (removal of the tumor with preservation of the nerve from which it arose). Although this type of removal is often practically achievable, and recurrence rates are low, some surgeons are dubious about the likelihood of preservation of nerve function.

Malignant PNSTs should be treated by wide surgical excision, but local recurrence is a common occurrence, and hematogenous metastasis occurs in at least half of treated cases. The tumor is resistant to radiotherapy and chemotherapy, and those occurring in NF-1 behave in a more aggressive fashion than those not associated with the syndrome. Overall, the 5-year survival rate for malignant PNSTs is 40 to 75%.

6.4 The Salivary Glands

6.4.0 Embryology and Anatomy of the Salivary Glands

◆ Key Features

- The salivary glands begin to form at 6 to 9 weeks gestation.
- The major salivary glands arise from ectodermal tissue.
- Salivary glands are composed of acini and ducts.
- The parotid gland is the largest of the salivary glands, and the submandibular glands are the second largest, followed by the sublingual glands.

◆ Embryology

The embryologic development of the salivary glands is the result of complex interaction between the oral epithelium and the underlying mesenchyme, with a contribution also from neural crest. The salivary glands share a common embryogenesis in that they develop from growths of oral epithelium into the underlying mesenchyme. The acini (secretory units) and the ductal system of each gland will eventually arise from these epithelial outgrowths, which are of ectodermal origin for the parotid glands, submandibular glands, and sublingual glands, and are of mixed ectodermal and endodermal origin for the minor salivary glands. The epithelial cells carry the information for the type of salivary secretions that will be produced by each future gland, while the mesenchymal cells contain the information for the branching pattern that eventually will be the morphologic signature of these glands. The stroma, which comprises the capsule of each gland as well as the septa that divide the gland into lobes and lobules, will develop from cranial neural crest cells.

The parotid anlagen appear first, between the fourth and sixth embryonic weeks, as solid epithelial placodes in the developing cheeks. The placodes for the submandibular glands appear later in the sixth embryonic week. During the seventh to eighth embryonic weeks, the sublingual gland anlagen arise from multiple epithelial placodes, lateral to the submandibular glands, and finally the minor salivary glands develop late in the 12th fetal week.

◆ Anatomy

Parotid Glands

The paired parotid glands are the largest of the major salivary glands and typically weigh 15 to 30 g. Located in the preauricular region and along the posterior surface of the mandible, each parotid gland is divided by the facial nerve into a superficial lobe and a deep lobe. The *superficial lobe*, overlying the lateral surface of the masseter, is defined as the part of the gland lateral to the facial nerve. The *deep lobe* is medial to the facial nerve and located between the mastoid process of the temporal bone and the ramus of the mandible. The parotid gland is bounded superiorly by the zygomatic arch. Inferiorly, the tail of the parotid gland abuts the anteromedial margin of the sternocleidomastoid muscle. This tail of the parotid gland extends posteriorly over the superior border of the sternocleidomastoid muscle toward the mastoid tip. The deep lobe of the parotid lies within the parapharyngeal space. The parotid duct (Stensen) secretes a serous saliva into the oral cavity. From the anterior border of the gland, it travels parallel to the zygoma, in an anterior direction across the masseter muscle. It then turns sharply to pierce the buccinator muscle and enters the oral cavity opposite the second upper molar tooth.

The submandibular gland is the second largest major salivary gland and weighs 7 to 16 g. The gland is situated in the *submandibular triangle*, its superior boundary is formed by the inferior edge of the mandible, and its inferior boundaries are formed by the anterior and posterior bellies of the digastric muscle. The *submandibular triangle* also contains the submandibular lymph nodes, facial artery and vein, mylohyoid muscle, and the lingual, hypoglossal, and mylohyoid nerves. The marginal mandibular branch of the facial nerve courses along the capsule of the gland laterally. Most of the submandibular gland lies posterolateral to the mylohyoid muscle. Often, smaller, tonguelike projections of the gland follow the duct, as it ascends toward the oral cavity, deep to the mylohyoid muscle (**Fig. 6.18**).

The submandibular gland has both mucous and serous cells that empty into ductules, which in turn empty into the *submandibular duct*. The duct exits anteriorly from the sublingual aspect of the gland, coursing deep to the lingual nerve and medial to the sublingual gland. It eventually forms the Wharton duct between the hyoglossus and mylohyoid muscles on the genioglossus muscle. The Wharton duct, the main excretory duct of the submandibular gland, is approximately 4 to 5 cm long, running superior to the hypoglossal nerve while inferior to the lingual nerve. It empties lateral to the lingual frenulum through a papilla in the floor of the mouth behind the lower incisor tooth. The openings for the sublingual gland, or the *sublingual caruncles*, are located near the midline of the sublingual fold in the ventral tongue.

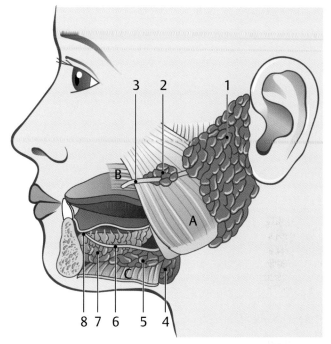

Fig. 6.18 The major salivary glands. Parotid gland (1) with small accessory gland (2) and Stensen duct (3). Submandibular gland (4) with uncinate process (5) and submandibular (Wharton) duct (6). Sublingual gland (7) with sublingual caruncle (8). A, masseter muscle; B, buccinator muscle; C, mylohyoid muscle. (Used with permission from Behrbohm H et al. *Ear, Nose, and Throat Diseases: With Head and Neck Surgery*. 3rd ed. Stuttgart/New York: Thieme; 2009:413.)

The sublingual glands, the smallest of the major salivary glands, typically weigh 2 to 4 g. Consisting mainly of mucous acinar cells, they lie as a flat structure in a submucosal plane within the anterior floor of the mouth, superior to the mylohyoid muscle and deep to the sublingual folds opposite the lingual frenulum. Several ducts from the superior portion of the sublingual gland either secrete directly into the floor of mouth or empty into the *Bartholin duct*, which then drains into the Wharton duct.

Approximately 1,000 minor salivary glands, ranging in size from 1 to 5 mm, line the oral cavity and oropharynx. The greatest number of these glands is in the lips, tongue, buccal mucosa, and palate. They can also be found along the tonsils, supraglottis, and paranasal sinuses. Each gland has a single duct, which secretes directly into the oral cavity; saliva can be serous, mucous, or mixed.

Arteries

The blood supply to the parotid gland is from branches of the *external carotid artery*. The external carotid courses superiorly from the carotid bifurcation and parallel to the mandible under the posterior belly of the digastric muscle. The artery travels medial to the parotid gland and splits into two terminal branches. The *superficial temporal artery* runs superiorly from the superior portion of the parotid gland to the scalp within the superior pretragal region. The *maxillary artery* leaves the medial portion of the parotid to supply the infratemporal and pterygopalatine fossae.

The *transverse facial artery* branches off the superficial temporal artery and runs anteriorly between the zygoma and parotid duct to supply the parotid gland and duct. The submandibular as well as the sublingual glands are supplied by the *submental* and *sublingual arteries*, branches of the lingual and facial arteries. The *facial artery* is the main arterial blood supply of the submandibular gland.

Veins

The retromandibular vein, formed by the union of the maxillary vein and the superficial temporal vein, runs through the parotid gland just deep to the facial nerve to join the external jugular vein. This vein is often crossed by the facial nerve branches.

Lymphatics

The parotid harbors two nodal layers, both of which drain into the superficial and deep cervical lymph systems. Approximately 90% of the nodes are located in the superficial layer between the glandular tissue and its capsule. The parotid gland, external auditory canal, pinna, scalp, eyelids, and lacrimal glands are all drained by these superficial nodes. The deep layer of nodes drains the gland, external auditory canal, middle ear, nasopharynx, and soft palate.

In contrast to the parotid gland, the lymph nodes draining the submandibular gland are located between the gland and its fascia but are not embedded in the glandular tissue. They lie in close approximation to the facial artery and vein at the superior aspect of the gland and empty into the deep cervical and jugular chains.

Nerves

Salivary flow is regulated predominantly by the autonomic nervous system. Although both sympathetic and parasympathetic stimulation produces saliva, the parasympathetic system is dominant. The glossopharyngeal nerve, cranial nerve (CN) IX, provides visceral secretory innervation to the parotid gland. The nerve carries preganglionic parasympathetic fibers from the inferior salivatory nucleus in the medulla oblongata through the jugular foramen. Distal to the inferior ganglion, *the tympanic nerve,* a branch of the glossopharyngeal nerve, enters the skull through the inferior tympanic canaliculus and into the middle ear to form the *tympanic plexus.* The preganglionic fibers course along as the lesser petrosal nerve into the middle cranial fossa and out the foramen ovale to synapse in the *otic ganglion.* Postganglionic parasympathetic fibers exit the otic ganglion beneath the mandibular nerve to join the auriculotemporal nerve in the infratemporal fossa. These fibers innervate the parotid gland for the secretion of saliva. Postganglionic sympathetic fibers innervate salivary glands, sweat glands,

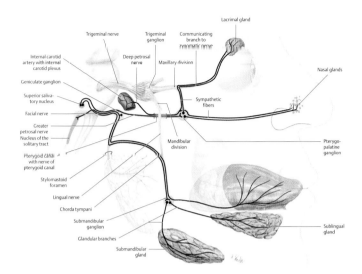

Fig. 6.19 The nervus intermedius supplies taste sensation to the anterior two-thirds of the tongue (chorda tympani nerve), preganglionic parasympathetic innervation to the submandibular, sublingual, and *minor salivary glands* (chorda tympani nerve via synapses in the submandibular ganglion), and preganglionic parasympathetic innervation to the nasal mucus glands and lacrimal glands (greater superficial petrosal nerve, via synapses in the pterygopalatine ganglion). (Used with permission from Gilroy AM, MacPherson BR, Ross LM. *Thieme Atlas of Anatomy, Head and Neuroanatomy.* 1st ed. Stuttgart/New York: Thieme;2007, illustration by Karl Wesker.)

and cutaneous blood vessels through the external carotid plexus from the *superior cervical ganglion.* Acetylcholine serves as the neurotransmitter for both postganglionic sympathetic and parasympathetic fibers (**Fig. 6.19**).

The submandibular as well as the sublingual glands are innervated by the secretomotor fibers of the facial nerve (CN VII). Parasympathetic innervation comes from the *superior salivatory nucleus* in the pons, passes through the nervus intermedius and into the internal auditory canal. The fibers are next carried by the *chorda tympani nerve* in the mastoid segment of CN VII, which travels through the middle ear and petrotympanic fissure to the infratemporal fossa. The *lingual nerve*, a branch of the mandibular division of CN V, then carries the presynaptic fibers to the *submandibular ganglion.* The postsynaptic nerve leaves the ganglion to innervate both the submandibular and sublingual glands to secrete serous (watery) saliva. The sympathetic innervation from the *superior cervical ganglion* accompanies the lingual artery to the submandibular tissue and stimulates glandular production of mucoid saliva.

Salivary Gland Secretory Unit

The salivary glands are made up of acini and ducts; together these constitute the secretory unit. The acini contain cells that secrete mucus, serum, or both. These cells drain into the intercalated duct, followed by the striated duct, and finally into the excretory duct. Myoepithelial cells surround the acini and intercalated duct and serve to expel secretory products into the ductal system. Basal cells along the salivary gland unit replace damaged elements. The combined salivary glands produce 1 to 1.5 L of saliva per day. About 45% is produced by the parotid gland, 45% by the submandibular glands, and 5% each by the sublingual and minor salivary glands (**Table 6.21**).

Table 6.21   Salivary gland secretions

Parotid gland secretion • Proteinaceous, watery, serous secretion • Two-thirds of salivary flow during gustatory and olfactory stimulation • Organic (proteins including enzymes) and inorganic materials are higher.
Submandibular gland secretion • High mucin content, viscous/serous secretion • Higher basal flow rate • Calcium is higher.
Sublingual gland secretion • Higher mucin content than submandibular gland • 5% of salivary flow
Minor salivary gland secretion • Purely mucous glands • 5% of salivary flow

Data from Witt RL, ed. *Salivary Gland Diseases: Medical and Surgical Management.* New York, NY: Thieme;2006.

6.4.1   Salivary Gland Disease

◆ Key Features

- Salivary gland disease may be infectious, inflammatory, noninflammatory, or autoimmune in nature.
- Salivary gland disease may be accompanied by a decrease in salivary flow.
- An underlying autoimmune condition and tumor must be ruled out.

Salivary gland disease may be infectious, inflammatory, noninflammatory, or autoimmune in nature.

◆ Infectious Diseases of the Salivary Glands

Acute Sialadenitis

Acute sialadenitis is an acute inflammation of a salivary gland. Several viral microorganisms have been identified as causative agents for infections of the salivary glands. The most common virus that causes sialadenitis is the mumps virus (Rubulavirus). Others include coxsackievirus, echovirus, influenza virus, and human immunodeficiency virus (HIV).

Signs and Symptoms

Symptoms of acute sialadenitis include acute painful swelling of the affected salivary gland (**Fig. 6.20**). At times only one gland is affected initially. There may be swelling of adjacent cervical lymph nodes. The duct orifice may be erythematous. Other symptoms include fever and trismus.

Differential Diagnosis

- Cervical lymphadenopathy
- Acute bacterial sialadenitis
- Inflammatory sialadenitis
- Abscess
- Tumor
- Odontogenic abscess
- Infection

Treatment Options

Treatment is supportive; it typically consists of fluid intake, sialagogues (such as lemon wedges), and analgesics.

Acute Bacterial Sialadenitis

Acute bacterial sialadenitis is a suppurative infection that most commonly infects the parotid glands in debilitated, dehydrated, or elderly patients. Acute bacterial sialadenitis is thought to be an ascending bacterial infection due to decreased salivary flow. Situations that cause a tendency for acute sialadenitis include diabetes mellitus, immunocompromised state, and poor

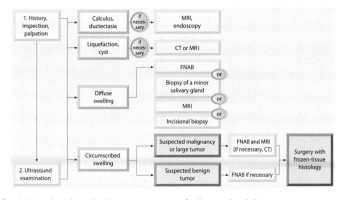

Fig. 6.20 Flowchart for the investigation of salivary gland disease. MRI, magnetic resonance imaging; CT, computed tomography; FNAB, fine-needle aspiration biopsy. (Used with permission from Probst R, Grevers G, Iro H. *Basic Otorhinolaryngology: A Step-by-Step Learning Guide*. Stuttgart/New York: Thieme; 2006:141.)

oral hygiene. Other rarer infectious causes of sialadenitis include tuberculosis, actinomycosis, syphilis, and HIV infection.

Signs and Symptoms

Symptoms include diffuse, painful swelling of the affected gland (**Fig. 6.21**). The skin over the gland may be warm, red, and tight. The orifice duct of the affected salivary gland may be red, and massage of the gland may express purulent material from the orifice. Trismus may be present.

Microbiology

The main causative pathogen is *Staphylococcus aureus*. Other bacterial organisms that may cause sialadenitis include *Streptococcus viridans*, *Haemophilus influenzae*, *Streptococcus pyogenes*, and *Escherichia coli*.

Treatment Options

Medical treatment includes antibiotics, hydration, sialagogues (such as lemon wedges), warm compresses, gland massage, and meticulous oral hygiene. If an abscess develops, incision and drainage should be performed with careful attention to the underlying facial nerve. The incision should be made in parallel to the branches of the facial nerve.

♦ Inflammatory Diseases of the Salivary Glands

Sjögren's syndrome

Sjögren's syndrome is an inflammatory disease of the exocrine glands. This autoimmune condition may cause chronic sialadenitis. Patients may develop a gradual decrease in salivary production. Xerostomia (dry mouth), xerophthalmia (dry eyes), and lymphocytic infiltration of the exocrine glands is

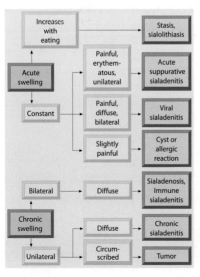

Fig. 6.21 Differential diagnosis of acute and chronic salivary gland swelling. (Used with permission from Probst R, Grevers G, Iro H. *Basic Otorhinolaryngology: A Step-by-Step Learning Guide.* Stuttgart/New York: Thieme; 2006:140.)

known as the sicca complex. The pathogenesis is antibodies directed against the antigens of the salivary duct epithelium, causing gland atrophy and interstitial lymphocystic infiltration

Epidemiology

The disease predominantly affects women.

Signs and Symptoms

Both parotid glands may be involved. Their consistency on palpation is doughy. There may be little or no pain or tenderness. Patients may have associated xerostomia, keratoconjunctivitis, lymphadenopathy, and polyneuropathies.

Labs

An elevated erythrocyte sedimentation rate (ESR) and the presence of auto-antibodies Sjögren's syndrome A (SS-A) and Sjögren's syndrome B (SS-B), rheumatoid factor, and antinuclear antibodies are indicators for the disease.

Other Tests

Biopsy of the minor salivary glands of the lip is diagnostic in 60 to 70% of the cases. Sialography, if performed, may demonstrate a leafless tree pattern.

Treatment Options

Treatment includes immunosuppressant therapy as well as symptomatic therapy with saliva substitutes and artificial tears as well as pilocarpine to augment salivary stimulation.

Complications

Complications of Sjögren's syndrome involving the salivary glands include dental caries. There is an increased incidence of non-Hodgkin lymphomas (NHLs) of the salivary glands among patients with Sjögren's syndrome.

Heerfordt's syndrome

Another cause of chronic sialadenitis is Heerfordt's syndrome, a form of sarcoidosis with enlargement of the parotid glands, mild fever, uveitis, and facial nerve palsy.

◆ Noninflammatory Salivary Disease

Sialolithiasis

Sialolithiasis (salivary stones or calculi) is a stone formation in the excretory duct system of the salivary glands. Sixty to 70% of these are located in the main duct of the gland; 70 to 80% occur in the submandibular gland; 20% occur in the parotid gland. A much smaller percentage may occur in minor salivary glands. Pathogenesis is ductal debris, and calcium phosphate coalesces due to infection, inflammation, or salivary stasis.

Epidemiology

Sialolithiasis typically affects adults; males are more commonly affected than females.

Signs and Symptoms

Symptoms vary according to the degree of obstruction and may include pain and swelling often while or after eating.

Differential Diagnosis

- Inflammation
- Infection
- Tumor

Imaging

Ultrasound may reveal the dilation of the duct system. Seventy to 80% of submandibular salivary stones and only 20% of parotid stones are radiopaque and may be seen on computed tomography (CT) imaging. Noncontrast CT imaging is preferable for detecting salivary stones.

Treatment Options

Typically, the treatment for sialolithiasis is surgical. Intraglandular stones in the submandibular gland typically result in the removal of the gland. Salivary stones that are located near the orifice may be manipulated out. Stones that are more proximal to the gland can be removed either endoscopically (if small enough) or through an incision through the duct system.

Complications

Complications include abscess formation and infection.

Ranula

Ranula is a sialocele of the sublingual gland typically found in the floor of the mouth. It represents a pseudocyst enlargement. The treatment is surgical excision or marsupialization.

6.4.2 Benign Salivary Gland Tumors

◆ Key Features

- Tumors of the salivary glands represent 2 to 4% of head and neck neoplasms.
- 70% of salivary gland tumors originate in the parotid gland.
- 85% of salivary gland tumors are pleomorphic adenomas (benign mixed tumors).
- Salivary gland tumors most often present as painless masses.
- The most common parotid mass in a child is a hemangioma.

Pleomorphic adenomas are the most common benign salivary gland tumors. They constitute 70% of parotid gland tumors and 50% of submandibular gland tumors. Pleomorphic adenomas are often located in the tail of the parotid gland. When they are found in the minor salivary glands, the hard palate is the site most frequently involved, followed by the upper lip. Warthin's tumors (papillary cystadenoma lymphomatosum) occur almost exclusively in the parotid gland. They account for 4 to 11.2% of all salivary gland tumors. These lesions can be multifocal and bilateral (10%) and are more common in individuals who use tobacco (**Table 6.22**).

Table 6.22 Classification of benign primary epithelial salivary gland tumors

Benign mixed tumor (pleomorphic adenoma)
Warthin's tumor (papillary cystadenoma lymphomatosum)
Oncocytoma (oxyphil adenoma)
Monomorphic tumors
Sebaceous tumors
Benign lymphoepithelial lesion
Papillary ductal adenoma (papilloma)

◆ Clinical

Signs

A painless mass can be felt in the affected salivary gland.

Symptoms

There is slowly increasing, painless swelling of the affected salivary gland. (Pain, rapid growth of long-standing benign parotid mass, and facial nerve paralysis should raise the suspicion of malignant disease; see **Chapter 6.4.3**.)

Differential Diagnosis

- Adenopathy of periparotid or perifacial lymph nodes
- Malignant salivary tumors
- Metastatic lesions
- Autoimmune, infectious, or inflammatory salivary gland lesions

◆ Evaluation

History

History should include questions about time course and onset of mass, pain, relationship of swelling to eating, xerophthalmia, known autoimmune conditions, weight loss, fever, night sweats, and infectious diseases.

Physical Exam

A full head and neck examination, including the salivary glands and the neck, and a bimanual examination of submandibular glands should be performed. Facial nerve function should be documented.

Imaging

Imaging studies are most helpful in the diagnostic evaluation. Ultrasound may help fine-needle aspiration biopsy (FNAB) localization. Magnetic resonance imaging (MRI) is the most sensitive test for establishing the borders of soft tissue tumor extension. Computed tomography (CT) is usually sufficient.

Labs

A white blood cell count should be ordered to investigate for any evidence of leukocytosis and neutrophilic shift, possible infectious process, or lymphoproliferative disease. A lymphoepithelial cyst or recurrent parotid abscess should prompt human immunodeficiency virus (HIV) testing.

Other Tests

FNAB findings provide evidence for a preoperative diagnosis.

Pathology

Pleomorphic adenomas are characterized by variable, diverse, structural histologic patterns. Frequently, they have growth patterns of sheets, strands, or islands of spindle and stellate cells, with a myxoid configuration occasionally predominating. Warthin's tumors are composed of an oncocytic epithelial component that can have a papillary, glandular–cystic, and/or solid growth pattern. Oncocytomas are composed of large oxyphilic cells (oncocytes) (**Fig. 6.22**, **Fig. 6.23**).

◆ Treatment Options

Medical

Medical therapy is appropriate for infectious and inflammatory processes. Radiotherapy is for nonoperative candidates with pleomorphic adenomas or recurrent multiple pleomorphic adenomas.

Surgical

Management of benign salivary gland tumors includes complete removal with an adequate margin of tissue to avoid recurrences. This involves superficial parotidectomy, total parotidectomy with preservation of facial nerve for deep lobe masses, or submandibular gland removal.

◆ Complications

During submandibular gland excision, unintentional injury may be inflicted on the lingual, hypoglossal, or mandibular (branch of the facial) nerve. Recurrence is usually caused by inadequate excision, tumor enucleation, or tumor spillage.

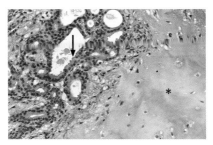

Fig. 6.22   Luminal structures lined with cells showing an apocrine phenotype (*arrow*) and cartilaginous stroma (*asterisk*). (Used with permission from Bradley PJ, Guntinas-Lichius O, eds. *Salivary Gland Disorders and Diseases: Diagnosis and Management*. Stuttgart/New York: Thieme;2011:33.)

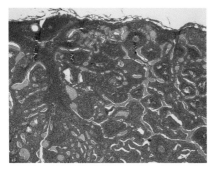

Fig. 6.23   Histology of Warthin tumor. These lesions show bilayered oncocytic epithelium and a dense, lymphoid stroma (hematoxylin/eosin, ×40). (Used with permission from Witt RL, ed. *Salivary Gland Diseases: Surgical and Medical Management*. New York, NY: Thieme; 2006:126.)

With parotidectomy, facial nerve paralysis (paresis) takes a few weeks to resolve spontaneously but can last months or be permanent. Reported rates of permanent postoperative facial nerve paresis range from 0 to 30%. Eye care is important until there is a return of facial nerve function.

Frey's syndrome (gustatory sweating) is caused by an aberrant connection of the postganglionic gustatory parasympathetic fibers to sympathetic fibers of the sweat glands of the overlying skin. It is best avoided by raising a thick flap during parotid surgery.

◆ Outcome and Follow-Up

Evaluate postoperative facial, hypoglossal, and lingual nerve function. Occasionally, transient facial nerve paresis occurs, but it usually resolves within weeks of surgery.

Outcome is typically excellent, and the recurrence rate is very low. Malignant degeneration to carcinoma ex pleomorphic adenoma occurs in 1.4 to 6.3% of untreated pleomorphic adenomas. Malignant degeneration is often associated with a prolonged history of untreated or recurrent pleomorphic adenoma.

6.4.3 Malignant Salivary Gland Tumors

◆ Key Features

- Malignant salivary gland neoplasms account for 0.5% of all malignancies.
- Malignant salivary gland neoplasms account for 3 to 5% of all head and neck cancer.
- The most common malignant major and minor salivary gland tumor is mucoepidermoid carcinoma.
- Numbness or facial nerve weakness and pain in conjunction with salivary gland mass suggest malignancy.

◆ Epidemiology

The frequency of malignant lesions varies by site. Approximately 20 to 25% of parotid tumors, 35 to 40% of submandibular tumors, 50% of palate tumors, and > 90% of sublingual gland tumors are malignant. Mucoepidermoid carcinoma is the most common malignant neoplasm of the salivary glands. Most cases originate in the parotid gland. Mucoepidermoid carcinoma is a malignant epithelial tumor that is composed of various proportions of mucous, epidermoid, intermediate, columnar, and clear cells. Microscopic grading of mucoepidermoid carcinoma is important to determine the prognosis. Mucoepidermoid carcinomas are graded as low, intermediate, and high based on the degree of epidermoid and mucinous cell populations.

Adenoid cystic carcinoma (formerly known as cylindroma) is a slow-growing but aggressive neoplasm with a remarkable capacity for recurrence. This is the most common malignant tumor of the submandibular and minor salivary glands and constitutes 4% of all salivary gland tumors. Morphologically, three growth patterns have been described: cribriform or classic pattern, tubular, and solid or basaloid pattern. This tumor has a propensity for perineural spread. Regardless of histologic grade, adenoid cystic carcinomas, with their unusually slow biologic growth, tend to have a protracted course and ultimately a poor outcome, with a 10-year survival reported to be < 50% for all grades. Many advocate following these patients for the duration of their lifetime, as recurrence can be quite late.

Acinic cell carcinoma is a malignant epithelial neoplasm in which the neoplastic cells express acinar differentiation. In Armed Forces Institute of Pathology (AFIP) data on salivary gland neoplasms, acinic cell carcinoma is the third most common salivary gland epithelial neoplasm; > 80% occur in the parotid gland, women are affected more than men, and the mean patient age is 44 years. Clinically, patients typically present with a slowly enlarging mass in the parotid region. Pain is a symptom in > 33% of patients. For acinic cell carcinoma, staging is likely a better predictor of outcome than histologic grading.

Carcinoma ex pleomorphic adenoma, also known as carcinoma ex mixed tumor or pleomorphic carcinoma, is a carcinoma that shows histologic evidence of arising from or in a benign pleomorphic adenoma. The neoplasm occurs primarily in the major salivary glands. Diagnosis requires the identification of benign tumor in the tissue sample. The incidence or relative frequency of this tumor varies considerably depending on the study cited.

Lymphomas of the major salivary glands are characteristically of the non-Hodgkin's lymphoma (NHL) type. In an AFIP review of case files, NHL accounted for 16.3% of all malignant tumors that occurred in the major salivary glands, and disease in the parotid gland accounted for ~ 80% of all cases.

Primary squamous cell carcinoma (SCC), also known as primary epidermoid carcinoma, is a malignant epithelial neoplasm of the major salivary glands that is composed of squamous (i.e., epidermoid) cells. Diagnosis requires the exclusion of primary disease located in some other head and neck site; indeed, most SCCs of the major salivary glands represent metastatic disease (**Table 6.23**).

Table 6.23 Classification of malignant primary epithelial salivary gland tumors

Mucoepidermoid carcinoma
Adenoid cystic carcinoma

Adenocarcinomas
• Acinic cell carcinoma
• Polymorphous low-grade adenocarcinoma
• Adenocarcinoma, NOS
• Rare adenocarcinomas
  o Basal cell adenocarcinoma
  o Clear cell carcinoma
  o Cystadenocarcinoma
  o Sebaceous adenocarcinoma
  o Sebaceous lymphadenocarcinoma
  o Oncocytic carcinoma
  o Salivary duct carcinoma
  o Mucinous adenocarcinoma

Malignant mixed tumors • Carcinoma ex pleomorphic adenoma • Carcinosarcoma • Metastasizing mixed tumor

Rare carcinomas
• Primary squamous cell carcinoma
• Epithelial-myoepithelial carcinoma
• Anaplastic small-cell carcinoma
• Undifferentiated carcinomas
  o Small-cell undifferentiated carcinoma
  o Large-cell undifferentiated carcinoma
  o Lymphoepithelial carcinoma
• Myoepithelial carcinoma
• Adenosquamous carcinoma

Abbreviation: NOS, not otherwise specified.

Malignant neoplasms whose origins lie outside the salivary glands may involve the major salivary glands by:

1. Direct invasion from cancers that lie adjacent to the salivary glands
2. Hematogenous metastases from distant primary tumors
3. Lymphatic metastases to lymph nodes within the salivary gland

Direct invasion of nonsalivary gland tumors into the major salivary glands is principally from squamous cell and basal cell carcinomas of the overlying skin. Prior exposure to ionizing radiation appears to substantially increase the risk for development of malignant neoplasms of the major salivary glands.

◆ Clinical

Signs and Symptoms

A painless swelling of the affected salivary gland is a sign of a salivary gland tumor. Approximately 10 to 15% of malignant parotid neoplasms present with pain. Occasionally, malignant salivary gland tumors may be characterized by rapid growth or a sudden growth spurt. Numbness or nerve weakness caused by nerve involvement and persistent facial pain are highly suggestive of malignancy. Depending on the site of the primary tumor, other symptoms include drainage from the ipsilateral ear, dysphagia, trismus, and facial paralysis. The overlying skin or mucosa may become ulcerated.

Differential Diagnosis

- Adenopathy of periparotid or perifacial lymph nodes
- Benign salivary tumors
- Metastatic lesions
- Autoimmune, infectious, or inflammatory salivary gland lesions

◆ Evaluation

History

History includes questions about time course and onset of mass, pain, facial weakness, weight loss, known autoimmune disease, fever, and night sweats.

Physical Exam

A full head and neck examination including salivary glands, neck, and a bimanual examination of submandibular glands should be performed. Cranial nerve (CN) function should be assessed.

Imaging

Imaging studies are helpful in the diagnostic evaluation. Ultrasound may help fine-needle aspiration biopsy (FNAB) localization. Magnetic resonance imaging (MRI) is the most sensitive test for establishing the borders of soft tissue tumor extension. Contrast-enhanced computed tomography (CT) is usually sufficient.

Other Tests

FNAB findings often provide evidence for a preoperative diagnosis,

Pathology

Salivary gland neoplasms show extreme histologic diversity. These neoplasms include malignant tumors of epithelial, mesenchymal, and lymphoid origin. There are several characteristic appearances that are notable. Mucoepidermoid carcinoma, as the name suggests, will have a combination of mucinous cells and squamous cells that become more de-differentiated in higher-grade tumors. Adenoid cystic carcinoma, especially the cribriform subtype, can have a "Swiss cheese" appearance on histology. Histologic grading (**Table 6.24**) of salivary gland carcinomas is important to determine the proper treatment approach. However, it is not an independent indicator of the clinical course and must be considered in the context of the clinical stage; see Staging of Malignant Salivary Gland Tumors (**Fig. 6.24**).

Table 6.24   Histologic grading of salivary gland carcinomas

Low-grade
• Acinic cell carcinoma
• Basal cell adenocarcinoma
• Clear cell carcinoma
• Cystadenocarcinoma
• Epithelial-myoepithelial carcinoma
• Mucinous adenocarcinoma
• Polymorphous low-grade adenocarcinoma
Low-, intermediate, and high-grade
• Adenocarcinoma, NOS
• Mucoepidermoid carcinoma
• Squamous cell carcinoma
Intermediate and high-grade
• Myoepithelial carcinoma
High-grade
• Anaplastic small-cell carcinoma
• Carcinosarcoma
• Large-cell undifferentiated carcinoma
• Small-cell undifferentiated carcinoma
• Salivary duct carcinoma

Abbreviation: NOS, not otherwise specified.

◆ Treatment Options

Medical

The use of chemotherapy for malignant salivary gland tumors remains under evaluation. Postoperative radiotherapy augments surgical resection, particularly for the high-grade neoplasms, when margins are close or

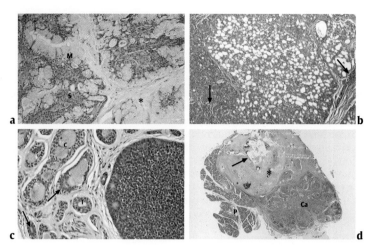

Fig. 6.24 **(a)** Slightly hematoxyphilic mucous cells (M), eosinophilic squamoid cells (S), and stromal pooling of mucosubstances (*asterisk*). **(b)** A microcystic acinic cell carcinoma (ACC) with stromal lymphoid aggregates (*arrows*). **(c)** Solid **(S)**, cribriform **(C)**, and tubular **(T)** arrangements, showing lumina lined with eosinophilic cells (*arrows*). **(d)** The "ghost" of a pleomorphic salivary adenoma (*asterisk*) with fragmented calcification (*arrow*). Ca, a malignant invasive component; P, parotid. (Used with permission from Bradley PJ, Guntinas-Lichius O, eds. *Salivary Gland Disorders and Diseases: Diagnosis and Management.* Stuttgart/New York: Thieme; 2011:36–38.)

involved, when tumors are large, or when histologic evidence of lymph node metastases is present. Fast neutron-beam radiation or accelerated hyperfractionated photon beam schedules have been reported to be more effective than conventional X-ray therapy in the treatment of inoperable, unresectable, or recurrent malignant salivary gland tumors.

Surgical

The minimum therapy for low-grade (and intermediate-grade mucoepidermoid carcinoma) malignancies of the superficial portion of the parotid gland is a superficial parotidectomy. For all other lesions, a total parotidectomy with facial nerve preservation is often indicated. The facial nerve or its branches should be resected if involved by tumor. Rarely, a mastoidectomy or temporal bone resection may be performed to obtain a negative margin on CN VII. Neck dissection may be performed, depending on tumor type and nodal involvement.

◆ Complications

Parotidectomy

Recurrence may be caused by inadequate excision, positive margins, or tumor spillage. Facial nerve paralysis and cosmetic deformity may need to be addressed surgically. CN dysfunction from the tumor and resultant surgery is a possible complication. Eye care is important in the presence of facial nerve paralysis.

◆ Outcome and Follow-Up

Early-stage low-grade malignant salivary gland tumors are usually curable by adequate surgical resection alone. The prognosis is more favorable when the tumor is in a major salivary gland. Large, bulky tumors or high-grade tumors carry a poorer prognosis. The prognosis also depends on the following: the gland in which they arise, histology, the grade, the stage, perineural involvement, and spread to adjacent structures, lymph nodes, or distant sites. The prognosis for any treated cancer patient with progressing or relapsing disease is poor, regardless of histologic type or stage. It is notable that adenoid cystic carcinoma can recur in a delayed fashion, with some recurrences occurring more than 10 years after treatment of the primary tumor.

◆ Staging of Malignant Salivary Gland Tumors

Primary Tumor (T)

TX: Primary tumor cannot be assessed

T0:   No evidence of primary tumor

Tis: Carcinoma in situ

T1:   Tumor ≤ 2 cm in greatest dimension without extraparenchymal extension

T2:   Tumor > 2 cm and ≤ 4 cm in greatest dimension without extraparenchymal extension

T3:   Tumor > 4 cm and/or tumor having extraparenchymal extension

T4:

   T4a: Moderately advanced disease; tumor invades the skin, the mandible, the ear canal, and/or the facial nerve

   T4b: Very advanced disease; tumor invades the skull base and/or the pterygoid plates and/or encases the carotid artery

*Extraparenchymal extension is clinical or macroscopic evidence of invasion of soft tissues. Microscopic evidence alone is not sufficient.

Regional Lymph Nodes (N)*

NX: Regional lymph nodes cannot be assessed

N0:   No regional lymph node metastasis

N1:   Metastasis to a single ipsilateral lymph node measuring ≤ 3 cm in greatest diameter and ENE negative

N2:   Further divided into three categories:

   N2a: Single ipsilateral lymph node > 3 and ≤ 6 cm and ENE negative (pathologic staging also includes a single ipsilateral or contralateral lymph node ≤ 3 cm and ENE positive)

   N2b: Multiple ipsilateral lymph nodes ≤ 6 cm and ENE negative

   N2c: Bilateral or contralateral lymph nodes ≤ 6 cm in greatest dimension and ENE negative

N3:   Now further divided into two categories:

   N3a: Metastasis to a lymph node > 6 cm, ENE negative

N3b: Metastasis to a single lymph node that is ENE positive (pathologic staging includes single lymph nodes that are ENE positive >3cm), or metastasis to multiple lymph nodes with any ENE positive

A designation of "U" or "L" can be attached to the N category to indicate nodes above ("U") or below ("L") the lower border of the cricoid. Similarly, clinical and pathologic ENE should be recorded as ENE (−) or ENE (+). Clinical and pathologic staging are similar with the differences noted in parenthesis.

*Superior mediastinal lymph nodes are considered regional lymph nodes (level VII). Midline nodes are considered ipsilateral nodes.

Distant Metastasis (M)

M0: No distant metastasis

M1: Distant metastasis

American Joint Committee on Cancer Stage Groupings of Malignant Salivary Gland Tumors (8th edition)

Stage 0 disease: Carcinoma in situ (TisN0M0)

Stage I disease: Includes only T1 N0 M0 tumors

Stage II disease: Includes only T2 N0 M0 tumors

Stage III disease: Includes T3 N0 M0 and T1 -3 disease that is N1 M0

Stage IVA disease: Includes T4a disease with N0-N2 M0 disease and T1-T3 disease that is N2 M0

Stage IVB disease: Includes T4b disease with any nodal disease or T1-T4a disease with N3 disease without distant metastases (M0)

Stage IVC disease: Any disease with distant metastases (M1)

See **Table 6.7** in Chapter 6.3.3.

6.4.4 Sialendoscopy

✦ Key Features

- Sialendoscopy utilizes tiny semirigid scopes to visualize salivary ducts for stone and foreign body removal, dilation of stenosis, and irrigation.
- Sialendoscopy is a relatively new procedure now rapidly gaining wide acceptance.

Traditional methods of treating nonneoplastic disorders of the salivary gland include watchful observation, medical treatment, surgical excision of the involved salivary gland, and sialendoscopy. The latter is a relatively new procedure that allows endoscopic transluminal visualization of major salivary glands and offers a mechanism for diagnosing and treating both inflammatory and obstructive pathology related to the ductal system.

Sialendoscopy is a minimally invasive gland-preserving technique for obstructive salivary disease. Technical advancements now allow working scopes that range from 1.1- to 1.6 mm external diameter with a working channel and an irrigation channel, and diagnostic scopes down to a 0.8-mm external diameter scope with only an irrigation channel. Scopes are inserted through the papilla of the duct of the submandibular and parotid glands and can access up to fifth-order branches. Wire baskets, microforceps, and balloons are employed for interventions.

◆ Clinical

Symptoms

- Chronic or recurrent swelling and pain of submandibular or parotid gland
- Swelling may follow eating and gradually resolve.

Signs

- Facial / neck swelling

Differential Diagnosis

- Sialolithiasis
- Salivary duct strictures
- Salivary duct foreign body
- Salivary duct mass

◆ Evaluation

Ultrasound in the setting of gland swelling will show an obstruction. Diagnostic sialendoscopy is the next step.

◆ Treatment Options

The procedure can be done under general or local anesthesia with sedation. A mouth prop is placed. Using loupes or a microscope, the papillary orifice is located, and duct probes of increasing diameters are placed through it to dilate the duct. The submandibular duct has a smaller opening than does the parotid duct, making it more difficult to access. A guidewire can also be placed and dilation done with a bougie or dilator. The scope can be inserted through the dilator, which makes its use advantageous. The scope contains a working channel and an irrigation channel. Irrigation is required because the duct walls are collapsed. If the goal is stone removal, the stone is visualized and a wire basket is passed through the working channel of the scope, advanced past the stone, opened, and manipulated to capture the stone. A papillotomy may be necessary to allow stone extraction. Larger stones may be debulked using a diamond bur or laser. Balloon catheters are available for stricture dilation.

Indications for sialendoscopy include:

- Sialolithiasis
- Noncalcified duct obstructions

- Recurrent sialadenitis
- Assessment of treatment outcomes

  Contraindications include acute suppurative sialadenitis.

◆ Postoperative Care

- Glands swell for 1 to 2 days postop, which may require analgesics.
- Stimulate salivary flow with gland massage and natural stimulants such as lemons.

◆ Complications

- Duct avulsion—requires an open procedure
- Duct perforation—a short-term stent can be placed with good results.
- Duct strictures—these can be dilated with a balloon catheter, or a stent placed.
- Hematoma—small ones will resolve spontaneously, large ones may need drainage.
- Injury to lingual nerve or facial nerve
- Failure of resolution is treated with open duct surgery, lithotripsy, or gland excision.

◆ Outcome and Follow-Up

A recent systematic review showed a success rate of 76% for stone removal, with incidence of gland extirpation 0 to 24.5%. When combined with surgical approaches, gland extirpation rate is 4.6%.

7 Endocrine Surgery in Otolaryngology

Section Editors

David Goldenberg

Neerav Goyal

Contributors

David Goldenberg

Bradley J. Goldstein

Neerav Goyal

7.0 Embryology and Anatomy of the Thyroid Gland

Key Features

- The thyroid is an H-shaped vascular gland located in the anterior lower neck just below the larynx.
- Its function is the synthesis and secretion of thyroid hormones thyroxine (T_4) and triiodothyronine (T_3).
- The isthmus overlies the second to fourth tracheal rings.
- The thyroid weighs, on average, 25 g in adults.
- A pyramidal lobe may be present as an extension of the embryologic thyroglossal duct (50%).
- The tubercle of Zuckerkandl is a lateral or posterior projection from the thyroid lobe.
- The thyroid gland is usually not visible externally; when it increases in size, it forms a characteristic swelling in the neck called a goiter.

Embryology

The human thyroid gland begins to develop at around 4 weeks after conception and moves down the neck while forming its characteristic bilobular structure, which is completed by the third trimester (**Fig. 7.1**).

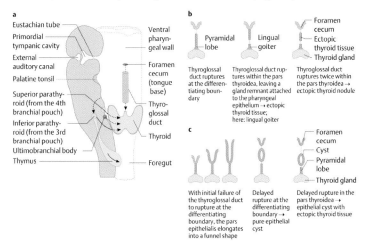

Fig. 7.1 (a–c) Embryology and malformations of the thyroid gland. (Used with permission from Probst R, Grevers G, Iro H. *Basic Otorhinolaryngology: A Step-by-Step Learning Guide.* Stuttgart/New York: Thieme; 2006:323.)

◆ Ligaments and Fascia

The thyroid gland is ensheathed by the middle layer of the deep cervical fascia. The posteromedial part of the gland is attached to the cricoid cartilage, first and second tracheal rings, by the posterior suspensory ligament (Berry ligament). Under the layer of cervical fascia the gland has an inner true capsule, which is thin and adheres closely to the gland.

◆ Thyroid Cells

The thyroid is made up of follicular and parafollicular cells (C cells; clear, light cells). Follicular cells are responsible for the formation of the colloid (iodothyroglobulin), whose function is to store thyroid hormones prior to their secretion). The parafollicular cells are scattered between the thyroid follicles and produce the hormone calcitonin, which is central to calcium homeostasis. The cells migrate from the neural crest and are most concentrated at the junction between the upper one-third and lower two-thirds of the lobes.

◆ Vascular Anatomy

Arteries

The principal arterial supply is from the superior thyroid artery (STA) and inferior thyroid artery (ITA). The STA originates from the external carotid artery. The ITA originates from thyrocervical trunk, which is a branch of the subclavian artery. The ITA serves as an important surgical landmark for the recurrent laryngeal nerve and parathyroid glands. Occasionally, the thyroidea ima artery supplies the thyroid isthmus directly from the innominate artery or aortic arch (1.5–12%).

Veins

There are the superior, middle, and inferior thyroid veins. The superior and middle thyroid veins drain into the internal jugular vein. The inferior thyroid vein drains into the brachiocephalic veins.

Lymphatics

The upper, middle, and lower deep cervical nodes receive lymph from the thyroid gland, as do the pretracheal and paratracheal nodes and the prelaryngeal (delphian) node.

◆ Nerves

The innervation of the thyroid gland itself derives from the autonomic nervous system.

- **Sympathetic**: superior, middle, and inferior sympathetic ganglia
- **Parasympathetic**: vagus nerves

The recurrent laryngeal nerve (RLN) does not innervate the thyroid gland itself: the RLN innervates all intrinsic laryngeal muscles except the cricothyroid muscle. The left RLN lies in the tracheoesophageal groove throughout its length. The right RLN lies laterally in the first part of its course but veers medially and ascends toward the gland (a slightly diagonal course). In rare cases (0.3–0.8% of people), the right RLN is nonrecurrent and comes directly off the vagus. The right nonrecurrent nerve is associated with a right subclavian artery arising directly from the aortic arch.

Landmarks for identifying the RLN during thyroid surgery include the following:

- The "Simon triangle" (the carotid triangle) is formed by the carotid artery, the trachea, and the inferior pole of the thyroid.
- The recurrent laryngeal nerve may be identified 0.5 cm below the inferior cornu of the thyroid cartilage.
- The "tubercle of Zuckerkandl" is a lateral or posterior projection from the lateral thyroid lobe that indicates the point of embryologic fusion of the ultimobranchial body and the principal median thyroid process. The RLN lies between the tubercle of Zuckerkandl and the trachea.
- The "Beahrs triangle" is formed by the RLN, the inferior thyroid artery, and the common carotid artery.

The superior laryngeal nerve is subdivided into external and internal branches. The external branch parallels the superior thyroid artery and descends to innervate the cricothyroid muscle. The internal branch parallels the superior thyroid artery and enters the thyrohyoid membrane to give sensation to the larynx above the goiter.

The nerve of Galen is an anastomosis between the sensory branch of the RLN and the internal branch of the superior laryngeal nerve.

7.1 Physiology of the Thyroid Gland

◆ Key Features

- The functional unit of the thyroid gland is the follicle (**Fig. 7.2**).
- Thyroid follicles are composed of a single layer of epithelial cells (thyroid follicular cells) surrounding a central space filled with colloid.
- The follicular cells synthesize Tg, a large tyrosine-rich glycoprotein, and secrete it into the lumen of the follicle; colloid is essentially a pool of Tg.
- Key thyroid hormones include thyrotropin-releasing hormone (TRH), thyroid-stimulating hormone (TSH), T_4, and T_3.
- Only 1% of total thyroid hormone is in the unbound or free state and available for metabolic purposes. The rest is bound to globulin, prealbumin, and albumin.
- Calcitonin is a peptide produced by the parafollicular cells of the thyroid gland. It reduces resorption of calcium in the bone and lowers the serum calcium.

◆ Thyroid Hormone Regulation

The hypothalamus secretes thyrotropin-releasing hormone (TRH), which passes via the portal venous system to the anterior pituitary. Here, it stimulates synthesis and release of thyroid-stimulating hormone (TSH). The TSH stimulates iodide trapping, release of thyroid hormones, and thyroid growth. The thyroid hormones exert negative feedback control of the hypothalamic-pituitary axis.

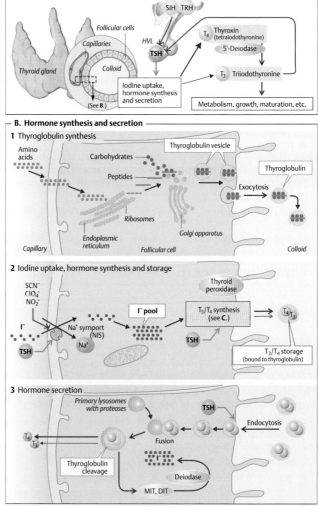

Fig. 7.2 **(a,b)** Physiology of thyroid hormone production and synthesis. (Used with permission from Silbernagl S, Despopoulos A. *Color Atlas of Physiology*. 6th ed. Stuttgart/New York: Thieme; 2009:289.)

◆ Steps in Thyroid Hormone Synthesis

1. Iodide uptake: The thyroid selectively concentrates inorganic iodine (iodide).
2. Organification: Iodine is produced by oxidation of iodide. Iodine reacts with tyrosine on the Tg first to produce monoiodotyrosine (MIT) and then diiodotyrosine (DIT).
3. Coupling: Coupled reactions between DIT lead to the formation of thyroxine (T_4), and those between DIT and MIT form triiodothyronine (T_3).
4. Storage: The T_4 and T_3 are stored as colloid, still a part of the Tg molecule.
5. Release: Endocytosis of the stored colloid leads to formation of colloid droplets (phagolysosomes) in which Tg is digested by proteases to release T_4, T_3, DIT, and MIT into the blood.

Note that thyroid peroxidase (TPO) catalyzes the oxidation of iodide and its transfer to tyrosine (organification) and coupling.

◆ Thyroid Hormones and Their Actions

The thyroid gland releases two hormones into the blood, mostly T_4 and some T_3. T_3 is the active hormone, whereas T_4 is the prohormone and converts to T_3 in many tissues of the body through a process called peripheral deiodination. Effects include:

- Calorigenesis: the thyroid hormones generate heat and increase oxygen consumption.
- Carbohydrate and fat metabolism
- Growth and development

7.2 Thyroid Evaluation

◆ Key Features

- Thyroid function tests are common procedures performed to determine how well the thyroid is functioning.
- Evaluation may include blood tests and imaging (ultrasound), nuclear thyroid scans, fine-needle aspiration and functional stimulation tests. Recently, molecular testing of thyroid cytology has been used in cases of indeterminate thyroid nodules.

◆ Thyroid Function Tests

T_4 and T_3 (Total)

Both T_4 (> 99%) and T_3 (~ 98%) are tightly bound to transport proteins in the plasma: thyroxine-binding globulin (TBG), thyroxine-binding prealbumin (TBPA), or albumin. Therefore, only 1% of the thyroid hormones are in the metabolically active "free" state. Assays of "total" T_4 or T_3 measure mainly the protein-bound hormone (plus the unbound or "free" hormone). Values may vary with conditions that affect protein concentration (**Table 7.1**). Because drugs and illness can alter concentrations of binding proteins, it is necessary to estimate free hormone concentrations.

Table 7.1   Conditions affecting protein concentration

Increased TBG (high T_4)	Decreased TBG (low T_4)
Pregnancy	Liver disease/kidney disease
Estrogens	Androgens
Oral contraceptive pills	Congenital TBG deficiency
Drugs: narcotics, clofibrate	Drugs: steroids, NSAIDs, ASA

Abbreviations: ASA, acetylsalicylic acid (aspirin); NSAIDs, nonsteroidal anti-inflammatory drugs; TBG, thyroxine-binding globulin.

Thyroid-Stimulating Hormone

The thyroid-stimulating hormone (TSH) assay is the screening test of choice for thyroid function. The very sensitive TSH assay (it measures TSH into very low ranges between 0.01 and 0.001 mU/L) is currently in wide use.

Free T_4 and T_3 (FT_4 and FT_3)

These assays measure the unbound, metabolically active thyroid hormones in the circulation (~ 0.0003 to total). Free thyroid hormone tests fall into two main categories: equilibrium dialysis (not affected by TBG abnormalities) and analogue assays (affected by protein binding but still superior to total T_3 and T_4 assays).

Thyroid Hormone Uptake Test

The thyroid hormone uptake test (or the T_3 resin uptake test) is inversely proportional to the protein-bound T_4; accordingly, T_3 resin uptake is low when T_4 protein binding is increased and high when protein binding is reduced. This measurement helps clinicians distinguish protein-binding disorders from true thyroid diseases.

Radioactive Iodine Uptake

Thyroid follicular cells have iodine pumps that trap iodine in cells for thyroid hormone synthesis. The activity of these pumps can be determined by measuring the radioactive iodine (RAI) uptake. Uptake of ^{131}I by the gland is measured after oral ingestion of RAI. The normal 24-hour RAI uptake is approximately 10 to 25% in the United States. This test is most useful in the differentiating of causes for thyrotoxicosis (**Table 7.2**).

Table 7.2 Different causes for thyrotoxicosis

High RAI uptake	Low RAI uptake
Graves' disease	Exogenous use of thyroxine (thyroiditis factitia)
Hot nodules Toxic multinodular goiter Solitary toxic adenoma	Destructive thyroiditis—subacute thyroiditis Postpartum Silent
TSH-secreting pituitary tumor	Iodine-induced thyrotoxicosis (contrast dye, diet, amiodarone)

Abbreviations: TSH, thyroid-stimulating hormone; RAI, radioactive iodine.

Thyroglobulin Measurements

Thyroglobulin (Tg) measurements are taken based on two indications:

1. Detection of residual or recurrent epithelial thyroid cancers (papillary, follicular, and Hurthle cell carcinomas) after thyroidectomy
2. Differentiation of thyroiditis factitia (Tg suppressed) from all forms of endogenous hyperthyroidism (Tg normal or high)

This test is not reliable in the presence of circulating anti-Tg antibodies. Other biochemical tests of thyroid function, such as TRH tests, have been used only rarely since the advent of the highly sensitive TSH assays (**Table 7.3**).

Table 7.3 Summary of thyroid function work-up

First test: TSH	Second test: free T_4	Clinical status
High	Low	Primary hypothyroidism
	Normal	Subclinical hypothyroidism
	High	Pituitary hyperthyroidism
Low	High	Thyrotoxicosis
	Normal	Subclinical hyperthyroidism
	Low	Pituitary hypothyroidism

Abbreviation: TSH, thyroid-stimulating hormone.

◆ Imaging

Thyroid Radionucleotide Study

A thyroid radionuclide study uses a gamma camera to obtain information on the size, shape, and position of the thyroid gland and distribution of administered isotope within it. It is rarely used for nodule diagnosis at this point. Scan may show a "warm nodule" against a normally active background, a hyperfunctioning "hot" nodule against a suppressed background (4% malignancy rate), or a hypofunctioning "cold" nodule (5–20% malignancy rate).

Ultrasound

High-resolution ultrasound is currently the imaging modality of choice for evaluation of thyroid nodular disease. Ultrasound may distinguish between a single node or a multinodular goiter and differentiate between solid and cystic lesions. Ultrasound can be used to guide a fine-needle aspiration biopsy (FNAB) when necessary. Doppler flow may show vascularity of a thyroid nodule.

Fine-Needle Aspiration Biopsy

FNAB is the gold standard assessment of a thyroid nodule. It has a 1 to 10% false-negative rate, depending on the experience of the cytologist. It is especially useful in the identification of papillary, medullary, and poorly differentiated carcinomas. It may also be used for diagnosing thyroid lymphoma, but it is not considered useful in distinguishing between follicular carcinoma and adenoma.

◆ Molecular Testing of Thyroid Aspirate

Approximately 25% of biopsy samples do not render diagnostic information and are classified as indeterminate. Indeterminate specimens are stratified by the Bethesda Classification system into three diagnostic categories:

- Category III: atypia/follicular lesion of undetermined significance
- Category IV: follicular neoplasm/suspicious for follicular neoplasm
- Category V: suspicious for malignancy

Two principal tests are currently marketed for use to improve the malignancy risk assessment of "indeterminate" thyroid nodules: "Rule In" and "Rule Out" tests that attempt to confirm or exclude, respectively, the presence of cancer within a thyroid nodule. The Rule In tests assess for the presence of single-gene point mutations (such as *BRAF* or *RAS*) or gene rearrangements (such as *RET/PTC, PAX8/PPAR*γ). The Rule Out test utilizes a proprietary gene expression classifier (RNA expression) specifically designed to maximize the ability to define a processes as benign. At present, molecular testing is meant to complement but not replace clinical judgment, ultrasound assessment, and visual cytopathology interpretation.

7.3 Thyroid Nodules and Cysts

◆ Key Features

- A thyroid nodule is a discrete lesion within the thyroid gland that is radiologically distinct from the surrounding thyroid parenchyma.
- Nodular disease of the thyroid gland is estimated to be present in 5 to 10% of the population.
- Thyroid nodules are more common in women.
- Less than 5% of thyroid nodules are malignant.

The prevalence of thyroid nodules is 2 to 6% by palpation, 19 to 35% with ultrasound, and 8 to 65% in autopsy data. The important question when a thyroid nodule is detected is whether the nodule is in fact malignant.

◆ Epidemiology of Nodules

Females are affected more than males. Nodule incidence increases with age and is increased in people with iodine deficiency and after radiation exposure. The prevalence of cancer is in thyroid nodules is higher in children, adults < 30 years or > 60 years old, patients with a history of head and neck radiation, and those with a family history of thyroid cancer. The prevalence of cancer may be lower in patients with multinodular goiters and autonomously hyperfunctioning ("hot") nodules.

◆ Clinical

The usual presentations of thyroid nodules are as a lump in the neck noted by the patient, as an incidental finding during routine physical examination, or during a radiologic procedure such as carotid ultrasonography or neck computed tomography (CT). Symptoms associated with increased risk of malignancy include a rapid increase in size, dysphagia, hoarseness (nerve involvement), and pain.

◆ Evaluation of Nodules

History

Pertinent history includes prior head and neck irradiation, thyroid carcinoma in a first-degree relative, rapid growth of the nodule, hoarseness, dysphagia, neck pain or pressure, and any symptoms of hyperthyroidism (e.g., due to an autonomous hot nodule) or hypothyroidism (e.g., due to Hashimoto's thyroiditis). Family history of pheochromocytoma, hyperparathyroidism, chronic constipation and diarrhea, hypertension may be indicative of a multiple endocrine neoplasia (MEN) syndrome.

Physical Exam

A complete physical exam focusing on the thyroid gland and adjacent cervical lymph nodes should be performed. The nodule should be palpated to note size, consistency, mobility, and tenderness. Vocal fold mobility (nasopharyngoscope) should be noted. Cancer may be suspected when nodules are > 4 cm in size, when they are fixed to the surrounding structures, or when there is associated lymphadenopathy or vocal fold paralysis.

Labs

Thyroid function tests should be obtained as part of the initial evaluation of a solitary thyroid nodule. Serum thyroglobulin (Tg) levels are not indicated in the evaluation of solitary thyroid nodule.

Imaging

- Nuclear imaging cannot reliably distinguish between benign and malignant nodules and is not required if nodules are present. However, in patients with a suppressed thyroid-stimulating hormone (TSH) level, a thyroid scan determines regional uptake or function and can be used as a secondary study.

- Diagnostic thyroid/neck ultrasound should be performed in all patients with a suspected thyroid nodule, nodular goiter, or radiographic abnormality suggesting a thyroid nodule incidentally detected on another imaging study.

- Diagnostic thyroid ultrasound will help to determine whether there is truly a thyroid nodule that corresponds to the palpable abnormality or a thyroid cyst; to look for other nonpalpable thyroid nodules that may also need to be biopsied and the location and the number of the nodules; and to guide fine-needle aspiration biopsy (FNAB) (**Table 7.4; Table 7.5; Table 7.6**).

Table 7.4   Ultrasound patterns of thyroid nodule and malignancy

High suspicion [malignancy risk 70–90%]:
Solid hypoechoic nodule or solid hypoechoic component of a partially cystic nodule with one or more of the following features: irregular margins, microcalcifications, taller than wide shape
Intermediate suspicion [malignancy risk 10–20%]:
Hypoechoic solid nodule without high-suspicion features
Low suspicion [malignancy risk 5–10%]:
Isoechoic or hyperechoic solid nodule, or partially (> 50%) cystic nodule, with eccentric solid area without high-suspicion features
Very low suspicion [< 3%]:
Spongiform or partially cystic nodules without high- or intermediate-suspicion features
Benign [< 1%]: Purely cystic nodules

Table 7.5   Sonographic features of thyroid nodule that warrant biopsy

	Threshold for FNAB
Solid nodule	
• With suspicious sonographic features	≥ 1.0 cm
• Without suspicious sonographic features	≤ 1.5 cm
Mixed cystic–solid nodule	
• With suspicious sonographic features	≥ 1.5–2.0 cm
• Without suspicious sonographic features	≤ 2.0 cm
Spongiform nodule	≥ 2.0 cm
Simple cyst	Not indicated
Suspicious cervical lymph node	FNAB node ± FNAB associated thyroid node(s)

Table 7.6   Bethesda Diagnostic Categories for thyroid cysts and nodules

Bethesda Diagnostic Category		**Risk of malignancy**	**Usual management**
I	Nondiagnostic or unsatisfactory	Cyst fluid only Virtually acellular specimen Other (obscuring blood, clotting artifact, etc.)	1 to 4%	Repeat FNAB with ultrasound guidance
II	Benign	Consistent with a benign follicular nodule (includes adenomatoid nodule, colloid nodule, etc.) Consistent with lymphocytic (Hashimoto's) thyroiditis in the proper clinical context Consistent with granulomatous (subacute) thyroiditis Other	0 to 3%	Clinical follow-up
III	Atypia of undetermined significance or follicular lesion of undetermined significance		5 to 15%	Repeat FNAB Molecular testing

(continued)

Table 7.6   Bethesda Diagnostic Categories for thyroid cysts and nodules *(Continued)*

IV	Follicular neoplasm of suspicious for a follicular neoplasm	Specify if Hurthle cell (oncocytic) type	15 to 30%	Molecular testing Surgical lobectomy
V	Suspicious for malignancy	Suspicious for papillary carcinoma Suspicious for medullary carcinoma Suspicious for metastatic carcinoma Suspicious for lymphoma Other	60 to 75%	Molecular testing Surgical lobectomy or Near-total thyroidectomy
VI	Malignant	Papillary thyroid carcinoma Poorly differentiated carcinoma Medullary thyroid carcinoma Undifferentiated (anaplastic) carcinoma Squamous cell carcinoma Carcinoma with mixed features (specify) Metastatic carcinoma	97 to 99%	Near-total thyroidectomy

- Thyroid sonography with survey of the cervical lymph nodes should be performed in all patients with known or suspected thyroid nodules.

- If serum TSH is low, a radionuclide thyroid scan may be used determine whether a nodule is "hot," "warm," or "cold"; a hot functioning nodule rarely harbors malignancy. Radionuclide scanning alone is not the most accurate technique to distinguish benign from malignant thyroid disorders.

- CT and magnetic resonance imaging (MRI) are used to evaluate adenopathy, multinodular goiters causing pressure symptoms, substernal goiter, airway and vascular displacement, and invasion of tumor. These studies, however, are not routinely employed.

- Consider a chest CT to evaluate displacement of trachea seen on plain chest radiograph.

- Focal ^{18}F-fludeoxyglucose (FDG)–positron emission tomography (PET) uptake within a sonographically confirmed thyroid nodule conveys an increased risk of thyroid cancer, and FNAB is recommended for those nodules > 1 cm.

Other Tests

Generally, only nodules > 1 cm should be further evaluated, since they have a greater potential to be clinically significant cancers. Occasionally, there may be nodules < 1 cm that require evaluation because of suspicious findings or history.

FNAB is the single most important procedure for differentiating benign from malignant thyroid nodules.

Other cytopathologic yield of FNAB includes uniform follicular epithelium and abundant colloid (suggesting nodular or adenomatous goiters), inflammatory cells (suggesting thyroiditis), papillary cells (psammoma bodies), giant cells (suggesting papillary carcinoma), amyloid deposits stained with Congo red (suggesting medullary carcinoma), and undifferentiated cells (suggesting anaplastic carcinoma).

Serum TSH is an initial screening test and should be checked in all patients with thyroid nodules. If TSH is low, a radionuclide thyroid scan should be obtained to determine whether the nodule is functioning, or hot (uptake is greater in the nodule than in the surrounding normal thyroid). Functioning nodules are rarely malignant and so do not need to be evaluated further with FNAB. Further evaluation and treatment of the hyperthyroidism may be indicated. If the TSH is normal or high, a thyroid scan is of little value and should not be done.

Serum Tg is not routinely recommended, since it can be elevated in most thyroid diseases and is an insensitive and nonspecific test for thyroid cancer (it is the most valuable test as a marker of recurrence in follow-up of thyroid cancer after surgical treatment followed by radioactive iodine [RAI] treatment; see **Chapter 7.8**).

If thyroiditis is suspected, free thyroxine (FT_4), triiodothyronine (T_3), erythrocyte sedimentation rate (ESR), anti–thyroid peroxidase (anti-TPO), and anti-Tg should be checked only if they are clinically indicated. They have no routine role.

◆ Thyroid Cysts

Most cystic nodules of the thyroid are degenerating benign adenomas. Cysts that have a partial solid component are more suggestive of malignancy.

7.4 Hyperthyroidism

◆ Key Features

- Hyperthyroidism is a hypermetabolic condition associated with elevated levels of free T_4, free T_3, or both.
- The incidence of hyperthyroidism is between 0.05 and 1.3%, with most cases consisting of subclinical disease.
- It is caused by excess synthesis and secretion of thyroid hormone by the thyroid.
- Hyperthyroidism's causes include diffuse toxic goiter (Graves' disease), toxic multinodular goiter, and toxic adenoma.

Thyrotoxicosis is the presence of an excess of thyroid hormone (T_4 and/or T_3) in the body, which may be due to overproduction of thyroid hormone by the thyroid gland, increased release of thyroid hormone in such conditions as thyroiditis, and exogenous ingestion of thyroid hormone preparations. Hyperthyroidism refers to causes of thyrotoxicosis in which the thyroid produces excess thyroid hormone.

◆ Clinical

Signs

Signs include sinus tachycardia, atrial fibrillation, hyperreflexia with rapid relaxation of tendon reflexes, tachycardia, lid lag and stare, hair loss, goiter, warm and moist skin, muscle weakness and wasting, and onycholysis.

Symptoms

Symptoms include fatigue, weakness, heat intolerance, weight loss with increased appetite, palpitations, diarrhea, oligomenorrhea or amenorrhea, insomnia, brittle hair, shakiness, difficulty concentrating, irritability, or emotional lability.

◆ Etiology

The etiology of thyrotoxicosis is broadly divided into two categories:

1. **Hyperthyroidism secondary to increased synthesis of hormone**. This condition is associated with high radioactive iodine uptake (RAIU). Causes include:

   A. *Graves' disease*: the most common cause of hyperthyroidism, discussed more fully later in this chapter

   B. *Toxic multinodular goiter:* arises in the setting of a long-standing multinodular goiter; usually affects patients > 50 years of age; occurs when certain nodules develop autonomous function

   C. *Toxic adenomas:* a single benign thyroid nodule (adenoma) that becomes autonomous

   D. *Iodine-induced hyperthyroidism:* can develop, though uncommonly, after an iodine load, such as following administration of contrast agents used for angiography or CT or iodine-rich drugs such as amiodarone

   E. *Thyroid-stimulating hormone (TSH)-producing pituitary adenomas*

2. **Hyperthyroidism secondary to thyroiditis (with release of preformed hormone into the circulation) or an extrathyroidal source of thyroid hormone**. This condition is associated with low RAIU. Causes include:

- *Thyroiditis:* painless and postpartum thyroiditis, subacute painful or de Quervain thyroiditis (see **Chapter 7.7**)
- *Exogenous and ectopic:* factitious ingestion; excessive thyroid hormone

Graves' Disease: Key Points

- 30 cases per 100,000 persons per year
- Female/male ratio of 10:1
- Peak age of onset 40 to 60 years
- Autoimmune condition with TSH-receptor antibodies (TSHR Abs, also called thyroid-stimulating immunoglobulins, or TSIs)
- Clinical evidence of Graves' ophthalmopathy in 25 to 30% of patients with Graves' disease
- The ocular manifestations of thyroid-associated ophthalmopathy include eyelid retraction, proptosis, chemosis, periorbital edema, and altered ocular motility.

Graves' Disease: Etiology

Infection, iodide intake, stress, smoking, female sex, pregnancy, and genetic predisposition (*HLA-DRB1,* and *HLA-DQB1)* appear to be associated with Graves' disease susceptibility. Iodine and iodine-containing drugs such as amiodarone may precipitate Graves' disease.

Graves' Disease: Signs and Symptoms

Graves' disease presents with symptoms typical of thyrotoxicosis: rapid heart rate, palpitation, nervousness, and tremor. It also has some unique features, including ophthalmopathy (a hallmark of Graves' disease, with exophthalmos [proptosis], lacrimation, gritty sensation in the eye, photophobia, eye pain, diplopia, or even visual loss), and pretibial myxedema (raised, hyperpigmented violaceous, orange-peel textured papules).

Physical Examination

The thyroid gland in Graves' disease generally is diffusely enlarged and smooth. Thyroid nodules may be present. There is widening of the palpebral fissures, tachycardia, hand tremor, proximal muscle weakness, brisk deep tendon reflexes, and warm, velvety skin. Physical findings may include ophthalmopathy, pretibial myxedema, and clubbing of fingers with osteoarthropathy (acropachy).

Differential Diagnosis

- Anxiety disorders
- Chronic autoimmune (Hashimoto's) thyroiditis
- Hyperemesis gravidarum
- Pituitary adenomas
- Pheochromocytoma struma ovarii
- Papillary thyroid carcinoma
- Cocaine abuse
- Wolff-Parkinson-White's syndrome

◆ Evaluation

Labs

The most reliable screening methods of thyroid function are:

- TSH level: TSH levels are suppressed.
- Free thyroid hormone (FT_4 and FT_3): Elevated FT_4 level with suppressed TSH level establishes the diagnosis. If TSH is suppressed, FT_4 is normal, and FT_3 is elevated, this is known as T_3 thyrotoxicosis.
- TSI: If elevated, TSIs confirm Graves' disease; however, it may be undetectable or absent.
- Anti–thyroid peroxidase (anti-TPO): Anti-TPO antibodies are usually elevated in Graves' disease and usually low or absent in toxic multinodular goiter and toxic adenoma. Anti-TPO may also be elevated in autoimmune-related thyroiditis.

Imaging

- RAI scanning and measurements of iodine uptake: Useful to differentiate overproduction of thyroid hormone from excess release due to thyroiditis or exogenous thyroid hormone ingestion. In Graves' disease, the RAI uptake is increased, and the uptake is diffusely distributed over the entire gland.
- Computed tomography (CT) or magnetic resonance imaging (MRI) of the orbits may be necessary in the evaluation of proptosis.

◆ Treatment Options

The treatment depends on the cause of thyrotoxicosis. If the cause is hyperthyroidism (overproduction of thyroid hormone), treatment includes symptomatic treatment or definitive treatment options, which include RAI ablation and antithyroid medications.

Medical

β-blockers such as propranolol or atenolol provide symptomatic relief in all types of hyperthyroidism. Consider anti-inflammatory therapy with nonsteroidal anti-inflammatory drugs (NSAIDs), and corticosteroids in refractory cases, in patients with thyrotoxicosis due to thyroiditis.

Antithyroid drugs are used for primary therapy of thyrotoxicosis, for attainment of euthyroidism in preparation for thyroidectomy, and for use in conjunction with radioiodine therapy in selected patients. These inhibit new thyroid hormone production. These include methimazole (Tapazole; King Pharmaceuticals, Bristol, TN) and propylthiouracil (PTU) if needed for patients with allergy to methimazole (except agranulocytosis), who are pregnant or breastfeeding, or have severe thyrotoxicosis or thyroid storm. As primary therapy, use antithyroid drugs alone for 12 to 18 months. Monitor for hepatic dysfunction and agranulocytosis.

[131]I radiotherapy is primary therapy for thyrotoxicosis due to Graves' disease, toxic multinodular goiter, or autonomously functioning thyroid nodules and in patients failing to achieve a remission after a course of antithyroid drugs.

For Graves' disease, 10 to 30 mCi RAI therapy is safe and effective. Hypothyroidism occurs over time in ~ 75% of patients. Permanent hypothyroidism is likely; pregnancy and breastfeeding should be avoided until after 6 to 12 months. It may precipitate new or worsened ophthalmopathy, especially in smokers. There is a slight risk of thyroid storm after treatment (see **Chapter 7.6**).

Surgery

Thyroidectomy or subtotal thyroidectomy is usually curative but results in iatrogenic hypothyroidism; risks include potential injury to parathyroids and recurrent laryngeal nerve. Orbital decompression may be necessary in patients with severe Graves ophthalmopathy.

◆ Outcome and Follow-Up

The outcome depends on the cause of hyperthyroidism and the treatment modality. Patients should be routinely followed by an endocrinologist taking a history, physical exam, and thyroid function tests.

7.5 Hypothyroidism

◆ Key Features

- Hypothyroidism is a common endocrine disorder resulting from deficiency of thyroid hormone.
- In primary hypothyroidism, the thyroid gland produces insufficient amounts of thyroid hormone.
- In secondary hypothyroidism, there is a lack of thyroid hormone secretion due to inadequate secretion of either thyroid-stimulating hormone (TSH) by the pituitary or thyrotropin-releasing hormone (TRH) by the hypothalamus.

Hypothyroidism is reduced production of thyroid hormone by the thyroid gland; it can be caused by disease of thyroid gland itself (*primary hypothyroidism*), or by deficiency of TSH due to disease of pituitary or hypothalamus (*secondary and tertiary or central hypothyroidism*). *Subclinical hypothyroidism* is a mild asymptomatic hypothyroidism, in which TSH is mildly elevated but thyroxine (T_4) or free thyroxine (FT_4) levels are normal.

◆ Etiology

Primary Hypothyroidism

Primary hypothyroidism accounts for ~ 99% of cases. Causes include:

- *Hashimoto's thyroiditis (chronic autoimmune thyroiditis):* This is the most common cause of hypothyroidism in iodine-sufficient regions of the world and is discussed in more detail later in this chapter.
- *Iatrogenic disease:* Causes include thyroidectomy, radioiodine treatment, or external radiotherapy.
- *Iodine deficiency or iodine excess:* Both can cause hypothyroidism. The most common cause of hypothyroidism worldwide is iodine deficiency.
- *Drugs:* Medications used to treat hyperthyroidism (such as methimazole or propylthiouracil [PTU]) can cause hypothyroidism. Other drugs that can cause hypothyroidism include amiodarone, lithium carbonate, interleukin-2, and interferon-α.
- *Transient hypothyroidism:* This can occur during the course of several types of thyroiditis, followed by recovery of thyroid function. Some patients who undergo subtotal thyroidectomy become hypothyroid after 4 to 8 weeks but recover several weeks or months later. This condition may also follow radioactive iodine (RAI) treatment for Graves' disease (see **Chapter 7.4**), when glands are not completely ablated by radioiodine and there is some remaining thyroid tissue.
- *Hypothyroidism in infants and children:* The most common causes of congenital hypothyroidism are agenesis and dysgenesis of the thyroid, but a few cases are delivered by mothers who were receiving an antithyroid drug for hyperthyroidism. Among children who become hypothyroid later, the most common cause is chronic autoimmune thyroiditis.

Central (Secondary and Tertiary) Hypothyroidism

Central (secondary and tertiary) hypothyroidism can have several causes.

- Most often the cause is a pituitary tumor (macroadenomas), pituitary surgery, or irradiation.
- Less common causes include head injury, postpartum pituitary necrosis (Sheehan's syndrome), pituitary apoplexy (bleeding in a pituitary tumor), hypophysitis, nonpituitary tumors such as craniopharyngiomas, and infiltrative diseases.

Tissue Resistance to Thyroid Hormone

Tissue resistance to thyroid hormone is rare.

◆ Epidemiology

Primary hypothyroidism is a common disease worldwide in both iodine-deficient and iodine-replete regions. The prevalence is 4 to 8% in the general population. It occurs more commonly in women, with a female to male ratio of 10:1. Mean age at diagnosis in women is 60 years, with increasing occurrence with advancing age. Mild hypothyroidism may exist in 7 to 15% of the elderly population.

The prevalence of central hypothyroidism in the general population is roughly 0.005%. The sex distribution is equal. It occurs with peaks in childhood and in adults 30 to 60 years old.

◆ Clinical

Deficiency of thyroid hormone causes a generalized slowing of metabolic processes and/or accumulation of matrix glycosaminoglycans in the interstitial spaces of many tissues.

Signs

Signs include slow movement, slow speech, delayed relaxation of tendon reflexes, bradycardia, dry and coarse and yellowed skin, puffy facies and loss of eyebrows, periorbital edema, and diastolic hypertension.

Symptoms

Symptoms include fatigue, weakness, myalgia, cold intolerance, weight gain, depression, cognitive dysfunction, mental retardation (in infants), constipation, menstrual irregularity, hair loss, and hoarseness.

Differential Diagnosis

- Laboratory confirmation of the diagnosis of hypothyroidism consists of measuring serum TSH and FT_4.
  - o Primary hypothyroidism is characterized by a high serum TSH concentration and a low serum FT_4 concentration. Patients with a high serum TSH concentration and a normal serum FT_4 concentration have subclinical hypothyroidism.
  - o Central (secondary and tertiary) hypothyroidism is characterized by a low serum T_4 concentration and a serum TSH concentration that is not appropriately elevated. In this setting, differentiation must be made between pituitary and hypothalamic disorders.
- Hyperlipidemia occurs with increased frequency in hypothyroidism; as a result, patients with dyslipidemia should be screened for thyroid dysfunction.
- Thyroid function should be measured in all patients with unexplained hyponatremia, as this is another laboratory manifestation of hypothyroidism.
- Thyroid function should also be measured in patients undergoing evaluation for high serum muscle enzyme concentrations or anemia.

◆ Treatment Options

- Start replacement therapy with L-thyroxine (Synthroid, AbbVie Inc., North Chicago, IL; Levothroid, Allergan, Dublin, Ireland; Levoxyl, Pfizer, New York, NY).
- The average replacement dose of T_4 in adults is ~ 1.6 µg/kg body weight per day (112 µg/day in a 70-kg adult). The initial dose can be the full anticipated dose in young, healthy patients.
- After initiation of T_4 therapy, the patient should be reevaluated and serum FT_4 and TSH should be measured in 3 to 6 weeks (depending upon the patient's symptoms) and the dose adjusted accordingly.
- The serum TSH concentration should be maintained between 0.5 and 3 mU/L.

- For monitoring therapy in patients with central hypothyroidism, serum FT_4 should be measured and maintained in the upper half of normal range.

Special treatment situations for hypothyroidism include:

- Elderly patients or those with known or suspected heart disease: These patients should initially be treated with low doses of levothyroxine 25 µg/day. The dose can be increased by 25 µg/day every 3 to 6 weeks until TSH is normal.
- Hypothyroidism during pregnancy: Women require more thyroid hormone during pregnancy.
- Surgical patients: Urgent surgery should not be postponed in hypothyroid patients. On the other hand, hypothyroidism should be corrected before elective surgery. Patients receiving chronic T_4 therapy who undergo surgery and are unable to eat for several days need not be given T_4 parenterally. If oral intake cannot be resumed in 5 to 7 days, then T_4 should be given intravenously. The dose should be ~ 50% of the patient's usual oral dose.

◆ Hashimoto's Thyroiditis

Hashimoto's thyroiditis (chronic autoimmune thyroiditis) is the most common cause of hypothyroidism in iodine-sufficient parts of the world. It is a disease predominantly of women, with a sex ratio of approximately 7:1. The clinical course of Hashimoto's thyroiditis is gradual loss of thyroid function. Histopathologic abnormalities include profuse lymphocytic infiltration, lymphoid germinal centers, and destruction of thyroid follicles.

Antibodies and antigen-specific T cells directed against thyroid antigens are the hallmark of Hashimoto's thyroiditis. Antigens include thyroglobulin (Tg), thyroid peroxidase (TPO, aka "microsomal" antigen) and the thyrotropin (TSH) receptor.

Uniformly, patients with Hashimoto's thyroiditis have high serum concentrations of antibodies to thyroglobulin (Tg) and thyroid peroxidase (TPO).

Treatment of Hashimoto's thyroiditis includes hormone replacement. Indications for surgery include a large goiter with obstructive symptoms; the presence of a malignant nodule, as demonstrated by cytologic examination; and the presence of a lymphoma primarily for diagnosis.

◆ Complications

Myxedema coma occurs in the setting of prolonged, untreated hypothyroidism. Usually it occurs in the elderly and is precipitated by intercurrent illness, surgery, or narcotic/hypnotic drugs. It is characterized by hypothermia, bradycardia, severe hypotension, seizures, and coma. Myxedema coma holds a poor prognosis with 20% mortality rate. These patients should be promptly treated with IV T_4, steroids, and supportive measures.

◆ Outcome and Follow-Up

The outcome depends on the cause of hypothyroidism and the treatment modality. Patients should be routinely followed by an endocrinologist taking a history, physical exam, and thyroid function tests.

7.6 Thyroid Storm

◆ Key Features

- Thyroid storm is a rare and potentially fatal complication of hyperthyroidism.
- Approximately 1 to 2% of patients with hyperthyroidism progress to thyroid storm.
- It usually occurs in patients with untreated or partially treated hyperthyroidism who experience a precipitating event such as surgery, infection, or trauma.

Thyroid storm is a state of severe thyrotoxicosis, in which there is an exaggeration of the manifestations of hyperthyroidism. It is a life-threatening condition.

◆ Etiology

Thyroid storm usually occurs in the setting of undiagnosed or inadequately treated thyrotoxicosis and an added precipitating event such as surgery (either thyroid or nonthyroid), infection, trauma, iodinated contrast dyes, and radioactive iodine (RAI) therapy.

◆ Clinical

The condition causes high fever (> 39°C or 102°F), tachycardia, cardiac arrhythmia, thromboembolic events, congestive heart failure, confusion, agitation, psychosis, extreme lethargy, coma, diarrhea, nausea and vomiting, and abdominal pain.

◆ Evaluation

The evaluation is mainly based on clinical presentation. Obtaining laboratory data is helpful, but waiting for these laboratories should not delay life-saving treatment.

Labs

Thyroid-stimulating hormone (TSH) may be undetectable; there is elevated FT_3 and FT_4, anemia, leukocytosis, hyperglycemia, azotemia, hypercalcemia, and abnormal function tests (LFTs).

◆ Treatment Options

The following are the immediate goals:

- To decrease thyroid hormone synthesis: propylthiouracil (PTU), methimazole
- To decrease thyroid hormone release: Iodine solution
- Blocking T_4-to-T_3 conversion: PTU, corticosteroids, propranolol
- Beta-adrenergic blockade: Propranolol

Remaining care is supportive, including treatment for fever with acetaminophen and cooling blankets, IV fluids, nutrition including glucose, thiamine, and treatment of the precipitating event. Consider monitoring the patient in an intensive care unit (ICU).

7.7　Thyroiditis

◆ Key Features

- Thyroiditis is an inflammation of the thyroid gland.
- Hashimoto's thyroiditis (chronic autoimmune thyroiditis) is the most common type.
- Other forms include postpartum thyroiditis, subacute thyroiditis (de Quervain), silent thyroiditis, drug-induced thyroiditis, radiation-induced thyroiditis, and acute thyroiditis.

Thyroiditis is a diverse group of disorders associated with inflammation of the thyroid gland. **Table 7.7** provides the main types of thyroiditis.

Table 7.7　The main types of thyroiditis

	Hashimoto's	Painless and postpartum	Subacute (painful)	Suppurative
Cause	Autoimmune	Autoimmune	Viral	Infectious
Clinical features	Painless, firm, bumpy, symmetric goiter (in 10% atrophied thyroid)	Painless, normal-size thyroid or diffuse goiter	Tender, firm goiter	Tender thyroid mass
Thyroid function	Hypothyroidism	Thyrotoxicosis, hypothyroidism, or both	Thyrotoxicosis, hypothyroidism, or both	Euthyroidism
Anti-TPO Abs	High titer, persistent	High titer, persistent	Low titer, absent or transient	Absent
ESR	Normal	Normal	High	High
24-hour RAI uptake	Variable	< 5%	< 5%	Normal

◆ Thyroiditis Associated with Pain and Tenderness

Subacute Thyroiditis

Also known as subacute nonsuppurative thyroiditis, de Quervain thyroiditis, and giant cell or subacute granulomatous thyroiditis, it is a self-limited inflammatory disorder and is the most common cause of thyroid pain.

Etiology

Subacute thyroiditis is most likely caused by a viral infection (coxsackievirus, mumps virus, influenza, echovirus, or adenovirus) or postviral inflammatory process. There is a strong association with *HLA-B35*.

Clinical

Many patients have a history of an upper respiratory infection preceding the onset of thyroiditis. Patients present with fever, malaise, extreme neck pain, swelling, or all of these. Pain may radiate to oropharynx or ears. Up to 50% of patients have symptoms of thyrotoxicosis.

Evaluation

On physical exam, the gland is extremely tender. In most patients, the painful thyrotoxic phase lasts 4 to 6 weeks followed by a hypothyroid phase lasting another 4 to 6 weeks followed by normalization of thyroid functions (recovery phase). Residual hypothyroidism persists in 5% of patients.

Initially, very high erythrocyte sedimentation rate (ESR), free T_3 (FT_3), and FT_4 (T_4 levels are elevated disproportionally to serum T_3) and thyroid-stimulating hormone (TSH) and radioactive iodine (RAI) uptake and the anti–thyroid peroxidase antibodies (anti-TPO Abs) are usually normal (thyrotoxic phase). As the disease progresses, FT_3 and FT_4 drop, TSH rises, and symptoms of hypothyroidism are noted. Later, RAI uptake rises, reflecting recovery phase.

Treatment Options

Treatment is symptomatic and includes pain control with NSAIDs, and β-blockers for control of hyperthyroid symptoms. For more severe thyroid pain, corticosteroids may be considered.

Infectious Thyroiditis

Infectious thyroiditis is also known as suppurative thyroiditis, acute suppurative thyroiditis, pyogenic thyroiditis, and bacterial thyroiditis.

Etiology

Infectious thyroiditis is usually caused by *Staphylococcus* and *Streptococcus*, but many other pathogens have also been implicated, including mycobacterial, fungal, and *Pneumocystis* infections. The disease typically occurs in immunocompromised, elderly, or debilitated patients.

Clinical

Patients present with acute illness, fever, chills, dysphagia, pain in the anterior neck, and swelling. On physical exam, the thyroid is tender.

Evaluation

FT$_3$, FT$_4$, and TSH are normal. Fine-needle aspiration biopsy (FNAB) with Gram stain and culture of the organism confirms diagnosis. Ultrasonography should be considered to confirm the presence of a single abscess. In most instances, rapid diagnosis and treatment are required.

Treatment Options

The condition is treated with antibiotics, with drainage in the case of an abscess.

Radiation Thyroiditis

Radiation thyroiditis may be caused by RAI given for treatment of Graves' disease (see **Chapter 7.4**). Patients present with mild thyroid pain and tenderness 5 to 10 days after receiving the RAI. Symptoms usually subside spontaneously in a few days to one week.

◆ Thyroiditis Not Associated with Pain and Tenderness

Hashimoto's Thyroiditis

Hashimoto's thyroiditis is also known as chronic autoimmune thyroiditis; see **Chapter 7.5**.

- Anti-TPO Abs: High titer, persistent
- ESR: Normal
- RAI uptake: Variable

Painless Thyroiditis

Painless thyroiditis (also known as silent thyroiditis, subacute lymphocytic thyroiditis, and lymphocytic thyroiditis) and postpartum thyroiditis are identical, except that the term "postpartum" is used for patients in whom painless thyroiditis develops within one year after delivery (or even after an abortion). Both account for 4.9% of all types of thyrotoxicosis.

Etiology

Chronic autoimmune thyroiditis is an autoimmune disorder due to lymphocytic infiltration of the thyroid gland.

Clinical

There is sudden onset of mild transient hyperthyroidism or hypothyroidism, which may be without localized pain. A nontender goiter may be present on physical exam.

Evaluation

The evaluation should include the patient's history and the results of thyroid function tests. Anti-TPO Abs are positive in 50% of patients. RAI uptake is low.

Note that postpartum thyroiditis must be differentiated from Graves' disease, which also commonly presents in women after delivery. RAI uptake can be obtained in women who are not nursing (low in thyroiditis and high in Graves' disease). Also check thyroid-stimulating immunoglobulin (typically positive in Graves'). In nursing mothers, thyroid ultrasound with Doppler flow may be helpful in differentiating these two conditions. Hypervascularity typically occurs with Graves' disease, whereas there is decreased vascularity in hyperthyroidism associated with postpartum thyroiditis.

Treatment Options
Patients with symptomatic hypothyroidism should be treated with levothyroxine for 2 to 3 months and then be reevaluated. In up to 25% of women with postpartum thyroiditis, hypothyroidism may be permanent.

Fibrous Thyroiditis

Fibrous thyroiditis (also known as Riedel thyroiditis [RT] and invasive thyroiditis) is characterized by extensive fibrosis of the thyroid gland that extends into adjacent tissues.

Etiology
The etiology of fibrous thyroiditis is unknown, but it may be related to a relatively new group of rare disorders, IgG4-related systemic disease (IgG4-RSD). Approximately one-third of patients with fibrous thyroiditis have an associated extracervical manifestation of multifocal fibrosclerosis.

Clinical
Patients present with a painless, hard, fixed goiter. Patients initially are euthyroid but may develop hypothyroidism after the gland becomes fibrosed. One distinguishing feature of RT is the absence of associated cervical adenopathy. However, accurate diagnosis of RT requires open biopsy.

Evaluation

- Anti-TPO Abs: Usually present
- ESR: Normal
- RAI uptake: Low or normal

Treatment Options
Treatment includes levothyroxine, corticosteroids, methotrexate, and surgery.

Drug-Induced Thyroiditis

Patients receiving interferon-α, interleukin-2, amiodarone, or lithium may develop painless thyroiditis.

7.8 Thyroid Cancer

◆ Key Features

- Well-differentiated tumors (papillary and follicular) are highly treatable.
- Undifferentiated tumors (medullary or anaplastic) are aggressive and have a poorer prognosis.
- Thyroid cancer affects women more than men.
- Solitary nodules are more likely to be malignant in the young and the elderly.

Most thyroid malignancies are well-differentiated cancers that originate from follicular cells (papillary and follicular carcinomas). Thyroid tumors can also originate from the other cell types in the thyroid gland, including the calcitonin-producing C cells (parafollicular cells), lymphocytes, other vascular components, and metastases from other organs (**Table 7.8**).

Table 7.8 Overview of thyroid cancers

Thyroid cancer	Type	Incidence	Cell origin	Mutations	Subtype	Treatment
Differentiated	Papillary carcinoma	80%	Endodermally derived follicular cell	*BRAF* 45%		Surgery and RAI
				RET/PTC 20%		
				RAS 10%		
				TRK < 5%		
	Follicular carcinoma	10%	Endodermally derived follicular cell	*RAS* 45%	Hürthle cell	Surgery and RAI
				PAX8-PPARγ 35%		
				PIK3CA < 10%		
				PTEN < 10%		
Undifferentiated	Medullary carcinoma	5–10%	Neuroendocrine-derived calcitonin-producing C cell	Familial forms *RET* > 95%		Surgery
				Sporadic *RET* 50%		

(continued)

Table 7.8 Overview of thyroid cancers *(Continued)*

	Anaplastic carcinoma	1–2%	Endodermally derived follicular cell	TP53 70%	Small-cell carcinoma	Surgery when possible Chemotherapy Radiation therapy
				β-catenin (CTNNB1) 65%		
				RAS 55%		
				BRAF 20%		
					Giant-cell carcinoma	
Others	Lymphoma	Rare	Intrathyroid lymphoid tissue	BRAF NRAS	Diffuse large B-cell lymphoma	Chemotherapy Radiation therapy

Abbreviation: RAI, radioactive iodine.

◆ Epidemiology

Thyroid cancer represents the most common endocrine malignancy, annual incidence being ~ 64,000 cases in the United States with approximately 2,000 deaths. The female/male ratio is ~ 2:1 to 4:1. The incidence of this malignancy has been increasing over the last few decades. Annual incidence increases with age, peaking by the fifth through eighth decades. Thyroid cancer is very rare in children < 15 years. Patients with a history of radiation administered in childhood have an increased risk of cancer as well as other abnormalities of the thyroid gland.

◆ Well-Differentiated Thyroid Carcinomas

Well-differentiated thyroid carcinomas originate from the thyroid follicular cells and include papillary and follicular carcinomas, as described subsequently. These respond to thyroid-stimulating hormone (TSH), concentrate iodine, and synthesize thyroglobulin (Tg), albeit less efficiently than normal thyroid tissue. Well-differentiated thyroid carcinomas are two to four times more common in females than males.

Specifically, molecular analyses have focused on a set of somatic alterations of genes in the mitogen-activated protein kinase (MAPK) pathway that are frequently present in carcinomas of the thyroid. These include point mutations of the *BRAF* and *RAS* genes and *RET/PTC* and *PAX8/PPARγ* chromosomal rearrangements. A V600E mutation in the *BRAF* gene has been identified as the most common genetic event in papillary thyroid carcinoma, occurring in 40 to 45% of cases.

Papillary Thyroid Cancer

Papillary thyroid cancer (PTC) is the most common type of thyroid malignancy. It has a female/male ratio of 2.5:1. The tumor generally grows slowly, and the overall prognosis is excellent.

Pathogenesis

Mutations or rearrangements in the genes encoding for the proteins in the MAPK pathway such as *RET/PTC, RAS,* or *BRAF* have been implicated in the development and progression of differentiated thyroid cancer. It has been thought that the *BRAF* mutation is associated with more aggressive tumors with higher rates of extrathyroidal extension, lymph node metastases, and recurrence; however, this remains controversial. A major advance in recent years has been the discovery of mutations that have prognostic value, such as *TERT* (telomerase reverse transcriptase) promoter mutations.

Epidemiology

PTC accounts for 80 to 90% of all thyroid cancers. Its peak incidence is between ages 30 to 50 years. Females are more commonly affected than males.

Risk Factors

- History of radiation exposure during childhood, such as that received as a treatment of childhood malignancies, is a risk factor. Prior to about 1960, external radiation to the head and neck was commonly used to treat a wide variety of conditions, including enlarged tonsils or thymus and even acne.
- History of thyroid cancer in a first-degree relative or a family history of a thyroid cancer syndrome is a risk factor.
- Suggestive signs of a nodule's being malignant include a rapid increase in its size, its fixation to surrounding tissues, new-onset hoarseness or vocal fold paralysis, and the presence of ipsilateral cervical lymphadenopathy.

Clinical Presentation

PTC typically presents as a painless discrete mass in the thyroid gland. These tumors may be multicentric. The tumor generally grows slowly and is late to break through the capsule of the gland. Once it has become extrathyroidal, however, it may ultimately become invasive. Nodal metastases appear classically in paratracheal nodes but may be present anywhere in the neck. Bilateral spread is found in 8% of patients. It usually spreads via the lymphatic system. It is not uncommon to find microscopic foci of papillary carcinoma at autopsy or incidentally in a thyroid removed for other indications.

Pathology

Characteristic cytopathologic features seen on fine-needle aspiration biopsy (FNAB) or after surgical resection are diagnostic, including psammoma bodies (layered accumulations of calcium); nuclei with empty centers (Orphan Annie nuclei, based on the comic-strip character Little Orphan Annie) and the formation of papillary structures.

Prognosis

With treatment, overall outcome is generally favorable. However, a small group of patients develop local recurrence and/or distant metastases. Features associated with increased risk of recurrence or mortality include age at diagnosis (age > 45 years), size of the primary tumor (> 2 cm), and the presence of soft tissue invasion and cervical lymph node or distant metastases.

Variants

PTC has several histologic subtypes, including a follicular variant, an oxyphilic variant, a solid or trabecular variant, and a clear cell variant. The follicular variant consists of several distinct subtypes. The diffuse follicular variant seems to present and behave in a more aggressive fashion.

Other biologically aggressive variants include a columnar variant, a tall cell variant, a diffuse sclerosing variant, and poorly differentiated carcinoma.

Follicular Thyroid Cancer

Epidemiology

Follicular thyroid cancer (FTC) is more common in the iodine-deficient regions of the world. It tends to occur in an older population, with a peak incidence between ages 40 and 60 years. Like most thyroid malignancies, FTC is more common in women (by about a 3:1 ratio).

Risk Factors

- Iodine deficiency may have a role in the pathogenesis, as there is a higher prevalence of FTC in iodine-deficient regions of the world, compared with iodine-sufficient regions.
- FTC is rarely associated with radiation exposure, *RET/PTC* mutations, or TSH receptor mutations.
- FTC has no association with familial syndromes.
- FTC may be associated with *RAS* mutations. *PAX8-PPARγ1* (a gene rearrangement) can be seen both in follicular adenomas and cancers.

Clinical Presentation

FTC typically presents as a painless solitary, mostly encapsulated nodule in the thyroid. FTC is more aggressive than PTC and usually spreads by hematogenous routes to bone or lung, and less commonly to brain and liver. It rarely invades lymphatics. The tumor is classified on the basis of degree of invasiveness into minimally invasive (encapsulated) or widely invasive. Metastases are more common with the widely invasive variant.

Diagnosis

FNAB cannot distinguish between follicular adenomas and carcinomas, because diagnosis of malignancy requires identification of tumor capsule and/or vascular invasion. Therefore, the actual diagnosis of follicular thyroid cancer is made on permanent pathologic evaluation of the thyroid specimen after surgery.

Prognosis

Factors associated with adverse prognosis in FTC include older age, distant metastases, large tumor size, vascular invasion, capsular extension, histologic grade (widely invasive variant, Hürthle cell, insular and trabecular variants), and male sex.

Variants

Clear cell tumor, oxyphilic cell type or Hürthle cell type, and insular carcinoma are FTC variants.

Treatment of Well-Differentiated Thyroid Carcinomas

The primary treatment is surgical, followed by referral to an endocrinologist for medical management. Radioactive iodine remnant ablation treatment may be given if needed; there should be lifelong follow-up and surveillance for recurrence. Surgical treatments include:

- Selected papillary carcinomas that are < 1 cm in a young patient without a history of radiation exposure may be treated with hemithyroidectomy and isthmectomy followed by close observation. All others should be treated with a near total thyroidectomy and removal of any involved lymph nodes in the central or lateral neck areas. Elective lateral neck dissection is not recommended.
- FTC is treated with a total thyroidectomy.
- Hürthle cell carcinoma is treated with a total thyroidectomy and neck dissection in cases with clinically positive lymph nodes.

Postoperative Complications of Well-Differentiated Thyroid Carcinomas

Permanent hypoparathyroidism, transient hypoparathyroidism, damage to the recurrent laryngeal nerve (hoarseness), and damage to the superior laryngeal nerve are possible postoperative complications.

Postoperative Management of Well-Differentiated Thyroid Carcinomas

Radioactive Iodine Remnant Ablation

All patients with FTC and those PTC patients who have features associated with increased risk of recurrence or mortality (see the discussion of Prognosis under Papillary Thyroid Cancer) may undergo radioactive iodine (RAI) remnant ablation (RAI treatment or ^{131}I remnant ablation). The RAI is taken up by the residual normal and tumor cells, leading to destruction or death of these cells. This not only reduces future recurrence risk but also facilitates surveillance for future recurrence. Before the treatment, plasma Tg is measured and a whole-body scan is performed after administration of a very small dose of RAI. Several days after the treatment, another whole-body scan is obtained (posttreatment scan).

Well-differentiated thyroid cancer has a reduced capacity to concentrate iodine compared with normal thyroid tissue. An elevated serum TSH stimulates the thyroid cancer cells to take up iodide enough to be detected by RAI imaging and synthesize and secrete Tg. TSH levels can be increased in two ways; one being withdrawal of thyroid hormone therapy. To achieve this, patients should be off of L-thyroxine (LT_4) for weeks prior to the whole-body scan (because of longer half-life). Alternatively, patients may be started on liothyronine (Cytomel, Pfizer Inc., New York, NY; or LT$_3$) for 4 weeks after surgery, stopping 2 weeks before the whole-body scan. This has a shorter half-life than L-thyroxine, and TSH levels rapidly rise after its discontinuation. Alternatively, the TSH level can also be increased by administration of recombinant human TSH (RhTSH; Thyrogen, Sanofi Genzyme, Cambridge, MA).

TSH Suppression Therapy

After the diagnostic whole-body scan or treatment, the patient is started on L-thyroxine. The goal is to suppress TSH as much as possible. This serves two purposes: maintaining the patient in a euthyroid state and suppressing TSH and growth of any residual thyroid, as most well-differentiated tumors are TSH-responsive.

Long-Term Follow-Up and Surveillance for Recurrence

A TSH-stimulated whole-body scan is done at 6- or 12-month follow-up. The TSH stimulation is achieved by either thyroid hormone withdrawal or Thyrogen injection (depending on the individual case). Based on the results of this scanning, the decision is then made whether further treatment with RAI is needed.

Tg is a very useful marker for detecting the recurrence of thyroid cancer. Levels are measured periodically both while on thyroid hormone suppression and prior to whole-body scanning on TSH stimulation. A rising Tg level raises suspicion for recurrence, indicating the need for further treatment through RAI or revision neck surgery.

Imaging, such as ultrasound and positron emission tomography (PET)–computed tomography (CT) scanning, is important for detecting recurrences.

Patients need periodic clinical follow-up to monitor for symptoms such as hoarseness, hemoptysis, pain, dysphagia, cough and dyspnea, recurrent mass, new-onset adenopathy, or a paralyzed vocal fold.

Other Therapies for Well-Differentiated Thyroid Carcinomas

External beam radiation may play a role in the treatment of non-RAI-avid tumors, gross residual tumor, and unresectable disease, as well as in nonsurgical candidates.

In general, thyroid cancers do not respond well to chemotherapy. A class of targeted drugs known as *kinase inhibitors* may help treat thyroid cancer cells with mutations in certain genes, such as *BRAF* and *RET/PTC*. Many of these drugs also affect tumor angioneogenesis. Some kinase inhibitors that have shown early promise against thyroid cancer in clinical trials include sorafenib (Nexavar, Bayer, Leverkusen, Germany), sunitinib (Sutent, Pfizer Inc., New York, NY), and vandetanib (Caprelsa, AstraZeneca, Cambridge, UK). Other options include clinical trials involving gene therapy and tumor redifferentiation agents.

◆ Other Forms of Thyroid Cancer

Anaplastic Thyroid Cancer

Anaplastic thyroid cancer, a poorly differentiated cancer, accounts for ~ 2% of all thyroid cancers. Anaplastic thyroid cancer is the most aggressive and lethal of human neoplasms. Median survival is 6 months, despite treatment.

Epidemiology

The annual incidence of anaplastic thyroid cancer is 1 to 2 cases per million. The female/male ratio is 1.2 to 3.1:1. A higher incidence has been reported in areas of endemic goiter. Anaplastic thyroid cancer may arise de novo, but dedifferentiation from long-standing differentiated thyroid carcinoma is also suspected. Anaplastic thyroid cancer is responsible for > 50% of the deaths per year attributed to thyroid cancer. It is often a disease of the elderly, typically presenting in the sixth or seventh decade of life.

Clinical Presentation

It usually presents with local symptoms caused by a rapidly growing thyroid mass and extensive local invasion. Distant metastases may occur early in the course of the disease to the lungs, liver, bones, and brain.

Diagnosis

Diagnosis is suggested by cytologic examination of cells obtained by FNAB or core biopsy, although it is not always diagnostic, in which case surgical pathology is needed to confirm the diagnosis. Histopathologically, atypical cells are seen that show numerous mitoses and form different patterns. Multinucleate giant cells, spindle-shaped cells, and squamoid cells usually predominate.

Treatment

Surgical treatment may consist of complete resection in selected individuals when possible, followed by a combination of chemotherapy and radiotherapy. Palliative therapy includes a tracheotomy and chemoradiation. Often, the tumor is not resectable at presentation, and surgery consists of a tracheotomy or cricothyroidotomy to prevent airway compromise.

Radiation therapy is indicated preoperatively to increase the tumor resectability rate, or postoperatively to enhance the effect of chemotherapy or to alleviate obstruction, but its efficacy must be balanced against its toxicity.

Several chemotherapeutic agents have been used with uniformly suboptimal results. Doxorubicin has been shown to be useful in some patients. Tyrosine kinase inhibitors (such as imatinib [Gleevec, Novartis, Basel, Switzerland], sunitinib, or sorafenib) are under evaluation for the treatment of ATC.

Medullary Thyroid Cancer

Medullary thyroid cancer (MTC) is a neuroendocrine tumor of the C cells (parafollicular cells) of the thyroid gland. Calcitonin is secreted by the tumor and is a useful marker for diagnosis and follow-up. MTC can be sporadic or familial.

Epidemiology

Seventy-five percent of MTCs are sporadic; the remainder are familial. There are three familial patterns of MTC: multiple endocrine neoplasia (MEN) 2A, MEN 2B, and familial MTC without other features of MEN. MTC is most aggressive in patients with MEN 2B.

Clinical Presentation

Medullary thyroid cancer typically presents as a painful hard nodule or mass in the thyroid gland or as an enlargement of the regional lymph nodes. Sometimes it comes to medical attention due to a metastatic lesion at a distant site.

Screening

RET proto-oncogene testing should be obtained in all patients with MTC. If the patient tests positive for the *RET* mutation, then genetic counseling and testing of family members should be offered. If screening is negative, no investigation of relatives is needed.

Pathology

Characteristic microscopic features are sheets of cells separated by a pink-staining substance that has characteristics of amyloid. Diagnosis can be confirmed by positive immunostaining of the tumor tissue for calcitonin and carcinoembryonic antigen. Preoperatively, patients should also be evaluated for hyperparathyroidism and for pheochromocytoma. Ultrasound or CT of the neck, a chest X-ray, and CT of the chest and upper abdomen should be obtained preoperatively to look for local and regional disease and distant metastases.

Treatment

Treatment is primarily surgical. Total thyroidectomy with removal of regional lymph nodes should be performed after excluding hyperparathyroidism and pheochromocytoma. In patients with MEN, surgery should be performed for pheochromocytoma prior to surgery for MTC. Patients with MEN often undergo prophylactic thyroidectomy in childhood to prevent the development of MTC.

Patients with MTC should receive a total thyroidectomy, a complete central neck dissection, and a lateral modified radical neck procedure on the side of the neck that harbored the tumor. Some recommend bilateral neck dissection. RAI is not a therapeutic option, because MTC does not take up iodine; therefore, it is imperative that surgery be thorough.

Postoperative Management

Patients should be started on thyroid hormone replacement (levothyroxine, LT_4) immediately after surgery. Because the C-cells are not stimulated by TSH, there is no role for TSH suppression.

Serum calcitonin and carcinoembryonic antigen (CEA) should be checked 6 months after surgery, to detect the presence of residual disease. An elevated basal serum calcitonin 6 or more months after surgery indicates residual disease.

Patients need continued follow-up with periodic physical examination and measurements of serum calcitonin and CEA. Patients with residual disease may benefit from radiotherapy. Vandetanib and cabozantinib (Cometriq, Exelixis, South San Francisco, CA) are tyrosine kinase inhibitors approved by the United States Food and Drug Administration (FDA) for progressive, metastatic medullary thyroid cancer. These agents target various tyrosine kinases, including MET, RET, and VEGFR-2.

Thyroid Lymphoma

Thyroid lymphomas are typical of the non-Hodgkin's lymphoma (NHL) type. Diffuse large-cell lymphoma is the most common type. Thyroid lymphoma may develop in the setting of longstanding Hashimoto's thyroiditis.

Epidemiology

Thyroid lymphoma represents approximately 2% of thyroid cancers. It is more common in women and usually presents in the sixth or seventh decade.

Clinical Presentation

Usually thyroid lymphoma presents as a rapidly enlarging goiter. Patients may experience symptoms or signs of compression of the trachea or esophagus, including dysphagia, dyspnea, stridor, hoarseness, and neck pain. On physical examination, the thyroid is usually firm, slightly tender, and is fixed to surrounding structures. It commonly extends substernally. It is not uncommon to see enlarged cervical or supraclavicular lymph nodes. Patients presenting with hoarseness usually have vocal fold paralysis.

In addition, 10% of patients have systemic (B) symptoms of lymphoma, including fever, night sweats, and weight loss (10% of body weight or more). Patients may also present with symptoms and signs of hypothyroidism or hyperthyroidism.

Diagnosis

An ultrasound of the thyroid gland should be performed. FNAB or core biopsy distinguishes thyroid proliferation from epithelial tumors and may differentiate lymphoma from chronic thyroiditis; often surgical specimens are required for diagnosis. Pathology, immunohistochemical staining, or flow cytometry may be necessary to establish monoclonality and characterize surface markers, especially to diagnose small cell lymphomas.

Staging includes physical examination, complete blood count (CBC), serum lactate dehydrogenase (LDH), B2 microglobulin measurements, liver function tests, bone marrow biopsy, and CT of the neck, thorax, abdomen, and pelvis, as well as an ^{18}F fludeoxyglucose (FDG)-PET-scan.

Treatment

Surgery is not the primary treatment and is typically used for diagnostic biopsy and surgical airway only. Treatment depends on extent of disease. If lymphoma is disseminated, chemotherapy is given. If disease is confined to the neck, treatment is guided by the histologic features of the lymphoma. Patients with large cell lymphoma are treated with chemotherapy with or without radiation. For patients with localized extranodal marginal zone lymphoma of the thyroid, follicular lymphoma, or small-cell lymphoma, radiotherapy alone may be adequate (**Fig. 7.3**).

◆ Staging of Thyroid Cancer

TNM and Stage Groupings

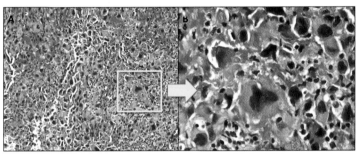

Fig. 7.3 Histology of anaplastic thyroid cancer (ATC). **(a)** Low-power view demonstrating abnormally shaped cells without papillary or follicular architecture. **(b)** High-power view demonstrating irregularly shaped cells and heterogeneity of nuclei, features typical of ATC. (Used with permission from Terris DJ, Duke WS, eds. *Thyroid and Parathyroid Diseases: Medical and Surgical Management*. 2nd ed. New York, NY: Thieme;2016:149.)

According to the American Joint Committee on Cancer 7th edition (AJCC), the TNM stage groupings for papillary and follicular carcinomas and variants are stratified by age into patients < 45 years of age and patients ≥ 45 years. In the 8th edition, effective January 2018, the age stratification is now < 55 years and ≥ 55 years. Tumor size and lymph node status are also considered in the TNM classification.

All categories may be subdivided into solitary tumor or multifocal tumor. With multifocal tumors, the largest one is used for classification. The lymph nodes must be specifically identified to classify regional node involvement.

Staging Thyroid Cancer Differentiated and Anaplastic (AJCC 8th edition)

Primary Tumor (T): Papillary, Follicular, Poorly Differentiated, Hürthle Cell, and Anaplastic Thyroid Carcinoma

TX: Primary tumor cannot be assessed

T0:   No evidence of primary tumor

T1:   Tumor ≤ 2 cm in greatest dimension limited to the thyroid

  T1a: Tumor ≤ 1 cm, limited to the thyroid

  T1b: Tumor > 1 cm but ≤ 2 cm in greatest dimension, limited to the thyroid

T2: Tumor > 2 cm but ≤ 4 cm in greatest dimension, limited to the thyroid

T3: Tumor > 4 cm limited to the thyroid or gross extrathyroidal extension invading only strap muscles

   T3a: Tumor > 4 cm limited to the thyroid

   T3b: Gross extrathyroidal extension invading only strap muscles (sternohyoid, sternothyroid, thyrohyoid, or omohyoid muscles) from a tumor of any size

T4: Includes gross extrathyroidal extension

   T4a: Gross extrathyroidal extension invading subcutaneous soft tissues, larynx, trachea, esophagus, or recurrent laryngeal nerve from a tumor of any size

   T4b: Gross extrathyroidal extension invading prevertebral fascia or encasing the carotid artery or mediastinal vessels from a tumor of any size

Note: All categories may be subdivided: (S) solitary tumor or (M) multifocal tumor (the largest tumor determines the classification).

Regional Lymph Node (N)

NX: Regional lymph nodes cannot be assessed

N0: No evidence of locoregional lymph node metastasis

   N0a: One or more cytologically or histologically confirmed benign lymph nodes

   N0b: No radiologic or clinical evidence of locoregional lymph node metastasis

N1: Metastases to regional nodes

   N1a: Metastases to level VI or VII (pretracheal, paratracheal, or prelaryngeal/delphian, or upper mediastinal) lymph nodes; this can be unilateral or bilateral disease

   N1b: Metastasis to unilateral, bilateral, or contralateral lateral neck lymph nodes (levels I, II, II, IV, or V) or retropharyngeal lymph nodes

Definition of Distant Metastasis (M)

M0: No distant metastasis

M1: Distant metastasis

American Joint Committee on Cancer Stage Groupings of Differentiated and Anaplastic Thyroid Cancer (8th Edition)

Differentiated: See **Table 7.9**. Anaplastic: See **Table 7.10**.

Histopathologic Type

- Papillary carcinoma
- Papillary microcarcinoma
  - Follicular variant
  - Solid variant

- o Hürthle cell variant
- Follicular carcinoma
  - o Encapsulated noninvasive
  - o Minimally invasive
  - o Widely invasive
- Hürthle cell carcinoma
- Poorly differentiated carcinoma (used for insular carcinoma as a subtype of poorly differentiated)
- Anaplastic carcinoma

Table 7.9 American Joint Committee on Cancer 8th edition stage groups, differentiated thyroid cancers

When age at diagnosis is...	and T is...	and N is...	and M is...	then the stage group is...
< 55 years	Any T	Any N	M0	I
< 55 years	Any T	Any N	M1	II
≥ 55 years	T1	N0/NX	M0	I
≥ 55 years	T1	N1	M0	II
≥ 55 years	T2	N0/NX	M0	I
≥ 55 years	T2	N1	M0	II
≥ 55 years	T3a/T3b	Any N	M0	II
≥ 55 years	T4a	Any N	M0	III
≥ 55 years	T4b	Any N	M0	IVA
≥ 55 years	Any T	Any N	M1	IVB

Used with permission from Amin MB, Edge S, Greene F, et al, eds. *AJCC Cancer Staging Manual* 8th Edition. New York: Springer; 2017.

Table 7.10 American Joint Committee on Cancer stage groups, anaplastic thyroid cancers

When T is...	and N is...	and M is...	then the stage group is...
T1–T3a	No/NX	M0	IVA
T1–T3a	N1	M0	IVB
T3b	Any N	M0	IVB
T4	Any N	M0	IVB
Any T	Any N	M1	IVC

Used with permission from Amin MB, Edge S, Greene F, et al, eds. *AJCC Cancer Staging Manual* 8th Edition. New York: Springer; 2017.

Medullary Thyroid Cancer

Primary Tumor (T)

TX: Primary tumor cannot be assessed

T0: No evidence of primary tumor.

T1: Tumor ≤ 2 cm in greatest dimension limited to the thyroid

    T1a: Tumor ≤ 1 cm in greatest dimension limited to the thyroid

    T1b: Tumor > 1 cm but ≤ 2 cm in greatest dimension limited to the thyroid

T2: Tumor > 2 cm but < 4 cm in greatest dimension limited to the thyroid.

T3: Tumor ≥ 4 cm or with extrathyroidal extension

    T3a: Tumor ≥ 4 cm in greatest dimension limited to the thyroid

    T3b: Tumor of any size with gross extrathyroidal extension invading only strap muscles (sternohyoid, sternothyroid, thyrohyoid, or omohyoid muscles)

T4: Advanced disease

    T4a: Moderately advanced disease; tumor of any size with gross extrathyroidal extension into the nearby soft tissues of the neck, including subcutaneous soft tissues, larynx, trachea, esophagus, or recurrent laryngeal nerve

    T4b: Very advanced disease; tumor of any size with extension toward the spine or into nearby large blood vessels, invading prevertebral fascia or encasing the carotid artery or mediastinal vessels

Regional Lymph Node (N)

NX: Regional lymph nodes cannot be assessed

N0: No evidence of locoregional lymph node metastasis

    N0a: One or more cytologically or histologically confirmed benign lymph nodes

    N0b: No radiologic or clinical evidence of locoregional lymph node metastasis

N1: Metastases to regional nodes

    N1a: Metastases to level VI or VII (pretracheal, paratracheal, or prelaryngeal/delphian, or upper mediastinal) lymph nodes; this can be unilateral or bilateral disease

    N1b: Metastasis to unilateral, bilateral, or contralateral lateral neck lymph nodes (levels I, II, II, IV, or V) or retropharyngeal lymph nodes

Distant Metastasis (M)

M0: No distant metastasis

M1: Distant metastasis

American Joint Committee on Cancer Stage Groupings of Medullary Thyroid Cancer (8th edition)

See **Table 7.11**.

Histologic Grade (G)

Grade is not used in the staging for MTC.

Table 7.11 American Joint Committee on Cancer stage groups, medullary thyroid cancers

When T is...	and N is...	and M is...	then the stage group is...
T1	N0	M0	I
T2	N0	M0	II
T3	N0	M0	II
T1–3	V1a	M0	III
T4a	Any T	M0	IVA
T1–3	N1b	M0	IVA
T4b	Any T	M0	IVB
Any T	Any T	M1	IVC

Used with permission from Amin MB, Edge S, Greene F, et al, eds. *AJCC Cancer Staging Manual* 8th Edition. New York: Springer; 2017.

7.9 Embryology, Anatomy, and Physiology of the Parathyroid Glands

There are four parathyroid glands (in two pairs), usually close to the upper and lower poles of the thyroid lobe.

◆ Embryology

The upper pair of parathyroid glands arises from the fourth branchial cleft and descends with the thyroid gland, usually at the cricothyroid junction. The lower pair arises from the third branchial cleft and descends with the thymus; the location of the lower parathyroids may be variable (**Fig. 7.4**). Ectopic parathyroids may be found anywhere along the pathway of descent of the branchial pouches. The (lower) parathyroid glands have been described in the carotid sheath, anterior mediastinum, and intrathyroid.

◆ Anatomy

Grossly the parathyroid glands are yellow-brown or caramel color, weighing 25 to 40 mg per gland. They each measure, on average, ~ 6 mm in length and from 3 to 4 mm in breadth and usually present the appearance of flattened oval disks.

◆ Histology

Parathyroid glands are composed primarily of chief cells and fat with a thin fibrous capsule dividing the gland into lobules; the glands may have a pseudofollicle pattern resembling thyroid follicles.

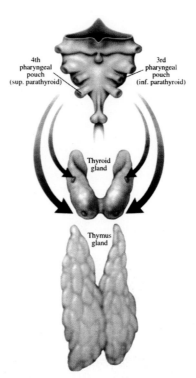

Fig. 7.4 Embryologic origin and descent of the *parathyroid* glands. (Used with permission from *Terris DJ, Gourin CG, eds. Thyroid and Parathyroid Diseases: Medical and Surgical Management.* New York, NY: Thieme; 2009:216.)

◆ Blood Supply

The arterial supply to the parathyroid glands originates from the superior and inferior parathyroid arteries, both of which usually arise from the inferior thyroid artery. Parathyroid glands do not receive nourishment from the adjacent thyroid gland.

◆ Physiology

Parathyroid glands help maintain serum calcium and phosphorus homeostasis in conjunction with calcitonin and vitamin D by secreting parathyroid hormone (PTH or parathyrin). PTH contains 84 amino acids and is cleaved in the liver to its active form, producing a biologically active N-terminal segment. Secretion of PTH is stimulated by low levels of ionized calcium and suppressed by high levels of ionized calcium. PTH binding to receptor sites results in cyclic adenosine monophosphate (cAMP) second-messenger system activation. Target end organs include the kidneys, skeletal bone, and the intestine. The half-life of PTH is a few minutes, which is clinically utilized to detect falling levels following a parathyroidectomy (**Fig. 7.5**).

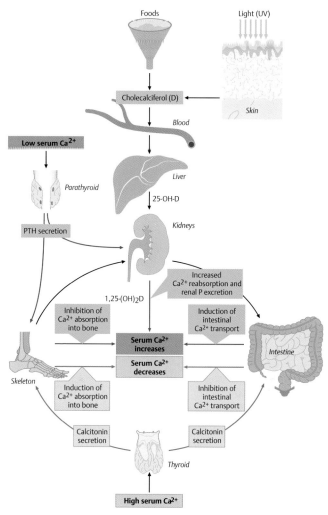

Fig. 7.5 Integration of vitamin D, *parathyroid* hormone, and bone mineral metabolism. Vitamin D precursors are produced in the skin from 7-deoxycholesterol by photocatalysis in the presence of ultraviolet radiation. The synthesis of 25-OH vitamin D, the storage form of the prohormone, to 1,25-(OH)$_2$ vitamin D, the active hormone, is under the control of *parathyroid* hormone. 1,25-(OH)$_2$ vitamin D increases calcium absorption from the gastrointestinal tract. Serum calcium and phosphate levels lead to the mineralization of new bone matrix and feedback on *parathyroid* hormone secretion. Higher levels of *parathyroid* hormone increase bone resorption when necessary to maintain normal serum calcium levels and stimulate the synthesis of 1,25-(OH)$_2$ vitamin D by the kidneys. (Used with permission from TannerThies R. *Physiology: An Illustrated Review*. New York, NY: Thieme; 2012:261.)

7.10 Hyperparathyroidism

◆ Key Features

- Hyperparathyroidism is caused by an excessive secretion of parathyroid hormone (PTH).
- Hyperparathyroidism is usually subdivided into primary, secondary, and tertiary hyperparathyroidism.
- Hyperparathyroidism results in elevated levels of plasma calcium by increasing the release of calcium and phosphate from bone matrix, increasing calcium reabsorption by the kidney, and increasing intestinal absorption of calcium.

Hyperparathyroidism (HPT) refers to the increased production of PTH by the parathyroid glands. There are three types of hyperparathyroidism: primary, secondary, and tertiary; these are described in subsequent paragraphs.

◆ Primary Hyperparathyroidism

Etiology

Eighty to 90% of hyperparathyroidism patients have single parathyroid adenomas, and up to 5% may have double adenomas. Diffuse hyperplasia of all four glands accounts for 6% cases of primary hyperparathyroidism (PHP). One to 2% of cases are due to parathyroid carcinoma.

The diffuse hyperplasia of all four glands can be sporadic or familial; occurring usually as a part of the multiple endocrine neoplasia (MEN) type 1 or 2 syndromes (**Table 7.12**). Other familial conditions associated with all-four-gland hyperplasia include familial hyperparathyroidism–jaw tumor syndrome and familial isolated hyperparathyroidism.

Familial hypocalciuric hypercalcemia is a rare, autosomal dominant disorder that should be included in the differential diagnosis of PHP. It is caused by mutations of the calcium-sensing receptor.

Table 7.12   Multiple endocrine neoplasia (MEN)

	MEN 1	MEN 2A	MEN 2B
Inheritance	AD	AD	AD
Clinical manifestations	PHP (95%) Pituitary tumors Enteropancreatic tumors	PHP (30%) MTC Pheochromocytoma Hirschsprung's disease Cutaneous lichen Amyloidosis	PHP (rare) MTC Pheochromocytoma Mucosal neuromas Intestinal Ganglioneuromatosis Marfanoid habitus

Abbreviations: AD, autosomal dominant; MTC, medullary thyroid cancer; PHP, primary hyperparathyroidism.

Epidemiology

Primary hyperparathyroidism can occur at any age, but the great majority of cases occur over the age of 45 years. Women are affected twice as often as men.

Clinical

Primary hyperparathyroidism is most often detected incidentally by routine biochemical screening. Most patients either are asymptomatic or experience subtle and vague symptoms such as fatigue, depression, difficulty in concentration, and generalized weakness.

Patients with primary hyperparathyroidism rarely present with classic symptoms and signs of hypercalcemia, as recalled by the famed mnemonic "painful bones, renal stones, abdominal groans, and psychic moans":

- Bones: The classic bone disease of PHP is osteitis fibrosa cystica, which is now rare in the United States. It presents with bone pain and/or pathologic fractures. A more common skeletal manifestation of PHP is a decrease in the bone mineral density (osteopenia), preferentially at the cortical sites (forearm and hip). The cause is prolonged PTH excess.

- Kidneys: Nephrolithiasis occurs in ~ 15 to 20% of patients with primary hyperparathyroidism. The cause is prolonged PTH excess. Hypercalciuria and chronic renal failure can also occur.

- Gastrointestinal: Hypercalcemia-associated symptoms include anorexia, nausea, vomiting, constipation, and peptic ulcer disease.

- Psychiatric and neurocognitive: Many patients may have depressed mood, lethargy, emotional lability, decreased cognitive function, and poor sleep. Frank psychosis is rare.

Often the presentation is much more subtle. Patients with familial hypocalciuric hypercalcemia are asymptomatic.

Parathyroid carcinomas are rare. Tumors may be large, palpable; PTH and calcium may be markedly elevated.

Evaluation

Patients suspected of having PHP should be referred to an endocrinologist for work-up and confirmation of the diagnosis.

Imaging

- Sestamibi scan: ^{99m}Tc sestamibi localizes to the mitochondria of parathyroid cells, which are rich in mitochondria. After injection, an image is taken at 10 to 15 minutes and again at 2 to 3 hours. The late phase is useful for the detection of adenomas. It has a sensitivity as high as 100%; specificity is at 90% (**Fig. 7.6**).

- Single proton emission computed tomography (SPECT) scan: The advantage of SPECT is that it portrays images in 3D and therefore may add localization to mediastinal lesions or ectopic adenomas in the carotid sheath. A hybrid SPECT/CT scan can further enhance localization by

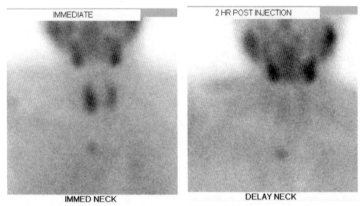

Fig. 7.6 Sestamibi scan shows small ectopic parathyroid adenoma in the right upper chest.

providing better resolution of surrounding structures. The fusion of CT with SPECT images allows combining the anatomic information from CT and the physiologic three-dimensional information from SPECT (**Fig. 7.7**).

- Ultrasound: Its advantage is ease of performance, low cost, and no radiation. Disadvantages include difficulty of localization of nonstandard locations, the potential of confusion with thyroid abnormalities, and interoperator variability.

- Parathyroid 4D-CT represents the latest technology in parathyroid imaging. The resolution of 4D-CT imaging is higher than that of any other type of parathyroid scan. The patient is given intravenous contrast. 4D-CT is most commonly performed with three phases: noncontrast, arterial, and delayed phase imaging. Images are then acquired with the CT scanner at very specific times when the contrast is maximally taken up by the parathyroid glands. (The fourth dimension here in the name is time.) 4D-CT has a higher radiation dose than scintigraphy.

- Selective venous sampling: The veins draining the parathyroid region can be sampled. A twofold gradient between PTH levels in the sampled vein versus the peripheral vein levels can help localize the parathyroid adenoma.

- Intraoperatively, localization, dye, or radioactive tracers may be used.

Labs

PTH levels can be elevated or normal. Serum calcium levels are generally elevated; however, 10 to 20% of patients with primary hyperparathyroidism have normal serum calcium concentrations (normocalcemic PHP). In some patients this may be due to coexisting vitamin D [25(OH)D] deficiency. Low serum phosphorus, increased 24-hour urinary calcium excretion, and elevated serum 1,25-dihydroxyvitamin D may be seen. Blood urea nitrogen and creatinine should be checked as well.

It is important to rule out familial hypocalciuric hypercalcemia, because the course of this disease is usually benign and parathyroidectomy is not

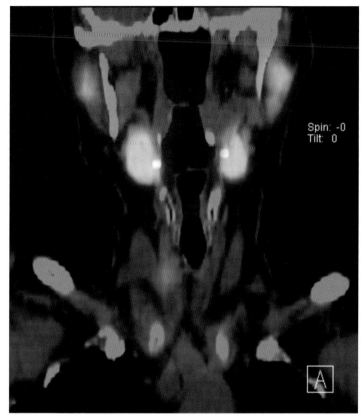

Fig. 7.7 SPECT/CT shows small ectopic parathyroid adenoma in the retromanubrial right upper chest.

indicated. Past medical history should be carefully obtained, as these patients are asymptomatic and have a history of elevated calcium levels since childhood. Their family members may have hypercalcemia as well. Their 24-hour urinary calcium excretion is low.

Secondary hyperparathyroidism should also be ruled out (either from a renal source or from decreased calcium absorption/intake or vitamin D deficiency).

Treatment Options

Medical

Medical treatment is indicated in patients who do not meet the criteria for surgery, refuse surgery, or are poor surgical candidates. This includes adequate hydration and moderate calcium intake ~ 1,000 mg/day. The calcium levels, renal function, and a dual-energy X-ray absorptiometry (DEXA) scan are periodically followed under the care of an endocrinologist. Medications used in the treatment of osteoporosis, such as bisphosphonates, may be useful. Calcimimetics such as cinacalcet (Sensipar, Amgen, Inc., Thousand Oaks, CA) lower PTH and calcium levels but are not yet FDA-approved for PHP.

Surgical

Surgery is curative and is indicated in all cases with symptomatic disease. Following are the indications of surgery in asymptomatic patients:

1. Serum calcium > 1.0 mg/dL above normal
2. Creatinine clearance reduced to < 60 mL/min
3. 24-hour urine calcium > 400 mg/dL
4. Age < 50 years
5. DEXA bone density scan with T score below –2.5 at any site
6. Patient requests surgery.

After surgery, 90% of patients' calcium levels normalize. Surgery consists of removal of the adenoma. Preoperative imaging localization enables guided and minimally invasive parathyroidectomy in most cases.

Occasionally parathyroid adenomas may be found in an ectopic site. Common ectopic sites include the thymus/mediastinum, transesophageal groove, retroesophageal, intrathyroidal, and the carotid sheath.

Surgery in Multigland Disease

1. Multigland diffuse hyperplasia does not localize with sestamibi. Remove enlarged glands and do an intraoperative parathyroid hormone assay.
2. Non-MEN familial hyperparathyroidism: Patients tend to be younger and more likely to have multiglandular disease and persistent or recurrent hyperparathyroidism after surgery. More aggressive than MEN 2a, this disease is more likely to be associated with profound hypercalcemia or hypercalcemic crisis. In a bilateral neck exploration, identify all four glands; perform a subtotal or total parathyroidectomy with thymectomy and autotransplantation of gland as needed.
3. MEN 1: Patients should have a bilateral neck exploration with identification of all four glands. It is controversial whether a subtotal or total parathyroidectomy should be performed.
4. MEN 2a: Pheochromocytoma should be ruled out prior to surgery. After a bilateral neck exploration, with ID of all four glands, remove only the enlarged glands.
5. Renal failure–induced hyperplasia occurs if medical therapy fails. After a bilateral exploration, a subtotal or total parathyroidectomy with auto-transplantation can be done.

◆ Secondary Hyperparathyroidism

Secondary hyperparathyroidism is a normal elevation in the PTH level secondary to renal failure, hypocalcemia, hyperphosphatemia, malabsorption, gastric bypass surgery, or vitamin D deficiency. Treatment consists of treating the initial cause of the secondary hyperparathyroidism.

◆ Tertiary Hyperparathyroidism

Tertiary hyperparathyroidism is due to prolonged hypercalcemia that causes parathyroid gland hyperplasia. Autonomous oversecretion of PTH by the parathyroid glands results in hypercalcemia. Most commonly seen after renal transplant for end-stage renal disease that is associated with severe secondary hyperparathyroidism. Treatment is usually surgical.

7.11 Hypoparathyroidism

◆ Key Features

- Hypoparathyroidism is caused by low circulating levels of parathyroid hormone or insensitivity to its action.
- The most common causes are iatrogenic (surgery) and autoimmunity.

◆ Etiology

- Iatrogenic (surgical): This is the most common cause of hypoparathyroidism. This may occur after surgery on the neck (thyroidectomy, parathyroidectomy, or neck dissection). It maybe transient with recovery within days to weeks, or it may be permanent. It usually occurs as a result of manipulation of blood supply to the parathyroid glands during surgery or injury to or removal of one or more parathyroid glands.
- Patient who have undergone gastric bypass are more susceptible to severe postthyroidectomy hypocalcemia.
- Hypoparathyroidism may also occur in the setting of "hungry bone syndrome" following surgery. In this case, bones readily take up calcium and phosphate. This is usually associated with severe preoperative hyperparathyroid bone disease.
- Autoimmunity: This occurs secondary to immune-mediated destruction of parathyroid glands. This may be acquired or familial.
- Hypoparathyroidism may occur due to abnormal development of the parathyroid glands. This is usually associated with DiGeorge's syndrome, which is a congenital abnormality of the third and fourth branchial pouches and results in the absence of parathyroid glands and thymus.
- Idiopathic hypoparathyroidism is more common in females and has been associated with anti–parathyroid hormone (PTH) antibodies.
- Hypoparathyroidism may result from the destruction of parathyroid glands by irradiation or infiltrative diseases (such as metastatic cancer and granulomatous disease) or storage diseases (such as Wilson's disease and hemochromatosis).

◆ Clinical

Signs and Symptoms

Patients present with symptoms and signs of hypocalcemia (see **Chapter 7.12**).

Differential Diagnosis

Hypoparathyroidism is usually associated with hypocalcemia (low serum calcium levels), hyperphosphatemia (high serum phosphate levels), and low or undetectable PTH levels. Note that, in contrast, "hungry bone syndrome" is associated with hypocalcemia and hypophosphatemia (low serum phosphate levels).

◆ Treatment Options

For management of acute hypocalcemia, see **Chapter 7.12**. Patients with hypoparathyroidism may require lifelong supplementation with calcium and vitamin D. The goal of treatment is to maintain serum calcium levels in the low normal range. Patients are given 1.5 to 2 g of elemental calcium in divided doses daily with meals to maximize absorption. Calcitriol (Rocaltrol; Hoffmann–La Roche, Basel, Switzerland) is usually given at a starting dose of 0.25 to 0.5 μg orally daily and titrated as needed. Renal function and calcium levels should be closely monitored in these patients.

Recombinant PTH (Forteo [teriparatide]; Eli Lilly & Co., Indianapolis, Indiana) may be another treatment option. In recent years, PTH replacement therapy has been shown in several studies to be an alternative to conventional treatment. PTH may abolish or reduce the need for calcium supplements and activated vitamin D analogues while maintaining eucalcemia.

7.12 Calcium Disorders

◆ Key Features

- Hypercalcemia can result when too much calcium enters the extracellular fluid or when there is insufficient calcium excretion from the kidneys.
- Hypocalcemia is less frequent than hypercalcemia.
- Hypocalcemia occurs in patients with renal failure, vitamin D deficiency, magnesium deficiency, acute pancreatitis, and with hypoparathyroidism and pseudohypoparathyroidism.

About 99% of the body's calcium is found in the bones. The remaining 1% is found in the extracellular fluid. Of this 1%, ~ 40% of calcium is bound to albumin, and 50% is in the free (unbound, active, or ionized) form. A basic metabolic panel and a comprehensive metabolic panel measure the total calcium levels (bound plus unbound), although it is the free (unbound) form that is most important.

◆ Control of Calcium Metabolism

Calcium is absorbed from the gut, stored in the bone, and excreted by the kidneys. Calcium levels are affected by the following:

- Parathyroid hormone (PTH): Decreased serum calcium levels lead to an increase in PTH, which in turn causes a release of bone calcium stores and decreased renal excretion of calcium.
- Vitamin D: PTH stimulates conversion of 25(OH)D into its active form [1,25-(OH)2D], which in turn increases calcium and phosphate absorption from the gut.
- Calcitonin. Calcitonin is synthesized in the C cells of the thyroid and causes a decrease in plasma calcium and phosphate levels.

◆ Hypocalcemia

Etiology

- Hypoparathyroidism: The most common cause is iatrogenic (surgery); see **Chapter 7.11**.
- Pseudohypoparathyroidism: An inherited disorder that is caused by resistance to PTH by target organs. Patients present in childhood. It is associated with hypocalcemia, hyperphosphatemia, and elevated PTH levels.
- Renal failure
- Vitamin D deficiency
- Hypomagnesemia
- Acute pancreatitis
- Hyperphosphatemia

Clinical

- Neuromuscular irritability: Patients may present with tingling, paresthesias in fingers and periorally, tetany, carpopedal spasm, seizures, irritability, and confusion.
  - Chvostek's sign: Gentle tapping over the facial nerve causes twitching of facial muscles.
  - Trousseau's sign: Carpopedal spasm after blood pressure cuff is inflated above patient's systolic blood pressure for 3 minutes.
- Cardiac manifestations: electrocardiogram changes—prolonged QT interval, heart failure, and arrhythmias
- Other manifestations include subcapsular cataracts, dry flaky skin, and brittle nails.

Evaluation

Serum albumin concentration should be measured in patients with hypocalcemia. When albumin is low, the calcium level should be corrected (adjusted) for the level of albumin (add 0.8 mg/dL Calcium for every 1.0

g/dL of albumin below 4.0 g/dL). Alternatively, a serum ionized calcium level should be obtained. Additionally, phosphate levels, intact PTH levels, magnesium levels, vitamin D levels, and creatinine levels should also be obtained.

Treatment Options

Treatment should be tailored to treat the underlying cause. Endocrine consult (or referral) should be considered.

- Acute hypocalcemia: Patients with symptomatic tetany, seizures, or stridor need immediate correction of hypocalcemia. Calcium is given as a slow IV bolus over 10 to 15 minutes because a rapid infusion may cause cardiac dysfunction. The patient should be in a monitored setting (telemetry). This may be followed by a slow calcium infusion over several hours. Serum calcium levels should be closely monitored during the IV infusion.
- Chronic hypocalcemia: Calcium and vitamin D supplementation are the mainstays of treatment. Daily divided doses of 1.5 to 2 g of elemental calcium are given with meals to maximize absorption. Vitamin D supplementation is given as ergocalciferol (vitamin D_2), which has a long duration of action, or calcitriol (Rocaltrol, Hoffmann–La Roche, Basel, Switzerland), which has a short duration of action.

◆ Hypercalcemia

Etiology

- Hyperparathyroidism is the most common cause of hypercalcemia; see **Chapter 7.10**.
- Malignancy is the second most common cause of hyperparathyroidism; it is commonly associated with solid tumors (e.g., breast, lung, ovary) and hematologic cancers (e.g., myelomas and lymphomas).
- Granulomatous disorders (such as sarcoidosis, tuberculosis)
- Milk alkali syndrome
- Paget's disease
- Multiple endocrine neoplasia (MEN) syndromes
- Thyrotoxicosis
- Medications: thiazides, vitamin A and D intoxication, lithium
- Immobilization

Clinical

See **Table 7.13**.

Evaluation

Labs should include intact PTH level, ionized calcium level, and vitamin D. If PTH levels are low and malignancy is suspected, parathyroid hormone–related protein (PTHrP) levels should be obtained. Other lab values should be obtained to diagnose the suspected underlying etiology.

Table 7.13 Signs and symptoms of hypercalcemia

Bones	Bone pain, muscle weakness, osteopenia/osteoporosis
Renal	Polyuria, polydipsia, nephrolithiasis, nephrocalcinosis, acute and chronic renal insufficiency
Gastrointestinal	Anorexia, nausea, vomiting, constipation, pancreatitis, peptic ulcer disease
Neurologic-psychiatric	Decreased concentration, confusion, fatigue, depression
Heart	Shortening of the QT interval, bradycardia, and hypertension

Treatment Options

Treatment should focus on the underlying etiology of hypercalcemia.

For acute severe hypercalcemia, the volume status should be assessed and the patient should be aggressively rehydrated with IV normal saline. Use with caution in patients with heart failure or renal failure to avoid fluid overload. The serum electrolytes, calcium, and magnesium levels should be monitored closely. Once the fluid deficit has been corrected, consider adding furosemide (loop diuretic). Bisphosphonates can be given, as these inhibit bone resorption by osteoclasts and are effective in lowering calcium levels to the normal range within 2 to 5 days. Calcitonin rapidly lowers serum calcium and can be administered subcutaneously as an adjunct.

For chronic severe hypercalcemia, the cause should be identified and treated accordingly (see **Chapter 7.10**). Bisphosphonates, gallium nitrate, or glucocorticoids can be used in the treatment of malignancy-associated hypercalcemia. Hypercalcemia associated with granulomatous diseases is also treated with glucocorticoids. If hypercalcemia is caused by medication overdose, then that medication should be stopped.

8 Pediatric Otolaryngology

Section Editor

Michele M. Carr

Contributors

Eelam A. Adil

Michele M. Carr

David Culang

Sharon L. Cushing

Carole Fakhry

David Goldenberg

Bradley J. Goldstein

Colin Huntley

Christopher K. Kolstad

Michael P. Ondik

Vijay Patel

Sarah E. Pesek

Christopher A. Roberts

Sohrab Sohrabi

Jonathan M. Sykes

8.1 Pediatric Airway Evaluation and Management

◆ Key Features

- The airway is relatively narrower and more tenuous in children.
- The potential for airway emergency is high.
- Many conditions causing respiratory distress in infants resolve spontaneously with growth.

The pediatric airway is proportionally smaller than that of the adult: the tongue is relatively larger and more anterior, the soft palate descends lower, the adenoid is larger, the epiglottis is omega-shaped, larger, and more acutely angled toward the glottis; the cricoid ring is narrower, the trachea is shorter and narrower, the surrounding soft tissue is looser, and cartilaginous structures are less rigid. Thus the pediatric airway is more prone to compromise by infection, inflammation, neoplasia, and normal breathing. Foreign body aspiration may be a life-threatening emergency. An aspirated solid or semisolid object may lodge in the airway. If the object is large enough to cause nearly complete obstruction of the airway, then asphyxia may rapidly cause death. Infants are at risk for foreign body aspiration because of their tendency to put everything in their mouths and because of immature chewing. Children may be asymptomatic. If present, physical findings may include stridor, fixed wheeze, or diminished breath sounds. If obstruction is severe, cyanosis may occur.

◆ Clinical

Signs and Symptoms

- Stridor: Harsh, high-pitched sound of turbulent airflow past partial obstruction in upper airway
  - Inspiratory stridor signifies supraglottic obstruction.
  - Biphasic stridor signifies glottic or subglottic obstruction.
  - Expiratory stridor signifies tracheal or large bronchial compression.
- Stertor: Low-pitched, snorting sound resulting from partial nasal/nasopharyngeal/hypopharyngeal obstruction
- Wheezing: A continuous whistling or musical sound on expiration from a small bronchiole constriction

For subjective assessment of respiratory distress, see **Table 8.1**. Indications for intubation for airway compromise include P_{AO_2} < 60 mm Hg with F_{IO_2} > 0.6 (without cyanotic heart disease), P_{ACO_2} > 50% (acute, unresponsive to other intervention), actual or impending obstruction, neuromuscular weakness (maximum negative inspiratory pressure over –20 cm H_2O, vital capacity < 12–15 mL/kg), and an absent cough/gag reflex.

Table 8.1 Subjective assessment of respiratory distress

	None	Mild	Moderate	Severe
Stridor	None	Mild	Moderate at rest	Severe on inspiration and expiration or none with markedly decreased air entry
Retractions	None	Mild	Moderate at rest	Severe, marked use of accessory muscles
Color	Normal	Normal	Normal	Dusky or cyanotic
Level of consciousness	Normal	Restless when disturbed	Anxious; agitated; restless when disturbed	Lethargic, depressed

Data from Davis HW, Dartner JC, Galvis AG, et al. Acute upper airway obstruction: croup and epiglottitis. *Pediatr Clin North Am* 1981;28(4):859.

Differential Diagnosis

- Supralaryngeal
  - Adenoid hypertrophy
  - Macroglossia
  - Mass (nasopharyngeal, base of tongue)
  - Choanal atresia
  - Foreign body
  - Cellulitis
  - Neck/pharyngeal abscess
- Laryngeal
  - Laryngomalacia (most common overall cause of pediatric stridor)
  - Vocal fold paralysis (unilateral often is iatrogenic or trauma-related, bilateral is often due to central nervous system [CNS] lesion or dysfunction).
  - Laryngeal web
  - Subglottic stenosis or hemangioma
  - Papillomata
  - Laryngeal cleft
  - Viral croup
  - Epiglottitis
  - Gastric reflux
- Tracheobronchial
  - Tracheomalacia

- Bronchomalacia
- Stenosis
- Vascular ring
- Airway foreign body
- Bronchitis
- Bronchiolitis
- Tracheoesophageal fistula (TEF)

✦ Evaluation

History

A thorough history of respiratory distress (cyanosis, apnea, dyspnea, retractions, grunting) including age of onset, frequency, degree, and rate of progression, ameliorating and exacerbating factors (including positional), as well as feeding difficulties and fevers, should be elicited. Difficult delivery, history of prematurity, and postpartum complications (asphyxia, duration of intubation) should be noted.

Physical Exam

On the physical exam, note respiratory rate, nasal flaring, intercostal and supraclavicular retraction, gasping, or respiratory fatigue. Examine the mouth using a tongue blade, unless epiglottitis is suspected. Auscultate the chest and neck. Note change in breathing when positioning child upright, supine, prone, and on each side. Visualize airway with flexible laryngoscope, unless epiglottitis is suspected. More severe cases may require bronchoscopy and possibly esophagoscopy. Bronchoscopy (rigid or flexible) may be both diagnostic and therapeutic (**see A1** in **Appendix A**).

Imaging

Upright anteroposterior (AP) and lateral soft tissue X-rays of the airway (ideally on full inspiration with head in extension) best evaluate the upper airway. Additionally, AP and lateral chest X-rays can detect extrinsic compression or evaluate for evidence of airway foreign body. If child has feeding difficulties, obtain a barium esophagram. Magnetic resonance imaging (MRI) with MR angiography (MRA) is a good alternative to angiography for vascular malformations. Obtain gastric emptying scans and esophageal pH monitoring if reflux is suspected.

For foreign body aspiration, employ posteroanterior inspiratory and expiratory chest radiography (to look for hyperinflation), computed tomography (CT), or fluoroscopy. Studies may be false-negative; if index of suspicion remains high, bronchoscopy in the OR is indicated.

Other Tests

Although pulmonary function testing with a flow-volume loop can help distinguish inspiratory versus expiratory as well as intrathoracic versus extrathoracic obstruction, the test requires a cooperative subject and is not often feasible in children < 6 years. Polysomnography is very helpful in the evaluation of possible pediatric sleep-related respiratory disorders; a differentiation between obstructive and central apnea can be obtained. This is highly recommended in children with a history of neurologic disorder.

◆ Treatment Options

Acute choking, with respiratory failure associated with airway foreign body obstruction, may be successfully treated at the scene using standard first aid techniques such as the Heimlich maneuver, back blows, and abdominal thrusts. Even in less urgent settings, expeditious removal of airway foreign bodies is recommended and a work-up may be performed.

Medical

Definitive management will of course depend upon the specific diagnosis. But in general terms, for the child with airway compromise, continuous monitoring with pulse oximetry is necessary. Supplemental humidified oxygen, racemic epinephrine, or heliox may be implemented. Systemic steroids are often employed.

Reflux medications such as lansoprazole (Prevacid, Takeda Pharmaceuticals USA, Deerfield, IL) to decrease gastric acid production, as well as metoclopramide (Reglan, Schwarz Pharma Inc., Milwaukee, WI) to promote gastric emptying, can help with reflux irritation of the airway. Upper respiratory infections should be empirically treated as an inpatient with ceftriaxone 75 mg/kg/day intravenously (IV), or comparable antibiotic covering *Streptococcus pneumoniae*, *Streptococcus pyogenes*, and *Haemophilus influenzae*.

Surgical

Again, definitive management will, of course, depend upon the specific diagnosis. In cases of severe compromise, pediatric tracheotomy may be necessary. In laryngomalacia, redundant laryngeal tissue can be excised, and aryepiglottic folds can be divided using endoscopic scissors or CO_2 laser. However, many cases of laryngomalacia may be managed with observation (see **Chapter 8.2**). Subglottic stenosis can be dilated or a cricoid split or cartilage graft reconstruction performed (see **Chapter 8.7**). Obstructing masses should be removed, if possible. Subglottic hemangioma management is discussed in **Chapter 8.14**.

◆ Outcome and Follow-Up

The child should be monitored closely overnight in case of bleeding or edema compromising airway. Oxygen saturation should be monitored. Specific conditions are discussed in detail in the following chapters.

Outcome depends on the diagnosis and management. The child can be followed with the usual well-child checks, and immunizations should be kept up to date.

8.2 Laryngomalacia

◆ Key Features

- Laryngomalacia is the most common cause of stridor in infants (accounts for ~ 75% of infantile stridor).
- Often self-limited; most patients are symptom-free by 12 to 24 months of age.
- Treatment for 90% of cases is expectant observation.
- Its etiology is unknown.

Laryngomalacia is a temporary physiologic dysfunction due to abnormal flaccidity of laryngeal tissues or incoordination of supralaryngeal structures.

◆ Epidemiology

Laryngomalacia is the most common congenital airway abnormality. Overall, laryngomalacia accounts for 60% of cases of chronic laryngeal stridor. It is more common among males than females (2:1). Concomitant airway abnormalities are found in 12 to 37% of patients. Comorbidities, including prematurity, cardiovascular malformation, and neurologic congenital or chromosomal abnormalities, are present in ~ 41% of patients.

◆ Clinical

Signs and Symptoms

Most commonly, patients present with intermittent inspiratory stridor that is relieved by neck extension and a prone position. Stridor is exacerbated by agitation. In extreme cases, patients become cyanotic, have a poor oral intake, have chest retractions, and develop pectus excavatum.

Differential Diagnosis

Other causes of stridor in the early pediatric age group include:

- Unilateral or bilateral vocal fold paralysis
- Laryngeal cleft
- Choanal atresia
- Airway hemangioma
- Laryngeal web
- Airway foreign body
- Acquired or congenital subglottic stenosis
- Craniofacial anomalies
- Glottic cysts
- Laryngeal reflux

- Saccular cyst
- Tracheomalacia
- Papillomatosis

Acid-reflux disorders (see **Chapter 5.5**) have been documented in up to 80% of patients with laryngomalacia.

◆ Evaluation

Physical Exam

An examination of any child with a possible breathing problem should discern whether there is an oxygenation problem, and if so, an oxygen requirement. In the physical examination, one should assess for the location of a possible obstruction and include auscultation, inspection for chest retraction, assessment for cyanosis and other anomalies such as micrognathia. To diagnose laryngomalacia and assess for other upper airway abnormalities, direct flexible endoscopic examination during respiration must be performed. Inward collapse of supraglottic structures is visualized on inspiration. The vocal folds are normal in appearance and motility.

Direct laryngoscopy and bronchoscopy in the operating room is the definitive evaluation.

Imaging

Radiologic examination is not generally necessary. However, if there is concern about dysphagia, barium swallow is helpful to assess esophageal function and to assess for evidence of vascular rings or other obstructive lesions or evidence of tracheoesophageal fistula (TEF).

Pathology

Histologically, submucosal edema and lymphatic dilatation are seen. Mechanisms of obstruction have been described by numerous authors, some of whom considered the occurrence of two or more synchronously as causal in airway obstruction. These factors include an inward collapse of aryepiglottic folds, an elongated epiglottis (flaccid) curled on itself, anterior and medial collapsing movements of the arytenoid cartilages, posterior and inferior displacement of the epiglottis, short aryepiglottic folds, and an overly acute angle of epiglottis.

◆ Treatment Options

Medical

If an infant has good progress, which is indicated by adequate weight gain and normal development, then surgical therapy is not necessary. Instead, supportive care can be the mainstay of treatment.

Surgical

In one series of 985 patients with laryngomalacia, 12% required surgical intervention. Patients who should be considered for surgical management are those with severe stridor and failure to thrive, obstructive apnea, weight loss, severe chest deformity, cyanotic attacks, pulmonary hypertension, or cor pulmonale. Supraglottoplasty is performed using carbon dioxide laser or laryngeal microscissors, or other cold instruments such as pediatric ethmoid through-cutting forceps. Most commonly, surgery involves removal of the prolapsing aryepiglottic fold with cuneiform cartilage or division of a tight, short aryepiglottic fold. Unilateral supraglottoplasty has been advocated by some to reduce the risk of supraglottic stenosis. If the epiglottis is displaced posteriorly, an epiglottopexy can be performed.

Potential complications include continued airway obstruction and posterior stenosis. In the event of continued airway obstruction, a tracheotomy may be necessary until the child "outgrows" laryngomalacia. The use of postoperative antibiotics has not been well evaluated in the literature and is controversial. Antireflux medications are used routinely.

◆ Outcome and Follow-Up

Supraglottoplasty relieves symptoms of airway obstruction in 90% of patients. Most infants require only a short hospital stay (1–3 days).

8.3 Bilateral Vocal Fold Paralysis

◆ Key Features

- Bilateral vocal fold paralysis is the second most common cause of infantile stridor.
- It typically requires a tracheotomy for maintenance of airway until vocal fold mobility returns or definitive airway surgery is performed.
- Acquired causes are most common, even in infants.

Bilateral vocal fold paralysis (BVFP) is a potentially lethal problem requiring aggressive management, typically tracheotomy, at least in the short term. Depending on the cause, spontaneous recovery can occur. Recovery, however, is generally a slow process, taking up to a year. A variety of surgical approaches to widen the airway have been described. Usually, however, the voice quality is degraded when there is an intervention to enlarge/improve the laryngeal airway.

◆ Epidemiology

Twenty-five percent of BVFP is congenital. Most of the remaining cases are late presentations of central lesions. Acquired cases are most likely to occur as a result of surgery in the chest or from forceps delivery or infections.

◆ Clinical

Signs

Vocal fold immobility can be seen using flexible laryngoscopy in the clinic. Stridor is a sign of BVFP.

Symptoms

- Stridor
- Typically a normal voice, episodic respiratory distress (e.g., with upper respiratory tract infections)
- Weak cough; aspiration if underlying cause is a neural lesion above the nodose ganglion (inferior ganglion of vagus nerve)

Differential Diagnosis

- Vocal fold fixation
- Laryngeal mass
- Laryngeal web

◆ Evaluation

Physical Exam

Assess for stridor, respiratory effort and rate, color, and weight (plot on a growth chart). Flexible laryngoscopy is mandatory: it may show twitching of cords with respiration; it typically shows paramedian vocal folds.

Imaging

Magnetic resonance imaging (MRI) should scan from skull base to mediastinum (to image the complete course of laryngeal nerves).

Other Tests

Tests depend on the clinical scenario. For example, consider audiometry if a central nervous system (CNS) disorder is present; consider a biopsy of nonvascular laryngeal mass lesion, if present.

Pathology

Congenital Causes

- Laryngeal anomalies, malformations
- CNS anomalies: Arnold-Chiari malformation, hydrocephalus, encephalocele, leukodystrophy, cerebral dysgenesis
- Peripheral neuropathy: neonatal myasthenia gravis, benign congenital hypotonia, Werdnig-Hoffmann's disease, Charcot-Marie-Tooth's disease, arthrogryposis, viral neuropathy
- Birth trauma, including perinatal hypoxia

Acquired Causes

- Sequelae of cardiac or esophageal surgery
- Neoplasia
- Infections
- Trauma

◆ Treatment Options

Medical

No medical treatment options are available other than supportive care initially to maintain ventilation and oxygenation during definitive treatment planning.

Surgical

- Tracheotomy and monitoring for spontaneous recovery (minimum of 1 year)
- Arytenoidopexy, endoscopic vocal fold lateralization procedures
  - Lateralization sutures passed through the vocal process and thyroid ala lateralize the vocal fold without mucosal destruction
- Arytenoidectomy
  - External approach (lateral cervical or via laryngofissure)
  - CO_2 laser via endoscopic approach
- Posterior cartilage graft
- Laryngeal reinnervation: not widely used in children

◆ Complications

Accidental tracheotomy displacement can be fatal in the early recovery period. Other complications related to laryngeal airway surgeries include dysphonia, aspiration in 4 to 6%, and dyspnea in 3 to 8% of patients undergoing arytenoid procedures. Other procedures have not been studied enough to ascertain their complication rates. Assessment for aspiration should be done preoperatively, as posterior glottic expansion surgery can increase risk of aspiration.

◆ Outcome and Follow-Up

Initially, the patient is monitored in an intensive care unit (ICU) setting with continuous pulse oximetry. Placement of "stay sutures" for any pediatric tracheotomy is mandatory. These two polypropylene (Prolene, Johnson & Johnson, Inc., Cincinnati, OH) sutures, placed through cartilage adjacent to the tracheal opening at the time of surgery and secured to the neck skin with Steri-Strips (3M, St. Paul, MN), greatly facilitate the replacement of a trachcotomy tube into the airway if there is accidental displacement. To help prevent displacement, the tracheotomy appliance should be secured to the skin with four sutures as well as the umbilical necktie.

Overall, arytenoidopexy and arytenoidectomy yield high rates of successful decannulation. Such patients require long-term follow-up.

8.4 Laryngeal Clefts

◆ Key Features

- Laryngeal clefts are a rare congenital anomaly.
- They are frequently associated with other anomalies.
- Clinical presentation varies with the extent of the cleft. The patient may have problems with the airway, feeding, and voice.
- Most clefts are short, but complete laryngotracheoesophageal clefts have a mortality rate greater than 90%.

Laryngeal clefts represent a rare cause of stridor. Failed fusion of the posterior cricoid lamina and incomplete development of the tracheoesophageal septum results in a laryngeal cleft, an abnormal communication of the larynx and esophagus. Laryngeal clefts are usually sporadic nonsyndromic congenital abnormalities. Most are associated with other nonsyndromic congenital abnormalities, including tracheoesophageal fistula (TEF), esophageal atresia, congenital heart disease, cleft lip and palate, micrognathia, glossoptosis, laryngomalacia, gastrointestinal and genitourinary anomalies. Rarely, they are attributable to a specific syndrome [Opitz-Frias's and Pallister-Hall's syndrome, VATER (vertebral defects, imperforate anus, tracheoesophageal fistula, and renal dysplasia) association].

◆ Epidemiology

Laryngeal clefts are rare. Congenital anomalies of the larynx are found in only 0.5% of the population, and clinically symptomatic laryngeal clefts constitute only 0.3 to 0.5% of all congenital laryngeal anomalies. Males are more likely to be affected than females (3:1). Thirty percent of laryngeal clefts are associated with maternal polyhydramnios. TEF is present in ~ 25% of patients with a laryngeal cleft and is associated with a higher failure rate of surgical repair.

◆ Clinical

Signs and Symptoms

There are no pathognomonic findings. Clinical symptoms depend on the extent of the cleft. Small clefts, whose anatomic involvement is limited to the interarytenoid musculature, present with stridor and feeding problems.

There may be coughing, choking, stridor, aspiration pneumonias, or cyanotic episodes. Occasionally, patients with small laryngeal clefts may be asymptomatic. However, the most severe clefts are accompanied by aphonia, severe upper airway obstruction, and respiratory distress. Stridor occurs due to anterior collapse of posterior supraglottic structures. Cyanosis and stridor are exacerbated with feeding. In utero, polyhydramnios due to impaired swallowing of amniotic fluid by the fetus is associated with laryngeal clefts.

Differential Diagnosis

- Subglottic stenosis
- Laryngomalacia
- Unilateral or bilateral vocal fold paralysis
- Subglottic hemangioma
- TEF

◆ Evaluation

Physical Exam

A full head and neck exam should be performed, including a fiberoptic airway exam. Attention should be directed at possible sources of airway symptoms, such as choanal atresia, craniofacial anomalies, laryngomalacia, and vocal fold motion impairment.

Laryngeal clefts must be visualized. Suspension microlaryngoscopy is used to visualize and palpate a laryngeal cleft. Palpation is performed on the lateral spread of the interarytenoid mucosa. The normal interarytenoid height from the vocal fold is 3 mm and is severely reduced in laryngeal clefts. Bronchoscopy and esophagoscopy are necessary to adequately assess the airway and to investigate concomitant anomalies (**Fig. 8.1**).

Imaging

Modified barium swallow and a chest radiograph should be performed. Aspiration with thin liquids is the most common finding. A fiberoptic endoscopic evaluation of swallowing (FEES) is helpful preoperatively.

Pathology

There are several classification schemes in the literature. Because of the rare nature of this disorder, there is no consensus, although the Benjamin/Inglis Classification is commonly used. This classification is based on the inferior extent of cleft:

- Type 1: Interarytenoid soft tissue cleft does not extend into cricoid cartilage.
- Type 2: The cleft extends into cricoid cartilage.
- Type 3: The cleft extends through the entire posterior cricoid cartilage.
- Type 4: The cleft extends into the thoracic trachea; it may extend to the carina.

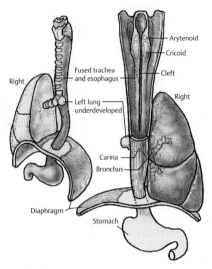

Fig. 8.1 Left anterolateral view and posterior view of type IV laryngotracheoesophageal cleft with left-side pulmonary agenesis and microgastria.

◆ Treatment Options

Medical

Speech and feeding therapy aimed toward decreasing aspiration may be used in conjunction with medical therapy if the cleft is short. For clefts that extend only through interarytenoid musculature but not into cricoid, antireflux therapy in conjunction with thickened diet may be sufficient to control symptoms. However, most clefts require repair. In general, any cleft associated with significant aspiration is repaired.

Surgical

The surgical approach should be individualized based on the symptoms, other associated findings on airway endoscopy, and type of cleft. The decision for surgical repair initially hinges on the extent of the cleft with respect to cricoid and its relationship with local anatomy. Endoscopic techniques may be feasible for type 1 and some type 2 clefts. However, if the cleft extends into inferior anatomic structures, open surgery is generally necessary. Type 3 and 4 clefts require open repair. This is also an option for patients who fail endoscopic management. Early repair is important to minimize irreversible pulmonary damage due to persistent aspiration.

Laryngeal clefts that extend into cricoid or trachea, without carinal involvement, are accessed via anterior laryngofissure to avoid neurovascular damage. Clefts that extend into the cricoid *and* involve carina require either a lateral pharyngotomy and lateral thoracotomy or an anterior laryngofissure and median sternotomy. Sternotomy requires cardiopulmonary bypass during the intrathoracic portion and perioperative tracheotomy. Clefts repaired via open approach in young children most often require tracheotomy. This likely is kept in place for an extended period, as these patients tend to have substantial tracheomalacia for several years.

◆ Complications

Potential complications include recurrent laryngeal nerve injury, mediastinitis, respiratory distress, and dysphagia. Mediastinitis must be aggressively treated with IV antibiotics. Positive pressure ventilation and pulmonary care are necessary for respiratory distress, although aggressive positive pressure ventilation may compromise the anastomosis in the airway. Dysphagia is a chronic problem; many patients require a feeding tube. Input from a skilled pediatric swallow therapist is necessary. Mortality associated with a type 4 cleft approaches 90%.

◆ Outcome and Follow-Up

Sedation and paralysis is employed in the early recovery period. Splinting is useful to maintain the neck in a neutral midline position. An oral or nasogastric tube is contraindicated; pressure compromises the anastomosis and may result in breakdown, tissue necrosis, and fistula formation. Antireflux medications and good pulmonary toilet are maintained. Enteral feeding is preferable (via jejunostomy or gastrostomy).

Outcomes vary greatly with the extent of anomaly, specific treatment, and possible comorbidities. For type 1 clefts repaired endoscopically, there is a 94% success rate reported in one series.

8.5 Tracheoesophageal Fistula and Esophageal Atresia

◆ Key Features

- Tracheoesophageal fistula (TEF) and esophageal atresia (EA) are the result of a congenital communication between the trachea and esophagus.
- EA is also present in most cases of TEF.
- These congenital anomalies present with respiratory and/or feeding difficulties in the newborn.

Congenital TEF and EA are common congenital anomalies that usually occur together. Most cases are diagnosed immediately following birth or during infancy due to the associated life-threatening complications. However, isolated TEF may escape diagnosis until later. Problems with growth and feeding, pulmonary complications, and gastroesophageal morbidity may result from the condition.

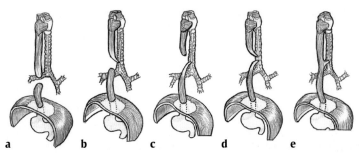

a   b   c   d   e

Fig. 8.2   Classification of tracheoesophageal fistula (TEF) and esophageal atresia (EA). **(a)** EA (Gross classification A, Vogt classification 2, approximate frequency 8%). **(b)** Proximal TEF with distal EA (Gross classification B, Vogt classification 3A, approximate frequency 0.8%). **(c)** Distal TEF with proximal EA (Gross classification C, Vogt classification 3B, approximate frequency 88.5%). **(d)** Proximal TEF and distal TEF (Gross classification D, Vogt classification 3C, approximate frequency 1.4%). **(e)** TEF without EA, or "H"-type TEF (Gross classification E, approximate frequency 4%).

◆ Epidemiology

TEF and EA in their various forms occur in ~ 1 in 3,000 live births, with a slight male predominance. In over 50% of cases, TEF and EA are linked with other defects, such as in the VACTERL (vertebral defects, imperforate anus, cardiac anomalies, TEF, renal dysplasia, limb defects) association, and with chromosomal anomalies.

◆ Clinical

Signs and Symptoms

A sign of the condition, though nonspecific, is polyhydramnios on prenatal ultrasound. Symptoms of TEF include recurrent chest infections, cyanosis and choking on feeding, and abdominal distension. When EA is also present, the patient will not be able to swallow saliva or feed and will drool excessively.

Differential Diagnosis

- Aspiration pneumonia
- Laryngeal cleft
- Tracheomalacia
- Esophageal stricture
- Esophageal diverticula
- Vascular ring
- Gastroesophageal reflux
- Other feeding problems

TEF and EA develop as a result of incomplete separation of the respiratory and digestive divisions of the primitive foregut. Several variants of TEF and EA have been described, but five types predominate, as shown in **Fig. 8.2**.

◆ Evaluation

Physical Exam

The exam is likely to be normal unless marked abdominal distension is present. Other congenital anomalies may be noted. Passage of a tube from the mouth to the stomach may be impossible in the presence of EA. The subsequent chest X-ray will typically show the tip of the catheter coiled in the proximal esophageal pouch.

Imaging

A chest X-ray will show gaseous distension of the bowel when TEF is present. There may be pulmonary changes from persistent respiratory infections. A contrast esophagram can be used to demonstrate an isolated TEF but may provide a false negative because of the slanted orientation of the fistulous tract. Abdominal ultrasonography is used to look for associated renal pathology. Echocardiography is used to examine the heart for any associated anomaly and to aid in planning surgical treatment. Bronchoscopy may help find the location of the fistula and guide operative strategy.

◆ Treatment Options

To prevent aspiration and gastric reflux, a sump catheter should be immediately placed into the upper esophageal pouch and connected to constant suction. The patient should be placed in a prone, head-up position.

Most infants undergo immediate primary repair. Reasons for the delay of surgical treatment include severe associated anomalies, severe pneumonia or respiratory distress, and a long gap between the esophageal pouches.

Repair consists of ligation of the fistula and primary esophageal anastomosis via a right posterolateral thoracotomy. If a right-sided aortic arch is present, a left thoracotomy is used. A cervical incision may be used if there is an isolated TEF. If more than two vertebral bodies separate the upper and lower esophageal segments ("long-gap"), extramucosal circular myotomies can be used. If the gap persists or if there are significant complications, then replacement of the esophagus is necessary.

If a patient cannot undergo immediate primary repair, then a gastrostomy may be used for gastric decompression and access for feedings.

◆ Complications

Anastomotic Leaks

Anastomotic leaks usually resolve with parenteral nutrition and posterior drainage. Repeat thoracotomy is required if healing does not occur.

Stricture

Stricture is usually treated with repeated dilatation.

Dysphagia

Peristalsis is abnormal in the vast majority of patients with a history of TEF or EA. Patients are advised to eat slowly and may need to avoid ingesting meats. Esophageal obstruction may occur, and foreign body removal may be required.

Acid Reflux Disorders

All patients should be placed on antireflux medical treatments, and these should be continued until at least the time when an upright posture is achieved. Antireflux surgery may be necessary in some cases.

Tracheomalacia

Treatment is generally reserved for those with "dying spells" or recurrent pneumonia. Aortopexy is generally employed. If this fails, tracheotomy may be required. Rarely tracheal stents are employed, but these are not used in infants and are uncommonly employed in young children.

Recurrent Tracheoesophageal Fistula

Recurrent TEF requires reoperation.

◆ Outcome and Follow-Up

Oral feeding is delayed until a contrast study done several days after the operation shows no leaks or narrowing around the anastomosis. In the case of isolated TEF repair, oral feeding can resume immediately if the integrity of the repair is certain. Complications occur relatively frequently following operative repair of TEF/EA, and one or more additional operations are needed in half the cases. Strictures are the most common complication, and a barium swallow or esophagoscopy is needed before hospital discharge in all patients.

Although complications occur relatively frequently, patients have an excellent chance of leading normal lives in the absence of severe associated anomalies. Inherent structural and functional defects in the trachea and esophagus result in significant respiratory and gastroesophageal sequelae, including poor growth, feeding problems, tracheomalacia, bronchomalacia, recurrent chest infections, and reflux. However, the frequency of such events appears to decrease significantly with age.

8.6 Vascular Rings

◆ Key Features

- The trachea and esophagus are completely or incompletely surrounded by vascular structures.
- Compression of the trachea, the bronchi, and/or the esophagus may occur.
- Most symptomatic malformations present during infancy or early childhood.

The term *vascular ring* refers to an aortic arch abnormality in which the trachea and esophagus are surrounded by vascular structures. It may be complete or incomplete. The greater the degree of compression the vascular ring causes, the more severe the symptoms are and the earlier they present. For symptomatic patients, treatment is generally surgical.

◆ Embryology and Anatomy

Vascular rings arise during embryonic development from the abnormal evolution of the arterial branchial arch system. In normal embryonic vascular development, ventral and dorsal aortae are connected by six pairs of aortic arches. The first, second, and fifth arches regress, as does a portion of the right fourth arch. This leaves the usual left aortic arch. Residual segments of the third, fourth, and sixth arches develop into the mature anatomy of the mediastinal vascular structures. Inappropriate persistence or development of segments leads to congenital aortic arch anomalies.

The most common vascular ring is a double aortic arch, accounting for 50 to 60% of symptomatic vascular rings. A right aortic arch with an aberrant left subclavian artery is the second most common, accounting for 12 to 25% of cases. Other vascular anomalies include a right aortic arch with mirror image branching and left ductus arteriosus, a pulmonary artery sling, an anomalous innominate artery, and left aortic arch anomalies.

◆ Epidemiology

At autopsy, 3% of the population has a congenital anomaly of the aortic arch system. Most are asymptomatic. Vascular rings account for less than 1% of congenital cardiovascular malformations.

◆ Clinical

Signs and Symptoms

Symptoms depend on the location and degree of vascular compression. Wheezing, stridor, aspiration, cyanotic or apneic attacks, and dysphagia are characteristic. Feeding may exacerbate stridor. Dysphagia is worsened by solid foods. Recurrent respiratory infections such as aspiration pneumonia may also be present.

Differential Diagnosis

- Asthma
- Tracheomalacia
- Bronchiolitis
- Laryngeal stenosis
- Congenital stridor
- Laryngeal web
- Croup
- Foreign body aspiration
- Laryngomalacia

◆ Evaluation

Physical Exam

Physical findings vary, often in accordance with the patient's history. Stridor is characteristically expiratory. It is often associated with cough, tachypnea, and rhonchi. Expiratory, high-pitched wheezes and intercostal retractions can also be appreciated. Patients may hold their neck in hyper-extension to alleviate respiratory distress. Respiratory findings typically do not improve with nebulized bronchodilator treatment and are worsened by exertion. Pulmonary infection may be the presenting symptom, especially in older children.

Imaging

A chest radiograph will reveal laterality of the aortic arch by typical contralateral deviation of the trachea. Two arches may be suspected if there is compression of the trachea at the level of the arches. On the lateral view, anterior tracheal compression may be evident. Tracheal constriction evidenced by narrowing or obliteration of the distal tracheal air column and lung hyperinflation may also be seen.

A barium esophagram is diagnostic in over 90% of patients with a vascular ring. With most aortic arch anomalies, a posterior indentation of the esophagus will be seen. Bilateral and posterior indentations are common in double aortic arch and both types of right aortic arch. Retroesophageal subclavian arteries will show slanted filling defects in the posterior esophagus. A pulmonary artery sling will typically show an anterior esophageal indentation. An anomalous innominate artery usually produces a normal esophagram.

Bronchoscopy is often the diagnostic technique of choice to evaluate structural and dynamic anomalies of the airway. Bronchoscopy can also evaluate the tracheobronchial tree for coexisting or intrinsic lesions such as tracheomalacia, stenosis, complete tracheal rings or aberrant bronchi. In many centers, MRI is becoming the diagnostic technique of choice. Sedation, airway management, and intubation may be challenging in the patient with signs and symptoms of airway compression.

CT may show location, degree, and extent of tracheal narrowing. It is faster and requires less sedation than MRI but is not as good at defining vascular anatomy unless CT angiography is obtained. Other disadvantages include exposure to ionizing radiation and IV contrast.

Frequently but not invariably, echocardiography can show the presence and define the anatomy of a vascular ring. It will show associated cardio-vascular anomalies and can be done at the bedside. It does not image the airways.

Cardiac catheterization with angiography provides a clear delineation of abnormal vessels and is helpful in evaluating associated congenital heart defects. With the advent of MRI, it is rarely necessary for isolated aortic arch anomalies.

Other Tests

Pulmonary function tests can be used in the evaluation of infants and children with suspected tracheal obstruction of vascular origin. The shape of partial expiratory flow-volume curve can help to localize the site and assess the severity of airway obstruction. Usually, pulmonary function testing cannot be obtained in children under age 6.

◆ Treatment Options

Medical

Asymptomatic or mildly symptomatic patients can be managed medically with humidification of inspired air, drainage of bronchial secretions, anti-biotics, and supplemental oxygen when needed, and a soft diet or tube feedings if dysphagia exists.

Surgical

Surgery is indicated in all patients with symptomatic vascular rings. Asymptomatic complete rings should undergo elective surgery if there is suspicion for progressive airway compromise. The goal of surgical treatment is to divide the compressive vascular ring, relieve tracheobronchial and esophageal compression, and maintain normal perfusion of the aortic arch. For a double aortic arch, the atretic or hypoplastic arch is divided along with the ligamentum or ductus arteriosus. For right aortic arch variants, the left ductus or ligamentum arteriosum is divided. If surgery is indicated for an anomalous innominate artery, the preferred treatment is aortopexy. For a pulmonary artery sling, the ductus or ligamentum arteriosum is divided and the left pulmonary artery is divided and reimplanted into the main pulmonary artery.

The approach is generally through a left posterolateral thoracotomy, but certain types of vascular rings require a right thoracotomy. A sternotomy incision is indicated for concomitant repair of intracardiac defects, or for the repair of pulmonary artery sling, or for repair of complete tracheal rings with slide tracheoplasty on cardiac bypass. Intraoperative bronchoscopy is helpful in evaluating the effects of surgery on airway patency; tracheomalacia will persist after repair but will usually improve with time.

◆ Complications

Tracheomalacia and Bronchomalacia

Prolonged intubation may be required to maintain airway patency in long-segment malacia but can lead to endoluminal airway complications such as granuloma formation. Endoluminal stenting procedures have also been described. Occasionally, reconstruction of the affected airway segment is required. Generally, with growth of the trachea and gradually increasing stiffness of the cartilage, symptoms are likely to improve. Tracheotomy may be needed to stent substantial tracheomalacia.

Recurrent Laryngeal Nerve Injury

In unilateral vocal fold paralysis, the need for intervention is based on the degree of hoarseness and the risk of aspiration. In bilateral fold paralysis, surgery is needed to alleviate glottic obstruction. Tracheotomy may also be required.

Chylothorax

This is an uncommon perioperative complication. Treatment of choice is implantation of a pleuroperitoneal shunt.

◆ Outcome and Follow-Up

Intensive respiratory care is always needed postoperatively. Humidified oxygen, antibiotic prophylaxis for pulmonary infections, frequent suctioning of tracheal secretions, and diligent chest physiotherapy are vital.

Major postoperative issues relate to concurrent cardiac defects and residual airway disorders. Successful tracheal extubation is possible in most patients. Successful repair of the vascular ring may not immediately relieve airway obstruction.

The patients who are asymptomatic or mildly symptomatic with incomplete rings are likely to improve with age. Of the patients who receive surgical repair, 95% are expected to survive, and most of them will become completely asymptomatic. However, persistence of various degrees and types of pulmonary function anomalies may be found in a significant number of patients.

8.7 Subglottic Stenosis

◆ Key Features

- The subglottis is the narrowest part of the infant airway.
- Acquired subglottic stenosis is most commonly found; the most common related factor is intubation.
- Subglottic stenosis of 70% or more of the lumen is associated with daily symptoms.

The subglottis, the narrowest part of the pediatric airway, is composed of a complete cartilaginous ring, the cricoid, and loose submucosa that swells when irritated (as in, for example, croup). It is the region most likely to be affected by pressure from a too-large or frequently moving endotracheal tube. Congenital subglottic stenosis most commonly results from an abnormally shaped cricoid, with intraluminal lateral shelves, resulting in an oval shape to the lumen. Intervention is individualized to the patient: sometimes a watch-and-wait approach works; other children benefit from some type of surgery.

◆ Epidemiology

Incidence is ~ 1.5 cases per million, but it occurs in 1 to 8% of neonates requiring intubation.

◆ Clinical

An abnormal, narrow airway causes stridor. It is, therefore, worth reviewing the typical dimensions of the "normal" airway (**Table 8.2**).

Table 8.2   Normal airway size by age

Age	Normal subglottic airway diameter (mm)	Expected endotracheal tube size	Expected bronchoscope size
Premature	3.5–4.5	2.5–3.0	2.5
0–3 months	5.0	3.5	3.0
3–9 months	5.5	4.0	3.5
9–24 months	6.0	4.5	4.0
2–4 years	6.5–7.0	5.0	4.0
4–6 years	7.5	5.5	5.0
6–8 years	8.0	6.0	6.0

Used with permission from Van de Water TR, Staecker H, eds. *Otolaryngology: Basic Science and Clinical Review*. Stuttgart/New York: Thieme; 2006:213.

Signs

The signs include stridor, respiratory distress, and typically a normal voice.

Symptoms

- Unsuccessful extubation of a patient in the neonatal intensive care unit (NICU)
- Stridor; may be biphasic, may present only with agitation
- Respiratory distress exacerbated by upper respiratory tract infection
- Recurrent croup
- Feeding problems
- Slow growth, failure to thrive

Differential Diagnosis

Other causes of stridor with normal voice include laryngomalacia, subglottic cyst, subglottic hemangioma, and tracheal stenosis.

◆ Evaluation

Physical Exam

Flexible laryngoscopy should be done to assess vocal fold movement. The subglottis is sometimes seen with this exam, but the scope should not be passed through the glottis because of the risk of inducing vasovagal reflexes. Bronchoscopy will show subglottic stenosis. The degree of narrowing and the length of the narrowed segment are important to measure.

The Cotton-Meyer grading system apparently correlates to symptoms and prognosis (**Table 8.3**). Grade I stenoses typically are asymptomatic unless there is an upper respiratory tract infection.

Table 8.3   Cotton-Meyer grading system for subglottic stenosis

Grade	Degree of narrowing
I	< 50%
II	50–70%
III	71–99%
IV	Total obstruction

Data from Myer CM, O'Connor DM, Cotton RT. Proposed grading system for subglottic stenosis based on endotracheal tube size. *Ann Otol Rhinol Laryngol* 1994: 108; 319.

Imaging

A soft tissue lateral X-ray, airway fluoroscopy, or computed tomography (CT) may show the subglottic anatomy. Note that airway fluoroscopy involves significant radiation exposure.

Other Tests

A complete evaluation for reflux (including a barium swallow, a gastric scintiscan, or a pH probe) may be helpful. Pulmonary function tests and video stroboscopy are indicated in cooperative older patients.

Pathology

Congenital subglottic stenosis may be cartilaginous or membranous (a thickened submucosa). The subglottis is the narrowest part of the pediatric airway in normal circumstances, so pressure necrosis from an endotracheal tube is more likely here than elsewhere in the airway. Acquired stenosis may be caused by mucosal necrosis with healing by granulation tissue and subsequent fibrosis, although deeper injuries including cartilage necrosis can occur. Factors related to injury include size of endotracheal tube, number of reintubations, tube movement, and tube material (polyvinyl chloride is considered safest).

◆ Treatment Options

Medical

Antireflux medications have a role in management. If an acid-reflux disorder is not diagnosed with traditional tests, prophylactic reflux medications should be given, especially if there is a suggestion of reflux laryngitis on examination.

Surgical

Dilation

Dilation is an option for mild soft stenosis.

Laser Division

Laser division (CO_2, argon, or potassium titanyl phosphate [KTP] laser) is an option for early stenosis (granulation tissue), crescent-shaped bands, and thin circumferential webs.

Cricoid Split

A cricoid split is indicated in neonates with solitary subglottic stenosis and failure to extubate. Traditionally, the criteria for the procedure are weight at least 1,500 g, no ventilator support for 10 days prior to repair, oxygen requirement less than 30%, no congestive heart failure in the month prior to the repair, no acute upper respiratory infection, and no antihypertensive medications required in the 10 days prior to extubation. Basically, the approach is like a tracheotomy, but the anterior midline incision in the trachea extends through the cricoid and the inferior part of the thyroid cartilage. An endotracheal tube is placed such that the incision is open by 2 to 3 mm and left in situ for 7 to 14 days, and steroids are used prior to extubation.

Laryngotracheoplasty

If more than 3 mm of circumference gain is needed, a cartilage graft is necessary. Auricular or costal cartilage may be used. Grafts can be placed anterior and posterior in the subglottis. Stenting is required if the posterior cricoid is divided; this may be achieved by endotracheal intubation for 1 to 2 weeks.

Only mature stenoses should be reconstructed with an open procedure. Cricotracheal resection is reserved for amenable airway lesions.

◆ Complications

Emergency complications can involve airway obstruction or respiratory problems. Causes include mucous plugs, granulation tissue, aspiration of stenting materials (if used), hematoma, hemorrhage into the airway, or pneumothorax. Treatment is aimed at the underlying problem. Treatment may require airway suctioning for mucous plugs; use of aerosolized steroids (e.g., dexamethasone 0.25 to 1.0 mg/kg per day to a maximum of 20 mg/d) to reduce granulations; chest tube placement for pneumothorax, hemorrhage, or hematoma; or return to the operating room for bronchoscopic or possible open treatments.

Other complications include cricoid split failure (repeat intubation for 72 additional hours with a half-size smaller tube; if that fails, then tracheotomy) and laryngotracheoplasty failure (infection may lead to graft necrosis, treated by antibiotics and revision surgery).

◆ Outcome and Follow-Up

A postoperative chest radiograph should always be obtained for open reconstructive procedures. Continuous O_2 saturation monitoring should be overnight; an intensive care unit (ICU) setting should be available for any open procedures. Sedation is required, but paralysis is not desired, so that in the event of accidental extubation, the child can make breathing efforts. Also, spontaneous ventilation is preferred because of improved airway clearance of secretions and decreased muscle weakness that can develop from not breathing for 7 to 10 days.

Humidification and chest physiotherapy are helpful. Racemic epinephrine may be used to treat postextubation edema. Steroids are judiciously avoided in patients with new cartilage grafts, as steroids may inhibit mucosalization and compromise neovascularity. Only one dose is given the morning of extubation.

Antireflux medications are typically employed. Prophylactic postoperative antibiotics are typically given. Management by a skilled pediatric intensivist is required, to reduce potential morbidities.

These children require long-term follow-up. Depending on the procedure employed and the patient's symptoms, serial bronchoscopy may be indicated.

8.8 Pierre Robin's Sequence

◆ Key Features

- Pierre Robin's sequence requires the presence of micrognathia, glossoptosis, and usually a cleft palate (frequently U-shaped).
- Infants present with airway obstruction, because the tongue falls into the pharyngeal airway, and feeding difficulties.
- Hearing loss is frequent as a result of otitis media (OM) with effusion (OME; 90%), middle ear anomalies (60%), and inner ear anomalies (40%).

Described first in 1891 by Lannelongue and Ménard, then further by Pierre Robin in 1923, the sequence requires the presence of micrognathia and glossoptosis. Most (90%) also have a cleft palate. Neonates have feeding difficulties. They have upper airway obstruction and are usually difficult to intubate. These children have a high incidence (up to 80%) of other systemic anomalies.

◆ Epidemiology

Incidence is 1 in 8,500 births. Up to 80% are syndromic, most commonly Stickler's syndrome (autosomal dominant; 1 per 10,000 incidence in the United States; flat midface, cleft palate, retinal detachment, cataracts, arthropathy) and velocardiofacial syndrome (autosomal dominant; cleft palate, cardiac anomalies, almond-shaped palpebral fissures, tubular nose, small mouth, learning disabilities). Some cases have autosomal recessive or X-linked inheritance.

◆ Clinical

Signs

- Micrognathia, glossoptosis, cleft palate
- Airway obstruction with desaturations
- Pinna abnormalities, OME may be associated

Symptoms

- Airway obstruction with stertor, cyanosis, respiratory failure
- Prone position may improve airway obstruction in mild cases.
- Failure to thrive

Differential Diagnosis

- Stickler's syndrome
- Velocardiofacial syndrome
- Fetal alcohol syndrome

- Treacher Collins's syndrome
- Nager's syndrome
- Beckwith-Wiedemann's syndrome

All of these syndromes are associated with Pierre Robin's sequence.

◆ Evaluation

The most important matter is to first ensure an adequate airway and feeding. Then one should determine whether there is an associated syndrome. Syndromic patients will generally require more involved interventions.

Physical Exam

A complete head and neck exam will reveal the signs of the sequence. A maxillary–mandibular discrepancy can be measured by placing the infant upright, passively closing the jaw, placing the wooden end of a cotton applicator on the anterior surface of the mandibular alveolar ridge in the midline, then marking where the anterior surface of the maxillary alveolar ridge falls. This measure can be used to monitor growth and surgical outcome.

Pinnae and tympanic membranes should be evaluated. A flexible laryngoscopy is required to rule out concomitant laryngomalacia.

Imaging

Imaging is not typically required to assess the airway obstruction. Imaging may be indicated to evaluate other anomalies coincident with the sequence.

Labs

Continuous monitoring and oxygen saturation monitoring in a neonatal intensive care unit (NICU) environment is required.

Other Tests

All children with Pierre Robin's sequence should have early vision and hearing screening, given the association with Stickler's syndrome. A sleep study may be indicated in mild cases. Bronchoscopy is indicated in severe cases.

Pathology

This sequence is initiated by mandibular hypoplasia in utero. Because of insufficient room in the mouth for the tongue, it remains positioned between the palatal shelves, preventing their normal fusion and leading to a cleft palate.

◆ Treatment Options

Medical

- Positioning: prone position works in about half of patients
- Nasopharyngeal airway
- Oral airway

- Short-term intubation
- Manage reflux

See Table 8.4.

Table 8.4 Strategies for treating airway obstruction in patients with Pierre Robin's sequence.

Prone positioning
Nasopharyngeal airway
Glossopexy, tongue–lip adhesion
Tracheotomy for severe obstruction, synchronous airway lesions, failure of other methods
Mandibular distraction osteogenesis

Surgical

About half of patients require surgery to support their airway.

Temporary Tongue–Lip Adhesion

This involves raising a flap on the inner lower lip and ventral tongue, suturing these together, and sometimes suspending a button placed on the tongue base via a suture that goes around the anterior mandible (this button stays in only for the first week). This brings the tongue forward. All this is taken down by the first year of life; by this time the mandible has usually grown enough that the airway is clear. Fifteen percent will fail and require a tracheotomy.

Mandibular Distraction Osteogenesis

Proximal and distal screws are placed into the mandible bilaterally, then an osteotomy is performed between them. An external device is attached to distract the mandibular segments gradually, typically 1 mm per day. The distractor needs to be left in place for 6 to 8 weeks for consolidation.

Tracheotomy

A tracheotomy is indicated in syndromic children, patients with aspiration, patients with reflux or severe sleep apnea, those with second sites of obstruction below the hypopharynx, and those who fail tongue–lip adhesion and/or distraction osteogenesis.

◆ Complications

- Tongue–lip adhesion: Dehiscence or failure to relieve airway obstruction is treated by either mandibular distraction or tracheotomy.
- Mandibular distraction osteogenesis: Pin tracks may become infected, loosening the pins, which will then require replacement; note also that

tooth buds may be damaged. Temporomandibular joint (TMJ) ankylosis and malocclusion problems may occur.

- Tracheotomy (see **A6 in Appendix A**)

◆ Outcome and Follow-Up

Infants require continuous close monitoring in an ICU setting. Initial feeding requires a nasogastric tube, and if there are no desaturations, trials of oral feeding start. Children may be discharged home once the airway and feeding are stabilized.

Elective repair of the cleft palate is also required, but management of airway obstruction takes priority. Nonsyndromic patients can generally undergo tracheotomy decannulation following palatoplasty, if standard decannulation criteria are met.

Nonsyndromic children, particularly those not requiring surgical intervention, do very well with catch-up growth and are likely to have a normal facial profile by age 5. Syndromic children are more likely to require multimodality treatment. Follow-up needs to continue only until the airway obstruction is resolved.

8.9   Genetics and Syndromes

Congenital anomalies, whether single or multiple, can be induced by environmental and teratogenic insults as well as chromosomal or single-gene defects. This chapter includes only the most common and relevant syndromes with associated craniofacial anomalies. The otolaryngologist may be primarily involved in managing the otolaryngologic manifestations of these syndromes but may also play an important role in the early identification and referral for genetic counseling in children with suspected genetic or syndrome features.

◆ Epidemiology

Major congenital anomalies diagnosed within the first year of life affect ~ 3% of neonates and congenital defects contribute to nearly 20% of infant deaths. Of the defects affecting children with multiple congenital anomalies, 62% are otolaryngologic in nature. In the case of multiple anomalies where the underlying cause has been identified, 84% have an otolaryngologic feature.

◆ Relevant Definitions

Association: Nonrandom occurrence of a pattern of anomalies that are not identified as a sequence or syndrome; for example, CHARGE (*c*oloboma of the eye, *h*eart defects, *a*tresia of the nasal choanae, *r*etardation of growth and/or development, *g*enital and/or urinary abnormalities, and *e*ar abnormalities and deafness) association.

Sequence: Pattern of multiple defects resulting from a single primary malformation or insult—e.g., Pierre Robin's sequence. The fact that a cluster of anomalies is defined as a sequence does not exclude Mendelian inheritance.

Syndrome: Cluster of anomalies in which all features are pathologically related; for example, Down's syndrome, fetal alcohol syndrome.

◆ Relevant Associations, Sequences, and Syndromes

- **Achondroplasia**
  - Inheritance: Autosomal dominant
  - Genetic loci: Spontaneous mutation leading to a defect in fibroblast growth factor receptor-3
  - General: Most common cause of short-limbed dwarfism; advanced paternal age is a risk factor
  - Relevant features: Frontal bossing, midface hypoplasia, obstructive sleep apnea
  - Associated features: Shortened limbs, long narrow trunk, lumbar lordosis, limited elbow extension, genu varum, compression of craniovertebral junction (can lead to central apnea and sudden death), hypotonia

- **Branchio-oculo-facial (BOF) syndrome**
  - Inheritance: Autosomal dominant
  - Genetic loci: Not yet identified
  - Relevant features: Branchial cleft sinuses, lacrimal duct obstruction, conductive hearing loss, pseudocleft of upper lip, auricular malformations (low-set, malformed)
  - Associated features: Low birth weight, growth and developmental delay, premature aging

- **Catel-Manzke's syndrome**
  - Inheritance: X-linked (speculated)
  - Genetic loci: Not yet identified
  - Relevant features: Cleft palate, micrognathia, auricular malformations
  - Associated features: Cardiac septal defect, growth delay, hyperphalangy (increased number of phalanges) of index finger

- **CHARGE association**
  - Inheritance: Sporadic
  - Genetic locus: 8q12.1, 7q21.1
  - General: Coloboma iris, heart defects, choanal atresia, retarded growth, genital hypoplasia, ear abnormalities
  - Additional relevant features: Auricular anomalies (prominent, folded ears, absent helix) conductive/sensorineural hearing loss, micrognathia, midface hypoplasia, dysphagia, short neck
  - Additional associated features: Short stature, ptosis, microphthalmos, omphalocele, cryptorchism, syndactyly, renal hypoplasia, delayed skeletal maturation, pituitary defects, hypocalcemia

- **Costello's syndrome**
  - Inheritance: Autosomal dominant and/or gonadal mosaicism
  - Genetic loci: *HRAS* or *KRAS* gene mutation on chromosome 11p15.5
  - Relevant features: Auricular malformations (low-set, thick lobes), oral, nasal, and anal papillomas
  - Head and neck features: Macrocephaly, epicanthic folds, coarse facial features, strabismus, thick lips, depressed nasal bridge, curly hair
  - Associated features: growth and developmental delay; hypertrophic cardiomyopathy; thin, deep-set nails; skin hyperpigmentation; deep plantar/palmar creases; short neck; tight Achilles tendons
- **Cri du chat syndrome**
  - Inheritance: De novo mutations most common, can result from unbalanced translocation/recombination in a parent (12%)
  - Genetic loci: Partial and variable deletion of short arm of chromosome 5
  - Relevant features: Narrowed endolarynx (diamond-shaped), persistent interarytenoid cleft, microcephaly, round face, hypertelorism, micrognathia, epicanthal folds, low-set ears
  - Associated features: Hypotonia, severe psychomotor and developmental delay
- **Down's syndrome**
  - Inheritance: Sporadic
  - Genetic loci: Trisomy 21
  - General: Most common genetic disorder associated with mental retardation and developmental delay; advanced maternal age risk factor (> 35 years); 1:800 live births
  - Relevant features: Microcephaly, midface retrusion, upslanting palpebral fissures, epicanthal folds, macroglossia, frequent OM with effusion, sleep apnea, auricular anomalies (small, low-set, overfolding of upper helices), middle and inner ear anomalies
  - Associated features: Congenital cardiac defects (40%), hypotonia, joint laxity, and underdeveloped cervical vertebra (risk of atlantoaxial subluxation/dislocation), flat occiput, three fontanels, excess nuchal skin, short stature, clinodactyly 5th digit, single palmar crease
- **Ectrodactyly–ectodermal dysplasia–clefting (EEC) syndrome**
  - Inheritance: Autosomal dominant (variable expression)
  - Genetic loci: 7q11.2-q21.3
  - Relevant features: Cleft lip and/or cleft palate; blue irides; lacrimal duct defects; blepharophimosis; partial anodontia; light, spare, thin, wiry hair
  - Associated features: Hyperkeratosis, hypotrichosis, hypohidrosis, hypoplastic nipples, anomalies of the extremities (syndactyly, ectrodactyly), genitourinary defects
- **Fragile X syndrome**
  - Inheritance: X-linked
  - Genetic loci: Xq27.3

- General: Second most common cause of genetic developmental delay
- Relevant features: Prominent ears, large jaw, long face, high-pitched speech
- Associated features: Mitral valve prolapse, behavioral disturbance, macroorchidism, joint hypermobility, pes planus

- **Fraser's (cryptophthalmos) syndrome**
  - Inheritance: Autosomal recessive
  - Genetic loci: *FRAS1* or *FREM2* gene 13q13.3, 4q21
  - Relevant features: Ear anomalies (aural atresia, cupped ears); laryngeal stenosis/atresia; hypoplastic, notched nares; bilateral cryptophthalmos; eyebrow anomalies
  - Associated features: Developmental delay (50%), partial cutaneous syndactyly, genital anomalies, renal hypoplasia/agenesis

- **Larsen's syndrome**
  - Inheritance: Autosomal dominant (known), possible recessive form speculated
  - Genetic loci: 3p21.1–p14.1
  - Relevant features: Cleft palate, flat facies, depressed nasal bridge, hypertelorism, prominent frontal boss
  - Associated features: Congenital joint dislocation; long, nontapering fingers with short fingernails; spinal deformities

- **Marshall's syndrome**
  - Inheritance: Autosomal dominant
  - Genetic loci: 1q21
  - Relevant features: Sensorineural hearing loss; short nose with flat nasal bridge and midface; anteverted nares; large eyes; prominent, protruding upper incisors
  - Associated features: Cataracts, myopia, short stature, calvarial thickening, spondyloepiphyseal abnormalities

- **Miller's syndrome (postaxial acrofacial dysostosis)**
  - Inheritance: Autosomal recessive
  - Genetic loci: Not yet identified
  - General: Facial features similar to Treacher Collins's syndrome with limb anomalies
  - Relevant features: Cleft lip and/or cleft palate; malar hypoplasia and/or vertical bony cleft; micrognathia; hypoplastic cup-shaped ears; down-slanting palpebral fissures, coloboma; ectropion
  - Associated features: Absence of fifth digit on all limbs, accessory nipples

- **Möbius's syndrome**
  - Inheritance: Sporadic
  - Genetic loci: 13q12.2–q13
  - Relevant features: Congenital cranial nerve VI and VII palsy, orofacial dysmorphism
  - Associated features: Limb malformations, developmental delay

- **Mucopolysaccharidoses**
  - General: Storage diseases secondary to lysosomal enzyme deficiencies
  - Examples: Hunter's, Hurler's, Morquio's, Sanfilippos, etc., syndromes
  - Relevant features: OME, sensorineural hearing loss, obstructive sleep apnea
  - Associated features: Developmental delay, short stature
- **Nager's syndrome (Nager acrofacial dysostoses)**
  - Inheritance: Autosomal dominant
  - Genetic loci: 9q32
  - General: Facial features similar to Treacher Collins with limb anomalies or deficiencies
  - Relevant features: Aural atresia, cleft palate, auricular malformations (low-set, rotated posteriorly), malar hypoplasia, high nasal bridge, down-slanting palpebral fissures, absence of lower eyelashes
  - Associated features: Hypoplasia of radial limbs; development and cognition normal
- **Noonan's syndrome**
  - Inheritance: Autosomal dominant
  - Genetic loci: 12q24
  - Relevant features: Neck webbing, auricular anomalies (low-set), down-slanting palpebral fissures, ptosis, hypertelorism
  - Associated features: Low posterior hairline, short stature, pectus excavatum, pulmonic stenosis, bleeding diathesis
- **Opitz's G syndrome (BBB syndrome)**
  - Inheritance: X-linked recessive and autosomal dominant
  - Genetic loci: 22q11
  - General: Midline defects
  - Relevant features: Cleft lip and/or cleft palate, laryngeal clefting, auricular anomalies (ears rotated posteriorly), micrognathia, flattened nasal bridge, anteverted nostrils, hypertelorism
  - Associated features: Developmental delay, hypospadias, cryptorchidism, hernias
- **Oro-facial-digital syndrome**
  - Inheritance
    - Type I: X-linked dominant, lethal in males
    - Type II: Autosomal recessive (speculated)
  - Genetic loci
    - Type I: Xp22.2–p22.3 CXORF5 gene
    - Type II: Not yet identified
  - Relevant features
    - Type I: Median cleft lip, cleft palate, bifid tongue, oral frenula and clefts, hypoplastic nasal alae, lateral displacement of inner canthi

- Type II: Midline partial cleft palate, cleft tongue, low nasal bridge, broad nasal tip, conductive hearing loss, lateral displacement of inner canthi
  - Associated features
    - Type I: Developmental delay (variable), asymmetric digits, polycystic kidney disease
    - Type II: Partial reduplication of the hallux and 1st metatarsal, bilateral polydactyly of the hands and polysyndactyly of the feet
- **Oto-palatal-digital syndrome**
  - Inheritance
    - Type I: X-linked (intermediate expression in female carriers)
    - Type II: X-linked (mild expression in female carriers)
  - Genetic loci
    - Type I: Xq28
    - Type II: Xq28
  - Relevant features
    - Type I: Moderate conductive deafness, cleft palate, frontal and occipital bossing, thickened frontal bone and skull base, hypertelorism, small mouth and nose
    - Type II: Conductive hearing loss, cleft palate, frontal bossing, auricular anomalies (low set, malformed), flat nasal bridge, micrognathia, small mouth, down-slanting palpebral fissures
  - Associated features
    - Type I: Broad distal digits with short nails, developmental delay, small stature and trunk, pectus excavatum
    - Type II: Late closure of fontanels, microcephaly, flexed overlapping finger, short broad thumbs and hallux, bowing of radius, ulna, femur and tibia, flattened vertebral bodies
- **Pierre Robin's sequence**
  - Genetic loci: 2q32.3–q33.2 (in some cases)
  - General: Up to 80% of children with Pierre Robin's sequence are also affected by a named syndrome (most commonly Stickler's).
  - Relevant features: Triad = glossoptosis, micrognathia, cleft palate; airway and feeding difficulty
  - Associated features: Developmental delay, hypospadias, cryptorchidism, hernias
  - For further information on Pierre Robin's sequence, see **Chapter 6.8**.
- **VATER association**
  - Inheritance: Sporadic
  - Genetic loci: No chromosomal anomaly identified
  - Relevant features: Malformation of the vertebrae, anus, trachea, esophagus, radial and renal structures
  - VACTERL association: As above, plus cardiac and limb anomalies

- **Velocardiofacial syndrome (Shprintzen's syndrome, 22q11 deletion syndrome)**
  - Inheritance: Autosomal dominant
  - Genetic loci: 22q11 deletion
  - General: 10% associated with DiGeorge's syndrome (hypocalcemia, thymic aplasia)
  - Relevant features: Velopharyngeal incompetence, high arched/cleft palate (overt or submucous), conductive hearing loss, square nasal root, prominent nasal dorsum, deficiency of nasal alae, retrognathia, medial displacement of carotid artery (25%)
  - Associated features: Mild developmental delay, short stature, cardiac defects (85%), increased risk of psychiatric disorders, slender hands/fingers
- **Van der Woude's syndrome**
  - Inheritance: Autosomal dominant
  - Genetic loci: 1q32 (incomplete penetrance)
  - Relevant features: cleft lip and/or cleft palate, lower lip pits, absent central/lateral incisors, canines, bicuspids
  - Associated features: Developmental delay, hypospadias, cryptorchidism, hernias

The following syndromes (of which hearing loss is a primary feature) are covered in **Chapter 8.12**:

- Alport's syndrome
- Apert's syndrome
- Branchio-oto-renal syndrome
- Connexin-26 deafness
- Crouzon's syndrome
- Goldenhar's syndrome
- Jervell and Lange-Nielsen's syndrome
- Neurofibromatosis (NF1 and NF2)
- Norrie's syndrome
- Osteogenesis imperfecta
- Oto-palato-digital syndrome
- Pendred's syndrome
- Stickler's syndrome
- Treacher Collins's syndrome
- Usher's syndrome
- Wildervanck's syndrome
- Waardenburg's syndrome
- X-linked hearing loss

◆ Evaluation

History

- Three-generation family history
- Parental consanguinity
- Parental ethnicity
- Maternal, paternal age
- Teratogen exposure
- Prior pregnancies, miscarriages, still births
- Illness during pregnancy

Physical Exam

A complete head and neck exam with a focus on dysmorphologic examination is needed. A general examination should be undertaken to identify syndromic features (see the foregoing for description of characteristic syndromic features).

Imaging

Specific imaging recommendations are based on associated features of specific syndromes. Computed tomography (CT) or magnetic resonance imaging (MRI) of the brain will often be undertaken.

Labs

- Karyotyping
- DNA analysis
- Molecular genetic testing
- Fluorescence in situ hybridization (FISH) evaluation
- Targeted studies for metabolic disorders

Other Tests

None are routinely done.

◆ Treatment Options

- Genetic counseling for patient and family
- Referral to medical and surgical specialists based on specific features of syndrome
- Developmental assessment

8.10 Diseases of the Adenoids and Palatine Tonsils

8.10.1 Adenotonsillitis

◆ Key Features

- Adenotonsillitis is most commonly viral in etiology.
- Bacterial etiology is similar to acute otitis media (OM):
  - Group A β-hemolytic *Streptococcus pneumoniae*
  - *Moraxella catarrhalis*
  - *Haemophilus influenzae*
- Chronic infection is typically polymicrobial.
- There is growing evidence for the role of biofilm.

Acute adenotonsillitis most commonly presents in children 5 to 10 years of age and young adults 15 to 25 years of age. The primary consideration in its accurate diagnosis and treatment is prevention of secondary complications particularly associated with group A β-hemolytic *Streptococcus pneumoniae*, including rheumatic fever and poststreptococcal glomerulonephritis. Suppurative complications avoided by early and appropriate management include peritonsillar abscess and deep neck space infection.

◆ Epidemiology

The average incidence of all acute upper respiratory infections is five to seven per child per year. It is estimated that children have one streptococcal infection every 4 to 5 years. Group A *Streptococcus* is isolated in 30.0 to 36.8% of children with pharyngitis, and asymptomatic carriage of group A *Streptococcus* is ~ 10.9% for children aged 14 or younger.

◆ Clinical

Signs

- Erythremic, exudative palatine tonsils
- Tonsilloliths
- Trismus
- Cervical adenopathy
- Palatal petechiae (infectious mononucleosis)

Symptoms

- Halitosis
- Sore throat
- Odynophagia

- Purulent rhinorrhea
- Postnasal drip
- Nasal obstruction
- Fever

Differential Diagnosis

- Adenotonsillar hypertrophy
- Acute pharyngitis (bacterial or viral)
- Peritonsillar abscess
- Infectious mononucleosis
- Lymphoma, leukemia, or other neoplasm (unilateral/asymmetric tonsillar enlargement)

◆ Evaluation

Physical Exam

In the head and neck exam, focus on examination of the oral cavity, inspection of palatine tonsils looking for enlargement, erythema, peritonsillar cellulitis, abscess, and exudates. Palpation of the neck is performed to assess for cervical adenopathy.

Imaging

Contrast-enhanced computed tomography (CT) if concerned about retropharyngeal or deep neck space infection.

Labs

Complete blood count (CBC) with differential; monospot, if clinically indicated.

Other Tests

Do a throat swab for culture and sensitivity and latex agglutination tests for group A β-hemolytic *Streptococcus.*

◆ Treatment Options

Medical

Analgesics and antipyretics are prescribed.

Relevant Pharmacology

Antibiotic therapies include:

- **Amoxicillin:** Penicillin-based β-lactam antibiotic with bactericidal action due to interference with bacterial cell wall synthesis
  - 45 mg/kg per day divided every 8 hours for 7 to 10 days
- **Amoxicillin + Clavulanate:** Clavulanate has itself little antibacterial action, but it is a potent β-lactamase inhibitor, protecting the penicillin-based antibacterial action.

o 45 mg/kg per day (amoxicillin component) divided every 12 hours for 7 to 10 days

- **Azithromycin:** Macrolide, semisynthetic derivative of erythromycin. Bactericidal action is through inhibition of protein synthesis via binding to the 50S ribosomal RNA subunit.
  o 10 mg/kg for 1 dose, then 5 mg/kg per day for 5 days
- **Cefuroxime axetil:** Second-generation cephalosporins' bactericidal action is due to the inhibition of peptidoglycan synthesis interfering with cell wall synthesis, similar to penicillin's.
  o 30 mg/kg per day divided every 12 hours for 7 to 10 days

Surgical

Surgery entails a delayed tonsillectomy and/or adenoidectomy for recurrent disease (**Table 8.5**). Currently, it is rare to perform a tonsillectomy in the setting of an acute infection (quinsy tonsillectomy). The presence of a peritonsillar abscess requires acute incision and drainage; removal of the tonsil to allow drainage is rarely needed.

Table 8.5   Adenotonsillectomy indications and contraindications

Absolute indications • Complication of sleep apnea secondary to tonsillar hypertrophy (i.e., cor pulmonale) • Suspected tonsil malignancy • Febrile convulsions secondary to tonsillitis • Tonsillar hemorrhage • Severe failure to thrive with enlarged tonsils
Relative indications • Obstructive sleep apnea • Recurrent acute tonsillitis • 5–7/yr for 1 yr • 5/yr for 2 yr • 3/yr for 3 yr • > 2 weeks of school missed over 1 yr • Peritonsillar abscess, persistent or recurrent • Chronic tonsillitis (throat pain, halitosis, cervical adenitis) • Severe odynophagia • Tonsillolithiasis (if severe, persistent) • Acquired dental or orofacial abnormalities • Chronic carrier of *Streptococcus* • Recurrent/chronic otitis media (adenoidectomy alone)
Contraindications • Cleft palate* • Velopharyngeal insufficiency* • Bleeding diathesis (unless correctible medically; e.g., von Willebrand patients can undergo surgery with appropriate treatment perioperatively)

*Relative contraindication for tonsillectomy, absolute contraindication for adenoidectomy (although partial adenoidectomy may be considered).

◆ Complications

See **Chapter 8.10.2** for a detailed discussion of complications. Primary tonsillar hemorrhage often requires operative management (0.5 to 2.2 per 100). Secondary (delayed) tonsillar hemorrhage is often managed conservatively with close observation (0.1 to 3 per 100).

◆ Outcome and Follow-Up

In the absence of complications in an otherwise healthy child, adenotonsillectomy is a same-day procedure with analgesia and possibly postoperative antibiotics depending on the technique and the surgeon's preference. Hospital admission criteria are also discussed in **Chapter 8.10.2**. Follow-up is 3 to 6 weeks after tonsillectomy and adenoidectomy.

8.10.2 Adenotonsillar Hypertrophy

◆ Key Features

- Adenoids and palatine tonsils are a common source of upper airway obstruction in childhood.
- Peak size is achieved by ~ 5 years of age.
- Airway compromise presents as obstructive sleep apnea (OSA).

Adenotonsillar hypertrophy leads to a spectrum of airway obstruction in children and is a common indication for surgery in the pediatric age group. Adenoids and palatine tonsils enlarge over the first to fifth years of life. Progressive involution occurs by 12 to 18 years of age, though the course is highly variable and is influenced by both allergy and the frequency of recurrent tonsillar and upper respiratory tract infections.

◆ Epidemiology

Adenotonsillar hypertrophy is the most common cause of sleep-related upper airway obstruction in children. Forty percent of children snore; the incidence of true obstructive apnea is estimated to be 3%.

◆ Clinical

Signs

- Mouth open posture
- Failure to thrive and feeding difficulties
- Hyponasal speech
- Adenoid facies (high arched palate, flattened midface, "allergic shiners," mouth-open posture)

- Behavioral disturbances
- Daytime somnolence

Symptoms

- Snoring and/or apneic pauses
- Restless sleep
- Choking or gagging noises while asleep
- Hyperactivity, attention deficit symptoms
- Enuresis
- Nasal obstruction

Differential Diagnosis

- Acute or chronic tonsillitis, adenoiditis (bacterial or viral)
- Acute pharyngitis (bacterial or viral)
- Peritonsillar abscess
- Infectious mononucleosis
- Lymphoma
- Other causes of upper airway obstruction include nasal polyposis, deviated nasal septum, rhinitis, and sinusitis (infectious, allergic, or nonallergic).

◆ Evaluation

History

History usually indicates irregular snoring with gasping or witnessed pauses and daytime somnolence. A history of behavior problems, attention deficit–hyperactivity disorder, and enuresis should be elicited. Any previous sleep studies should be reviewed. It is important to ask for any family history of known bleeding disorders, or a patient or family history of abnormal bruising or bleeding.

Physical Exam

Complete head and neck exam with focus on:

1. Assessment of the status of the middle ear (there is an increased incidence of acute OM and OME with adenoid hypertrophy)
2. Examination of the oral cavity, inspection, and grading of palatine tonsils: grade 1 (tonsils within the tonsillar pillars), grade 2 (< 50% obstruction), grade 3 (> 50% obstruction), grade 4 (where tonsils abut in the midline)
3. Exclusion of obvious craniofacial malformation or syndromic features; assess for cleft palate

Consider the direct examination of adenoid size using small flexible fiberoptic scope, especially in the cooperative child.

Imaging

Consider a lateral neck plain film to assess the size of the adenoid pad.

Labs

A complete blood count (CBC) should be done, with partial thromboplastin time (PTT) and prothrombin time/international normalized ratio (PT/INR) tests preoperatively if there is any family history or suspicion for potential coagulopathy. A platelet function test (PFA-100 analyzer) is a rapid inexpensive screen for platelet dysfunction, although it is nonspecific. A positive test should prompt von Willebrand studies and a referral to hematology.

Other Tests

Nasal endoscopy should be performed to assess the degree of nasopharyngeal obstruction. Rhinomanometry is rarely used to assess the degree of nasal obstruction.

An otherwise generally healthy child with parents who provide a good description of irregular snoring with gasping, pausing, or choking noises, and an exam that reveals obvious obstructive hypertrophy, does *not* need a polysomnography; proceed with an adenotonsillectomy. If the child has an unconvincing exam or the parents cannot provide a good history, polysomnography is helpful. If the child has other comorbidities, and *especially* if the child has neurologic problems, polysomnography is important, as central rather than obstructive apnea may be occurring. Central apnea will not be improved by an adenotonsillectomy.

Pathology

Hyperplasia of the lymphoid tissue of the adenoids and tonsils is found.

◆ Treatment Options

Medical

- Watchful waiting
- Topical nasal steroids
- Antibiotics may shrink tonsils occasionally
- Continuous positive airway pressure (CPAP) for OSA (see **Chapter 1.3**)

Surgical

The surgical procedures employed include adenoidectomy, tonsillectomy, and adenotonsillectomy. For instrumentation, most surgeons currently use the electrocautery. Also, some surgeons perform cold dissection, use a bipolar radiofrequency ablation device (coblation), or use a microdébrider for so-called intracapsular or subtotal tonsillectomy. Other devices have been introduced and marketed but are less widely used.

◆ Complications

Bleeding

The most common significant complication is postoperative hemorrhage, which occurs at a rate of 2 to 3%. The patient/family must understand risk of delayed bleeding and the need to present to the emergency department promptly if there is any bleeding. Children in rural areas should not be allowed to be more than 30 minutes from a hospital for 2 weeks.

Bleeding may be classified as intraoperative, primary (occurring within the first 24 hours), or secondary (occurring between 24 hours and 10 days). Primary tonsillar hemorrhage (0.5–2.2 per 100) often requires operative management. This is due either to a failure to control a vessel that was likely in spasm or to an unrecognized clotting problem, typically platelet dysfunction.

Secondary (after first 24 hours) tonsillar hemorrhage (0.1–3 per 100) is often managed conservatively with close observation. This is most common at ~ 1 week postoperatively.

Recurrent secondary hemorrhage should prompt a thorough hematologic evaluation and mandates admission with close observation based on concern for a possible "sentinel" bleed (**Table 8.6**).

Table 8.6   Management options for posttonsillectomy bleeding

If active bleeding, go directly to the operating room for definitive control.
If inactive or scant bleeding: Admission with 24-hr observation. If rebleed, go to operating room. If no bleeding for 24 hr, discharge.
All patients: Check hemoglobin, hematocrit, PT, PTT. Establish intravenous access, hydrate.
Possible measures to control mild/scant bleeding in emergency department: silver nitrate or other chemical cautery

Abbreviations: PT, prothrombin time; PTT, partial thromboplastin time.

Other Complications

In some studies respiratory compromise is the most frequent complication occurring in children after tonsillectomy. The risk of respiratory complications is 4.9 times higher in those who have obstructive sleep apnea than in children who do not. Early postoperative airway obstruction may require humidified oxygen, steroids, and reintubation. Chronically obstructed patients are at risk of postoperative pulmonary edema, diagnosed with physical exam and chest radiography. This may require furosemide, humidified oxygen, chest physiotherapy, positive end expiratory pressure ventilation, and reintubation.

Postoperative dehydration may require readmission. Treat with intravenous (IV) hydration, antiemetics, analgesia as needed, and parental education.

Nasal reflux is commonly mild and resolves; if severe or persistent, this may be difficult to correct. Speech therapy can be helpful.

Nasopharyngeal stenosis/scarring is uncommon and extremely difficult to correct. Prevention is best.

Airway fire: This should be extremely rare. One should check for cuff leak before operating; should not leak below 20. Communicate with the anesthesiologist, and be sure F_{IO_2} is kept less than 40%. If there is a fire, then immediately extubate, turn off all the oxygen, and reintubate.

◆ Outcome and Follow-Up

Close postoperative monitoring in children with OSA, given the risk of ongoing or worsening apnea in the immediate postoperative period. Following tonsillectomy, children with a positive preoperative sleep study and/or any children 3 years or younger are typically observed overnight with continuous pulse oximetry, although there is a lack of consensus on this issue.

Other measures: Liquid/soft diet for 2 weeks postoperative. Pain management is important to enable the patient to maintain adequate hydration. Although there is no consensus, a recommended combination is acetaminophen liquid up to 15 mg/kg/ dose three or four times daily, using plain oxycodone liquid 0.1 mg/kg/dose (5 mg maximum) every 4 hours as needed for breakthrough pain. Separating the acetaminophen and the opioid enables the patient to minimize opioid use in many cases. Nonsteroidal anti-inflammatory drugs (NSAIDs) are avoided out of concern for platelet inhibition, although some studies suggest this does not increase bleeding risk. Oral liquid antibiotic is used for 1 week postoperatively, usually amoxicillin if the patient is nonallergic. Intraoperatively, a single dose of dexamethasone 0.5 mg/kg IV is helpful to reduce postoperative pain and swelling; the dose is typically 4 to 12 mg.

Continued routine follow-up if conservative treatment approach adopted. Repeat sleep study may be considered 3 to 6 months postoperatively if symptoms persist. Follow-up is scheduled 3 to 6 weeks after adenotonsillectomy.

Adenotonsillectomy achieves a 90% success rate for childhood sleep-disordered breathing. Of all tonsillectomies and adenoidectomies performed in the United States each year, 75% are performed to treat sleep-disordered breathing.

8.11 Congenital Nasal Obstruction

◆ Key Features

- Congenital nasal obstruction can range in severity from a mild irritant to a life-threatening condition with potentially devastating consequences in the neonate.
- The most common cause of congenital nasal obstruction is simple inflammation of the nasal mucosa, which may be managed using conservative therapies.
- Treatments for congenital nasal obstruction include observation, medications, and surgical interventions.

Congenital nasal obstruction is an uncommon yet important clinical entity to recognize, given the fact that newborns are obligate nasal breathers for the first several months of life. As a result, persistent nasal obstruction requires timely evaluation such that the appropriate medical and/or surgical therapies can be promptly initiated.

◆ Clinical

Signs and Symptoms

Signs include apnea, collapse of lateral nasal wall, cyclical cyanosis, a mass within the nose, mucous crusting, mucosal edema, nasal flaring, poor weight gain, respiratory distress, retractions, septal deviation, and/or stertor.

The timing, onset, and laterality of symptoms can provide clues to the etiology of the observed nasal obstruction. Symptoms include aerophagia, difficulty sleeping, dyspnea, epiphora, failure to thrive, feeding difficulties, grunting, hyponasal cry, rhinorrhea, and snoring.

Differential Diagnosis

- Congenital
  - Choanal atresia (see **Chapter 8.18**)
  - Piriform recess stenosis
  - Midnasal stenosis
  - Midfacial hypoplasia
  - Dacryocystocele
- Inflammatory
  - Gastroesophageal reflux
  - Neonatal rhinitis
  - Conchal hypertrophy
- Infectious
  - Congenital sexually transmitted diseases
    - Chlamydia
    - Gonorrhea
    - Syphilis
- Maternal
  - Estrogenic stimuli
- Metabolic
  - Hypothyroidism
- Midline nasal masses (see **Chapter 8.16**)
  - Encephalocele
  - Glioma
  - Nasal dermoid
  - Thornwaldt cyst
- Neoplasms
  - Teratoma
  - Hamartoma

- o Hemangioma (see **Chapter 8.14**)
- o Lipoma
- o Lymphangioma (see **Chapter 8.14**)
- o Lymphoma
- o Neurofibroma
- o Rhabdomyosarcoma
- Traumatic
  - o Septal deviation

◆ Evaluation

Physical Exam

- Anterior rhinoscopy
- Flexible nasopharyngoscopy
- Indirect mirror

Syndromes and Associations

Several etiologies of nasal obstruction may present with concurrent developmental abnormalities that may require further assessment, including a genetic evaluation. Congenital nasal obstruction has been described secondary to abnormal embryologic development in association with Crouzon's, Pfeiffer's, Apert's, Treacher Collins's, Down's, and fetal alcohol syndromes and CHARGE association (see **Chapter 8.9**). Neonates may present with respiratory difficulties due to numerous pathophysiological mechanisms; with regards to nasal obstruction, hypoplasia of the maxilla and nasal atresia are the primary contributory factors. As a result, many infants with craniofacial anomalies require placement of a tracheostomy at some point in their life.

Imaging

Computed tomography (CT) will provide excellent characterization and definition of the bony and cartilaginous structures of the nose. If there are concerns that the nasal mass may be contiguous with the cerebrum, then magnetic resonance imaging (MRI) is also indicated to determine the extent of intracranial involvement.

Pathology

Dacryocystocele is caused by lacrimal duct imperforation at the level of the valve of Hasner (lacrimal fold); this promotes a proximal valvelike obstruction at the junction of the lacrimal sac and common canaliculus. This presents as facial swelling and epiphora with either a bluish cystic mass at the level of the medial canthus or an intranasal bulge below the inferior concha.

Midnasal stenosis is due to bony overgrowth midway through the intranasal cavity. This presents as a narrowed midnasal passage with loss of visualization of the middle concha.

Neonatal rhinitis is an idiopathic disorder multifactorial in etiology (viral, inflammatory, vascular, drug-related, trauma, etc.). This presents as bilateral congestive nasal mucosa and mucus secretion with conserved nasal permeability.

Piriform recess stenosis is caused by bilateral bony overgrowth of the medial nasal processes of the maxilla. This presents as a narrowed anterior nasal passage with bilateral medial bony thickening.

Septal deviation is often caused by facial trauma, typically observed in infants born via spontaneous vaginal delivery, resulting from direct pressure across the maxilla during parturition. This presents as a deviated nasal tip with an angulated columella and a flattened, asymmetric nasal ala.

Conchal hypertrophy can be caused by either bony or mucosal overgrowth secondary to mucosal inflammation, leading to unequal airflow through the nasal passages. This presents as nasal mucosal edema, crusting, and septal deviation.

◆ Treatment Options

Therapies for congenital nasal obstruction include observation, medical, and surgical interventions. In general, severe obstruction may necessitate endotracheal intubation or tracheostomy until further surgical intervention can be performed depending on the infant's overall clinical condition and associated anomalies.

Medical

Nasal stenosis, including piriform recess and midnasal stenosis, usually responds to conservative management, including gentle suctioning and humidification with saline drops, topical steroids (dexamethasone ophthalmic solution, beclomethasone, or fluticasone), and occasional topical decongestants (oxymetazoline 0.025%). Conservative management of dacryocystoceles includes warm compresses, gentle massage, and nasal decongestants. Finally, management of neonatal rhinitis and conchal hypertrophy consists of nasal decongestants, nasal irrigations, and topical steroids.

Surgical

Surgical intervention is usually indicated in infants with respiratory distress unresponsive to conservative measures, or failure to thrive. Symptomatic dacryocystoceles can be treated with endoscopic resection or marsupialization with possible probing of the duct and dacryocystorhinostomy with stenting in order to maintain patency. For midnasal stenosis, surgical dilation can be considered in patients with respiratory failure. Similarly, in severe cases of piriform recess stenosis, a surgical approach utilizing a sublabial incision to access the inferolateral piriform recess and opening it with a diamond bur will widen the bony nasal inlet. For conchal hypertrophy not amenable to medical therapies, intramural cautery or submucosal resection can be employed. Conversely, formal surgical repair for septal deviation should not be necessary in infancy because of the relative plasticity of the nasal subunits. This is usually deferred to late childhood.

◆ Complications

Surgical complications include bleeding, infection, midface hypoplasia, nasolacrimal duct injury, restenosis, and tooth bud dysgenesis.

◆ Postoperative Care

Topical nasal saline drops or irrigations twice a day should be performed to promote postprocedure healing. Gentle suctioning will remove any intranasal crusts or mucus that impede nasal airflow. Humidification is helpful in maintaining the health and integrity of the nasal mucosa.

◆ Outcome and Follow-Up

Patients should be monitored at regular intervals to assess for interim changes, response to medical and/or surgical therapies, and resolution of symptoms.

8.12 Pediatric Hearing Loss

◆ Key Features

- Age at identification has significantly decreased since the advent of newborn hearing screening.
- Early identification and treatment of hearing loss is essential to obtain an optimal outcome.
- Connexin-26–related deafness is the most common cause of inherited hearing loss.
- Acquired hearing loss often occurs within the antenatal period.
- Perinatal history is the key to identifying risk factors for both congenital and acquired hearing loss.

The onset of hearing loss in children regardless of etiology often occurs prior to the development of language. The disorders causing both congenital and acquired hearing loss range from the simple and common to the rare and complex. The list of potential diagnoses in this chapter is not exhaustive; additional syndromes with hearing loss as a minor characteristic can be found in **Chapter 8.9**. For the purpose of this chapter, we will examine hearing loss using the structure seen in **Fig. 8.3**, with the caveat that some diagnoses may fall under more than one category.

◆ Epidemiology

Hearing loss is the most common congenital sensory deficit, with an estimated incidence of 2 per 1,000 children. Likewise, acquired loss is

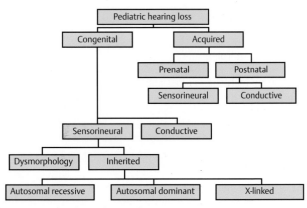

Fig. 8.3 Types of pediatric hearing loss.

exceedingly common, with most children experiencing at a minimum a transient conductive hearing loss (CHL) due to chronic serous otitis. An estimated 50% of childhood sensorineural hearing loss (SNHL) is due to genetic factors, with this proportion increasing with the ongoing detection of new mutations. Genetic causes may eventually account for a large proportion of the hearing loss currently labeled as unknown in etiology. For cases of congenital hereditary hearing loss, about two-thirds are nonsyndromic. In the setting of genetic-related deafness, most cases (70–80%) are autosomal recessive, roughly 20% are autosomal dominant, and the remainder are due to X-linked chromosomal or mitochondrial anomalies. About 50% of the cases of congenital SNHL are considered nonhereditary (i.e., acquired), and most of these are due to TORCHES (*to*xoplasmosis, *r*ubella, *c*ytomegalovirus, *h*erpes simplex *e*ncephalitis, and oto*s*yphilis) infections, sepsis, or severe prematurity.

◆ Clinical

Signs

- Speech delay or regression of speech
- Vestibular dysfunction
- Delays in ambulation
- Gait disturbances
- Otorrhea

Symptoms

- Hearing loss (may be progressive or fluctuating)
- Tinnitus
- Vertigo
- Otalgia
- Aural fullness

◆ Congenital Sensorineural Hearing Loss

Dysmorphologies

Most cochlear dysmorphologies are membranous in nature (80–90%) and not identifiable on computed tomography (CT); the remainder have a discernible bony anomaly that is identifiable on CT imaging.

Mondini Deformity
- Incomplete partition of cochlea
- Autosomal dominant
- Unilateral or bilateral hearing loss may be progressive or fluctuating (interspersed with normal hearing).
- CT: Cystic dilation of cochlea with absence of modiolus, enlarged vestibular aqueduct, semicircular canal anomalies
- Associated with Pendred's, Waardenburg's, and Treacher Collins's syndromes and branchio-oto-renal syndrome (described subsequently)

Michel Aplasia
- Autosomal dominant
- Anacusis
- CT: Absent cochlea and labyrinth, hypoplasia of petrous pyramid

Alexander Deafness
- Autosomal recessive or sporadic inheritance
- Most common inner ear aplasia
- High-frequency loss with residual low-frequency hearing
- Aplasia of cochlear duct (membranous defect)
- CT: No characteristic features
- Associated with congenital rubella and Jervell and Lange-Neilsen's, Usher's, and Waardenburg's syndromes

Scheibe Aplasia
- Autosomal recessive
- Most common inner ear dysplasia
- Partial to complete aplasia of cochlea and saccule (pars inferior) with normal semicircular canals and utricle (pars superior)
- CT: No characteristic features (membranous defect)
- Associated with Usher's and Waardenburg's syndromes

Enlarged Vestibular Aqueduct
- Most common radiologic deformity of the inner ear
- Progressive SNHL that may be sudden or stepwise decrease
- Can occur in isolation or with Mondini deformity
- Associated with progressive and/or fluctuating vestibular dysfunction and Pendred's syndrome
- Associated with perilymph gusher

Bing-Siebenmann Dysplasia
- Rare, complete dysplasia of membranous labyrinth

Inherited Disorders

Autosomal Recessive

Connexin 26

- Chromosomal mutation on 13q11
- Most common genetic cause of deafness (> 50% of recessive nonsyndromic hearing loss)
- Most commonly autosomal recessive (90 mutations identified)
- Can be autosomal dominant (nine mutations identified)
- Quantitative and qualitative defects in protein coding for gap junctions (GJB2), which are responsible for maintaining endolymphatic potential in the cochlea [K^+], caused by the gene mutation
- 35delG the most common mutation (however, > 100 mutations have been identified)

Usher's Syndrome

- Chromosome arm 14q (type I), chromosome arm 1q32 (type II)
- SNHL, retinitis pigmentosa with or without mental retardation, and cataracts

  See **Table 8.7**.

Table 8.7   Classification of Usher syndrome

Type	Sensorineural hearing loss	Vestibular function	Blindness
I	Profound	Areflexia	Early adulthood
II	Moderate to severe	Normal	Midadulthood
III	Progressive	Progressive	Variable

Pendred's Syndrome

- Chromosomal mutation on 7q coding for pendrin (sulfate transporter)
- *SLC26A4* the most common mutation
- Defect in tyrosine iodination
- Severe to profound SNHL
- CT: Mondini deformity or isolated enlarged vestibular aqueduct
- Associated with euthyroid multinodular goiter in childhood

Jervell and Lange-Nielsen's Syndrome

- Chromosomal mutation on 11p15 as well as 3, 4, 7, 21
- Bilateral SNHL
- Long Q-T syndrome (treated with β-blockers)

Goldenhar's Syndrome

- Hemifacial microsomia
- Chromosomal mutation on 9
- Developmental anomalies of the first and second branchial arches affecting facial nerve, stapedius muscle, semicircular canals, and oval window
- Associated with preauricular tags, pinnae anomalies, aural atresia, facial asymmetry, colobomas, and mental retardation

Autosomal Dominant

Waardenburg's Syndrome

- Chromosomal mutation on 2q and 14q
- Unilateral or bilateral SNHL and/or vestibular dysfunction
- Associated with pigment anomalies (white forelock, heterochromia iridum [different colored irises]), telecanthus, synophrys (unibrow), skeletal anomalies, Hirschsprung's disease

Stickler's Syndrome

- Progressive arthroophthalmopathy
- Chromosomal mutation on 6p and 12q
- Variable expression
- Progressive SNHL and/or conductive loss (eustachian tube dysfunction due to cleft palate)
- Associated with myopia and/or retinal detachment, cataracts, Pierre Robin's sequence, marfanoid habitus, joint hypermobilization, and early arthritis

Treacher Collins's Syndrome

- Mandibulofacial dysostosis
- Chromosomal mutation on 5
- Conductive hearing loss: EAC atresia, ossicular malformations, replacement of tympanic membrane with bony plate
- Sensorineural hearing loss: widened cochlear aqueduct
- Associated with aberrant facial nerve, auricular anomalies, preauricular fistulas, mandibular hypoplasia, coloboma, palate defects, and downward-slanting palpebral fissures

Branchio-Oto-Renal Syndrome

- Chromosome mutation on 8q
- *EYA1* and *SIX1* mutations have been identified.
- Developmental anomalies of the branchial arches and kidneys
- Variable SNHL
- CT: Possible Mondini deformity
- Associated with auricular deformities, preauricular pits, fistulas, tags, mild renal dysplasia progressing to agenesis

Neurofibromatosis

- Neurofibromatosis type 1 (NF1): Long arm of chromosome 17; 5% risk of unilateral vestibular schwannoma
- Neurofibromatosis type 2 (NF2): Long arm of chromosome 22; frequently bilateral vestibular schwannomas, multiple meningiomas
- Progressive profound SNHL due to acoustic neuroma
- Associated with café-au-lait spots, groin/axillary freckling, cutaneous, central nervous system (CNS) and peripheral nerve neurofibromas, Lisch nodules (eye hamartomas), and pheochromocytomas

Apert's Syndrome

- Acrocephalosyndactyly
- Chromosomal mutation on 10
- Autosomal dominant or sporadic inheritance
- CHL due to stapes fixation
- CT: patent cochlear aqueduct, large subarcuate fossa
- Associated with syndactyly, midface anomalies including hypertelorism, proptosis, saddle nose deformity, high-arched palate, trapezoid mouth, and craniofacial dysostosis

Crouzon's Syndrome

- Craniofacial dysostosis
- Chromosomal mutation on 10q; CHL to aural atresia and ossicular deformities
- Associated with cranial synostosis, small maxilla, hypertelorism, exophthalmos, prognathic mandible, and short upper lip

Osteogenesis Imperfecta

- Chromosomal mutation on 5p or 17q
- Typically autosomal dominant inheritance, although a familial recessive form has been described
- Disorder of type I collagen (quantitative and qualitative collagen defect); progressive conductive, mixed, or sensorineural hearing loss
- Associated with hypermobility of joints and ligaments, bone fragility, and blue sclera

X-Linked

Alport's Syndrome

- Chromosome Xq, some autosomal dominant mutations in chromosome 2q
- Abnormality of type IV collagen formation in basement membrane
- Progressive SNHL due to degeneration of organ of Corti and stria vascularis within first decade
- Associated with progressive nephritis (hematuria, proteinuria, chronic glomerulonephritis, uremia), myopia, and cataracts

- *Oto-Palato-Digital Syndrome (see also* **Chapter 8.9**)
- CHL due to ossicular malformations
- Associated with cleft palate, broad fingers and toes, hypertelorism, mental retardation, and short stature

Norrie's Disease

- Chromosomal mutation on Xp11
- Progressive SNHL (in one third of patients; in second or third decade)
- Rapidly progressive blindness (bilateral pseudoglioma, exudative vitreo-retinopathy, and ocular degeneration)

Wildervanck's Syndrome

- Dominant X-linked
- SNHL (one third of cases)
- Associated with CN VI paralysis and Klippel-Feil syndrome (fusion of cervical vertebrae)

X-Linked Hearing Loss

- Chromosomal mutation on Xq
- Rare syndrome with mixed hearing loss due to stapes fixation and peri-lymph gushers

◆ Congenital Conductive Hearing Loss

Atresia

Atresia may be unilateral or bilateral.

Syndromic

Treacher Collins's syndrome, Apert's syndrome, Crouzon's syndrome, oto-palato-digital syndrome, osteogenesis imperfecta, X-linked hearing loss (see foregoing syndrome descriptions)

◆ Acquired Hearing Loss

Acquired hearing loss is often due to prenatal or perinatal insult, such as infection.

Acquired Prenatal

Infection *before* birth results in hearing loss.

Rubella
- Hair cell loss, atrophy of the organ of Corti, thrombosis of stria vascularis
- Severe to profound SNHL and/or delayed endolymphatic hydrops
- Associated with mental retardation, lower limb deformities, anemia, cataracts, cardiac malformations, microcephaly, and thrombocytopenia

Syphilis

- *Treponema pallidum*
- Often fatal
- Profound SNHL (within first 2 years, or in second or third decade)
- Hennebert's sign (nystagmus with fluctuating pressure on external auditory canal [EAC] in the presence of an intact tympanic membrane—in delayed congenital syphilis)
- Delayed endolymphatic hydrops
- Penicillin for acquired infection and/or corticosteroids for SNHL

Cytomegalovirus (CMV)

- Mild to profound SNHL
- May be unilateral and/or progressive
- Associated with hemolytic anemia, microcephaly, mental retardation, hepatosplenomegaly, cerebral calcifications, and jaundice

Hypoxia

- SNHL and/or auditory neuropathy
- Risk factors include birth anoxia, postnatal hypoxia and/or ventilatory support, and extracorporeal membrane oxygenation (ECMO).

Hyperbilirubinemia

- SNHL and/or auditory neuropathy

Acquired Postnatal

Infection or injury *after* birth results in hearing loss.

Sensorineural Loss

Meningitis

- SNHL typically bilateral, permanent, profound to severe (15–20% of cases)
- Onset of SNHL early in this disease
- Bacterial etiology: *Haemophilus influenzae* (most likely to cause hearing loss), *Streptococcus pneumoniae* (most common cause of meningitis in children; most likely to cause labyrinthine ossification)
- Access of bacteria and their toxins to inner ear likely via the cochlear aqueduct and the internal auditory canal (IAC)
- Possible role of inflammatory, hypoxic injury to neural elements
- Repeated auditory brainstem response assessment starting early in the course of disease
- CT: May have labyrinthine ossification. Lateral semicircular canal is often first to ossify. If child medically stable and fulfills audiologic candidacy, cochlear implantation should occur immediately (≤ 6 weeks) if scan shows fibrosis, because once the cochlea has ossified, implantation then requires cochlear drill-out, allowing only a partial electrode, portending a poorer outcome.

Trauma

- Possible temporal bone fracture
- SNHL due to fracture through otic capsule, stapes subluxation with perilymphatic leak, or excessive displacement and shearing of basilar membrane (leads to a high-frequency loss)
- CHL due to soft tissue and debris in the EAC, tympanic membrane perforation (20–50%), hemotympanum (20–65%), ossicular dislocation or injury (incus most commonly dislocated, more commonly associated with longitudinal fracture)
- Associated with facial nerve injury, vertigo, and posttraumatic benign paroxysmal positional vertigo

Auditory Neuropathy/Dyssynchrony

- Disorder of central processing
- Poor discrimination scores out of keeping with pure tone thresholds (absent auditory brainstem response, normal otoacoustic emissions [OAEs])
- Risk factors include hyperbilirubinemia, hypoxia or mechanical ventilation, low birth weight, congenital anomalies of the CNS, Stevens-Johnson's syndrome
- May accompany neurologic diagnosis (Friedrich's ataxia, Ehlers-Danlos's syndrome, Charcot-Marie-Tooth's syndrome)
- Most commonly acquired, although inherited variants exist
- May perform well with cochlear implantation due to suprathreshold synchronous stimulation it supplies to auditory nerve

Conductive Loss

- Cholesteatoma
  - Ossicular erosion leading to maximal conductive loss
- Tympanic membrane perforation
  - CHL (30–50 dB)
  - Successful repair may not improve hearing.
  - Perforation due to acute OM, chronic OM, barotraumas, complication of tympanostomy tube insertion or middle ear surgery
  - Should obey water precautions, particularly in bath water and lake water
- Chronic serous otitis
- Trauma
  - See full description under sensorineural loss.
- Ear foreign body
  - See **Chapter 3.1.4**.

◆ Evaluation

Physical Exam

See **Chapter 3.4.2** for pediatric audiologic assessments. A complete head and neck exam should include otoscopy, pneumatoscopy, Rinne and Weber tuning fork tests if age-appropriate, and inspection of the auricle and preauricular skin for pits or tags. A clinical examination of the vestibular system appropriate for the child's age should be undertaken, as well as a general examination to identify syndromic features (see preceding discussions for differential diagnosis for characteristic syndromic features) (**Table 8.8**).

Table 8.8   Suggested evaluation for congenital sensorineural hearing loss

Syndromic   • Refer to geneticist.   • Consider: electrocardiography, urinalysis   • Other imaging as directed by specific syndrome
Nonsyndromic   • Tests for possible acquired causes: • RPR/FTA-ABS   • TORCH IgM assay   • Genetic testing: testing for known common connexin mutations; various genetic panels (such as CapitalBioMiamiOtoArray; MiamiOtoGenes) others
All   • CT of temporal bone   • Referral to ophthalmology   • Serial hearing testing to follow possible progression

Abbreviations: CT, computed tomography; IgM, immunoglobulin M; RPR/FTA-ABS, rapid plasma reagin/fluorescent treponemal antibody absorbed; TORCH, toxoplasmosis, rubella, cytomegalovirus, herpes simplex encephalitis, and otosyphilis.

Imaging

High-resolution CT of the temporal bones will identify cochleovestibular anomalies. Consider magnetic resonance imaging (MRI) with attention to the IAC to examine for the presence and size of the auditory nerve, white matter changes due to sequelae of prematurity, CMV, hyperbilirubinemia, or in cases of neurofibromatosis.

Labs

- Pendred's syndrome: thyroid-stimulating hormone (TSH) test
- Alport's, branchio-oto-renal syndrome: urinalysis, BUN (blood urea nitrogen), creatinine
- TORCH: IgM assay (toxoplasmosis, syphilis, rubella, CMV, herpes simplex)
- Rubella: Viral culture of amniotic fluid, urine, and throat
- Syphilis: fluorescent treponemal antibody absorbed (FTA-ABS), Venereal Disease Research Laboratory (VDRL) test

Other Tests

- Repeated audiometric assessment with tympanometry appropriate for age (**Table 8.9**)
- Assessment of visual acuity due to exponential increase in morbidity in presence of dual sensory impairment
- Genetic evaluation, counseling: connexin-26, syndromic and/or inherited loss
- Jervell and Lange-Nielsen's syndromes: Electrocardiogram to detect prolonged Q-T interval
- Pendred's syndrome: thyroid ultrasound
- Branchio-oto-renal syndrome: renal ultrasound, pyelogram

Table 8.9   Audiometric assessment by age

Birth to 6 months • Behavioral observation audiometry • Otoacoustic emission • Auditory brainstem response
6 months to 3 years • Visual response audiometry • Otoacoustic emission • Auditory brainstem response
3–6 years • Conventional play audiometry
> 6 years • Standard audiometry

◆ Treatment Options

Medical

Appropriate and timely fitting of amplification (by 6 months if identified by newborn hearing screening) with a frequency modulation (FM) system or tactile aids. An auditory verbal therapist or a total communication program, including American Sign Language (ASL) where appropriate, should be considered. Liaise with the school, teachers, and the educational audiologist.

Surgical

- Tympanostomy tubes: Mixed loss due to chronic serous OM
- Cochlear implantation for profound bilateral SNHL (see **Chapter 3.5.4**)
- Bone-anchored hearing aid for aural atresia, chronic OM (see **Chapter 3.5.5**)
- Surgical correction of atretic ear and canal
- Middle ear exploration and/or ossiculoplasty, tympanoplasty for suspected congenital or acquired conductive loss
- Auditory brainstem implant (see **Chapter 3.5.5**) for:

○ Bilateral acoustic neuroma in NF2
○ Cochlear or auditory nerve agenesis (i.e., Michel aplasia)

◆ Complications

Treat TM perforation due to chronic OM or as a complication of tympanostomy tube insertion with delayed tympanoplasty once a dry ear is established. Treat OM aggressively with antibiotics and tympanostomy tubes in children following cochlear implantation due to risk of meningitis.

◆ Outcome and Follow-Up

Postoperatively, apply analgesia and/or systemic antibiotics where the auditory prosthesis has been placed. Children receiving cochlear implantation should receive pneumococcal and meningitis vaccination as prophylaxis prior to implantation. Ongoing and repeated audiologic assessment should be maintained with attention to the child's speech and language development.

With a child with tympanostomy tubes, follow up every 6 months until the tubes have extruded and the myringotomy site has closed without reaccumulation of effusion.

8.13 Infectious Neck Masses in Children

◆ Key Features

- Cervical lymphadenitis is the most common infectious neck mass in children, but an abscess is also a possibility.
- The age of the patient, the location, and the time frame to development of adenitis are important clues to the underlying etiology.
- The diagnosis is commonly based on history and physical exam, not laboratory findings.
- Medical management is appropriate for many causes.

Enlarged or inflamed lymph nodes are the cause of 95% of pediatric neck masses. A thorough physical examination is necessary because the lymph node groups are associated with different diseases, which will dictate proper management. Most of the lymphatics from the head and neck region drain to the submaxillary and deep cervical lymph nodes, explaining why these nodes are most commonly affected by cervical lymphadenitis. In the absence of cervical adenopathy, enlargement of the supraclavicular nodes can be indicative of thoracic or abdominal disease. The most common causes of isolated right supraclavicular node enlargement are Hodgkin's and non-Hodgkin's lymphoma. Isolated enlargement of the left supraclavicular nodes is most commonly associated with intraabdominal tumor or inflammation (Troisier sign).

◆ Etiology

The underlying etiology of cervical lymphadenitis can be predicted based on the patient's age. In neonates, group B streptococci are the most common cause of lymphadenitis. *Staphylococcus aureus* is usually the causative organism in patients 2 months to 1 year old. Along with *Bartonella henselae* (cat-scratch disease) and nontuberculous mycobacteria, *S. aureus* is also a common cause in 1- to 4-year-old patients. These organisms can be the cause of cervical adenitis in older patients along with tuberculosis, anaerobic bacteria, and toxoplasmosis. The timeframe is also an important factor to consider when determining the etiology of cervical adenitis. Acute bilateral disease is usually a response to acute pharyngitis but can also occur with Epstein-Barr virus, cytomegalovirus, herpes simplex virus, roseola, and enteroviruses. Acute unilateral lymphadenitis commonly presents with an associated cellulitis and is typically caused by *S. aureus, Streptococcus pyogenes*, and group B streptococci. Subacute or chronic unilateral lymphadenitis is much less common. It can be due to cat-scratch disease, mycobacterial infection, or toxoplasmosis.

◆ Clinical

Signs

A thorough physical examination is essential. Note the size, location, laterality, firmness, and number of nodes. Erythema and tenderness are also important signs. Associated illnesses such as pharyngitis or systemic infection need to be noted.

Symptoms

Patients can present with unilateral or bilateral neck swelling, with or without any other symptoms. Tenderness of the affected nodes is commonly associated with acute infection.

Differential Diagnosis

Infectious causes are the most common. Malignancy is an important consideration in patients with no other signs of infection, with recent weight loss or fevers, or with isolated supraclavicular involvement. Noninfectious causes are much less common and include Kawasaki's disease, sarcoidosis, sinus histiocytosis, histiocytic necrotizing lymphadenitis, and Kimura's disease.

◆ Evaluation

Physical Exam

Cervical lymphadenitis typically presents with acute unilaterally or bilaterally enlarged (> 3 cm) and tender lymph nodes in the jugulodigastric area. Atypical mycobacterial infection generally presents with an enlarged, erythematous single mass, distinct from reactive adenopathy or fluctuant abscess.

Imaging

Imaging is not necessary if cervical lymphadenitis is suspected based on history and physical exam findings. If there is concern for tuberculosis or an abscess, an ultrasound or computed tomography (CT) of the neck can be performed. Cervical lymphadenitis will manifest as enlarged, enhancing nodes with low central attenuation if necrosis is present. Tuberculosis-infected lymph nodes will have thick peripheral enhancement on contrasted CT, low central attenuation, a relative lack of fat stranding, and calcification.

Labs

Complete blood count (CBC) is useful for determining whether the enlarged lymph nodes are secondary to systemic infection. Other laboratory studies, including Gram staining, acid-fast staining, and culture, can be done if aspiration is undertaken. Perform cat-scratch titer or monospot if infection is suspected.

Other Tests

Fine-needle aspiration biopsy (FNAB) can be both diagnostic and therapeutic. Obtain the aspirate from the largest, most fluctuant node using a 23- or 20-gauge needle. Gram stain, acid-fast stain, and culture should be obtained. The etiology is discovered in 60 to 90% of patients who undergo needle aspiration. Excisional biopsy is indicated if the node is hard, is fixed, fails to regress following aspiration or antibiotic use, enlarges, or is associated with fever or weight loss or if the diagnosis is uncertain. Biopsy of more than one node is preferable. Placing a portion of the specimen in a flow cytometry medium is important if lymphoma evaluation is required.

Pathology

Pathology varies depending on the underlying etiology.

◆ Treatment Options

Medical

Patients who have asymptomatic, small (< 3 cm), bilaterally enlarged cervical lymph nodes can be observed. If mass persists or enlarges over several weeks, biopsy is warranted. Those with signs and symptoms typical of acute bacterial lymphadenitis (large, tender, erythematous unilateral node with no systemic symptoms) can be treated empirically for *S. aureus* and *S. pyogenes* with amoxicillin-clavulanate, cephalexin, or clindamycin. If cellulitis is present or if the patient is having severe symptoms, parenteral nafcillin, cefazolin, or clindamycin is appropriate. When lymphadenitis is secondary to dental infection, anaerobic infection should be suspected, and clindamycin or penicillin plus metronidazole is effective. Azithromycin, trimethoprim-sulfamethoxazole, or rifampin is effective early in the course of disease in preventing abscess formation if cat-scratch disease is suspected.

Relevant Pharmacology

- Amoxicillin-clavulanate: Amoxicillin binds to penicillin-binding protein thereby preventing bacterial cell wall synthesis. Clavulanate inhibits β-lactamases, which increases amoxicillin's spectrum of activity. Dosing is based on the amoxicillin component.

  < 3 months old: Total dose is 30 mg/kg/day. Divide dose and administer twice daily using the 125 mg/5 mL suspension. Children < 40 kg: 25 to 45 mg/kg/day divided every 12 hours using either 200 mg/5 mL or 400 mg/5 mL suspension. Alternatively, 200- or 400-mg chewable tablets can be used. Children ≥ 40 kg and adults, 875 mg twice daily

- Clindamycin: This antibiotic inhibits bacterial protein synthesis by binding to bacterial 50S ribosomal subunits.
  - Children < 16 years
    Oral: total dose of 8 to 25 mg/kg/day in 3 or 4 divided doses
    Parenteral: 15 to 20 mg/kg/day
  - Adults
    Oral: 300 mg three times daily
    Parenteral: 1.2 to 1.8 g/day in two to four divided doses

- Trimethoprim-sulfamethoxazole: Both agents inhibit bacterial folic acid production. Trimethoprim inhibits dihydrofolic acid reduction, and sulfamethoxazole interferes with dihydrofolic acid. Dosing is based on trimethoprim component.
  - Children > 2 months
    Total dose: Trimethoprim 8 to 12 mg/kg/day in divided doses every 12 hours or 20 mg/kg/day in divided doses every 6 hours for serious infections
  - Children > 40 kg or adults
    Oral: Trimethoprim 160 mg every 12 hours
    Parenteral: Trimethoprim 2 mg/kg every 6 hours

Surgical

Incision and drainage is useful if there is an abscess, especially due to *S. aureus* or *S. pyogenes*. If a mycobacterial or *Bartonella henselae* infection is suspected, then FNAB is preferable to avoid fistula formation. Most cases of cat-scratch fever are managed medically. Incision and drainage are reserved for cases progressing to abscess formation. Surgical excision or curettage is effective if nontuberculous mycobacterial infection is the cause. Removal of the largest node and necrotic nodes is sufficient, because the remaining adenopathy will resolve spontaneously.

◆ Complications

Infection control is essential if a postoperative complication occurs. Empiric use of broad-spectrum antibiotics is appropriate. Further care depends on the type of complication. Internal jugular venous thrombosis can be managed with anticoagulation. Abscess is treated with incision and drainage.

◆ Outcome and Follow-Up

The patient can return home after incision and drainage or surgical excision, but close monitoring is necessary because of the potential complications. Mediastinal abscesses, purulent pericarditis, thrombosis of the internal jugular vein, pulmonary emboli, or mycotic emboli are all rare, but serious, complications.

Cervical lymphadenitis resolves completely in the majority of patients who receive appropriate antibiotic therapy. No further follow-up is necessary unless the patient's symptoms do not improve or if they worsen.

8.14 Hemangiomas, Vascular Malformations, and Lymphatic Malformations of the Head and Neck

◆ Key Features

- Hemangiomas, vascular malformations, and lymphatic malformations of the head and neck are common congenital and neonatal abnormalities.
- Vascular tumors are classified into hemangiomas and vascular malformations.
- Accurate diagnosis is the key to prognosis and treatment plan.
- Accurate diagnosis is based on natural history and key clinical features.

Vascular tumors are common pediatric anomalies and may develop throughout the head and neck. They are divided broadly into hemangiomas and vascular malformations, each with a distinct natural history. Lymphatic malformations (or lymphangiomas) are defects in the lymphatic system that present as swellings or nodules in the skin or mucous membranes of the head and neck. The malformation of lymphatic tissue causes an accumulation of fluid, which accounts for the clinical presentation.

◆ Epidemiology

Infantile hemangiomas occur in up to 12% of all children. They are more common in females than males, at a ratio of 3:1, and more common in European Americans. Sixty percent of hemangiomas are located in the head and neck, including the upper aerodigestive tract, and 80% occur as single lesions.

Vascular malformations are divided into lymphatic malformations, capillary malformations or portwine stains, venous malformations, and high-flow arteriovenous malformations (AVMs). Lymphatic malformations are further divided into microcystic lymphatic malformations and macrocystic lymphatic malformations involving the soft tissue of the neck. Vascular malformations have no gender or racial predilection and most commonly occur in the head and neck. Lymphatic malformations represent 6% of benign cervicofacial tumors of childhood; they are seen in fewer than 2.8 per 1000 people. Patients with Down's, Turner's, or fetal alcohol syndrome have a higher incidence of lymphatic malformations.

◆ Clinical

Signs and Symptoms

Hemangiomas

Infantile hemangiomas are generally not present at birth and first appear during the first 6 weeks of life. Hemangiomas go through predictable phases of growth. The initial proliferative phase occurs over the first year, is characterized by rapid growth, and is followed by the involution phase with subsequent regression. Complete involution occurs in 50% of children by 5 years of age, 70% of children by 7 years of age, and 90% of children by 9 years of age.

Vascular Malformations

Vascular malformations are by definition present at birth but may go unrecognized. They grow proportionately with the child and may present throughout childhood or early adulthood. Hemangiomas are firm; vascular malformations are easily compressible. They may involve the facial skeleton and abruptly increase in size with acute hemorrhage or infection, puberty, or pregnancy.

Lymphatic Malformations

Lymphangioma circumscriptum presents as a nodular mass with a red, wartlike appearance. They are typically asymptomatic, but bleeding or drainage of fluid may occur.
Cavernous lymphangioma (cystic hygroma) presents as a painless subcutaneous swelling or nodule and can rapidly enlarge with infections.

Differential Diagnosis

The key to diagnosis is to differentiate between hemangiomas and vascular malformations. Diagnosis can generally be made on the clinical history and physical exam alone. Lymphatic malformations presenting as cystic lesions within the neck must be differentiated from other congenital cystic lesions, including branchial cleft cysts (discussed in **Chapter 8.15**).

◆ Evaluation

History

In the patient history, the timing of the development of the lesion is important, particularly whether it was present at birth. Also note the growth rate of the lesion.

Physical Exam

A complete head and neck exam should focus on the character of the lesion. Children with hemangiomas in the chin and chest are more likely to have concurrent airway lesions, including subglottic hemangiomas. Noisy breathing in these children must be evaluated with laryngoscopy and likely with bronchoscopy.

Imaging

Imaging is generally unnecessary for diagnostic purposes but may be warranted in children with multiple cutaneous hemangiomas, who are more likely to have concurrent visceral lesions. Magnetic resonance imaging (MRI) may be useful, particularly in the preoperative setting, to determine the extent of soft tissue involvement. Imaging may also be helpful in the evaluation of a child with cutaneous hemangioma and noisy breathing. Flow voids are indicative of high-flow lesions.

Pathology

Pathologic exam also helps to differentiate between hemangioma and vascular malformation. Hemangiomas are characterized by proliferating endothelial cells and are positive for GLUT1, helping to differentiate them from other vascular tumors. Hemangiomas grow by cellular hyperplasia; vascular malformations grow by hypertrophy.

◆ Treatment Options

Hemangiomas

Expectant management is recommended for most hemangiomas. Intervention is indicated for lesions threatening the airway or vision and may be considered for bleeding and infection or progressive disfigurement. Tracheotomy is sometimes required to manage the airway of a child with a subglottic hemangioma.

The first-line therapy for hemangiomas is propranolol, a nonselective β-blocker. Side effects or lack of response to propranolol therapy are rare, but selective β-blockers may be used if side effects are noted due to the nonselective nature of propranolol. Topical β-blocker therapy with timolol ophthalmic gel is commonly used for superficial, localized hemangiomas.

Corticosteroids were previously used as first-line therapy for hemangiomas. However, the short- and long-term complications associated with corticosteroid therapy have limited their use. Corticosteroids are often reserved for patients with contraindications to β-blocker therapy or as an acute therapy for patients being started on β-blocker therapy.

Interferon has been used with success but is associated with neurologic complications. The use of various lasers may be considered. Surgery may be appropriate, but must be considered carefully.

Vascular Malformations

Vascular malformations are not expected to involute, and so the decision to treat is less controversial. Tracheotomy may be required for large cystic hygromas. Sclerotherapy with OK-432 (picibanil) has shown success, though OK-432 remains an experimental treatment modality. There are other older sclerotherapy agents used widely with success, such as ethanol.

Argon lasers and dye lasers are used in the treatment of capillary malformations or portwine stains (see **Chapter 6.3.14**). Complete surgical resection, with the consideration of preoperative embolization, is required in the treatment of AVMs.

Lymphatic Malformations

Surgical management of lymphatic malformations may be considered, although the lesion may involve vital structures and complete resection may not be appropriate.

◆ Complications

Complications of enlarging vascular tumors and surgical intervention depend on the size and location of the lesion. Functional and cosmetic factors must be considered in both the decision to treat and the extent of treatment.

◆ Outcome and Follow-Up

Hemangiomas initially managed expectantly must be monitored closely, as even lesions not involving the airway or orbit may cause significant stress to parents during the proliferative phase. Untreated vascular malformations must be similarly monitored as they grow proportionally with the child. Large lymphatic malformations can require multiple surgeries, require tracheotomy, and cause significant morbidity.

8.15 Branchial Cleft Cysts

◆ Key Features

- Branchial cleft cysts represent the most common noninflammatory lateral neck masses in children.
- Definitive treatment is complete surgical excision.

Branchial cleft cysts are composed of remnants from any of the first five branchial arches, which give rise to head and neck structures (**Table 8.10**). Branchial cleft cysts may be associated with a fistula or sinus tract. Cysts may have different locations and characteristics depending on their branchial cleft of origin.

◆ Epidemiology

Branchial cleft cysts are common; they are responsible for 33% of congenital neck masses and 17% of pediatric neck masses. Most branchial cleft cysts are derived from the second branchial arch apparatus; 1% of cysts are derived from the first branchial arch. Third-arch cysts are reported; fourth-branchial-cleft cysts are extremely rare.

Table 8.10 Structures that arise from differentiation of branchial arches

Arch	Nerve	Structure	Muscle	Artery
First	Trigeminal	Mandible, body of incus, head and neck of malleus, major salivary glands, tympanic membrane, eustachian tube	Masticator muscles, tensor tympani, anterior belly of digastric	Facial
Second	Facial (CN VII), vestibulocochlear (CN VIII)	Two-thirds of long process of incus, manubrium of malleus, crura and head of stapes, styloid, lesser cornu of hyoid, upper body of hyoid, tonsil	Platysma, muscles of facial expression, stapedius, posterior belly of digastric	Stapedial
Third	Glossopharyngeal (CN IX)	Greater cornu of hyoid, thymus, inferior parathyroid, body of hyoid	Superior constrictors	Internal carotid
Fourth	Vagus (CN X)	Thyroid cartilage, epiglottis, superior parathyroid	Inferior constrictor, laryngeal musculature	Aortic arch, right subclavian
Fifth	Spinal accessory (CN XI)	Arytenoid cartilage, cricoid cartilage, lungs	Portion of laryngeal musculature	Pulmonary ductus

Used with permission from Van de Water TR, Staecker H. *Otolaryngology: Basic Science and Clinical Review*. Stuttgart/New York: Thieme;2006:208. *Abbreviation:* CN, cranial nerve.

◆ Classification

First branchial arch abnormalities can be classified as type 1 or 2:

- Type 1 abnormalities are of ectodermal origin and are lined by epidermoid elements. They lie parallel to the external auditory canal in the preauricular area. They may be associated with a fistula or sinus tract that may end in the middle ear or external auditory canal.

- Type 2 abnormalities are more common than type 1. They are of ecto-dermal and mesodermal origin and consist of squamous epithelium and adnexal structures. An external opening may be present, leading to a cyst or sinus tract that courses through the parotid gland. Patients often present with otorrhea unresponsive to typical treatment. Note that this tract may be closely associated with the facial nerve at the stylomastoid foramen.

Second-branchial-arch remnants, the most common branchial anomaly, present as a painless mass or dimple below the angle of the mandible, at the anterior border of the sternocleidomastoid muscle. They may present as a cyst or may have a tract ending at the tonsillar fossa. The tract, if present, traverses the carotid bifurcation (**Fig. 8.4**).

Third- and (especially) fourth- and fifth-branchial-cleft remnants are much more rare; they may have a long tract looping deep to the carotid artery and ending in the region of the piriform.

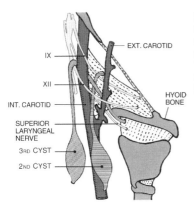

Fig. 8.4 Relationship of second- and third-branchial-cleft anomalies to the carotid artery and cranial nerves. (Used with permission from Van de Water TR, Staecker H. *Otolaryngology: Basic Science and Clinical Review*. Stuttgart/New York: Thieme; 2006:209.)

◆ Clinical

Signs and Symptoms

Branchial cleft cysts often present as lateral painless masses and may enlarge after an upper respiratory infection. If there is an external sinus or fistula opening, there are troublesome mucus secretions; recurrent infections are common. Larger branchial cysts may compress the airway causing stridor, dyspnea, or dysphagia.

Differential Diagnosis

- Branchial cleft cyst or sinus
- Lymphatic malformation
- Hemangioma
- Ectopic thymus

- Lipoma
- Thymic cyst
- Parotid cyst
- Pseudotumor of infancy
- Malignant tumor
- Laryngocele

◆ Evaluation

History

The timing of the development of the lesion is important, particularly whether it was present at birth. Also, note the growth rate, size fluctuation, and history of infection or drainage.

Physical Exam

During the head and neck exam, note the size, the precise location of the mass, the presence or absence of a dimple or opening, and quality (firm, soft, etc.). Assess for possible other congenital anomalies or syndromic features.

Imaging

Branchial abnormalities are visualized using computed tomography (CT) with contrast; if a sinus or fistula is present, contrast fistulography and barium swallow esophagography may demonstrate the path of the abnormality.

Pathology

Branchial cleft cysts arise from residual embryonic tissue from the branchial clefts or pouches (**Table 8.10**).

◆ Treatment Options

Medical

If the branchial cyst is infected, treatment with intravenous (IV) antibiotics is indicated before surgical excision.

Surgical

The treatment of choice for branchial cleft cysts is surgical excision. Excision of a Type 1 first-branchial-cleft cyst may include the cartilage of the external auditory canal. For Type 2 first arch, total parotidectomy with facial nerve dissection may also be needed.

Second-, third-, fourth-, and fifth-branchial-cleft cysts are excised through horizontal neck incisions. "Stepladder" incisions may be needed to excise a tract. The relationship of the tract to carotid and cranial nerves is predictable and must be understood. If a lesion is a true third-branchial cyst, it may present as a thyroid cyst, in which case hemithyroidectomy is performed.

Other treatments such as radiation or sclerosing agents do not provide a cure for branchial cysts and increase the risk of recurrence.

◆ Complications

Bleeding or hematoma can be prevented using electrocautery on small blood vessels and silk ties on larger vessels. Recurrence of branchial cleft cysts can occur if there is incomplete excision of the mass. Injury to the facial nerve may occur during the excision of a first-branchial-cleft cyst. Damage to associated neurovascular structures may occur during the excision of a second- or third-branchial abnormality.

◆ Outcome and Follow-Up

If facial nerve dissection was performed, then assess function in the early postoperative period. A Penrose or suction drain is recommended for any extensive dissection. Antibiotics are necessary if the aerodigestive tract was entered or if the cyst was infected. Postoperative care is otherwise routine.

8.16 Congenital Midline Neck Masses

◆ Key Features

- Thyroglossal duct cysts, dermoid cysts, and lipomas are common midline congenital masses.
- Thyroid cancer can develop from a thyroglossal duct cyst, rarely.
- Treatment requires complete surgical excision.

Thyroglossal duct cysts are midline masses that may appear anywhere between the base of the tongue and the thyroid gland. Dermoid cysts typically present in the submental area of the neck but can appear in other areas of the head and neck. Lipomas are derived from adipose tissue and present as soft painless masses that may occur anywhere in the body.

◆ Epidemiology

Thyroglossal duct cysts are the most common congenital neck mass, present in 7% of the population. Lipomas are the most common soft tissue tumor. They may occur at any age but are common after age 40.

◆ Clinical

Signs and Symptoms

Thyroglossal duct cysts are firm, mobile typically midline masses and can appear anywhere along the path of the thyroid's descent. They can be off-midline. They will elevate upon protrusion of the tongue or swallowing and are usually asymptomatic. However, large cysts, or those in the base of the tongue, can compress the airway, causing dysphagia and respiratory difficulties. Cysts can become infected and may also enlarge after an upper respiratory infection.

Dermoid cysts are attached to and move with the skin. They are usually located in the submental area. They do not move upon swallowing or protrusion of the tongue. They are typically asymptomatic unless infected.

Lipoma presents as a soft, movable lump under the skin. They occur in the neck but also in multiple tissues and locations throughout the body.

Differential Diagnosis

- Thyroglossal duct cyst
- Dermoid cyst
- Lipoma
- Enlarged thyroid isthmus
- Pyramidal lobe of thyroid
- Plunging ranula
- Thyroid nodule/cyst
- Sebaceous cyst
- Teratoma
- Cervical thymic cyst

◆ Evaluation

Physical Exam

During the full head and neck exam, note the location, the quality of the mass, its size, and its motion with skin or swallowing. Assess for possible other congenital anomalies.

Imaging

Ultrasound of the thyroid is mandatory to document thyroid tissue in its normal location, as a thyroglossal duct cyst may rarely contain all functioning thyroid tissue. Ultrasound may be sufficient to diagnose a thyroglossal duct cyst and differentiate it from ectopic thyroid. If the diagnosis is unclear, computed tomography (CT) or magnetic resonance imaging (MRI) will usually differentiate thyroglossal duct cyst, dermoid, and lipoma.

Pathology

Thyroglossal duct cysts arise from remnants of the thyroid gland as it descends from the foramen cecum during embryologic development (**Fig. 8.5**). Dermoid cysts are epithelial-lined cavities containing adnexal structures. They result from epithelium becoming enclosed in tissue during embryological development. Lipomas are benign, subcutaneous masses derived from adipose tissue.

◆ Treatment Options

Medical

If the cyst is infected, treatment with intravenous (IV) antibiotics is indicated before surgical excision.

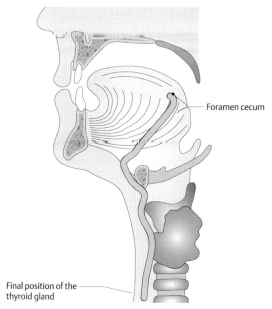

Fig. 8.5 Drawing of the lateral neck showing the path of descent of the thyroid anlage. Thyroid duct cysts, fistulae, and ectopic thyroid tissue can occur anywhere along the course of this duct. (Used with permission from Mafee MF, Valvassori GE, Becker M. *Imaging of the Head and Neck,* 2nd ed. Stuttgart/New York: Thieme;2005:837.)

Surgical

Thyroglossal duct cysts are excised through a transverse incision at the level of the hyoid bone. The center of the hyoid bone is removed to include a tract entering the base of the tongue (Sistrunk's procedure) to minimize recurrence. Avoiding lateral dissection will minimize the possibility of injury to the hypoglossal nerves.

Dermoid cysts and lipomas are excised through a simple transverse neck incision positioned in accordance with the location of the mass.

◆ Complications

Bleeding or hematoma can be prevented using electrocautery on small blood vessels and silk ties on larger vessels. Damage to superior laryngeal nerves or the hypoglossal nerve is also possible. Incomplete excision of the thyroglossal duct increases the risk of recurrence.

◆ Outcome and Follow-Up

The incision should be drained with a Penrose or suction drain. Specimen should be sent to pathology to rule out neoplasm. Prophylactic antibiotics should be given if the excised cyst was infected.

8.17 Congenital Midline Nasal Masses

◆ Key Features

- The most common congenital midline nasal masses are gliomas, encephaloceles, and dermoids.
- The most common of these is the dermoid, derived from ectodermal embryonic tissue.
- A glioma consists of central nervous system (CNS) tissue at the nasal dorsum; it is congenital and not a true neoplasm.
- Meningoceles and encephaloceles do communicate with the ventricles and contain cerebrospinal fluid (CSF).
- Teratomas are true neoplasms arising from totipotent cells; half of all head and neck teratomas occur in the nose.

Gliomas, meningoceles, encephaloceles, dermoids, and teratomas exist in the differential diagnosis of the congenital midline nasal mass. A dermoid cyst is a congenital benign neoplasm containing keratinizing squamous epithelium and adnexal skin structures, may be located anywhere from the columella to the nasion, and often presents as a dimple on the nasal bridge. The dermoid may involve only skin and nasal bone, or it may have a true dural connection. Nasal gliomas lack a direct connection to the CNS and contain heterotopic glial elements in a fibrillar stroma, of varying growth rate. Encephaloceles are continuous with the CNS. Sincipital encephaloceles present in the nasal dorsum or forehead region, basal encephaloceles in the nasopharynx. Encephaloceles may include meningoceles (containing only meninges), encephalomeningoceles (containing brain also), and encephalo-meningocystoceles (including part of the ventricular system). Midline nasal masses should never be biopsied in the outpatient setting or without prior imaging studies.

◆ Epidemiology

Congenital midline nasal masses occur in 1 in 20 to 40,000 live births. Ten percent of dermoids occur in the head or neck, and 10% of these occur in the nose. Encephaloceles occur in 1 in 1,250 to 2,000 live births; 40% have other abnormalities. Occipital encephaloceles are most common in North America (75%), although sincipital ones are most common in Southeast Asia.

◆ Clinical

Signs

Dermoids are typically anywhere along the midline of the nose and are firm, noncompressible, and nonpulsatile. A nasal dermoid sinus or cyst presents with a dimple containing a hair follicle. Rarely, the nasal base is widened. Encephaloceles are soft, bluish, compressible, pulsatile, and may transilluminate. Gliomas are smooth, firm, noncompressible, and nontransilluminating. All may be associated with a cranial defect, although this is most common with an encephalocele.

Symptoms

Masses may be intranasal or extranasal.

Differential Diagnosis

- Nasal obstruction
- Hypertelorism
- Epiphora
- Infection (local or meningitis)

◆ Evaluation

Physical Exam

- Internal and external nasal exam
- There may be a positive Furstenberg test in encephaloceles (mass expands with jugular vein compression).
- Exam for other possible congenital anomalies

See **Table 8.11**.

Table 8.11 Clinical approach to congenital midline nasal mass

Evaluation • Head and neck exam • Location, size, quality of mass • Evidence of other congenital anomalies
Furstenberg test • Possible meningocele or encephalocele (enlargement of mass with jugular compression)
Imaging • CT and/or MRI
Presumptive diagnosis • Treatment planning; neurosurgical consult if evidence of CSF connection

Abbreviations: CSF, cerebrospinal fluid; CT, computed tomography; MRI, magnetic resonance imaging.

Imaging

Computed tomography (CT) with contrast; if there is any hint that the mass may be continuous with the CNS, magnetic resonance imaging (MRI) is also required. Ossification of the anterior cranial base is variable in children under 5 years.

Pathology

These masses may result from a failure of complete involution of a dural diverticulum that protrudes through the fonticulus nasofrontalis and typically forms the foramen cecum.

- Dermoid: A cyst lined with squamous epithelium, along with hair and sebaceous glands
- Glioma: Astrocytes, neuroglial fibers, and S-100 positive
- Encephalocele: A nonneoplastic mature neuroglial tissue with meninges

◆ Treatment Options

Small superficial dermoids may be removed via a nasal dorsum incision. A sinus should be removed with an elliptic incision. Other dermoids may require an external rhinoplasty approach and, sometimes, a bicoronal flap if there is extension to the cranial base. For large dermoids, calvarial bone may be needed for reconstruction of cranial base defects.

External gliomas also require an elliptic skin incision or external rhinoplasty approach. Internal gliomas are usually lateral and can be removed through a lateral rhinotomy incision. In either case, if a CSF leak is encountered, a bifrontal craniotomy or an endoscopic CSF leak repair is necessary. This may necessitate collaboration with neurosurgical colleagues for repair.

Encephaloceles require neurosurgical collaboration, and likely a bifrontal craniotomy to maximize visualization. Repair of defects requires temporalis or pericranial flaps for a watertight closure. Extracranial repair is similar to that for gliomas.

◆ Complications

A CSF leak may require lumbar drainage and another patch procedure. Local wound infection or meningitis will require antibiotic therapy:

- Antibiotic coverage for meningitis (see also **Chapter 3.2.3**):
  - Cefotaxime, intravenous (IV), every 4 hours or ceftriaxone, IV, every 12 hours plus ampicillin, IV, every 6 hours
- Alternative if there is drug resistance:
  - Vancomycin (child 15 mg/kg, IV, every 6 hours) plus cefotaxime or ceftriaxone plus ampicillin

Incomplete dermoid or glioma excision will lead to recurrence or fistula formation and require a wide local excision with reconstruction.

◆ Outcome and Follow-Up

Typically, patients are observed in a neurologic intensive care unit (ICU) setting, except for minor external excisions. Patients should be monitored for complete healing and infection.

8.18 Choanal Atresia

◆ Key Points

- Choanal atresia occurs in ~ 1 in 5,000 to 8,000 births.
- Bilateral atresia is more common and is associated with other anomalies (e.g., CHARGE association).
- Endoscopic techniques have greatly improved the safety of the transnasal approach.

Choanal atresia is a congenital condition in which one or both of the choanae are replaced with a bony or mixed bony and membranous wall. Unilateral atresia usually presents later in life, while bilateral atresia is detected at birth. Bilateral atresia can often be medically managed with the use of a McGovern nipple while allowing growth in preparation for repair. The most common repair options include the transnasal and transpalatal approaches. The most frequent complication of repair is restenosis.

◆ Epidemiology

Choanal atresia is relatively rare, only occurring in 1 in 5,000 to 8,000 births. It is almost twice as common in females as in males; 65 to 75% of cases are unilateral. The right choana is more commonly affected. Nearly 75% of bilateral atresias are associated with other disorders, including Treacher Collins's syndrome, DiGeorge's sequence, Apert's syndrome, trisomy 18, and CHARGE association.

◆ Clinical

Signs

Bilateral atresia will most often present in newborns with cyanotic spells relieved by crying and worsened with feeding. Unilateral atresia may present later in childhood with unilateral thick nasal secretions similar to sinusitis.

Symptoms

Bilateral disease will present at birth with difficulty breathing. Unilateral disease may present in older children and may be associated with history of nasal congestion.

◆ Differential Diagnosis

Bilateral

- Congenital nasal piriform aperture stenosis
- NOWCA (nasal obstruction without choanal obstruction)
- Midnasal stenosis
- Choanal stenosis

Unilateral

- Sinusitis
- Nasal foreign body
- Nasal septal deviation
- Choanal stenosis

◆ Evaluation

Physical Exam

Examination of the nares will reveal thick mucous secretions. Commonly, the diagnosis is made after failure to pass a soft suction catheter into the nasopharynx. A flexible endoscope can also be used to assess choanal patency.

Imaging

Computed tomography (CT) provides the most reliable method of diagnosis. Axial images show narrowing of the choanal orifice or widening of the posterior vomer. Approximately 30% of atresias will be purely bony in nature, and 70% will be mixed bony and membranous.

Pathology

There are multiple theories, one of which is that the atresia is due to the persistence of the buccopharyngeal membrane.

◆ Treatment Options

Medical

Initially, an oral airway or a McGovern nipple may be used to maintain an airway. Stimulating the infant to cry will also provide temporary relief. Endotracheal intubation is often appropriate.

Surgical

- *Transnasal approach*: Puncture of the atretic plate using a curved trocar or urethral sound, followed by drilling of the vomer, hard palate, and pterygoid plate. This is usually done with the use of a 120° endoscope in the nasopharynx to provide visualization. Blind use of a trocar is to be avoided. Stents may be placed at the completion of the procedure. Advantages include its ability to be performed in infants and its relatively short operative time. Disadvantages include difficulty in preserving mucosal flaps with the use of the drill. Some surgeons advocate the use of laser (CO_2 or Nd-YAG) with the transnasal approach.
- *Transpalatal approach*: Creation of a palatal flap followed by removal of palatine bone, atretic plate, and vomer. Stents may be placed. Advantages include better visualization, the ability to create lining flaps, and reduced duration of stenting. Disadvantages include oronasal fistula and palatal growth disturbance, with risk of crossbite or midface retrusion.
- *Transantral approach*: Primarily used in revision cases. The choana is opened widely to include the maxillary sinus.

- *Transeptal approach*: Primarily used in unilateral atresia. Removal of posterior septum creates a passage to bypass the atresia.
- The endoscopic technique (nasal or retropalatal), with or without powered instrumentation, offers excellent visualization with great ease in removing the bony choanae. Microdébriders may provide clearer operative fields and causing less tissue trauma for experienced surgeons. Carbon dioxide and potassium titanyl phosphate (KTP) lasers are sometimes used. The use of mitomycin C topically as an adjunct to the surgical repair of choanal atresia may offer improved patency results.

◆ Outcome and Follow-Up

Postoperative care should include daily suctioning of stents, serial endoscopy, and dilation. The rate of restenosis varies widely, with reports between 50 and 100%. Both transnasal and transpalatal approaches seem to have similar rates of restenosis.

8.19 Cleft Lip and Palate

◆ Key Features

- Group 1: Cleft lip
  - Unilateral or bilateral
  - Complete (extension to nasal floor)
  - Incomplete (muscle diastases: vermillion to bridge of tissue at nasal sill)
- Group II: Cleft palate
  - Unilateral or bilateral
  - Secondary palate only
- Group III: Cleft lip and cleft palate
  - Complete cleft palate (both primary and secondary palate)
- Group IV: Cleft palate
  - Unilateral or bilateral
  - Primary palate only

Cleft lip and cleft palate can be classified as syndromic (15–60%) or nonsyndromic. Syndromic associations include Apert's, Stickler's, Treacher Collins's, and Waardenburg's syndromes. Cleft lip with or without cleft palate is believed to be genetically distinct from isolated cleft palate. Nonsyndromic clefts may be secondary to exposure to teratogens (e.g., ethanol, anticonvulsants, steroids, vitamin A excess). Likewise, maternal and intrauterine factors such as gestational diabetes, smoking, or amniotic bands may play a role.

Typically, cleft palate management is done by a team including surgeons, dentists, orthodontists, speech pathologists, and audiologists.

◆ Embryology of the Lip and Palate

The palate is embryologically divided into the primary (the maxillary alveolus and palate anterior to the incisive foramen), and secondary (originating posterior to the incisive foramen and terminating at the uvularis) components. Fusion of the paired median nasal prominences (MNPs) gives rise to the primary palate. This process initiates the separation of the oral from the nasal cavity. The coalescence of the MNPs forms the central maxillary alveolar arch, central and lateral incisors, anterior hard palate, premaxilla, philtrum of the upper lip, columella, and nasal tip. The genesis of the central upper lip occurs in association with the primary palate. The frequent association of these deformities is not unexpected. The remainder of the upper lip, lateral to the philtrum, is formed by fusion of the paired MNPs medially with the maxillary processes laterally.

Formation of the secondary palate is initiated by contact of the nasal septum to the lateral palatal shelves at the incisive foramen. The medialization of the palatal shelves then occurs in an anterior to posterior direction. The midline tongue represents a barrier to this medialization. Development of the mandible results in anterior displacement of the tongue, allowing normal growth of the palatal shelves. Failure of this process results in the Pierre Robin's sequence (micrognathia, relative macroglossia, and U-shaped cleft palate); see also **Chapter 8.8**.

There is not only an embryologic structural division of the palate, but a temporal one as well. The primary palate forms during weeks 4 to 7 of gestation. The secondary palate begins development after completion of the primary palate and occurs during weeks 8 to 12 of gestation.

◆ Epidemiology

Cleft lip and palate are the most common congenital malformations of the head and neck. The incidence of cleft lip with or without cleft palate in the United States is 1:1,000 newborns and varies according to race, with the highest incidence in Native Americans and a male/female ratio of 2:1. The incidence of cleft palate is 1:2,000 and is equal across ethnic groups, with a male/female ratio of 1:2.

◆ Clinical

Signs

See the classification of defects noted under Key Features. Signs of submucous cleft palate include:

- Bifid uvula
- Zona pellucida
- Notched hard palate

Symptoms

The symptoms are feeding difficulties with nasal regurgitation.

Differential Diagnosis

Associated syndromes include:

- Pierre Robin's sequence: Micrognathia, glossoptosis, and U-shaped cleft palate
- Stickler's syndrome: Retinal detachment, cataracts, and early arthritis
- Treacher Collins's syndrome: Eyelid colobomas, middle ear ossicular abnormalities, and malformation of facial bones
- Apert's syndrome: Acrocephaly, fused digits, and stapes fixation

◆ Evaluation

Physical Exam

- Determine type of defect:
  - Unilateral, bilateral, median
  - Complete (extension to nasal floor) or incomplete (submucosal)
  - Primary (anterior to incisive foramen) or secondary (posterior to incisive foramen)
- Look for associated defects:
  - Facial defects: telecanthus, maxillary/malar hypoplasia, nasal deformities, facial nerve paralysis
  - Otologic anomalies, which should be examined if they exist
  - Synostoses
- Determine presence of associated syndrome. Apert's, Stickler's, Treacher Collins's, Waardenburg's syndromes, and Pierre Robin's sequence are associated with cleft palate.
- Cleft lip nasal deformity

Dehiscence of the orbicularis oris muscle results in its abnormal, nonanatomic insertion laterally onto the ala and medially onto the columella. The subsequent muscular tension produces a characteristic nasal deformity. The nasal tip and columella are deflected to the noncleft side. The cleft-side ala is positioned laterally, inferiorly, and posteriorly. The cleft nostril is widened and horizontally oriented. The septum is bidirectionally affected. Whereas the caudal aspect deflects toward the noncleft side, the remainder of the cartilaginous and bony septum deflects toward the cleft side. This results in decreased air entry through both nasal passages.

The bilateral cleft nasal deformity is dependent on the severity of the individual sides. If both sides are equally involved, the nasal tip is typically midline, poorly defined, and frequently bifid. Both sides are composed of obtuse domal angles and widened, horizontally oriented nostrils. The alae are both positioned laterally, inferiorly and posteriorly. The septum is midline. If there is asymmetry of the cleft lip, deformities of the nasal tip, columella, and septum are deviated to the less affected side; however, the deflection is less apparent than it would be with a normal side.

Imaging

Adjunctive imaging may be required for the investigation of syndromic etiology.

Other Tests

Close audiologic monitoring is warranted given the increased incidence of acute otitis media (OM) and serous OM due to eustachian tube dysfunction in this population.

◆ Treatment Options

Medical

- Parental counseling
- Ensure adequate feeding and nutrition
  - Cleft lip and alveolus—often feed normally by bottle or breast
  - Complete cleft lip or palate—often have feeding problems initially
    - Inability to generate sufficient seal around the nipple
    - Increased work of feeding and swallowing of air
    - Specialty nipple may be required
      - Preemie nipple
      - Haberman feeder
      - Mead-Johnson cross-cut nipple
      - Squeeze bottle nurser
    - Palatal prosthesis for wide clefts for continued feeding difficulties

Surgical

- Lip adhesion
  - Converts a complete cleft lip into an incomplete cleft lip
  - Performed at 2 to 4 weeks of age
  - Allows definitive lip repair to be performed under less tension at 4 to 6 months of age
  - Criteria:
    - Wide unilateral complete cleft lip and palate where conventional lip repair would produce excessive incisional tension
    - Symmetric wide bilateral complete cleft lip with prominent premaxilla
    - Converts an asymmetric bilateral cleft lip to a symmetric cleft lip
  - Disadvantage: Scar tissue that may later interfere with definitive surgical management of the lip
- Cleft lip repair
  - "Rule of tens" for timing of cleft lip repair
    - Age ≥ 10 weeks
    - Weight ≥ 10 lb
    - Hemoglobin ≥ 10 g

- o Surgical approaches:
  - ■ Millard rotation advancement technique (**Fig. 8.6**)
  - ■ Tennison-Randall: Single triangular flap interdigitation (**Fig. 8.7**)
  - ■ Bardach: Double triangular flap interdigitation
  - ■ Straight line closure (uncommon)

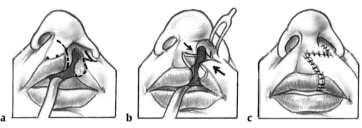

Fig. 8.6 (**a,b,c**) Millard rotation advancement lip repair.

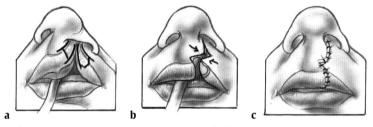

Fig. 8.7 (**a,b,c**) Tennison-Randall triangular flap lip repair.

- • Cleft palate repair
  - o The exact timing of surgical closure of cleft palate is controversial.
  - o There is a balance between establishing the velopharyngeal competence necessary for speech and the potential negative influence of early repair on maxillofacial growth and occlusion.
  - o It is usually performed between 9 and 16 months of age.
  - o Surgical approaches:
    - ■ Schweckendiek: Closure of soft palate only
    - ■ Von Langenbeck: Two bipedicle mucoperiosteal flaps are created by incising along the medial cleft edges and along the posterior alveolar ridge from the maxillary tuberosities to the anterior level of the cleft. They are mobilized medially and closed in layers (**Fig. 8.8**).
    - ■ Bardach: Two-flap palatoplasty for complete cleft palate repair
    - ■ Furlow palatoplasty: Double Z-plasty for secondary cleft palate repair (**Fig. 8.9**)
    - ■ V-Y pushback technique for secondary cleft palate repair
  - o Tympanostomy tubes are commonly inserted at the time of palate repair.

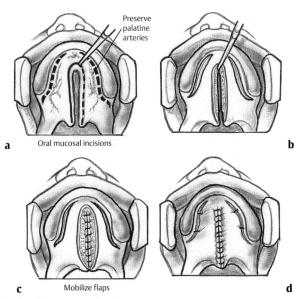

Fig. 8.8 (a–d) Von Langenbeck repair.

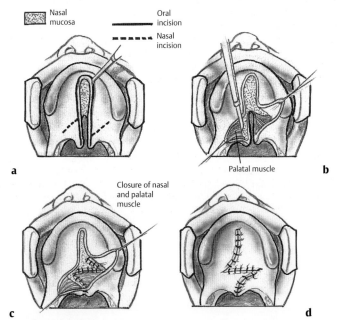

Fig. 8.9 (a–d) Furlow palate lengthening procedure ("double opposing Z-plasty").

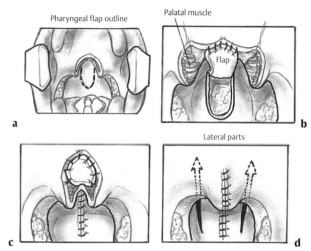

Fig. 8.10   **(a–d)** Palatal flap.

◆ Complications

Primary or secondary hemorrhage is uncommon but may require a return to the OR for management. Oronasal fistula is managed with secondary repair. Velopharyngeal insufficiency is failure of closure of the velopharyngeal sphincter, resulting in incomplete separation of the nasal cavity from the oral cavity. During speech, air leaks into the nasal cavity, resulting in hypernasal vocal resonance and nasal emissions. During feeding, it can result in nasal regurgitation of food. Treatment options may include speech therapy, palate lengthening (**Fig. 8.9**), a palatal flap (**Fig. 8.10**), and augmentation of the posterior pharyngeal wall.

◆ Outcome and Follow-Up

Postoperative care should include pain control, the establishment of a feeding plan, and monitoring of the airway. Routine surgical follow-up is required for cleft repairs at 4 weeks with growth and feeding assessment. Ongoing evaluation and management of the middle ear in combination with audiologic assessment should be completed every 6 months. There should be a referral to a speech therapist for assessment and therapy.

9 Facial Plastic and Reconstructive Surgery

Section Editor
Jessyka G. Lighthall

Contributors
Daniel G. Becker
Ara A. Chalian
Donn R. Chatham
John L. Frodel Jr.
David Goldenberg
Bradley J. Goldstein
Robert M. Kellman
Ayesha N. Khalid
Christopher K. Kolstad
Theda C. Kontis
J. David Kriet
Phillip R. Langsdon
Jessyka G. Lighthall
E. Gaylon McCollough
Michael P. Ondik
Stephen S. Park
Francis P. Ruggiero
John M. Schweinfurth
Dhave Setabutr
Scott J. Stephan
Jonathan M. Sykes
Travis T. Tollefson
Robin Unger
Jeremy Watkins

9.1 Craniomaxillofacial Trauma

For ear and temporal bone trauma, see **Chapter 3.1.2**. For laryngeal fractures, see **Chapter 5.1.2**. For neck trauma, see **Chapter 6.1.4**.

9.1.1 Nasal Fractures

◆ Key Features

- Nasal fractures are the most common head and neck fracture.
- They have aesthetic and functional implications.
- Septal hematoma should be recognized early and managed immediately.
- Closed reduction may reduce the need for delayed treatment.
- Open reduction may be necessary.
- Even if no surgical intervention is initially planned, the patient should be reevaluated in 1 to 2 weeks after any traumatic swelling has resolved.
- Cartilaginous injury, persistent deformity, or persistent nasal obstruction may require delayed functional septorhinoplasty.

The clinical presentation of a nasal fracture may include a history of nasal trauma with associated pain, edema, epistaxis, change in external nasal appearance, nasal airway obstruction, and infraorbital ecchymosis. Imaging is not necessary to diagnose a nasal fracture but may be indicated to rule out other injuries. Deformities that are not immediately identified may become obvious as edema resolves. Treatment may be immediate or delayed based on history, exam, and patient desires. Even if immediate intervention is performed, appropriate follow-up is necessary to identify persistent deformities or nasal obstruction.

◆ Epidemiology

Nasal fractures are cited as the most common type of facial fracture, accounting for approximately half of all facial fractures. These injuries occur largely in the younger, physically active segments of the population and predominantly in males. The most common mechanism is blunt trauma (e.g., accidents, assault, sports), although these fractures also occur via penetrating and high-energy injuries. Nasal fractures occur not only in isolation but also frequently in conjunction with more extensive facial fractures.

◆ Evaluation

A detailed history on mechanism of injury, patient symptoms, associated complaints, premorbid status of the nose, and a general health history should be obtained.

Physical examination is critical in the diagnosis of nasal fractures and may be facilitated if the nose is decongested. Visual inspection, manual palpation, and anterior rhinoscopy are essential. Nasal endoscopy may be performed to increase the acquisition of meaningful clinical data when necessary (**Fig. 9.1**).

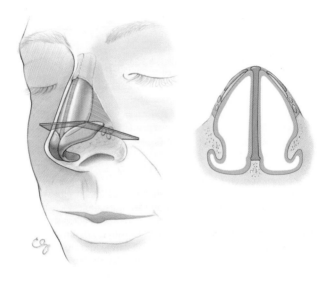

Fig. 9.1   Cross-section of the nose. Note the supporting soft tissue structures and attachment to the lateral nasal wall. Preservation of the lower portion of the lateral bony nasal wall is critical to preventing nasal airway narrowing postoperatively. (Used with permission from Papel ID, ed. *Facial Plastic and Reconstructive Surgery*. 4th ed. New York, NY: Thieme; 2016:439.)

After a focused facial trauma exam to rule out associated injuries, the nose should be examined. The integrity of the nasal skin should be assessed. Often, nasal edema limits visual examination. Palpation of the nose is critical to making the correct diagnosis. All aspects of the nose should be evaluated. Globally, the examiner should determine whether the nose is straight, whether there is a deviation, or whether other dorsal deformities exist (e.g., C-shaped deformity, saddle deformity, etc.). Palpation of the nasal bones will identify fracture of the bony pyramid as a segment versus more complex comminuted injuries. The examiner should assess rotation, projection, and tip and sidewall support. Anterior rhinoscopy must be performed to assess the status of the septum. Determining the status of the septum is frequently underemphasized; however, appropriate appreciation and management of septal injuries is essential to the restoration of optimal nasal function and appearance. The examiner should look for and document the presence or absence of a septal hematoma. If present, it should be expeditiously and appropriately managed.

Photographs should be taken, similar to the views obtained for rhinoplasty evaluation. Planar radiographs and computed tomography (CT) rarely add more valuable data than those obtained through the physical examination and medical history unless an associated injury is suspected based on exam (e.g., telecanthus, dystopia).

◆ Treatment Options

Observation

If minimal displacement of the nasal bones, minimal soft tissue injury, and minimal compromise of the nasal airway exists, observation is appropriate. Patients should be followed within 1 to 2 weeks once edema has resolved to confirm that no posttraumatic deformity exists.

Closed Manipulation

In the case of obvious bony deviation or more severe nasal bone or septal injuries, a closed reduction, with or without splinting, may be warranted. This may be performed under local or general anesthesia, based on patient and surgeon preference. Manipulation is typically performed within 2 to 3 days of injury prior to bony healing of the fracture. During closed reduction, the patient's fractured nasal bones and septum are mobilized and reduced digitally. This may be aided with the use of blunt instruments such as the Boies elevator or Ashe forceps. Traditional closed manipulation is best applied in patients who have actual subluxation or displacement of the nasal bones without comminution of the nasal bones themselves. However, closed reduction may be attempted in the latter case with the use of intranasal and extranasal stabilization.

Modified Open Reduction with Osteotomies

The modified open technique is a limited version of an open technique in which intranasal incisions are made for the introduction of osteotomes. Such patients frequently benefit from manipulation of the nasal bones into position after undergoing bilateral micro-osteotomies. As with closed manipulation, the position of the septum may impede the success of this technique. A secondary procedure may then be necessary or other treatment offered.

Open Nasal/Septal Repair

The open nasal/septal repair refers to an aggressive approach to the acute management of complicated injuries using existing lacerations or external and intranasal incisions. With this approach the surgeon can reduce, graft, and fixate fractured anatomic components under direct visualization.

Formal Septorhinoplasty

Formal septorhinoplasty after nasal fracture is employed in two general clinical situations. Septorhinoplasty may be used as a delayed primary treatment for late patient presentation or persistent deformity and/or obstruction after a period of fracture observation. It may also be used as a secondary procedure after initial acute management with persistent deformity or obstruction. Precise treatment plan is selected based on anatomic diagnosis of persistent deformities and may include osteotomies and repositioning of the bony pyramid, septoplasty, and grafting.

◆ Outcome and Follow-Up

Up to half of untreated nasal fractures require delayed surgical intervention. Immediate closed manipulation reduces the need for delayed intervention in appropriate cases. After nasal bone reduction, externally stabilizing dressings should be applied similarly to standard rhinoplasty care, and the patient should avoid activities that may lead to nasal trauma for 4 to 6 weeks. When there have been significant septal injuries, internal soft Silastic splints may provide stabilization and aid in the prevention of synechiae. Nasal bones may be supported by intranasal supports placed under the nasal bones. Packing is rarely necessary. Patients should be followed until healing is complete with satisfactory functional and aesthetic results.

9.1.2 Naso-Orbito-Ethmoid Fractures

◆ Key Features

- A naso-orbito-ethmoid fracture is a severe injury involving depression of nasal bones into ethmoids with associated medial orbital wall fracture.
- It is secondary to a high-energy mechanism; often associated with intracranial and other severe injuries.
- Treatment requires open reduction with internal fixation (ORIF).

Naso-orbito-ethmoid (NOE) fractures result from a high-energy injury, such as a motor vehicle accident. Accordingly, multiple serious injuries are often present, requiring neurosurgery, ophthalmology, and otolaryngology, and/or facial plastic surgery care. Treatment is directed at minimizing complications and achieving adequate functional and cosmetic repair.

◆ Epidemiology

NOE fractures result from severe trauma to the frontal and midface region. The most common mechanism is a motor vehicle accident with an unrestrained driver. Seatbelt and airbag use has reduced its incidence in recent decades to approximately 5% of all facial fractures in adults and around 15% in children.

◆ Clinical

Signs and Symptoms

Often, patients with NOE fractures have other life-threatening injuries due to the high-energy mechanism and require initial trauma evaluation and stabilization. These fractures rarely occur in isolation, and the most common concomitant facial injuries include frontal sinus fractures and LeFort pattern midface fractures. Eye and brain injuries are common. Concurrent ocular injury, such as globe rupture, lens dislocation, retinal detachment, or vitreous hemorrhage, occurs in ~ 30% of patients. Patients may have cerebrospinal fluid (CSF) leakage due to disruption of the anterior skull base. Typical associated signs and symptoms include severe epistaxis, CSF rhinorrhea, diplopia, epiphora, facial lacerations and severe facial pain. The typical facial deformity resulting from disruption of the ethmoids and medial canthal tendon attachments includes flattening of the nasal dorsum, upward tip rotation with loss of projection, and increased interpupillary distance (traumatic telecanthus).

Differential Diagnosis

It is important to differentiate NOE fractures from isolated nasal fractures (see **Chapter 9.1.1**), orbital fractures (see **Chapter 9.1.3**), and fractures that involve only the ethmoid air cells. Computed tomography (CT) imaging allows rapid, definitive diagnosis.

◆ Evaluation

History

The mechanism of injury will help determine possible injuries and severity. Often, the patient may be unable to provide history because of loss of consciousness, altered mental status, or intubation/sedation.

Physical Exam

Exam, as with all traumas, begins with ABCs (airway, breathing, circulation). Care must be taken to protect the cervical spine until it has been cleared. Head and face are inspected and palpated for ecchymoses, soft tissue injuries, skeletal stability, and bony step-offs. Telecanthus results from NOE fractures. The average intercanthal distance ranges from 25 to 35 mm; this is usually 50% of interpupillary distance. A distance of ≥ 40 mm is considered diagnostic of telecanthus (**Fig. 9.2**).

The medial canthal tendon attachment is easily evaluated with the "bowstring" test (**Fig. 9.3**). While palpating the tendon insertion at the lacrimal crest, the examiner retracts the lower lid laterally. If the tendon insertion is intact, the examiner will feel it tighten like a bowstring. Ideally, the nose should be decongested to allow for an intranasal exam. With use of a headlight and speculum, clots and blood are suctioned and mucosal tears,

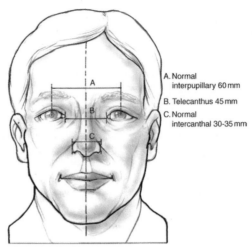

Fig. 9.2   The normal intercanthal distance and telecanthus. (Courtesy of the AO Foundation/AO Surgery Reference.)

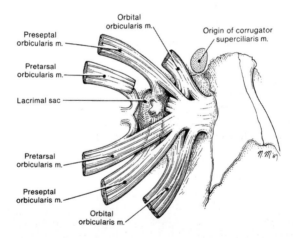

Fig. 9.3   The medial canthal tendon. (Used with permission from Papel ID, ed. *Facial Plastic and Reconstructive Surgery.* 4th ed. New York, NY: Thieme; 2016:816.)

position of the septum, and possible hematomas are noted. Clear fluid may represent a CSF leak. A drop of this fluid on gauze may reveal a "halo sign" indicative of CSF and suggesting concomitant anterior skull base disruption. As globe injuries are common, a thorough ophthalmologic evaluation should be performed.

Imaging

Thin-cut multiplanar CT is the most useful imaging study. Fractures of the facial and nasal bones are readily visualized, with excellent detail of the medial orbital walls and lacrimal region. The integrity of the skull base may be assessed, as well as the presence of pneumocephalus or other intracranial injury. NOE fractures can be categorized according to the degree of commi-nution at the medial canthal tendon insertion:

- Type I: Large central fragment
- Type II: Comminution of central fragment but not involving the tendon
- Type III: Comminution involving lacrimal fossa and tendon attachment site with tendon laceration

Labs

Lab studies may be indicated, including complete blood count (CBC), pro-thrombin time (PT), partial thromboplastin time (PTT), serum electrolytes, β-2-transferrin analysis of clear nasal drainage, and a toxicology screen.

◆ Treatment Options

Treatment of an NOE fracture typically requires ORIF once the patient is sta-bilized. For relatively limited fractures, an external ethmoidectomy incision may afford adequate exposure. Often the surgeon may take advantage of large lacerations for bony exposure. However, a coronal incision is generally used and affords excellent exposure to the NOE region and allows treatment of upper facial skeleton (frontal bone or frontal sinus) injuries. Stabilization of the central fracture fragment, to which the medial canthal tendon is attached, is achieved with plating to stable bone, especially in type I and II injuries. Transnasal wiring is often necessary to achieve an adequate result, especially in type III injuries, in which severe comminution is present with detachment of the medial canthal tendon. Many surgeons advocate slight initial overcorrection. Bone grafting may be necessary.

◆ Outcome and Follow-Up

Patients are often admitted secondary to their severe concomitant injuries for multidisciplinary treatment. The need for perioperative antibiotics is controversial. Frequent vision examinations are performed following repair of orbital fractures, and neurologic checks are performed for concomitant skull base and intracranial injuries. Infection, hematoma, or vision change requires prompt attention to correct underlying issues. Possible complica-tions of NOE fractures and their treatment include persistent telecanthus, nasal deformity, CSF leak, intracranial infection, standard postoperative complications, and unrecognized concomitant frontal sinus outflow tract injury with chronic frontal sinusitis or mucocele. Some authors recommend annual evaluation with CT scan to rule out the latter.

9.1.3   Zygomaticomaxillary and Orbital Fractures

◆ Key Features

- Zygomaticomaxillary complex (ZMC) fractures are the most common facial fractures after nasal bone fractures.
- ZMC fractures involve disruption of the maxillofacial buttresses.
- Features of an orbital floor blowout fracture may include enophthalmos, V_2 numbness, diplopia, and an orbital rim fracture.
- The fractured ZMC is most often displaced posteriorly and inferiorly.

Midface fractures require high force and may lead to aesthetic and functional deficits. Zygomaticomaxillary complex (ZMC) fractures are considered tetrapod fractures if they involve the zygomaticomaxillary, frontozygomatic, zygomaticotemporal, and zygomaticosphenoid sutures. Undiagnosed orbital or ZMC fractures may lead to delayed functional and aesthetic deficiencies. Treatment often requires surgical intervention with open reduction and internal fixation.

◆ Epidemiology

ZMC fractures often occur in conjunction with orbital fractures. Zygoma fractures are most common in men (in the third decade) and are most commonly caused by blunt force trauma from sports injuries, motor vehicle accidents, or assault. Up to 30% of midface and periorbital fractures have a concomitant orbital injury.

◆ Clinical

Signs and Symptoms

Patients suffering ZMC or orbital fractures typically present with a history of blunt trauma with development of periorbital edema or ecchymosis, lacerations, pain, vision changes, trismus, facial deformity. Numbness of the ipsilateral upper lip, gum, nostril, and cheek is common due to fractures through the infraorbital foramen because of injury to cranial nerve (CN) V_2 (the maxillary nerve). Orbital signs include chemosis, subconjunctival hemorrhage, proptosis, enophthalmos, and diplopia. Entrapment of the inferior rectus muscle in an orbital floor fracture results in diplopia due to impaired extraocular muscle function. Palpation of the zygoma may show stepoffs, mobility, or crepitus. Malocclusion may result from either a mobile midface (Le Fort) fracture or a concomitant mandible fracture. A depressed zygoma fracture may cause trismus by compressing the coronoid.

Differential Diagnosis

The spectrum of fractures in the zygoma, maxilla, and orbital bones can range from isolated to complicated, from severely displaced to greenstick, and from simple to comminuted. Classification should begin with assessing for midface instability, which would indicate a Le Fort fracture (see **Chapter 9.1.5**). Assessment of the seven bones that constitute the orbit (lacrimal, palatine, frontal, ethmoid, zygomatic, maxillary, and sphenoid) most often reveals fractures at the weakest bones: the lamina papyracea (ethmoid) and orbital floor (maxilla). Imaging is critical for appropriate diagnosis.

◆ Evaluation

Physical Exam

As with any trauma patient, establishing the ABCs and obtaining cervical spine clearance should be the first priority. The full head and neck examination must include cranial nerve testing, an ophthalmologic evaluation, and a maxillofacial skeletal assessment. Le Fort fractures have palatal mobility, which can be examined by grasping the upper teeth and pulling the maxillary arch forward and inferiorly. Finger palpation for step-off deformities of the orbital rims, zygoma, nasal bones, and frontozygomatic suture can help determine the site of fractures, although edema may make this difficult. The dermatome of CN V_2 should be tested and documented. Extraocular movement and vision testing may demonstrate diplopia or an entrapped inferior rectus muscle.

Forced duction testing may be performed by topically anesthetizing the conjunctiva with tetracaine drops, grasping the episcleral tissue in the fornix (near the inferior oblique insertion) with fine forceps, and testing the mobility of the globe for restriction that could indicate an impinged inferior oblique muscle in an orbital floor fracture. Facial nerve function should be assessed, especially when overlying lacerations are present. An ophthalmologic consult is often performed prior to fracture repair. Retinal detachment or retrobulbar hematoma may preclude immediate surgery or require orbital decompression, respectively.

Imaging

Fine-cut multiplanar maxillofacial computed tomography (CT) scan is the gold standard. Three-dimensional reconstruction, if available, enables an easy assessment of any displacement of the ZMC. Additionally, sagittal or parasagittal cuts improve evaluation of the orbital floor in conjunction with the coronal views. The pterygoid plates and zygomatic arches are best seen on axial films; the orbital rims, floor, and cribriform plate require coronal cuts. Subcutaneous air or intraconal air is often seen with both ZMC and orbital fractures. Foreign bodies or bone fragments near the optic nerve should be identified on CT to prevent damage during fracture reduction. For orbital floor fractures, bone and periorbital disruption should be assessed. The degree of floor disruption, amount of soft tissue herniation, and signs of entrapment should be evaluated. For zygoma fractures, imaging will enable more specific classification of the ZMC fracture, determine the severity of the fracture pattern, and assess the degree and direction of displacement.

◆ Treatment Options

Minimally displaced fractures can be managed with observation. Patients should be followed until full resolution of edema to confirm the absence of functional or aesthetic deficiencies. Isolated zygomatic arch fractures may be treated with a transoral (Keen), temporal (Gilles), percutaneous, or, rarely, coronal approach (comminuted fractures).

Displaced ZMC fractures should be repaired with open reduction and internal fixation. Approaches often include a combination of transoral (to address the maxillary buttress), lower eyelid (orbital rim and floor), and upper eyelid (frontozygomatic) approaches. Additionally, lacerations may be used to assess the fractured segments. Severe fractures may require a coronal approach for repair. Typically two- to four-point fixation with wires or miniplates to stabilize the ZMC is required.

Significant controversy exists regarding the need for operative repair of orbital floor fractures. In general, large fractures with significant soft tissue herniation, immediate enophthalmos, muscle entrapment, or a persistent oculocardiac reflex are indications for surgery. Transconjunctival, transcutaneous lower lid, and transantral/endoscopic approaches may be used based on surgeon experience and fracture characteristics. Basic tenets are to reduce herniated soft tissue and to restore normal orbital volume by reconstructing the orbital floor. Many types of implant materials are available for floor and wall reconstruction.

◆ Complications

Increased intraocular pressure from an orbital hemorrhage can cause vision loss from the injury itself or as a complication of repair. Prompt treatment includes immediate lateral canthotomy and cantholysis, intravenous (IV) steroids (methylprednisolone), ophthalmology consult, and an urgent CT scan. Orbital decompression may be necessary. The most common complications of orbital floor repair are inadequate fracture reduction with subsequent enophthalmos or diplopia, eyelid malposition, corneal abrasion, chronic lower eyelid edema, and chemosis. Complications after ZMC repair include poor reduction with cosmetic deformity and flattening of the malar eminence, intraoral wound dehiscence, and hardware complications (loosening, palpability, exposure).

◆ Outcome and Follow-Up

The use of perioperative antibiotics and steroids is controversial. Strict precautions for no nose blowing should be enforced to prevent subcutaneous and intraorbital air. Patients should be followed until good functional and aesthetic results are confirmed.

9.1.4 Frontal Sinus Fractures

♦ Key Features

- Frontal sinus fractures represent 5 to 15% of all craniomaxillofacial fractures and the third most common facial fracture.
- A primary cause is high-velocity blunt force found in motor vehicle accidents (60–70% of frontal sinus fractures) and assault.
- These fractures range from simple nondisplaced anterior table fractures to comminuted ones involving brain injury and cerebrospinal fluid (CSF) leak.
- It is critical to assess the frontal sinus outflow tract (FSOT).
- Long-term follow-up is the key to early diagnosis of mucocele formation.

The paired frontal sinuses are housed completely within the frontal bone. The frontal bone forms the upper facial skeleton and is closely related to the brain, orbits, and nasal cavities. The frontal sinus is absent at birth and develops in childhood due to pneumatization of the frontal bone, creating a mucosa-lined sinus with an anterior and a posterior bony table. It is bordered by the orbit inferolaterally and by the dura, cribriform plate, and frontal lobes of the brain posteriorly, and it connects to the intranasal cavity inferiorly via the FSOT. Displaced frontal sinus fractures may result in forehead deformities, traumatic injury to the brain, CSF leak, and FSOT obstruction.

♦ Epidemiology

The frontal bone has the highest tolerance of direct blunt force of the facial bones, with the anterior table typically able to withstand 800 to 2,200 lbs. of force (3,600–9,800 N) (**Fig. 9.4**). Because of its greater thickness compared with the posterior wall, a force strong enough to fracture the anterior table will usually fracture the posterior table and cause damage to the outflow tracts. Due to the high energy required to fracture the sinus, concomitant facial fractures occur in ~ 65% of individuals. Male-to-female ratio is 8:1. Although these fractures can occur at any age, the highest incidence occurs during the third decade of life.

♦ Clinical

Signs and Symptoms

Patients with frontal sinus fractures frequently have other associated facial fractures and severe intracranial or other injuries. Depending on the degree of force, patients may or may not have been conscious during the event and may have suffered significant head trauma. Those who are conscious during the inciting event and remain so will likely complain of frontal pain; forehead swelling, lacerations, and paresthesia may also be present. Obvious

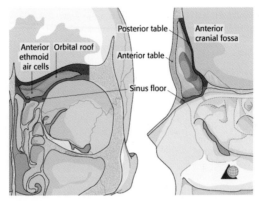

Fig. 9.4   Anterior and lateral views of the frontal sinus demonstrating a thick anterior table and relatively thin posterior table. The floor of the sinus forms the medial portion of the orbital roof. The posterior table forms a portion of the anterior cranial fossa. The anterior table forms part of the forehead, brow, and glabella. (Courtesy of the AO Foundation/AO Surgery Reference.)

forehead deformity may be noted, including significant depression, step-offs, and palpable crepitus, but typically the diagnosis is best characterized via a computed tomography (CT) scan. Epistaxis or CSF discharge may also be evident from the nose or wound.

Differential Diagnosis

Frontal sinus fractures should be distinguished from simple lacerations and contusions of the forehead. Frontal bone fractures can occur without involvement of the sinus, and CSF rhinorrhea is also seen in other isolated facial fractures. Adjacent facial structures must be evaluated for traumatic involvement (zygomaticomaxillary, orbital, naso-orbito-ethmoid [NOE], and skull base fractures).

◆ Evaluation

Physical Exam

It is critical to evaluate the ABCs (airway, breathing, circulation), provide cervical spine stabilization until cleared, and obtain a detailed trauma history and exam. Neurologic and visual status evaluation should be done as soon as potentially life-threatening injuries are addressed. Patients commonly have periorbital edema or ecchymosis, other maxillofacial skeletal instability, or traumatic telecanthus if an NOE fracture is present. Lacerations need to be thoroughly irrigated and probed for evidence of any foreign body or brain tissue. CSF rhinorrhea or otorrhea should be considered if any clear discharge is present.

Imaging

All patients with suspected frontal sinus fractures should undergo a fine-cut multiplanar maxillofacial CT scan. Axial images will allow good visualization of the anterior and posterior tables of the frontal sinus as well as of evidence of pneumocephalus. Coronal views allow visualization of the FSOT, the cribriform plate, and the floor of the frontal sinus, and 3D reconstructions should be requested if available. In general, a displacement of the posterior table of more than one thickness of adjacent bone is considered significant.

Labs

No specific laboratory tests are required for these patients; however, appropriate screening tests (complete blood count [CBC], chemistry, coagulation studies, drug screening, β-transferrin of nasal fluid if CSF leak is suspected) are often obtained during the initial trauma evaluation and may identify conditions warranting treatment.

◆ Treatment Options

The use of antibiotic prophylaxis for frontal sinus fractures is controversial. The evaluation of the patients should be directed at an assessment of whether the dura needs to be repaired, whether the outflow tracts have remained sufficiently functional, and whether there is a significant deformity. The concepts of importance in frontal sinus fracture repair are preventing intracranial infection, preventing frontal sinus disease (such as sinusitis) and mucocele formation, and producing a cosmetically acceptable outcome.

Nondisplaced fractures of the anterior table without evidence of FSOT obstruction and no forehead deformity should be treated nonoperatively. Apart from this fracture, there is no apparent consensus regarding treatment.

The management of frontal sinus injury is evolving, but the goals as just listed have been fairly constant. The management options may include sinus reconstruction and preservation, cranialization of the sinus, and obliteration. Preservation is usually considered in patients with more limited injuries and CT evidence of patent outflow tracts. Cranialization is performed when there has been comminution of the posterior table, necessitating dural repair, and damage to the outflow tracts. Cranialization involves removal of the posterior table of the sinus, removal of all sinus mucosa, obliteration of the outflow tracts, and, typically, placement of a pericranial flap to separate the intracranial and intranasal cavities. Obliteration of the sinus is performed in similar situations as cranialization, but rather than removing the posterior table of the sinus, the surgeon "obliterates" the sinus cavity with fat or other material.

Surgical access for frontal sinus fractures is best made with a coronal flap approach, a supraorbital brow incision, or an existing laceration. Minimally fragmented fractures can be sufficiently reduced with miniplates. Technological advancement now allows for the use of endoscopic assistance to avoid external scars and to avoid frontal sinus fat obliteration by endoscopically opening the nasofrontal outflow tract widely and permanently.

◆ Complications

Complications may include injury to sensory or motor nerves that typically improves over 3 to 12 months, though permanent injury may occur. Persistent CSF leak, FSOT obstruction, chronic frontal sinusitis, frontal sinus mucocele, pneumocephalus, and intracranial infection may occur from the injury or as a result of treatment. Persistent cosmetic deformity, palpable or visible hardware, and scar complications are also a concern.

◆ Outcome and Follow-Up

The patient should be followed closely for the first several months, with particular attention paid to follow-up CT to evaluate for mucocele development. The time frame for mucocele development can range from 2 months to many years, and thus long-term follow-up, while difficult, is necessary.

9.1.5   Midface Fractures

◆ Key Features

- Midface fractures typically result from high-energy blunt trauma, such as motor vehicle accidents and altercations.
- The mass, density, and speed of the striking object will affect the type and the severity of the facial injury.
- Suspect associated ocular, intracranial, and cervical spine injuries.

The midface transmits masticatory forces to the skull base through a series of three paired vertical pillars, or buttresses, of thickened bone: the zygomaticomaxillary (lateral), nasomaxillary (medial), and pterygomaxillary (posterior) buttresses (**Fig. 9.5**). These buttresses are essential for proper facial form and function. The horizontal buttresses also provide facial shape and include the frontal bar and supraorbital rims, the infraorbital rims with nasal bones, and the hard palate. Damage to the midface may involve fractures of any of these buttresses and requires high-force injury.

Proper realignment of the vertical buttresses is critical in establishing premorbid dental occlusion, facial height, and projection. Proper alignment of the orbital rims and maxillary alveolus (palatal fractures) is essential for establishing facial width, while the zygomatic arches play a key role in restoring both facial projection and width.

In 1901, René Le Fort described three predominant types of midface fractures, which he classified as follows (**Fig. 9.6**):

- Le Fort I fractures (horizontal) extend above the dental apices from the zygomaticomaxillary buttress through the nasomaxillary buttress, piriform aperture, and nasal septum.
- Le Fort II fractures (pyramidal) extend through the zygomaticomaxillary buttress, inferior orbital rim and orbital floor, the frontal process of the maxilla, and through the nasofrontal suture.
- Le Fort III fractures (craniofacial disjunctions) follow a fracture pattern extending from the nasofrontal suture along the medial orbital wall, then

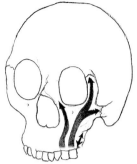

Fig. 9.5 Masticatory forces are transmitted through the zygomaticomaxillary (lateral), nasomaxillary (medial), and pterygomaxillary (posterior) buttresses to the skull base. (Used with permission from Stewart MG, ed. *Head, Face, and Neck Trauma: Comprehensive Management.* New York, NY: Thieme;2005:78.)

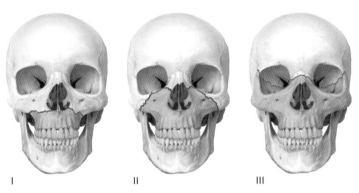

| I | II | III |

Fig. 9.6 Le Fort classification of midfacial fractures (I, II, III). The framelike construction of the facial skeleton leads to characteristic patterns of fracture lines in the midfacial region. (From THIEME Atlas of Anatomy, Head and Neuroanatomy, ©Thieme 2010. Illustration by Karl Wesker.)

traversing the orbital floor and lateral wall before extending through the zygomaticofrontal suture and zygomatic arch.

◆ Epidemiology

Most midface fractures occur in young males and account for 6 to 25% of facial fractures. Motor vehicle collisions and assaults are the most common mechanisms of injury. In older patients, motor vehicle collisions and falls are the typical cause.

◆ Clinical

Signs and Symptoms

Patients typically present with a history of high-force traumatic facial injury and may complain of pain, malocclusion, trismus, hypoesthesia, or diplopia. Examination often reveals periorbital ecchymosis, facial and oral mucosal edema, facial asymmetry, epistaxis, mobility of the midface, malocclusion (anterior open-bite deformity), or dental injury. Less commonly, cerebrospinal fluid (CSF) rhinorrhea and changes in visual acuity or restriction of extraocular motion are observed. Airway distress associated with severe injuries and decreased level of consciousness associated with intracranial injury may also be present. Inquiry should be made as to preinjury malocclusion or orthodontic/orthognathic treatment if possible.

Differential Diagnosis

Malocclusion is also seen in isolated dentoalveolar fractures and mandible fractures. Adjacent facial structures must also be evaluated for traumatic involvement (mandible, zygomaticomaxillary, naso-orbito-ethmoid [NOE], frontal sinus, and skull base fractures).

◆ Evaluation

Physical Exam

As with all trauma patients, the initial evaluation should include a detailed systemic examination using the advanced trauma life support protocol, and then a complete head and neck examination is performed. Airway compromise secondary to mucosal trauma and edema or profuse hemorrhage is possible, requiring securing of the airway. The patient's facial region should be thoroughly inspected and palpated for any bony step-offs. Midface mobility is assessed by applying traction to the maxillary central incisors and alveolus with one hand while stabilizing the forehead with the other. All teeth should be accounted for, and if any are fractured or missing, a chest radiograph should be performed to make sure the missing teeth did not enter the airway. A complete cranial nerve (CN) examination is critical. In the midface, injury to the maxillary division of the trigeminal nerve (CN V_2) is common, and facial nerve (CN VII) injury is also possible. Any deficits are documented prior to surgery. Visual acuity and extraocular motion are evaluated and ophthalmologic consultation obtained if these are abnormal or if ocular injury is suspected. Intranasal examination should assess for septal hematoma, septal perforation, and CSF rhinorrhea.

Imaging

All patients with suspected midfacial fractures should undergo a fine-cut multiplanar computed tomography (CT) scan with 3D reconstruction if available. High-quality reformatted coronal images are acceptable when cervical immobilization prevents direct coronal imaging. Many surgeons now routinely obtain CT images immediately postoperatively to confirm anatomic reduction and plating of the fractures. This is extremely useful in panfacial or comminuted fractures.

Labs

No specific laboratory tests are required for this patient population; however, appropriate screening tests (complete blood count [CBC], chemistry, coagulation studies, drug screening) are often obtained during the initial trauma evaluation and may identify conditions warranting treatment.

Other Tests

When CSF rhinorrhea is suspected, β-2 transferrin testing should be performed on the nasal fluid to confirm the diagnosis.

◆ Treatment Options

The goal of treatment is restoration of preinjury function and facial aesthetics. Treatment within the first 7 to 14 days of injury allows tissue edema to subside and lessens the likelihood of aesthetic and functional deficits, which are challenging to correct after delay.

Medical

Midface fractures that are nondisplaced, stable, and accompanied by normal occlusion can be observed, but the mainstay of treatment for all other midface fractures is surgical.

Surgical

Historically, midfacial fractures were managed with a prolonged course of maxillomandibular fixation (MMF) and/or suspension wires. Continued mobility of the fracture lines with this type of treatment led to a high incidence of residual bony and soft tissue deformity. As such, the standard treatment for displaced, mobile, or comminuted midface fractures is now open reduction and internal fixation (ORIF).

Operative treatment begins with exposure of all fracture lines using surgical approaches that may include gingivolabial (maxillary face and buttresses), transconjunctival or subciliary (orbital rim and floor), upper blepharoplasty (zygomaticofrontal and zygomaticosphenoid sutures), and coronal (zygomatic arches, frontal bone, and NOE area) incisions. The maxilla is then disimpacted and proper occlusion reestablished with MMF.

Reduction of all fractures is then performed along with internal fixation with titanium miniplates along the medial and lateral buttresses and along the inferior orbital rims, zygomaticofrontal sutures, zygomatic arches, and glabellar region as indicated. Consideration should be given to primary bone grafting when interfragmentary gaps > 5 mm are present. Miniplates (typically 1.5–2.0 mm) are used for medial and lateral buttresses. Microplates (1.0–1.3 mm) are used on the inferior orbital rim, and the zygomaticofrontal suture is treated with 1.3- to 1.5-mm plates. Although rigid or semirigid plating has greatly improved our ability to treat these injuries, the surgeon must be meticulous in achieving correct anatomic reduction and use exacting technique when adapting the plate to the bone to avoid "fixing" the patient in the wrong position. Most patients are released from MMF at the conclusion of surgery, although arch bars may be left in place for guiding elastics (occasionally useful with severe edema).

◆ Complications

Complications may include injury to sensory or motor nerves. It is essential to document nerve function prior to surgery. Most patients with sensory change will see improvement over the next 3 to 6 months. Temporary paresis of the temporal branch of the facial nerve may be seen if prolonged retraction during a coronal approach is required, but with careful exposure and surgical technique, permanent injury is rare.

Malocclusion should be noted postoperatively and surgical technique reviewed. CT may be helpful in determining the cause of the malocclusion, and if fracture malalignment is noted, reexploration should be considered, with revision reduction and plating prior to fracture union. Guiding elastics may assist in very minor dental malocclusions but cannot correct grossly malaligned fractures. Persistent facial deformity after bony union may require complex revision surgery with osteotomies or custom implant placement.

Lower eyelid malposition is largely avoided with gentle tissue handling and meticulous surgical technique. Ectropion is more common with transcutaneous than transconjunctival approaches, though entropion may be observed after transconjunctival approaches (rare). Massage is useful in the postoperative period if lower eyelid retraction is noted. More severe malpositions may require surgical intervention.

Other incisional problems include dehiscence, local infection, hypertrophy, and alopecia and are treated as indicated. Hardware exposure, infection, and loosening may require surgical removal after bony union is achieved. Hardware may be palpable. Nonunion and malunion are rare in midface fractures.

◆ Outcome and Follow-Up

The patient is admitted after surgery and monitored for airway status, visual change, hemorrhage, and pain control. Intermittent ice application is useful in decreasing edema, as is elevation of the head of the bed. The patient is instructed in oral hygiene consisting of frequent mouth rinses and gentle brushing, especially after meals. Diet should consist of soft foods for approximately 6 weeks, and then a normal diet may be resumed. Cutaneous sutures are removed ~ 7 days after surgery. Intraoral incisions are closed with resorbable sutures and do not require removal.

The patient should be followed closely for the first several weeks, with particular attention given to occlusal status and eyelid position. Long-term follow-up should also be scheduled, but it can sometimes be challenging in this patient population.

9.1.6   Mandible Fractures

◆ Key Features

- Pain and malocclusion are common findings in mandible fractures.
- Dentoalveolar trauma is often associated.
- Favorable fractures may be treated with closed reduction.
- Open reduction with internal fixation (ORIF) is often required for complex, comminuted, or multiple fractures.

Mandible fractures are common after facial trauma. Diagnosis can often be made by clinical exam, although confirmatory imaging evaluation is required. Fractures often traverse the alveolus, creating intraoral communication with the fracture site, which leads to contamination of fractures by oral flora. Antibiotic use is controversial. Repair is aimed at restoring premorbid occlusion, reestablishing anatomic alignment of the bone fragments, and ensuring healing with minimal morbidity. Mandible fractures are classified as favorable or unfavorable for healing (**Fig. 9.7**).

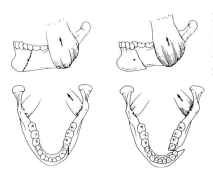

Fig. 9.7 Favorable and unfavorable mandible fractures. (Used with permission from Papel ID, ed. *Facial Plastic and Reconstructive Surgery.* 3rd ed. New York, NY: Thieme;2009:1002.)

◆ Epidemiology

Most mandible fractures are the result of interpersonal trauma or motor vehicle accidents; they typically occur in the third and fourth decades of life. In the elderly, falls become a more common cause, and in younger children sports activities and motor vehicle accidents are most prevalent.

Most studies indicate that the condylar/subcondylar complex is most frequently fractured, followed by the symphyseal region from canine to canine (**Fig. 9.8**). The mandibular angle region is next, followed by the body region. Fractures of the vertical ramus (excluding subcondylar fractures) occur less frequently, and coronoid process fractures are distinctly uncommon. There is some controversy regarding location frequency.

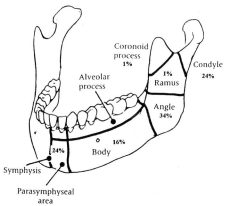

Fig. 9.8 Anatomy of the mandible, with relative incidence of fracture sites. (Used with permission from Papel ID, ed. *Facial Plastic and Reconstructive Surgery.* 3rd ed. New York, NY: Thieme;2009:1001.)

◆ Clinical

Signs

Malocclusion, with or without trismus, may be present. Edema and ecchymosis may be seen both intraorally and extraorally. Loose or fractured teeth should be identified, and attempts should be made to account for missing teeth (intruded teeth may occasionally be mistaken for avulsions). Intraoral lacerations are common at fracture sites. Paresthesia over the chin indicates injury to one or both inferior alveolar nerves.

Symptoms

Most patients with mandible fractures present because of pain or malocclusion, both of which tend to interfere with eating. It is important to establish what the patient's premorbid occlusion was, if possible. Other complaints include oral bleeding, facial swelling, loose teeth, jaw mobility, chin numbness, and trismus.

Differential Diagnosis

If the patient is (or was) unconscious, the nature of the trauma may be difficult to determine. Swelling and muscle injury may masquerade as a fracture. A patient with a serious dental infection, with or without a history of trauma, may have clinical findings of pain, trismus, and malocclusion, which may make it difficult to determine whether a fracture is present. Dislocation of the temporomandibular joints may present with similar symptoms. Other maxillofacial injuries should also be ruled out.

◆ Evaluation

Physical Exam

An initial trauma survey and complete head and neck exam should be performed. If any concern for airway compromise, the airway should be secured. Examine for swelling, tenderness, and ecchymosis. Warmth and fever would be signs of infection, usually seen when presentation is delayed. Examination of the mandible itself might reveal mobility of fragments (to bimanual palpation), trismus, and malocclusion. The occlusion class is based on the relationship of the retrobuccal cusp of the upper first molar to the buccal groove of the lower first molar:

- Class I occlusion (normal): The mesiobuccal cusp of the maxillary first molar occludes exactly with the mandibular first molar buccal groove.
- Class II occlusion: The mesiobuccal cusp is mesial or anterior to the mandibular first molar buccal groove.
- Class III occlusion: The mesiobuccal cusp is distal to the buccal groove.

See **Fig. 9.9**. Also look for loose, cracked, avulsed, and/or impacted teeth. A cranial nerve (CN) exam may show mandibular nerve (CN V_3) hypoesthesia on one or both sides.

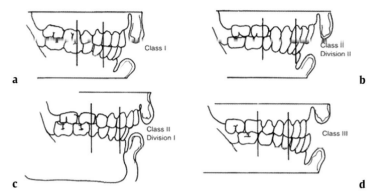

Fig. 9.9 Variants of adult occlusion. **(a)** Class I occlusion or ideal occlusion. **(b,c)** Variants of Class II occlusion. **(d)** Class III occlusion. (Used with permission from Papel ID, ed. *Facial Plastic and Reconstructive Surgery.* 4th ed. New York, NY: Thieme;2016:836.)

Imaging

Plain films are rarely used. A panoramic oral X-ray (Panorex, Dental Imaging Technologies Corp., Hatfield, PA) or fine-cut multiplanar computed tomography (CT) scan (maxillofacial, mandible, or Panorex) should be obtained. Some fractures may be difficult to visualize on Panorex, and in most settings a CT scan is easily acquired and becoming the study of choice.

Labs

No specific labs are required; however, standard preoperative labs may be obtained prior to surgical intervention (complete blood count [CBC], chemistry, coagulation studies, toxicology screen).

Pathology

Pathology studies are generally not applicable, unless there is a concern about a pathologic fracture in a patient with another underlying disease, or in a case of delayed management or complications of prior management, in which there may be concern for posttraumatic mandibular osteitis or osteomyelitis.

◆ Treatment Options

Medical

Nondisplaced, nonmobile favorable fractures without malocclusion can be managed nonsurgically. The patient is maintained on a mechanical soft diet. The patient should be seen after 1 to 2 weeks to ensure patient compliance and that the fracture is healing uneventfully. Any change in occlusion status will require additional treatment.

Subcondylar fractures with minimal displacement and without malocclusion may be managed with physiotherapy and exercises.

For both of the situations just mentioned, mouth-opening exercises are important to prevent trismus.

Relevant Pharmacology

Antibiotic prophylaxis is controversial. Despite a lack of good evidence to support their use, most patients are treated at some point in their care with an antimicrobial agent (preoperatively, perioperatively, or postoperatively). Actively infected wounds should be treated with an antibiotic that covers common oral flora with culture-directed antibiotics if possible. Patients with osteomyelitis may require débridement and prolonged intravenous antibiotics.

Surgical

There are three basic surgical approaches to mandible fractures: (1) placement of oral appliances and application of rigid maxillomandibular fixation (MMF; also called closed reduction, rigid fixation); (2) placement of oral appliances and the use of training elastics (nonrigid MMF; also called nonrigid closed reduction); and (3) open reduction of the fractures, generally used with rigid fixation of the fragments (ORIF).

The most common appliances used for MMF in the United States today are Erich arch bars. These are generally fixed to the teeth with wires and are equipped with small hubs to allow the placement of wires or elastic bands for rigid and nonrigid MMF, respectively. In the past couple of decades, multiple other techniques for MMF have been developed, including intermaxillary screws and multiple hybrid MMF systems that use screws rather than wire fixation of an arch bar. MMF is generally reserved as a solitary treatment option for uncomplicated, isolated, or favorable fractures as well as unilateral subcondylar fractures. MMF is often used intraoperatively to obtain and maintain occlusion prior to rigid fixation.

ORIF may be performed via either intraoral or extraoral approach. "Load-sharing" repairs are generally used when the bone being repaired is solid enough to provide a buttress, so that fixation can be placed in a biomechanically advantaged fashion that takes advantage of the naturally occurring forces of muscle function and mastication. This can be accomplished using the "Champy" technique, with miniplates placed along ideal lines of osteosynthesis with monocortical screws to avoid injury to tooth roots and the inferior alveolar nerve. This technique is commonly used in angle fractures. Two plates or two lag screws are generally used in the symphyseal and parasymphyseal regions, a single plate is commonly used along the mandibular body, and one or two plates are used for angle fractures. Compression plates can be used along the symphysis and body (not at the angle) as well, but this requires that bicortical screws be placed along the inferior border, so tension band plates or arch bars must be applied to avoid distraction of the alveolar portion of the fracture.

"Load-bearing" repairs are used when there is inadequate bone to form a buttress and share in the load. This requires the placement of longer, stronger reconstruction plates fixed with bicortical screws along the inferior border of the mandible. At least three and preferably four screws should be placed on either side of the fracture. Load-bearing reconstruction plate repairs are indicated to span areas of mandibular deficiency, such as defects, areas of comminution, atrophic mandibles (edentulous patients), and areas involved with infection (or previous nonunion). The reconstruction plate is also a fallback technique for any mandible fracture, particularly in the angle region after loss of an impacted third molar. Fractures of the condylar neck should be opened if there is significant foreshortening of the ramus of the mandible or persistent malocclusion. The endoscopic approach allows a mostly transoral repair of selected subcondylar fractures. Open reduction of condylar head fractures remains quite controversial.

Finally, external fixation with placement of a percutaneous external fixator device may be required in severe injuries, significant comminution, or with nonunion/hardware infection.

◆ Complications

A rigidly fixed malreduction should be reoperated, unless there are extenuating circumstances, because MMF cannot repair it. Wound infections should be drained and managed expectantly. Loose hardware must be removed. Failure of fixation requires reoperation, and if infection has developed, a stronger, load-bearing repair will be necessary. Nerve injuries (motor and sensory) should be documented.

◆ Outcome and Follow-Up

Routine wound care is indicated. Oral hygiene must be maintained, and antiseptic oral rinses are commonly used several times daily and after meals. A liquid diet is preferred initially, and this is advanced to a mechanical soft diet as tolerated. The use of postoperative imaging to ensure satisfactory reduction of fractures is controversial. If there is any concern for persistent malocclusion or hardware complication, imaging should be obtained. If satisfactory rigid fixation has been accomplished, MMF will not be necessary. After 1 week, trismus should be treated with mouth-opening exercises. Patients treated with rigid MMF are generally sent to the floor and discharged with wire cutters, in case they need to urgently release the MMF.

Patients should be followed closely for the first 6 weeks. At this point, most fractures are stable enough to allow removal of the arch bars. After this, patients should be followed until normal function is ensured.

9.1.7   Burns of the Head, Face, and Neck

◆ Key Features

- Head and neck burns are commonly associated with inhalation injuries.
- Burns may be due to direct contact with flame, hot water, steam, electrical injury, or chemicals such as bleach.
- Respiratory complications and sepsis can lead to mortality.
- Head and neck soft tissue damage requires consideration of aesthetic units for optimal reconstruction.

◆ Epidemiology

In the United States, more than 400,000 burn injuries require medical treatment annually, with over 40,000 hospital admissions. The majority of burn admissions are to burn centers that can provide specialized care.

◆ Clinical

Burns are classified by the total percentage of the body surface area involved, and the depth of tissue damage. In the adult, the head and neck represent approximately 9% of the total body surface area (head 7%, neck 2%). This same region in the neonate is approximately 19% of the total body surface area. The depth of the burn is estimated from clinical observations of the appearance, sensitivity, and pliability of the wound (**Fig. 9.10**).

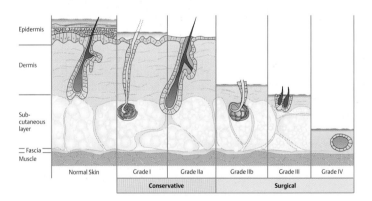

Fig. 9.10   Burn depth and skin layer involvement. (Used with permission from Ernst A, Herzog M, Seidl RO. *Head and Neck Trauma: An Interdisciplinary Approach.* Stuttgart/New York, NY: Thieme;2006:30.)

Signs and Symptoms and Classification

First-degree burns involve only the epidermis. The wounds are erythematous, dry, and not blistering. Such injuries are painful, since sensitive nerve endings are intact, but typically heal in 5 to 10 days.

Second-degree burns involve the epidermis and extend into the dermal layer. They are moist, may blister, and are painful, because uninjured nerve endings are irritated. They are usually hyperemic but may be pale if the injury extends deep into the dermis or if underlying edema has compromised the blood supply.

Third-degree burns appear pale to brown and leathery or carbonaceous black; they are avascular and result from coagulation necrosis of the entire dermis and all deep epidermal elements. Third-degree burn wounds of the head and neck are often accompanied by inhalation injuries and may result from prolonged contact with the flaming environment.

Fourth-degree burns affect all layers of the skin and also structures below the skin, such as tendons, bone, ligaments, and muscles. These burns may not be painful, owing to destruction of nerve endings (**Table 9.1**).

Table 9.1 Classification of burn wounds based on degree of severity

Burn degree	Description
First degree	Damage is limited to the uppermost layers of the epidermis. The result is redness, swelling, tautness, and pain. Spontaneous wound healing through epidermal regeneration and without scar formation.
Second degree	Thermal damage (coagulation, scabbing) extending into the dermis. Serous exudate elevates the upper layer of skin, causing the formation of burn blisters. Wounds are highly painful, because nerve endings are intact. The moist wound bases are at high risk of contamination. Healing may occur spontaneously, from uninjured cutaneous appendages.
Third degree	Full-thickness necrosis; wound base is dry, charred black or with white eschar. Sensation is completely lost. These wounds do not bleed, as vessels have been destroyed.
Fourth degree	Injury to muscle and bone tissue in addition to skin.

Adapted with permission from Ernst A, Herzog M, Seidl RO. *Head and Neck Trauma: An Interdisciplinary Approach*. Stuttgart/New York, NY: Thieme;2006:29.

◆ Evaluation

The otolaryngologist is often involved in caring for severe burn patients to evaluate and manage inhalation injuries. In addition, head and neck/facial plastic surgeons may manage head and neck soft tissue burn reconstruction.

History

History may be helpful in guiding management. Pertinent factors include timing, mechanism, loss of consciousness, and typical factors such as comorbidities.

Physical Exam

Physical examination should be directed to evaluation of injury to the head, neck, and respiratory tract.

Exam for Inhalation Injuries

Burns sustained from confined spaces, or associated with loss of consciousness or intoxication, favor inhalation injury. Inhalation injury has a significant impact on the survival of burn patients. It has three components: upper airway swelling, acute respiratory failure, and carbon monoxide intoxication. Facial, perioral, or neck burns; singeing of nasal hair; oropharyngeal edema; and charring constitute evidence that injury to the respiratory tract may have occurred. Tachypnea, dyspnea, or prolonged expiratory phase may indicate respiratory involvement. Burns of the upper airway are similar to cutaneous burns with reddening, edema, and soot on the oral and pharyngeal mucosa and upper airway passages. Stridor, hoarseness, and dysphonia are evidence of injury already present at the trachea. Fine rales, expiratory wheezes, decreased breath sounds, and increased resonance or dullness to percussion are typically late findings. Fiberoptic laryngoscopy and bronchoscopy may be performed and can assess the extent of airway injury and assist with intubation. Hypoxia due to carbon monoxide occurs rapidly, but subsequent signs develop slowly, affecting the supraglottic within the first day and the more distal airways within 1 to 3 days. Serial exams are, therefore, mandatory.

Exam for Head and Neck Tissue Injuries

The auricle is the most commonly involved site, followed by the nose. The head and neck injury sites are evaluated and categorized in terms of aesthetic units. Key functional sites include the eyelid, the mouth, and the nares. In addition, neck burns may present challenges in terms of potential tracheotomy placement.

Labs and Other Tests

Ongoing pulse oximetry and cardiac monitoring are performed for all patients with significant thermal burns. Laboratory studies typically obtained in burn patients may include complete blood count (CBC), electrolytes, blood urea nitrogen (BUN), creatinine, glucose, venous blood gas (VBG), and carboxyhemoglobin. Arterial blood gas (ABG), chest radiograph, and an electrocardiogram (ECG) are obtained in any patient at risk for inhalation injury. Standard pulse oximetry is *not* reliable with significant carbon monoxide toxicity, and ABGs must be followed.

◆ Treatment Options

The initial management of a severely burned patient is similar to that of any trauma patient. Burn patients should be systematically evaluated using the methodology of the American College of Surgeons Advanced Trauma Life Support course. A modified "advanced trauma life support" primary survey is performed, with particular emphasis on assessment of the airway and breathing. Burned areas should be cooled immediately using cool water or saline soaked gauze. Cooling is especially effective in the first 20 to 30 minutes after being burned.

Inhalation injury remains a leading cause of death in adult burn victims On presentation, burn patients should receive 100% oxygen through a humidified nonrebreather mask. Direct inspection of the oropharynx and larynx should be performed. If there is any concern about the patency of the airway, then intubation is the safest policy. Indications for intubation (often nasotracheal) include hypoxemia, evidence of progressive airway compromise (especially supraglottic edema on fiberoptic exam), or decreased mental status. Early conversion to tracheotomy may be beneficial if prolonged support is anticipated, especially if evidence of significant airway injury is found by exam, the patient is extensively burned, or there is difficulty controlling agitation. Tracheotomy through healthy tissue or graft is preferable than through eschar, which may cause increased infection. Serial bronchoscopic pulmonary toilet and removal of debris, secretions, and sloughing may be necessary.

Fluid management is paramount; however, fluid resuscitation can potentially exacerbate laryngeal swelling. Therefore, intubation should not be delayed if inhalation injury or developing respiratory distress is suspected. Intravenous access should be established with two large-bore cannulas, preferably placed through unburned tissue. A resuscitation regimen should be determined and initiated, usually following the Parkland formula or a similar algorithm: (Volume [mL] = 4× body weight [kg] × percent body area burned × 100) using crystalloid (lactated Ringer's) replacement, with half the volume given during the first 8 hours. Subsequently, adding colloid may be helpful. A urinary catheter is important in all adults with injuries covering > 20% of total body surface area to monitor urine output, which should be 0.5 to 1 ml/kg per hour. Patients with large area burns should receive intravenous morphine at a dose appropriate to body weight.

Burn patients should then undergo a burn-specific secondary. Persons with facial burns should undergo a careful examination of the corneas as well, with ophthalmology consultation.

Specific Treatment

First-degree burns typically heal within a week. Second-degree burns require gentle cleaning and cool compresses; after blisters rupture, they are débrided of nonviable skin and treated with topical ointments. A wide range of topical medications are available, including simple petrolatum, various antibiotic-containing ointments and aqueous solutions, and débriding enzymes. Common topical antimicrobials include mafenide acetate, aqueous 0.5% silver nitrate, and silver sulfadiazine. Third-degree burns are cleaned and initially débrided, then covered with topical antimicrobial ointment initially. For deep burns, the main options are twice daily (BID) cleaning, until granulation bed may be grafted, or early eschar excision and grafting. Tetanus prophylaxis should be given.

Wound membranes are dressings that provide transient physiologic wound closure. These membranes convey a degree of protection from mechanical trauma, via vapor transmission characteristics similar to skin, and a physical barrier to bacteria. Options include porcine xenograft, split-thickness allograft, and various semipermeable membranes such as AlloDerm (BioHorizons, Birmingham, AL) or Integra Bilayer Wound Matrix (Integra LifeSciences, Plainsboro, NJ).

Burns to head and neck anatomic structures require specific attention. Reconstruction should be performed while considering the facial a*esthetic units,* similar to the ideas guiding other facial reconstruction techniques, such as Mohs defects. Deep burns to the eyelids should be excised and grafted early to prevent cicatricial ectropion and corneal exposure. Ophthalmic antimicrobial ointments are necessary. Perioral wounds may require wedge or shield excision and closure. Large burns may need skin grafting as well as advancement of intraoral mucosa to reconstruct a vermilion. Auricular burns require local ointment and débridement but need to be treated with minimal local pressure. Chondritis (with fluctuance and pain) and infection are potential problems, requiring intravenous (IV) antibiotics and removal of necrotic cartilage. Late reconstruction is then performed. Nasal burns may also require complex reconstruction for loss of cartilaginous support. Nasotracheal tubes may require attention to prevent worsening of nostril rim injuries.

Neck burns may lead to several problems that need attention. The compressive effect of a full-thickness burn to the neck may contribute to airway compromise. Without tracheostomy, tight neck eschar accentuates airway edema and contracts the neck into flexion, further compromising the airway. A vertical incision through the eschar, from the sternal notch to the chin, helps maintain a patent airway. Tracheotomy issues have already been discussed.

◆ Complications

- Sepsis
- Infection
- Multiple organ failure
- Scarring
- Contracture
- Tracheotomy problems, such as tracheoesophageal fistula or stenosis

◆ Outcome and Follow-Up

Mortality for burns has decreased over recent decades to approximately 3,800 per year in the United States.

9.2 Facial Paralysis, Facial Reanimation, and Eye Care

◆ Key Features

- No single modality is universally appropriate for all afflictions of facial nerve function.
- Etiology of the paralysis, oncologic status, type of injury, and location of injury all contribute to the selection of the most appropriate treatment methods.
- Eye protection is critical.
- Close patient follow-up and counseling are necessary.

An extensive list of possible etiologic factors for facial paralysis exists. This may be narrowed based on clinical history and exam to direct further work-up. Treatment options may include medical therapies, rehabilitation, static procedures, dynamic procedures, and reanimation. Close follow-up and the setting of realistic expectations are important.

◆ Epidemiology

Facial paralysis may affect individuals of any age but is more common in the fifth to sixth decade. Females are more commonly affected than males.

◆ Clinical

Signs

Facial weakness may occur in select or all branches of the facial nerve. Decreased blink reflex, incomplete eye closure, or lower eyelid rounding may be observed. Deviation of nasal base and philtrum, loss of melolabial fold definition, or a drooped oral commissure are common. Patients may have periauricular vesicles, a body rash, or other neurologic deficits.

Symptoms

A detailed history is the key to identifying the etiologic cause of the facial weakness. A history of preceding illnesses, surgery, or trauma should be elucidated. Travel patterns, particularly in locations endemic with Lyme disease, or a tick bite may be reported. Facial weakness may be described as rapid onset (< 72 hours), delayed onset, progressive, fluctuating, unilateral, or bilateral. It may involve the entire hemiface or select branches. Associated pain or mass raises a concern for malignancy. A full assessment of other neurologic symptoms and a general review of systems should be undertaken.

Differential Diagnosis

There are a myriad of potential causes of facial paralysis. Bell's palsy (idiopathic) is the most common cause and is generally self-limited, with the majority of patients showing complete resolution (see **Chapter 3.1.3**). Other common causes are viral reactivation (Bell's palsy, Ramsay Hunt's syndrome), infection (Lyme disease, otitis media), or injury. Facial paralysis due to nerve injury may be iatrogenic or traumatic.

Intracranial nerve injuries most commonly occur during resection of vestibular schwannoma or other cerebellopontine angle (CPA) tumors. The incidence of facial nerve injury following CPA tumor surgery is reported to be 2.3%. Intratemporal facial nerve injury is usually encountered in patients following external head trauma with skull base fractures or iatrogenic injury during or following otologic surgery. Most temporal bone fractures result from motor vehicle accidents and violent encounters. Seven to 10% of these fractures result in facial nerve dysfunction, with paralysis more common in transverse fractures. Extratemporal injury to the facial nerve may occur during parotid surgery, temporomandibular joint procedures, or facelift procedures or following traumatic lacerations of the face. Patients at higher risk for facial nerve injury during parotid surgery include children and those undergoing a total parotidectomy. The differential may be narrowed by history, exam, and studies as indicated.

◆ Evaluation

Physical Exam

A general neurologic evaluation, complete head and neck exam, and a detailed cranial nerve exam should be performed, as findings may help narrow the differential diagnosis. At a minimum, the degree of facial impairment should be graded by the House–Brackmann Facial Nerve Grading System (**Table 3.3** in **Chapter 3.1.3**), although more detailed and updated grading systems now exist (**Table 9.2**; **Fig. 9.11**).

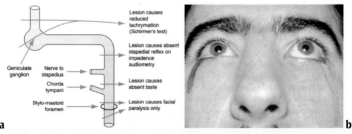

Fig. 9.11 Tests of facial nerve involvement. The level of involvement of the facial nerve in facial palsy can be determined by: **(a)** taste (electrogustometry—if taste is absent or impaired, then the lesion is proximal to the chorda tympani); stapedial reflex (impedance audiometry); or **(b)** lacrimation (Schirmer test litmus paper is placed under the lower lid; if the facial nerve lesion is proximal to or involves the geniculate ganglion, the tears are reduced). These tests are reliable in traumatic section of the facial nerve to detect the level of injury, but in Bell's palsy, these tests are of little value. (Used with permission from Bull TR, Almeyda JS. *Color Atlas of ENT Diagnosis.* 5th ed. New York, NY: Thieme;2010:103.)

Table 9.2   The Sunderland classification of nerve injury

	Type of injury and functional consequence	Structures involved	Management	Prognosis
Class I	Neuropraxia/ compression resulting in temporary dysfunction of Na+ channels, preventing transmission of nerve impulses	Myelin sheath	Watchful waiting ± steroids	Likely full recovery within weeks to months
Class II	Typically a crush or displacement of bony fragments resulting in axonotmesis, with preservation of individual endoneurial channels, resulting in Wallerian degeneration	Myelin, axons	Watchful waiting ± steroids	Likely full recovery over months
Class III	Laceration/ischemic injury resulting in neurotmesis and Wallerian degeneration	Myelin, axon, endoneurium	Surgical repair using suture or fibrin glue	Full recovery unlikely
Class IV	Laceration/ischemic injury resulting in neurotmesis and Wallerian degeneration with damage extended to fascicles, but preservation of the epineurial sheath	Myelin, axon, endoneurium, perineurium	Surgical repair using suture or fibrin glue	Full recovery unlikely
Class V	Laceration/ischemic injury resulting in complete discontinuity of proximal neural elements from distal elements, causing neurotmesis and Wallerian degeneration	Myelin, axon, endoneurium, perineurium, epineurium	Surgical repair using suture or fibrin glue	Full recovery unlikely

Data from Sunderland S. *Nerve Injuries and Their Repair: A Critical Appraisal*. Edinburgh/New York, NY: Churchill Livingstone;1991.

Imaging

Imaging is not routine for all patients, but computed tomography (CT) or magnetic resonance imaging (MRI) may be appropriate, based on history and exam. Facial paralysis in association with other neurologic deficits may warrant imaging to evaluate for stroke or intracranial tumor. Recurrent facial paralysis warrants imaging, typically an MRI scan of the internal auditory canal. Facial paralysis with facial pain or a mass warrants a CT scan or MRI of the face/neck to evaluate for malignancy. Other imaging tests will be performed when clinically indicated.

Labs

Lab studies are not routinely performed on all patients at initial presentation. Specific labs may be ordered based on the clinical scenario and include a complete blood count (CBC), C-reactive protein [CRP], autoimmune labs (antineutrophil cytoplasmic antibody [ANCA], rheumatoid factor [RF], antinuclear antibody [ANA]), tests for syphilis, Lyme titers, glucose, and human immunodeficiency virus (HIV).

Other Tests

The use of electrodiagnostic testing (typically electroneurography [ENoG]) is used in select situations for prognosis and occasionally treatment planning. It is helpful > 72 hours after onset of paralysis and within two weeks. If an ENoG shows > 90% degeneration of the facial nerve, a confirmatory electromyelogram is typically then performed. If this shows no motor unit potentials, a facial nerve decompression may be considered.

◆ Treatment Options

Medical

If a specific clinical diagnosis is not suggested based on history or exam, most authors recommend an initial treatment with a high-dose steroid taper and antiviral therapy, although the latter is controversial. If an underlying disease is identified based on additional studies or findings, then treatment of the underlying disorder is appropriate (doxycycline for Lyme disease, antiretrovirals for HIV, immune modulators for autoimmune disease).

Surgical

The options (in order of preference) for restoration of function following total unilateral facial paralysis are as follows:

1. Spontaneous facial nerve regeneration (observation)
2. Facial nerve neurorrhaphy (facial nerve anastomosis)
3. Interpositional graft (cable graft)
4. Nerve crossovers (anastomosis to other motor nerves)
5. Muscle transfer
6. Static procedures

Dynamic Procedures/Reanimation
● *Facial Nerve Neurorrhaphy*

If the nerve has been completely disrupted, then direct neurorrhaphy is the most effective way to reanimate the paralyzed face. The interrupted neural pathway can be reestablished either by direct anastomosis or by inserting a graft between the disrupted segments. Some of the key points in nerve repair are early identification, evaluation of nerve condition, and tension-free anastomosis. The best time to perform surgery is within the first 72 hours, before degeneration has occurred and while the distal nerve can still be stimulated, although success with exploration and repair has been noted up to several months after injury. It may be necessary to reroute the nerve within the temporal bone or to gain extra length by releasing the nerve. Factors that influence the success of repair include tension, the character of the wound, the presence of scar tissue, and time lag to repair.

The surgical suturing technique for nerve repair requires magnification, either with loupes or a surgical microscope. The nerve endings should be freshened with a new scalpel blade. At this point, axoplasm may be seen oozing from the proximal stump. Number 8–0 to 10–0 nylon sutures with a 75- or 100-micron needle should be used.

If possible, three or four simple sutures should be placed about the circumference of the epineural layers to achieve adequate union (**Fig. 9.12**).

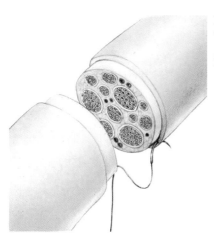

Fig. 9.12 Epineural nerve repair. (Used with permission from Papel ID, ed. *Facial Plastic and Reconstructive Surgery 4th Edition*. New York, NY: Thieme;2016:738.)

● *Interpositional Graft*

In cases where patients have undergone prior surgery or have had part of their facial nerve sacrificed or avulsed as a result of severe trauma, direct nerve repair is impossible and interposition of a nerve graft is required. This technique is reserved for cases in which direct nerve repair would result in excess tension or when there is loss of nerve tissue.

The great auricular nerve is the most commonly used donor nerve, especially when the nerve graft required is small. Advantages include its proximity to the operative field and ease of exposure (**Fig. 9.13**). If more nerve tissue is required, then the sural nerve may be harvested.

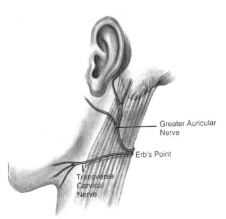

Fig. 9.13 Greater auricular and transverse cervical nerve grafts. (Used with permission from Burgess LPA, Goode RL. *Reanimation of the Paralyzed Face*. New York, NY: Thieme;1994:18.)

Greater Auricular Nerve

Erb's Point

Transverse Cervical Nerve

- *Nerve Crossovers*

This technique is used when direct suturing or cable grafting is not feasible, as is often the case after removal or obliteration of proximal or intratemporal portions of the facial nerve. It is particularly useful to treat facial paralysis resulting from intracranial or intratemporal disorders or surgery. These techniques are relatively simple and require one suture line. They provide a powerful source for reinnervation, although the results are not always consistent or predictable. Nerve crossovers most commonly utilize the hypoglossal nerve, the accessory nerve, or, more recently, the masseteric nerve. As the masseteric nerve is within the operative field, is easy to identify, and produces less morbidity than other nerve sources, it is becoming the donor nerve of choice.

Another technique is the "babysitter" graft. In this technique, the hypoglossal nerve and facial nerve are anastomosed with the interposition of a free nerve graft, end-to-end to the peripheral facial nerve stump and end-to-side to the hypoglossal nerve. This technique is typically used in candidates for cross–facial nerve grafting.

Cross–facial nerve grafting is a technique that uses the contralateral normal facial nerve to innervate certain facial muscles on the paralyzed side. This technique should be considered an alternative to hypoglossal or accessory nerve grafting. It should not be performed as long as spontaneous regeneration is still possible or in cases in which direct or cable grafting of the facial nerve is possible.

● *Muscle Transfer Techniques*

Muscle transfer techniques are used when neural techniques are unsuitable. Patients with longstanding facial paralysis (> 2 years) are unlikely to benefit from any of the reanimation procedures just discussed. Severe fibrosis occurs in the distal neuromuscular unit, along with atrophy of the facial musculature, making reinnervation unlikely.

○ Regional Muscle Transfer

Muscle transfer techniques entail transplanting a new neuromuscular unit into a region of the paralyzed face. This may be done in conjunction with a nerve graft or a crossover implanted in the transferred muscle. The two basic techniques to accomplish this are regional muscle transposition and a free-muscle transfer.

Regional muscle transfer is usually used to reanimate the lower third of the paralyzed face. The new neuromuscular unit is composed of the transposed muscle with its original nerve supply. Muscles available for these procedures include the masseter, temporalis, and digastric. It should be remembered that in all muscle transfer procedures, overcorrection is desired.

○ Temporalis Tendon/Muscle Transfer

In an attempt to enable some dynamic control of the oral commissure and smile symmetry, a temporalis muscle or tendon transfer may be performed. The temporalis muscle may be used to elevate the corner of the mouth. It classically was performed by exposing the insertion in the temple, folding a segment of the muscle over the zygomatic arch, and securing the muscle to the oral commissure. This technique is losing favor because of the secondary deformity of temporal hollowing and a visible bulge over the zygomatic arch. If used, most providers now favor the temporalis tendon transfer, which incorporates a transoral or transcutaneous incision followed by a coronoidectomy and detachment of the temporalis tendon. The tendon is then secured to the oral commissure musculature. This technique is also used less frequently as reinnervation techniques have gained popularity.

○ Free-Muscle Transfer

The ideal situation for use of an innervated vascularized muscle free flap for facial reanimation is the large defect seen following a radical parotidectomy. This flap would be used for both reanimation and soft tissue defect reconstruction. The free-muscle flap may also be used in cases of long-term paralysis in which considerable muscle atrophy or soft tissue contracture has taken place. The most commonly used free flaps for facial reanimation are the gracilis muscle, the inferior rectus abdominis muscle, and the latissimus dorsi muscle.

Static Procedures

Many procedures do not restore dynamic function of the face or reinnervate the face but allow static improvement in the appearance and function. Static treatments may be used in conjunction with dynamic or reinnervation procedures.

● *Tarsorrhaphy*

Tarsorrhaphy is an effective method of eye protection in patients with facial nerve paralysis and mild lagophthalmos. Functional and cosmetic drawbacks are associated with this type of procedure. A central tarsorrhaphy completely impairs vision and is not cosmetically acceptable as a permanent procedure.

● *Wedge Resection and Canthoplasty*

Wedge resection of the lower lid with canthoplasty is an effective and relatively simple procedure. It is particularly effective when lower lid laxity is mild. In cases with severe lid laxity or ectropion, a canthoplasty procedure is recommended.

● *Gold or Platinum Weights*

The gold or platinum weight implant is a very simple procedure that offers consistently satisfactory results. A gold weight lid load can be placed under local anesthesia and takes advantage of the relaxation of the levator that occurs with attempted eye closure and gravity. The weight in the upper eyelid passively closes the lid. Gold has been the material of choice for lid weighting because of its high density, relative inertness, and color, which blends with most skin tones. In recent years, platinum has become more frequently used, as the same density weight is available in a lower profile form and may have lower levels of complication.

Complications of weight insertion include extrusion, position shift, infection of the graft, contact allergy to gold, and overclosure of the eyelid.

● *Palpebral Spring Implant*

In cases in which there is poor levator action, a palpebral spring implant may prove more efficacious. However, this technique is technically more difficult and has a higher extrusion rate. The palpebral spring is basically a piece of wire and is therefore subject to possible complications, such as breakage, wearing out, migration, extrusion, and infection.

● *Lower Eyelid Shortening*

Lower eyelid weakness, rounding, and ectropion cause epiphora, worsening asymmetry, and increased scleral exposure. A lower eyelid tightening (canthopexy) or shortening procedure may be performed.

They may be performed under local anesthesia. A lateral canthotomy and inferior cantholysis are performed, and the anterior and posterior lamellae are denuded off the tarsus in addition to the superior epithelial surface. The bare tarsus may be trimmed to shorten the lower lid; then the lateral canthal attachment is recreated by securing it more superiorly to the Whitnall tubercle (marginal tubercle of the zygomatic bone), with improved lower lid apposition to the globe. The lateral canthal angle must be reestablished with a buried suture from the lateral inferior to lateral superior lid gray line.

Complications include ocular injury, recurrent lower lid rounding and ectropion, and abnormal rounding of the lateral canthal angle.

- *Static Sling*

This procedure allows static elevation of the corner of the mouth, creation of a nasolabial fold, and correction of alar collapse with improved symmetry at rest. Autologous tensor fasciae latae is the material of choice, though many authors report use of acellular dermal matrix, cadaveric tissue, or other implants.

Although variations on this procedure exist, in general two to three strips of suspension material are secured to a neo-nasolabial fold and alar base after elevation of a skin flip, then secured to the deep temporal fascia. Overcorrection is typically used, as recurrence has been noted with time.

Complications include infection, necessitating removal of suspension material, and persistent or worsening asymmetry.

- *Temporalis Sling*

The temporalis muscle may be used in similar fashion as a static sling to elevate the corner of the mouth. It is performed by either exposing the insertion in the temple and folding a segment of the muscle over the zygomatic arch and securing the muscle to the oral commissure. This technique is losing favor because of the secondary deformity of temporal hollowing and a visible bulge over the zygomatic arch.

- *Temporalis Tendon Transfer*

In an attempt to allow some dynamic control of the oral commissure and smile symmetry, a temporalis tendon transfer may be performed. This technique incorporates a transoral or transcutaneous incision followed by a coronoidectomy and detachment of the temporalis tendon. The tendon is then secured to the oral commissure musculature. This technique is also utilized less frequently, as reinnervation techniques are gaining popularity.

- *Ancillary Techniques*

Facial nerve paralysis may be associated with involuntary facial movements after partial or complete recovery or after reinnervation procedures (synkinesis). These signs may be due to aberrant regeneration of the facial nerve. Botulinum toxin (Botox, Allergan, Dublin, Ireland) induces a temporary and reversible neuromuscular blockade and thus is useful in alleviating synkinesis. Highly selective neurectomies and select myectomies (e.g., platysmectomy) might be also be useful.

◆ Eye Care

Paralysis of the upper branches of the facial nerve results in disorders of the eyelid and lacrimal function. Sequelae include incomplete closure of the eye with corneal exposure, lower lid ectropion with epiphora, decreased tear production, and loss of the corneal "squeegee" effect. These factors contribute to inadequate corneal protection, which can result in exposure keratitis, corneal ulceration, and blindness. Management of the eye in a patient with facial paralysis begins with supportive care to protect the cornea. This includes mainly moisturizing the eye and preventing exposure. These measures should be adequate in cases that are temporary or partial. Artificial tears are commonly used to keep the eyes moist. Ointments should be supplemented, especially at night before sleep. Closure of the eye can be achieved by carefully taping both the upper and lower lids. A clear humidity chamber provides moisture and protects the eye from trauma and foreign bodies.

◆ Outcome and Follow-Up

Facial rehabilitation is critical to optimizing results after reanimation procedures and in preventing and decreasing synkinesis. This ideally involves a therapist with specialized training in facial rehabilitation. Techniques used include facial muscle relaxation, stretching, and biofeedback. The goals of reanimation are facial symmetry, eye closure, oral competence, and voluntary movement. None of the described procedures can completely restore the paralyzed face to its normal function. Some synkinesis and residual weakness may persist, yet significant improvements in both function and appearance can be accomplished if the goals of reconstruction are kept in mind. However, patients require long-term follow-up for monitoring of outcomes, with additional procedures as necessary.

9.3   Facial Reconstruction

9.3.1   Skin Grafts

◆ Key Features

- A skin graft retains an important role in oral cavity reconstruction and cutaneous facial defects.
- The skin grafts can be either split thickness (STSG) or full thickness (FTSG).
- Complete immobilization of the graft in the early postoperative period is critical.

The skin is the largest organ of the human body, representing ~ 16% of the total body weight. Skin transplanted from one location to another on the same individual is termed an autogenous graft or autograft. Despite the development of sophisticated reconstructive methods utilized after ablative surgery, such as microvascular free flaps, much simpler approaches to reconstruction continue to be appropriate in many cases. Skin grafting in particular remains an excellent option for defects of the oral cavity, face, and scalp.

◆ Anatomy and Physiology

From superficial to deep, layers include the epidermis, the dermis, and the subcutaneous tissue. The epidermis constitutes ~ 5% of the skin; the remaining 95% is dermis. The epidermis is further divided into the superficial stratum corneum (no nuclei), stratum lucidum, stratum granulosum, and stratum basale. The dermis is further divided into the more superficial papillary dermis and the deeper reticular dermis, which contains hair follicles and sebaceous glands.

STSGs are composed of epidermis and a variable portion of the dermis. FTSGs include the epidermis and the entire dermis. The thickness of STSGs typically used ranges from ~ 0.012 to 0.018 inches (0.3–0.45 mm). Although thinner STSGs contract more, they "take" more consistently; thicker grafts contract less but are also more prone to fail. The thickness of FTSGs depends on the thickness of the donor site skin.

Skin graft healing is considered a three-step process. In the first stage, *imbibition*, the graft derives its nutrients from the underlying recipient bed. During the second stage, *inosculation*, preexisting blood vessels in both the graft and the recipient bed meet and form a network. Healing is completed by *neovascularization*, wherein new vessels form within the graft and grow into the underlying tissue.

Properties of the recipient bed are critical to skin graft healing. Skin grafts will "take" on most well-vascularized tissue, including granulation tissue, muscle, fat, perichondrium, periosteum, and cancellous bone. Conversely, skin grafts will not survive on naked cortical bone or bare cartilage (i.e., tissues without their periosteum or perichondrium). Actively infected tissue should not be skin grafted. Radiated tissue is also a much less favorable recipient bed.

◆ Indications

Common settings for skin grafting in head and neck surgery include oral cavity defects after cancer resection, cutaneous defects of the face after lesion excision or trauma, closure of free flap donor sites (radial forearm, fibula, etc.), and the framework elevation step of microtia repair.

◆ Operative Technique

Split-Thickness Skin Graft

Typically, the donor site of choice is the upper thigh (thick skin, relatively flat surface). To minimize donor site morbidity the scalp may also be used. An STSG is typically harvested with a pneumatic dermatome (e.g., Zimmer Air Dermatome, Zimmer, Warsaw, IN). The donor site is shaved, prepped, and draped, then cleaned of prep solution and lubricated (saline or mineral oil depending on model of dermatome). The donor site is held taut while the dermatome engages the skin at a 45° angle, then it is dropped slightly lower. The graft is harvested with steady and even pressure. A gauze soaked in 1/200,000 epinephrine is applied to the donor site to achieve hemostasis. The donor may be dressed in several ways, such as with Tegaderm (3M, St. Paul, MN) for 7 to 10 days or until reepithelialization is complete.

The recipient site is then prepared by ensuring meticulous hemostasis to prevent hematoma formation and loss of graft apposition. The skin graft is applied to the recipient site with the epidermis facing out, then sutured into place with absorbable stitches, ensuring good apposition with the recipient bed. A skin graft may be meshed to provide coverage of a greater surface area at the recipient site, with expansion ratios generally ranging from 1:1 to 6:1. This also allows egress of fluid that would otherwise collect underlying the graft. A bolster (e.g., Xeroform [Medtronic, Minneapolis, MN]) is applied to maintain apposition of the graft and recipient bed, secured with tie-over sutures for ~ 7 days.

Full-Thickness Skin Graft

FTSGs may be harvested from essentially any area; however, it is important to approximate a color and texture match to the recipient site if possible. Common donor sites include the post- or preauricular area and the supraclavicular neck. Chest wall and groin donor sites are common in microtia reconstruction. Grafts are typically designed in fusiform fashion to facilitate primary closure. The borders of the graft are incised sharply with a scalpel. The edges of the graft are held with a skin hook, and the remainder of the graft is elevated in a subdermal plane from underlying subcutaneous tissue using a knife or sharp scissors. The graft is thoroughly defatted with scissors or a knife prior to inset. Donor site hemostasis is secured with cautery, and elevation of surrounding skin flaps with primary closure is achieved. The graft is then trimmed and inset similar to an STSG as previously described (**Fig. 9.14**).

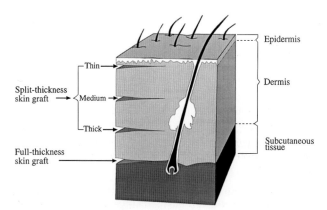

Fig. 9.14 Various skin graft thicknesses taken from the skin. (Used with permission from Papel ID, ed. *Facial Plastic and Reconstructive Surgery*. 4th ed. New York, NY: Thieme; 2016:605.)

◆ Complications

The major complication of skin grafting is partial or complete graft loss. Reasons for graft failure include hematoma, seroma, infection, and inadequate stabilization. Discoloration at the STSG donor site is to be expected, and skin grafts may have a "patch" appearance due to color or texture mismatch, shininess of the graft site, and volume differences.

◆ Postoperative Care

Feeding via a nasogastric feeding tube may be considered for oral cavity skin graft placement. Bolsters may be left in place for 3 to 10 days.

Management of the STSG donor site is quite variable; this area may be a source of discomfort for the patient. The STSG donor site epidermis regenerates by secondary epithelialization from the wound edges and from migration of dermal cells originating in the shafts of hair follicles as well as adnexal structures remaining in the dermis.

9.3.2   Local Cutaneous Flaps for Facial Reconstruction

◆ Key Features

- Local flaps are generally classified by the method of transfer.
- A defect analysis should be done systematically to achieve best results.
- Flap design must consider vectors of tension, resultant scars, and areas from which to recruit.

Cutaneous defects can arise from a host of different causes, but skin cancer remains the most common etiology in the Caucasian population. Local facial flaps are widely used for defects that are too large for primary closure or second-intention healing. They remain the workhorse for facial reconstruction.

◆ Defect Evaluation

When analyzing a cutaneous defect of the face, there is a series of steps that one should go through to help identify the optimal flap or, more importantly, which flaps will create significant problems, such as distortion, asymmetry, or functional issues.

- First, "immobile landmarks" of the face must be considered, including the hairline, vermilion border of the lip, and alar rim. These critical structures must remain undisturbed by scars as well as by flap tension.
- Second, the areas of optimal tissue recruitment surrounding the defect should be assessed.

- Third, the preexisting lines of the face and their orientation around the defect are evaluated. These include the visible wrinkles, relaxed skin tension lines (RSTLs), and borders of the aesthetic units. The face is separated into distinct aesthetic units such as the forehead, temple, nose, eyes, cheek, lips, and chin. When possible, it is best to place incisions along the margins of the aesthetic units and use flaps that lie within the same aesthetic unit as the defect.
- Finally, it is necessary to consider the resultant scars and vectors of tension of the given flap. For every flap design, one should be able to anticipate the exact orientation of the final scars and attempt to design the flap in a way that best conforms to the third step, having the scars lie within or parallel to the RSTLs. Moreover, one must anticipate the vectors of tension for each flap with respect to the landmarks noted in the first step. The flap should not create distortion of critical adjacent landmarks. Ideally, the greatest tension from the flap will align with the lines of maximal extensibility, which generally run perpendicular to the RSTLs.

◆ Flap Nomenclature

The different systems for classification of local flaps include tissue content, proximity of the flap, blood supply, and method of tissue transfer, the last two of which are the principal methods of nomenclature. The blood supply within a flap can be *random* (based on the rich dermal plexus of the face), can have an *axial pattern* (supplied by numerous larger-caliber vessels in the dermis and subcutaneous layer, which are arranged in an axial pattern along the flap), or can be *pedicled* (maintained by larger, named vessels). The other system is based on the method of tissue transfer (**Table 9.3**).

Table 9.3   Chart of local flaps

Advancement flaps   • Simple   • Unipedicled (U-plasty)   • Bipedicled (H- or T-plasty)   • V-Y island flap   • Cheek advancement flap
Pivotal   • Rotation   • Transposition   • Interposition   • Interpolated
Hinged

Advancement flaps refer to skin paddles that are mobilized in a linear vector to resurface a given defect. They create no distortion to the adjacent tissues, although standing cutaneous deformities may occasionally arise and require excision. Such flaps are rarely used in their truest form but rather follow the natural skin lines. They are further subclassified based on their vascular pedicle, be it a unilateral pedicle, a bipedicle, or a subcutaneous pedicle (island flap). The maximum length-to-width ratio for an advancement flap is typically 4:1.

The remaining method of tissue transfer is the *pivotal flap*, in which the tissue transposition has a rotational element as well. A true *rotation flap* moves tissue along the circumference of a circle, around a single, fixed pivot point, such as a scalp rotation flap. Most other flaps have a combined advancement and rotational element to them. A *transposition flap* involves mobilizing tissue over an incomplete bridge of skin (e.g., rhombic and bilobed flaps). *Interposition flaps* are similar to transposition flaps but include elevation of the incomplete skin bridge to the site of the donor defect, such as a Z-plasty. Finally, *interpolated flaps* move the skin paddle and pedicle over an intact skin bridge with its pedicle base removed from the defect. These interpolated flaps are two-staged flaps that require a secondary pedicle division, usually 3 weeks later. The forehead flap is such an example.

◆ Advancement Flaps

The most simple advancement flap is the lateral undermining and mobilization along the margin of a defect with primary closure. When closing a defect primarily, the apices of the defect should be less than 30° to avoid a standing cutaneous deformity. Traditional *unipedicled* (U-plasty) and *bipedicled* (H-plasty) advancement flaps without any rotational component have a narrow indication such as in closure of forehead and lip defects. These flaps are used when minimal tension is desired perpendicular to the direction of advancement to avoid distortion of adjacent anatomic landmarks such as the eyebrow. Secondary defects created along the axis of advancement can be addressed by the "halving technique," direct excision of the standing cutaneous deformity, or by advanced excision of a Burrow triangle (**Fig. 9.15**).

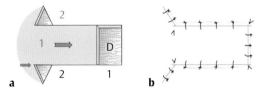

Fig. 9.15 Unipedicled advancement flap (U-plasty). **(a)** Unilateral advancement with direct excision of standing cutaneous deformity (Burow triangle). **(b)** Closure of defect. (Used with permission from Weerda H. *Reconstructive Facial Plastic Surgery: A Problem-Solving Manual.* 2nd ed. Stuttgart/New York: Thieme;2015:21.)

The leading edge of any advancement flap is the point of maximum tension. One can often design the flap such that the parallel resultant scar lies within the wrinkles or RSTLs of the facial aesthetic unit. The *V-Y island* advancement flap is a unipedicled triangular flap based on a subcutaneous pedicle that is mobilized in a linear vector toward the defect. The V-Y flap creates minimal distortion around the primary defect, but its reach is limited by the subcutaneous pedicle (**Fig. 9.16**). It is well suited for small defects of the upper lip and medial cheek that are in proximity to important anatomic landmarks.

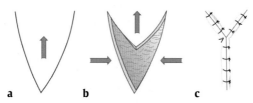

Fig. 9.16   V-Y island advancement flap. **(a)** Two unilateral advancement flaps around primary defect with minimal distortion to surrounding structures. **(b)** The triangular flap is based on a subcutaneous pedicle. **(c)** Defect closed with resultant Y-shaped scar on each side of defect. (Used with permission from Weerda H. *Reconstructive Facial Plastic Surgery: A Problem-Solving Manual.* 2nd ed. Stuttgart/New York: Thieme;2015:22.)

◆ Pivotal Flaps

The *rotation flap* is a pivotal flap mobilized along a curvilinear incision around a fixed point used for tissue that is not extensible, such as the scalp. Two standing cutaneous deformities are created and can be directly excised. The ratio between the peripheral arc of the flap and diameter of the defect is generally 4:1, but rotation flaps on the scalp often require a 6:1 ratio. The *cheek flap* is a combination advancement and rotation flap. The large area from which skin is recruited, together with the natural extensibility of cheek skin, make this flap particularly apt for large defects of the medial cheek. Resultant scars can be camouflaged along the melolabial fold, lower eyelid, and preauricular crease. It is imperative to avoid inferior tension on the eyelid by placing anchoring stitches between the periosteum of the malar eminence and infraorbital rim and the undersurface of the flap.

◆ Transposition Flaps

A *transposition flap* mobilizes a broad-based skin paddle over an incomplete bridge of skin (as opposed to the interpolated flap, which crosses a complete bridge of skin). The *rhombic flap* is a precise mathematical design that leaves minimal tension or distortion around the defect. The point of greatest tension and its vector are consistent and should be oriented along a line of maximal skin extensibility, perpendicular to RSTLs. This point should be secured with a long-lasting buried suture (**Fig. 9.17**). Small modifications in design, such as a narrower arc of rotation, can reduce the amount of tension from the donor site and distribute this to the tissues surrounding the defect.

The *bilobed flap* is a double transposition flap that minimizes distortion at the primary site by distributing the soft tissue tension over the perimeter of two separate flaps. As such, it is ideal for use near immobile anatomic structures such as the alar rim. Refinement of the bilobed flap design has

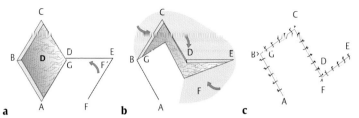

Fig. 9.17 Limberg rhombic transposition flap. **(a)** The flap is designed with 60° and 120° angles. **(b)** The flap is elevated in a subcutaneous plane and transposed into the defect. The arrows indicate areas of maximal tension after flap transposition. **(c)** Resultant scar. (Used with permission from Weerda H. *Reconstructive Facial Plastic Surgery: A Problem-Solving Manual.* 2nd ed. Stuttgart/New York: Thieme;2015:26.)

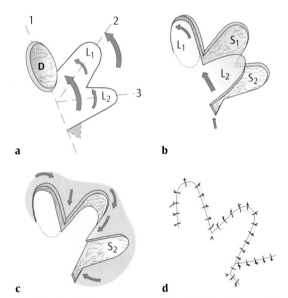

Fig. 9.18 Bilobed double transposition flap. **(a)** The flap is designed with adjacent flaps rotated 90° to 100°. Two wedges are excised to avoid standing cutaneous deformities. **(b)** Inset of flaps and resultant scar. The secondary donor site is closed primarily with a linear scar that can be oriented to run along borders of an aesthetic subunit. **(c)** The surrounding skin is mobilized, and all secondary defects are closed. **(d)** Appearance after closure of all defects. (Used with permission from Weerda H. *Reconstructive Facial Plastic Surgery: A Problem-Solving Manual.* 2nd ed. Stuttgart/New York: Thieme;2015:25.)

led to a tighter arc of rotation, reducing the standing cutaneous deformity. Each flap is usually separated by a 45° arc of rotation rather than 90° (**Fig. 9.18**). The primary lobe should be aggressively thinned to minimize the amount of pincushioning that typically occurs. The bilobed flap is excellent for repair of nasal tip defects up to 1.5 cm in diameter but can also be used for reconstruction of cheek defects away from the central face.

The *melolabial flap* is another transposition flap adjacent to the nose and lips, which provides a source of well-vascularized, color-matched skin for reconstruction of the nasal ala, sidewall, and lips. It can be based inferiorly or superiorly, but the aesthetic junction between the cheek and nose is often blunted.

The two-staged *melolabial flap* and the *forehead flap* are interpolated flaps commonly used in reconstruction of larger defects of the nose. In general, nasal defects > 2.5 cm in diameter, defects with denuded bone or cartilage, or wounds in irradiated fields are best reconstructed by heartier flaps such as these. With its ancient history, the forehead flap remains a robust and versatile flap and the workhorse technique for major nasal repair. The pedicle is based over the medial eyebrow area, centered on the consistent supratrochlear artery, which captures the perfusion pressure from the area rich in collaterals. The pedicle is kept narrow (i.e., < 1.5 cm) to facilitate rotation. The pedicle can be based on the ipsilateral side of the nasal defect for greater inferior reach, or on the contralateral side for reduced torsion on the pedicle base and visual obstruction to the patient. The donor site defect is closed primarily, and the pedicle division and flap inset is performed after 3 weeks.

◆ Complications

As for any surgical procedure, knowing the possible complications, ways to avoid them, and how to manage them when they arise is as important to success as the actual technique itself. Flap ischemia, obstructed venous outflow, infection, bleeding, and wound dehiscence are the principal complications. Flap ischemia and necrosis are dreaded complications and are related to both tension and impaired vascular perfusion. Flap tension can be attributed to insufficient undermining, flap distension from edema or hematoma, or excessive rotational or linear advancement. Flap perfusion is usually robust in the head and neck, but it may be compromised by smoking. Patient counseling for (at least) perioperative smoking cessation is critical to avoid complications. Good flap inflow with compromised venous outflow (venous congestion) in pedicled flaps may progress to ultimate flap failure. Rarely, medical leeching is necessary to salvage a flap with venous congestion.

Wound infection is not common in local flaps of the head and neck, but it can be devastating to the survival of the flap when present. Complications range from prolonged wound healing to scar widening, or even to complete flap necrosis. Hematomas can be destructive to a flap by several mechanisms: space-occupying tension, hemoglobin-derived free radical tissue injury, subdermal fibrosis, and an ideal medium for bacterial infection. Wound dehiscence can occur as a result of all the aforementioned complications. However, dehiscence may also result from local trauma or dynamic movement of a flap.

◆ Summary

Facial defects arise from a variety of causes, such as trauma, skin cancer, and congenital lesions. Their repair remains a challenging part of head and neck surgery, as it calls on precise technical skills, attention to details, a three-dimensional perspective for planning, and a creative and artistic element. Developing an algorithm for evaluating facial defects can be useful in terms of avoiding pitfalls such as significant asymmetry, functional issues, or unfavorable scars. Most local skin flaps are versatile and predictable. Familiarity with a host of designs can prove to be a tremendous asset in facial reconstruction.

9.3.3 Microvascular Free Tissue Transfer

◆ Key Features

- Free tissue transfer offers options to enhance surgical outcomes with improved function, appearance, and quality of life in head and neck cancer and trauma surgery.
- Free tissue transfer techniques require analysis of the defect, available donor sites, and the overall health, function, and rehabilitation potential of the patient.
- Common free tissue transfer donor sites used in head and neck surgery include myocutaneous and myofascial tissue from the radial forearm, latissimus dorsi, rectus abdominis, and lateral thigh; enteral sites such as the jejunum; and osseocutaneous flaps such as the fibula, lateral scapula, and iliac crest.

The decision to use a particular donor site for correction of a defect must account for the extent and functional sequelae of cancer or injury, characteristics of the defect itself, and aesthetic outcomes of a given flap. In addition, the treatment plan, patient's prognosis, general functional status and comorbidities, patient and family motivation, and rehabilitation options should be considered in detail. Consideration of relevant clinical concerns supports the physical examination and defect analysis to select a donor site. Free tissue transfer techniques require specialized training, appropriate clinical resources and equipment, and a well-educated interdisciplinary team.

◆ Epidemiology

Free tissue transfer is appropriate for patients of all ages who are physiologically and functionally suited to longer single or staged surgeries and will participate in necessary rehabilitation to make full use of the microvascular reconstruction. Free flaps are most often used for postablative indications, with posttraumatic defects the second major indication.

◆ Clinical

Patients who incur or suffer a head and neck defect that alters anatomic form, affects function of critical structures, and negatively changes appearance and quality of life may benefit from free tissue transfer.

Symptoms

Patients will typically complain of symptoms associated with their primary malignancy site (dysphagia, dysarthria, mass, odynophagia) or trauma (bleeding, deformity, pain, etc.). For planning reconstruction, it is critical to obtain a detailed medical history to assess the appropriateness for microvascular free tissue transfer. A history of peripheral vascular disease, coronary artery disease, uncontrolled diabetes, Raynaud's syndrome, radiation therapy to the recipient site, tobacco abuse, or prior vascular procedures may guide additional physical examination or vascular studies or alter the reconstructive options.

◆ Evaluation

Physical Exam

Specific donor tissues are variable, and donor sites are chosen based on recipient site requirements, such as the need and types of surface to be reconstructed, the need for bulk, and the need for bone or lubrication. Potential donor sites are then examined for vascular supply, anatomic suitability and anomalies, and age-related changes or tissue changes due to comorbid disease. Perfusion and adequacy of vascular donor sites as well as the remaining vascular anatomy in the defect are site specific.

Imaging

Use of imaging in free tissue transfer is controversial and is largely based on surgeon preference. Imaging for free tissue transfer may include an angiogram (formal, computed tomography angiogram [CTA], or magnetic resonance angiogram [MRA]) to gauge vascular competency of the donor or recipient site vessels. Site-specific computed tomography (CT), magnetic resonance imaging (MRI), or positron emission tomography (PET)/CT scans may be obtained to assess extent of disease and predict surgical defect and involvement of surrounding tissues in the field of resection. Noninvasive Doppler ultrasonography may also be used to assess lower extremity vascularity prior to fibula flap harvest.

Labs

Laboratory assays are somewhat dependent on comorbid disease, although standard preoperative evaluation with complete blood count (CBC), chemistries, albumin, prealbumin, coagulation panels, and/or a type and screen may be performed. In patients with diabetes a serum glucose and HbA1c should be obtained. Some surgeons will also evaluate status of tobacco abuse by obtaining serum cotinine levels.

Other Tests

An Allen test should be performed to assess the competency of the ulnar and radial artery contributions to the distal vascular arch prior to radial forearm free tissue transfer.

◆ Treatment Options

Medical

Medical therapeutics for free tissue transfer includes management of anti-coagulation to ensure flap patency and control of comorbid disease.

Relevant Pharmacology

Multiple pharmacologic interventions have been described, but no consensus exists regarding perioperative anticoagulation to maintain arterial or venous patency. Unfractionated heparin may be used in intermittent subcutaneous (SQ) injections or continuous intravenous (IV) drip postoperatively. Some patients are given aspirin, other platelet function inhibitors, or other inhibitors of the coagulation cascade. Streptokinase may be used in relevant flap vessels for flap salvage in anastomotic thrombosis.

Surgical

The most commonly used flaps are of fasciocutaneous or myocutaneous origin. Common myocutaneous or fasciocutaneous donor sites used for reconstruction of soft tissue defects include the radial forearm, rectus abdominis, latissimus dorsi, and anterolateral or lateral thigh. Among these options, the radial forearm free flap offers significant advantages in tissue characteristics, including pliability, thinness, and size to meet many head and neck reconstructive needs. The pedicle of this flap is often particularly long and of large caliber. When additional bulk is needed, the anterolateral thigh or other myocutaneous flaps may be used.

Repair of the pharynx may benefit from use of a tubed flap or an enteral flap. The jejunum and lateral gastric border flaps offer different advantages with pliability and tubed inset; however, secretion production may be of variable benefit for lubrication. The resultant wet speech may be perceived as a significant disadvantage. Harvesting these flaps risks more complications with breach of the abdomen and necessitates use of two surgical teams.

Bone defects, especially of the mandible, require osseocutaneous flaps from donor sites that offer good bone stock in lengths matched to the adult mandible. Both the lateral scapular border and the fibula can be successfully used. The scapula proves a more difficult site, as it requires repositioning the patient and may necessitate two surgical teams. Further, the scapula in women may offer limited or thin bone supply, which will suffice to correct a large mandibular defect. The scapula flap is associated with transient rotator cuff dysfunction at the least, and the fibula with potential foot drop or vascular sequelae.

The surgery and intraoperative care are focused on ablative procedures or preparation of the traumatic defect, flap harvesting, and final inset of the free tissue flap in the recipient site. Identifying the pedicle and recipient vessels, limiting ischemic time, and achieving anastomosis are critical elements of successful outcome. Anastomosis is performed in either end-to-end or end-to-side fashion. End-to-end using large-caliber, healthy vessels is preferred. End-to-side anastomosis may have associated difficulties.

◆ Complications

Complications of free tissue transfer include ischemia and necrosis of the flap from arterial or venous thrombosis. Monitoring flap perfusion is critical to early identification of thrombosis. If recognized early and managed promptly (< 6 hours), compromised flaps have a 75% salvage rate when taken back to the operating room. Reexploration of the site is often necessary to pinpoint thrombosis and perform thrombectomy and possible anastomotic revision. Some skin and soft tissue may necrose despite thrombectomy and successful salvage. Wound care to promote healing by secondary or tertiary intention is needed in these cases. Overall free flap failure rates are between 2 and 8% in most recent studies.

Oropharyngeal and laryngeal reconstructions risk fistula formation with or without anastomotic thrombi. Early feeding in oropharyngeal reconstruction is controversial. There is limited research to guide definitive choice of postoperative day to feed, but extended delay may result in nutritional depletion. Fistula formation is often preceded by tenderness, warmth, and erythema. These signs warrant immediate attention and opening of the incision to relieve compression as indicated by the physical examination. Further, oral feeding should stop, with exclusive use of enteral nutritional support to circumvent use of the oropharynx. Salvage, fistula, and wound care protocols are useful adjuncts to support best practice and good patient outcomes. Donor site complications are rare, are site-dependent, and include foot drop in fibula free flap harvest and tendon exposure in forearm or fibula donor sites. Rehabilitation with involvement of physical and occupational therapy optimizes patient outcomes when donor site complications occur.

◆ Outcome and Follow-Up

Monitoring the free flap during the postoperative phase is critical to ensuring flap survival. Techniques to monitor the free flap depend on the tissue composition and location of the flap. Specific monitoring techniques include evaluation of color, capillary refill, turgor, surface temperature, presence of bleeding, skin graft adherence, and auditory assessment of blood flow (Doppler). It is important to protect of the flap vascular supply (e.g., avoiding compression or flexion in the region of anastomosis). Other flap monitoring techniques that have been commonly used include implantable Doppler evaluation and monitoring tissue oxygenation.

Optimal patient outcomes are a functional, healthy free tissue transfer to restore the defect identified for reconstruction; restoration of function and appearance to the extent possible with the tissue used and the defect corrected; and patient and family satisfaction with regional and overall patient function, quality of life, and caregiver burden.

Follow-up is predicated on expected cancer and trauma protocols and includes flap healing, function, and late complications such as scarring, tethering, and ischemia.

9.3.4 Bone and Cartilage Grafts

◆ Key Features

- Bone grafts are used primarily for structural reconstruction of the craniomaxillofacial skeleton in select cases.
- The most commonly used bone graft is from the calvarial skull, followed by use of bone from the iliac crest, tibial region, and rib.
- Cartilage grafts are most commonly used for rhinoplasty, nasal reconstruction, and auricular reconstruction but have also been described for use in other areas such as orbital and eyelid reconstruction.
- The most common sources for cartilage grafting are the nasal septum, concha of the ear, and costal cartilage.

Bone and cartilage grafting remain key components in reconstructive surgery of the craniomaxillofacial skeleton, nose, and ears. Although alloplastic implants have supplanted the use of bone and cartilage in some regions, bone and cartilage remain the mainstays in certain reconstructive areas. Bone is essential for structural reconstruction such as in the mandible and along the buttresses of the maxilla in trauma and oncologic situations, whereas cartilage remains most commonly used in the both primary and secondary rhinoplasty as well as in reconstruction of the nose after cancer and reconstruction and in ear reconstruction. It is also sometimes used as a spacer graft in areas such as the lower eyelid.

◆ Epidemiology

Rhinoplasty is commonly performed for aesthetic and functional indications, and nasal reconstruction is commonly necessary after cancer ablation and traumatic defects of the nose. Ear reconstruction is most commonly due to a congenital deficiency (microtia) or due to resection of cutaneous malignancy. These reconstructions utilize cartilage grafts frequently to obtain an optimal aesthetic and functional result. In addition, bone grafts, either as free grafts or vascularized grafts, are often utilized in primary and secondary reconstruction of traumatic defects and after ablation of head and neck cancer.

◆ Clinical

A clinical history and patient exam should be performed, with a focus on their chief complaint. The necessity for bone or cartilage grafting will be guided based on etiology of deficiency, history of prior trauma or surgery, presence or absence of normal anatomy, and other patient factors. As bone and cartilage grafts require a vascular supply for survival, patient characteristics that may influence graft take should be assessed, such as tobacco abuse, vascular insufficiency, history of radiation, or poorly controlled diabetes.

Patient Assessment

Calvarial bone is still a common source for maxillofacial trauma reconstruction. Although other bony defects in acute trauma may be reconstructed with alloplastic materials (e.g., absence of bone along the infraorbital rim), bone is often preferred. In acute mandibular trauma with defects, such as avulsive bony loss, the choice for bone grafting is more commonly the iliac crest with a combination of cortical and cancellous bone. Cartilage grafts are particularly useful in nasal reconstruction to augment existing anatomy or replaced missing structural support. In ear reconstruction, rib is the most commonly used cartilaginous source and often requires a staged procedure.

◆ Evaluation

In acute maxillofacial trauma, radiographic evaluation may show comminuting segments of bone or obvious bone loss that suggest the need to plan for bone grafting in the preoperative setting. Fine-cut multiplanar computed tomography (CT) scans with 3D reconstructions, when available, will guide these decisions.

Cartilage grafts are commonly used in primary or secondary reconstruction of the nose and ear, with the donor site being determined by the characteristics and volume of cartilage required for the reconstructive effort. The most important feature is whether structural or contour reconstruction is necessary. With structural reconstruction, the grafting material of choice is septal cartilage followed by costal cartilage, whereas contour reconstruction can be achieved with both septal and conchal cartilage.

◆ Treatment Options

Calvarial Bone

The most common bone graft used in the midface and upper maxillofacial skeleton is that of calvarial bone. Calvarial bone is harvested most commonly as a split graft in the parietal skull region away from danger areas such as the coronal and temporal suture lines and away from the midline, where the underlying sagittal sinus exists. The anatomy of the skull is such that there is an outer and an inner cortex of bone (called the outer and inner tables, respectively) of varying degrees of thickness. A key feature to harvesting calvarial bone grafts is awareness of the underlying dura.

A variety of techniques have been described for the harvest of calvarial bone grafts, but the basic technique involves drilling a trough to expose the presumed cancellous layer between the outer cortex and the inner cortex of bone. The graft shape is outlined as this trough is created. Then either a wide curved osteotome or a sagittal or reciprocating saw can be used to elevate the bone graft within the diploic or cancellous layer. It is essential that the surgeon is aware of being in the correct plane at all times; as a rule, an assumption can be made that one is through the inner table if the osteotome or saw moves more freely than expected. After the first graft is elevated, subsequent grafts are commonly much more readily elevated as the surgeon has a better idea of the depth of the outer cortex, and further graft harvesting is also facilitated by the greater ease of placement of the osteotome due to the widening of the trough allowed by the harvest of the first bone. Alternatively, a split calvarial graft may be obtained from full-thickness frontal or cranial bone on the back table.

Iliac Crest

The most common graft areas of harvest for the mandible are cortical and cancellous bone grafts from the inner aspect of the iliac crest. This region is approached through an incision over the iliac crest with direct dissection down to the iliac crest. Great care should be taken to reflect the tissues in this region for later precise soft tissue repositioning. A section of the inner iliac crest is removed, followed by the harvest of cancellous bone using curettes. If only cancellous bone is used, the cortical segment is replaced and positioned usually with wires or strong sutures, and the soft tissue muscle elements are resecured to the region.

Alternatively, a less invasive approach involves a small incision dissection down through periosteum and making a small window of exposed bone. Trephines are then used to obtain cores of cancellous bone with minimal cortical bone disruptions and less postoperative pain.

Tibial Bone Grafts

Tibial bone grafts are used by some surgeons and are harvested at the region of the lateral epicondyle just inferior and lateral to the patella. A small incision is made in this region, and dissection is carried through periosteum to expose cortex. A small bony window may then be created with osteotomes, followed by harvest of cancellous bone with curettes. The cortical window may then be replaced and the wound closed. There are no functional deficits and minimal donor site pain with this technique; however, a smaller volume of cancellous bone can typically be harvested from this donor site than from iliac crest.

Cartilage Grafts

Nasal septal grafts are commonly harvested as part of the routine septoplasty or easily obtained during nasal reconstruction. The key when harvesting septal cartilage for grafting, however, is to harvest as large a piece of quadrangular cartilage as one unit while leaving an adequate dorsal and caudal strut.

Conchal cartilage can be harvested either through a lateral (inside the antihelical rim) or by a medial (postauricular) incision. Through either approach, an incision is made in the conchal cartilage, leaving a several-millimeter rim along the antihelix to maintain persistence of the structure of the ear, followed by an incision that may extend as far as the external auditory canal anteriorly and to the extent of the inferior crus of the ear superiorly in the cymba conchae. A curvilinear-shaped piece of cartilage is routinely removed for this purpose. The incision is closed, and then, because of the dead space created by the harvest of this cartilage, either a through-and-through bolster or a quilting suture is placed.

Costal cartilage is harvested classically through an inframammary incision in the region of the seventh and eighth ribs. However, the length and location of incision will vary based on the amount of cartilage needed, the curvature desired, and whether a cartilaginous or osseocartilaginous rib is desired. Depending on the amount of cartilage needed, after dissection through the chest and intercostal muscles, either a partial outer cortex section of cartilage is sharply removed or careful subperichondrial dissection around the cartilage is performed. The muscle layers are carefully reapproximated, as is the skin, and a pressure dressing is applied. The use of a pain pump is common.

◆ Complications

Complications in calvarial graft harvesting generally occur at the time of harvest, such as intracranial entry with a dural tear or brain injury. Neurosurgery evaluation may be required, but small tears can generally be managed by simple reapproximation of the dura and suture closure. One should vigilantly observe for any signs of postoperative subdural or extradural cerebrospinal fluid (CSF) or blood collection. Hematomas can occur in the subcutaneous region of the scalp and iliac crest as well as in the chest region, so pressure dressings or suction drains are often used. With respect to iliac crest bone grafting, postoperative pain may result in gait disturbance, and this is a common reason this donor site is avoided. Use of a minimally invasive approach and trephination has been shown to have less pain associated. Occasionally, chronic chest wall pain may be observed with rib harvest.

As with any septal surgery, septal perforation is a concern with cartilage graft harvesting, and standard techniques for mucosal coverage are essential.

The most common complication with a conchal graft harvest is mild deformity because of a slight collapse of the ear along with scar deformities. Finally, with respect to rib or costal cartilage graft harvesting, the most common adverse sequela is a slight depression in the region of the graft harvest along with the scar in this region. An acute complication is pleural entry and subsequent pneumothorax. If pleural entry is diagnosed at the time of positive-pressure breathing intraoperatively, a drainage tube under suction is placed in the pleural cavity through the tear, and suction is applied while closure is being performed; the tube is then withdrawn during a positive-pressure breath. A postoperative X-ray is always taken and will determine whether there is a postoperative pneumothorax or hemothorax. The latter situation may require chest tube drainage, but this is quite rare.

As these grafts require vascular ingrowth for survival, there is a risk of graft failure, particularly in smokers or patients who are radiated or have poorly controlled diabetes. Infection of grafts may lead to graft loss, as may excess tension of the skin soft tissue envelope due to pressure necrosis.

Cartilaginous grafts may exhibit some warping. Graft extrusion is uncommon, although this may occur with cantilevered dorsal nasal grafts if excess tension exists or in auricular reconstruction after trauma.

◆ Outcome and Follow-Up

The donor sites for bone grafts are generally treated like any other wounds, with adequate cleaning and moist wound care. Outcomes with bone grafting are generally favorable, particularly when rigid fixation is used. This is based on long-term follow-up over at least several months as well as determination of the rigidity of the region as based on function of the mandible and maxilla. When complications occur in terms of poor healing, it is generally manifested by pain, mobility, and even infection, thus necessitating further intervention. Resorption of bone can occur with rigid fixation; this is relatively unusual.

9.3.5   Incision Planning and Scar Revision

◆ Key Features

- Incision planning and scar revision requires an understanding of facial anatomy and aesthetics and of advanced principles of wound healing.
- Patients who have been injured may bear psychologic trauma induced by the initial event or the resulting deformative scar.
- Timing of scar revision is important and depends on a variety of factors, including type and location of injury.
- The relaxed skin tension lines (RSTLs) represent the directional tendency of the skin to be more or less extensible, depending on the axis.

Incisions heal best when oriented with RSTLs and closed without tension. Scar revision is generally performed when the scar is mature (~ 6–12 months) and involves reorienting the scar into the RSTLs, resurfacing, or reducing the scar into shorter segments. Steroid injection for hypertrophic scars and keloids should be performed within the first month if scars are inflamed, painful, or persistently firm.

Improperly oriented incisions and wounds are more likely to be noticeable, so whenever possible, they should be oriented into the RSTLs (**Fig. 9.19**). These lines are perpendicular to the pull of the underlying muscles (except around the eye) and are best found by pinching the skin. Incisions should be placed into the hairline whenever possible except low on the forehead of males (due to male pattern baldness). Incisions in concave areas should be interrupted to avoid scar contracture. Scars > 2 cm in length, > 2 mm in width, or with abnormal contours can usually be improved. Common revision techniques include reorientation, irregularization, resurfacing, and direct excision.

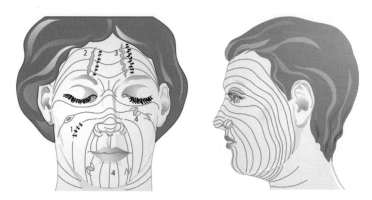

Fig. 9.19   Relaxed-skin tension lines (RSTLs) with elliptical excision in the RSTLs. (Used with permission from Weerda H. *Reconstructive Facial Plastic Surgery: A Problem-Solving Manual.* 2nd ed. Stuttgart/New York: Thieme;2015:10.)

✦ Epidemiology

Adverse scarring may result from many sources, including trauma, inflammation (e.g., acne, abscess), and radiation or may be iatrogenic. Scarring itself may be ideal, or the scar may have adverse features that create functional or aesthetic deficiencies. In such cases, scar revision may be appropriate.

✦ Clinical

Signs and Symptoms

Most scars are physically asymptomatic. Patients may present with pruritus, pain, or limitation of movement secondary to contractures. Scarring in certain areas of the face can contribute to functional problems, especially around the eyes or mouth. Care should be taken in performing scar revision in smokers, and an assessment of comorbidities (diabetes, autoimmune/inflammatory disorder, use of immune modulators) should be obtained to minimize complications.

Differential Diagnosis

It is important to rule out other types of skin lesions, such as infection, manifestations of systemic disease, and cutaneous malignancy. Adverse scarring from hypertrophic scarring or keloids requires special treatment consideration.

✦ Evaluation

Physical Exam

The etiology (**Table 9.4**), size, location, and orientation of the scar are the most important features when planning revision. Scar revision should not be performed until the scar is mature—that is, white as opposed to red and without any surrounding inflammation or induration. Maturation typically requires 6 to 12 months. Significant excision or reorientation cannot be performed if the skin is under considerable tension. Skin type also determines the propensity of the scar to pigment or heal favorably.

Table 9.4 Etiology of unfavorable scar formation

Genetic Fitzpatrick skin types III and above; darker skin types tend to hyperpigment
Iatrogenic Excessive trauma to the wound edges, failure to approximate wound edges at an identical level, and failure to sufficiently evert wound edges at the time of closure
Circumstantial Poor location or orientation of the wound, perioperative trauma, and postoperative mismanagement
Idiopathic

Pathology

Hypertrophic scars tend to be erythematous and firm and exhibit pruritus. They are elevated and remain within the original scar boundary. Pathologic evaluation shows collagen fibers arranged in a more wavy pattern, parallel to the surface with nodular myofibroblasts and vertically oriented vessels.

A keloid also tends to be raised but grows beyond the original scar boundary and may expand to surrounding tissue. In contrast to hypertrophic scars, keloids tend to show a thickened, hyalinized collagen (keloid collagen), abundant vasculature, a disarray of fibrous tissue, and a tonguelike advancing edge on pathologic analysis.

◆ Treatment Options

In general, the most straightforward option for a scar that is directed opposed to the RSTLs is to relocate the scar into an RSTL, into a hairline such as the brow, or into junctions of facial subunits such as the nasolabial fold. Wide scars that are favorably located may be simply excised or serially excised into a border or RSTL. Elongated scars or wide flat surfaces, such as the forehead and cheek, can be irregularized using a W-plasty, geometric broken-line closure (GBLC), or compound Z-plasty. GBLC is often considered a technically more difficult but better technique for longer scars. The idea of these techniques is to place as many segments as possible into the RSTLs for camouflage.

Z-plasty can be used to reorient the scar 90° into an RSTL or to increase the length of a contracture up to 125% (**Fig. 9.20**). The traditional Z-plasty consists of three incisions of equal length and two 60° angles with the central limb of the scar to be excised. Raising the resultant triangular skin flaps in the subcutaneous plane allows the tips to be transposed, resulting in a new central limb perpendicular to the original. Z-plasty is a useful technique to decrease webbing (medial canthal, alar base, oral commissure).

Where the size and elasticity of the scar preclude closure without distortion of nearby structures, tissue expansion or serial excision may be

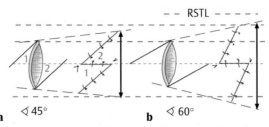

Fig. 9.20 Simple Z-plasty. **(a)** The scar, which crosses the RSTLs almost at right angles, is excised and dispersed with a 45° Z-plasty. Flaps 1 and 2 are transposed, causing a slight lengthening of the tissue in the direction of the arrow. **(b)** Transposing flaps 1 and 2 in a 60° Z-plasty produces even greater tissue lengthening (*arrow*). (Used with permission from Weerda H. *Reconstructive Facial Plastic Surgery: A Problem-Solving Manual.* 2nd ed. Stuttgart/New York: Thieme;2015:13.)

required. Resurfacing by dermabrasion or laser may be useful for uneven scars, multiple scars, or scars that cover a broad, flat area where excision is not practical. Combinations of the techniques mentioned more often lead to the best results.

◆ Outcome and Follow-Up

Scars should be followed closely to ensure that inflammation and induration improve within 1 to 2 weeks and that they gradually soften and become less red. Intralesional triamcinolone acetonide (10 mg/mL) can be injected monthly until the scar is stable. Recent literature has suggested that 5-fluorouracil may also be helpful when injected into scars. Patients should massage the scar several times daily and keep it covered with silicone sheeting or ointment as much as possible. Reducing sun exposure and using sunscreen are important adjuncts. Furthermore, limiting tension on the wound by keeping a new scar taped for up to 6 weeks can also be helpful in certain situations.

9.4 Cosmetic Surgery

9.4.1 Neurotoxins, Fillers, and Implants

◆ Key Features

> - Neurotoxins improve wrinkles by weakening selected muscles of facial expression.
> - A variety of filler materials have been developed to restore facial volume loss and treat moderate to severe facial folds and wrinkles, as well as volumize the lips.
> - Fat grafting is a surgical procedure that can restore facial volume loss to the aging face.
> - Alloplastic implants are used to achieve predictable structural volume changes for osseous cheek and chin deficiencies.

Restoring volume and structural support to the face can be achieved by a variety of surgical and nonsurgical procedures. In the last 20 years, the popularity of minimally invasive procedures for facial rejuvenation has skyrocketed, making them a billion-dollar industry. Although new injectable products are being developed, none give the permanent results that can be achieved with surgery.

◆ Epidemiology

The aging face results from a combination of facial lipoatrophy and volume loss, bone resorption, and loss of skin elasticity. Office-based procedures to improve the signs of facial aging include the use of neurotoxins and fillers to improve wrinkles and restore loss of subcutaneous fat pads. Surgical options for volume replacement include fat grafting to improve loss of soft tissue volume and solid facial implants to improve structural support.

◆ Clinical

Patients who present for correction of the aging face are focused primarily on the perceived effects of gravity and wrinkles, whereas volume deficiency or lipoatrophy is perhaps the single most important manifestation of the aging process. Injectable fillers have gained popularity in that they can easily be administered in an office setting, and many fillers now last up to 1 to 2 years. Fat grafting also restores facial volume and can provide a permanent correction of volume deficiency. Alloplastic implants are used more effectively to provide structural volume changes to individuals with related anatomic deficiencies, especially alloplastic chin augmentation for microgenia or permanent volume restoration in the malar region.

◆ Evaluation

Cosmetic rejuvenation of the face must address the skin, muscles, volume loss, and structural components. Fine lines and wrinkles may be best addressed with skin care and neurotoxins, whereas areas of volume loss can be treated with filler materials or fat transfer. The strategic areas for volume correction include the temporal hollow, inferior orbital rim, naso-jugal groove, nasolabial folds, anterior and lateral cheeks, prejowl sulcus, anterior chin, lips, and lateral mandible. When considering alloplastic chin augmentation, the patient's dentition should be carefully evaluated to determine whether orthotic or orthognathic procedures are more appropriate. The adjunctive use of fillers, fat grafting, or implants to optimize surgical results from face lifting, blepharoplasty, or rhinoplasty should also be assessed.

◆ Treatment Options

Medical

Neurotoxins

Botulinum toxin A (BoNT-A) is the most commonly used neurotoxin cosmetically and diminishes facial wrinkles by preventing the contraction of selected muscles of facial expression (**Table 9.5**).

Table 9.5 Neurotoxins

Generic name	Trade name	Typical dosing	Facial injection areas (FDA-approved)
Onabotulinumtoxin-A	Botox[†]	20 Botox units (BU)	Glabella, crow's feet
Abobotulinumtoxin-A	Dysport[*]	60 Dysport units (DU)	Glabella
Incobotulinumtoxin-A	Xeomin[§]	20 Xeomin units (XU)	Glabella

[*]Galderma, Lausanne, Switzerland
[†]Allergan Inc., Dublin, Ireland
[§]Merz, Frankfurt am Main, Germany

BoNT-A inhibits muscle contraction by preventing release of acetylcholine at the neuromuscular junction. Inhibition of certain muscles can allow the actions of opposing muscles to be accentuated and can result in lifting of the brow or elevation of the corners of the mouth. Common areas of "on label" FDA-approved areas of use include the glabella (procerus and corrugator muscles), crow's feet (orbicularis oculi muscles), whereas "off-label" or non-FDA-approved areas of injection include the forehead (frontalis muscle), wrinkled chin (mentalis muscles), and oral commissure elevation (depressor anguli oris muscles) (**Fig. 9.21**). Maximum effect after BoNT-A injection may take 3 to 7 days, and results will last approximately 3 to 4 months.

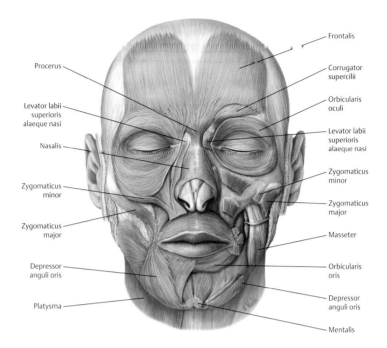

Fig. 9.21 The muscles of facial expression. (From THIEME Atlas of Anatomy, Head and Neuroanatomy, ©Thieme 2010. Illustration by Karl Wesker.)

Injectable Fillers

Injectable fillers are used in an office setting to restore facial volume loss and to elevate ptotic tissues, to some degree (**Table 9.6**). The hyaluronic acid fillers compose the majority of the fillers because of their softness, ease of injection, and reversibility with hyaluronidase (H-ase). These fillers differ by their amount of lift and range from thin consistencies for fine lines to more globular, thicker products used to improve more significant volume loss. Most fillers contain lidocaine, and injections are well tolerated. Topical anesthetic and regional blocks can also be used to improve patient comfort.

Surgical

Fat Grafting

Autologous fat grafting is a surgical procedure that can be used to restore volume to the aging face. Fat may be harvested from the lower abdomen, hips, and thighs. Tumescent anesthesia is infiltrated and fat is harvested using blunt-tipped cannulas using hand suction to minimize injury to the adipocytes. The harvested fat is then separated either by gravity separation or by centrifugation and placed into 1-mL syringes for injection into volume-deficient areas of the face.

Table 9.6 Injectable fillers

Filler	Trade names	Characteristics	Longevity
Hyaluronic acid (HA)	Restylane-L*, Juvederm Ultra XC[†], Juvederm Ultra Plus XC[†], Belotero[§]	Moderate thickness, used for moderate to severe folds and wrinkles and lip augmentation	8–12 months
	Restylane Lyft*, Juvederm Voluma[†]	Thicker products used for midface volumization and deeper folds	1–2 years
	Restylane Refyne*, Restylane Defyne*	More elastic properties, designed for circumoral folds and wrinkles	10–12 months
	Restylane Silk*, Juvederm Volbella[†]	Thin consistency, for lips and fine lines	4–6 months
Calcium hydroxylapatite (CaHA)	Radiesse+[§]	Thick calcium-based product, contraindicated for lips	10–12 months
Polymethylmethacrylate (PMMA)	Bellafill[‡]	Permanent microspheres in a bovine collagen base, skin test required, contraindicated for lips	Permanent filler—results improve over time
Poly-L-lactic acid (PLLA)	Sculptra*	Collagen-stimulating product, requires multiple injections, contraindicated for lips and around eyes	1–2 years

*Galderma, Lausanne, Switzerland
[†]Allergan Inc., Dublin, Ireland
[§]Merz, Frankfurt am Main, Germany
[‡]Suneva Medical, Santa Barbara, CA

Implants

The surgical technique for implant placement will vary based on recipient site, patient factors, and implant material. The most commonly used permanent solid implants are made from silicone, polyethylene, or expanded polytetrafluoroethylene, and most are preformed and sized to treat the desired anatomic region. Facial implants can be used to augment the chin, malar, or submalar regions. Placement of these three implant types can be performed via an intraoral incision and the implant placed into a subperiosteal pocket. The implant may be secured with suture or screws, if desired. In addition, custom implants based on patient imaging are often used for posttraumatic, iatrogenic, or congenital skeletal deficiencies.

◆ Complications

Neurotoxins

The most common complication from BoNT-A use is spread to an adjacent muscle. When treating the glabella with BoNT-A, spread of the product to the levator palpebrae superioris muscle will result in upper lid ptosis. There is no antidote to this complication, but the ptosis will resolve on its own in about 2 weeks. Use of an α-adrenergic agonist drop such as apraclonidine (Iopidine, Novartis, Basel, Switzerland) will stimulate the Müller muscle (superior tarsal muscle) and improve lid elevation until the levator muscle regains function.

Injectable Fillers

Minor risks of injectable fillers include bleeding, bruising and lumpiness, all of which are self-limited. The different filler types can be used simultaneously on the same patient without issue. Hyaluronic acid is the only reversible injectable filler; it can be eliminated in less than a day with injectable H-ase (Vitrase, ISTA Pharmaceuticals Inc., Irvine, CA). Some of the HA products can look blue under the skin (known at the Tyndall effect) when placed too superficially. This can be treated by dissolving the product with H-ase or by inserting a needle into the area of concern and expressing product through the needle tract.

Infection and biofilm formation have been described as complications of filler injections, but fortunately these are rare. The most serious complication of filler injections is vascular compression or embolization, which may result in tissue necrosis, and even blindness. Some feel that the use of cannulas for injection will minimize vascular injuries. When blanching of an anatomic region is seen during filler injections, injections should be stopped immediately, the area massaged and warm compresses placed. H-ase should be injected into the area and topical nitropaste used for maximal vasodilation.

Fat Grafting

Survival of transplanted fat is not 100%, and some patients will require more than one fat transfer procedure. Fat placed too superficially can produce visual or palpable lumps. Contour problems that arise with fat grafting are difficult to manage and may need to be camouflaged with additional fat or fillers, and lumps may need to be excised.

Implants

Complications following alloplastic implants include asymmetry, malposition, infection, and extrusion. Such complications may require implant removal and subsequent reinsertion.

◆ Outcome and Follow-Up

Neurotoxins

The cosmetic benefits from neurotoxin injections last on average 3 to 4 months. Patients find that in some cases, they can go longer between injections because once the BoNTA wears off, they learn to stop using the muscles that were injected.

Injectable Fillers

The duration of filler results depends on both the type of filler used and the location of the injection. Fillers tend to last longer in areas of the face with less movement, such as the temples and lower lids. Patients on average return every 6 to 12 months to augment their filler results.

Fat Grafting

It takes about 3 to 4 months for final assessment of fat survival after fat grafting. Patients may be satisfied with their results or may elect to have another fat grafting procedure. Injectable fillers can also be used in lieu of more surgery, to enhance their volumization.

Implants

Edema may be prolonged after facial implant placement, but at 3 to 4 months the final results should be evident and long-lasting.

9.4.2   Rhytidectomy

◆ Key Features

- Reversing the undesirable signs of the aging face has become important in societies worldwide.
- Although many techniques have been described to lift sagging facial tissues, some are more effective and long-lasting than others.
- Recommendations should be modified to address the problems specific to each patient.
- Postoperative results of a rhytidectomy (also called rhytidoplasty or facelift procedure) should be designed to produce a "natural" and "unoperated" appearance.

◆ Epidemiology

All human faces sag with aging. The skull becomes smaller, and fat is redistributed from the cheeks into the jawline and neck. As facial skin loses its elasticity, it responds to the downward forces of gravity. Prolonged stress, sun exposure, and illness seem to speed up the aging process, making the person appear older than he or she actually is.

◆ Clinical

Signs and Symptoms

Patients in their late forties may present with early sagging of the cheeks and deepening of the melolabial creases. With each decade, the conditions worsen, resulting in drooping of the forehead, lateral brows, cheeks, and neck. Facial rhytides (wrinkles) become more pronounced with each passing year, especially in the areas of facial animation.

In some patients, the platysmal muscles in the midline of the neck become separated and migrate laterally, producing vertical banding from the clavicle to the submental region. Many patients develop submental fat pads. Sagging and bulging tissues of the upper and lower lids are generally seen as well.

Differential Diagnosis

It is important to remember that surgery can reposition drooping tissues and remove loose skin; for facial rhytides, however, a resurfacing procedure is generally required. Dermabrasion, chemical peeling, or laser resurfacing can provide more permanent results in wrinkled skin. In general, unless it takes 2 weeks for a resurfaced area to heal, minimal long-term improvement is expected.

Botulinum neurotoxin and injectable fillers provide only temporary improvement and must be repeated several times each year (see **Chapter 9.4.1**). Injectables are not recommended for pronounced rhytides. Fat or fascial grafting may provide more permanent improvement in deep folds and creases.

◆ Evaluation

Physical Exam

Five facial regions should be examined for ptosis and loss of elasticity: forehead, temporal, cheek, neck, and submental areas. Special attention needs to be paid to the upper and lower lid areas as the forehead, brows, temporal, and cheek tissues are lifted. Some of the loose tissues in the upper lid may be improved by forehead and brow lifting; lifting the cheeks may accentuate loose skin in the lower lid regions.

The lower cheeks and neck should be examined to determine whether liposuction should be included in the treatment plan. If sagging muscles are present, then they must be lifted and secured with several sutures that produce fascia-to-fascia closures.

All branches of the facial nerve should be examined preoperatively to ensure full function. Photographs taken during facial expression maneuvers are helpful for documentation.

Imaging

Unless an underlying bony deformity is suspected, no imaging examinations are recommended for rhytidectomy.

Labs

Metabolic profiles, bleeding studies, and urinalysis are standard preoperative tests. For patients over the age of 40 (or high-risk patients), electrocardiography (ECG) is recommended. Medical clearance from the patient's personal physician is also recommended.

Other Tests

The value of quality photographic documentation before elective facial plastic surgery cannot be overemphasized. Photographs should be taken from frontal, oblique, and lateral positions, bilaterally.

◆ Treatment Options

The "facelift procedure" is not a single operation but *a series of procedures*, each designed to lift, reposition, and tighten redundant skin, muscles, and fat in the face and neck. A variety of approaches have been described, and new ones seem to arise almost daily. Surgical approaches to the aging face vary among surgeons. Some advocate ultraconservative techniques, meaning limited incisions in front of (and behind) the ear, minimal undermining of the skin, and no imbrication suturing of facial muscles and their enveloping fascia. In many cases, lifting is achieved only by lifting skin.

Other surgeons advocate more radical techniques, involving incisions from the occipital region, around the ear, into the hairline and across the head to join with those of a similar nature on the opposite side of the face and neck. In some cases extensive submental muscle and fat work is performed under the chin as a "routine" part of facelifting. The face and neck skin may be freed from ear to ear, connecting the flaps under the chin, and deep dissection may extend beneath the superficial musculoaponeurotic fascia, identifying the various branches of the facial nerve. Liposuction of the lower face and neck may also be added if indicated (see **Chapter 9.4.9**).

In recent years, minimally invasive techniques have been on the rise. Many of those, however, have been abandoned rather quickly because results appear to be short-lived.

◆ Complications

Complications of rhytidectomy include the following:

- Hematoma (most common complication after rhytidectomy)
- Nerve injury (permanent motor nerve paralysis occurs at a rate of 0.5 to 2.6%; the marginal branch is most commonly injured)
- Infection (rarely severe)
- Skin flap necrosis (more common in smokers and in patients with longer and thinner flaps)
- Hypertrophic scarring (predisposing factors for hypertrophic scarring include race, ethnicity, and skin type or family history)

- Alopecia and hairline/earlobe deformities (may be caused by excessive tension on suture lines and are often transient)
- Parotid gland pseudocyst (may occur after trauma to the parotid gland when raising the superficial musculoaponeurotic system flap)

◆ Outcome and Follow-Up

Postoperative care for rhytidectomy is similar to that for managing major flap reconstructions following head and neck cancer or trauma. Subcutaneous drains, negative-pressure vacuum systems, subcutaneous tissue sealants, or pressure dressings may be used to minimize the occurrence of postoperative bleeding.

Flaps should be monitored for vascularity and possible accumulation of body fluids between skin and underlying tissues. Hematomas and seromas should be evacuated as soon as possible.

Avoidance of undue tension on suture lines is important to minimize scarring. Sutures or staples should be removed within ~ 7 days. Preoperative and perioperative antibiotics are optional.

Patients should be counseled to avoid nicotine and other vasoconstricting agents during at least the first 2 postoperative weeks. Time-release niacin and topical nitroglycerin paste are often helpful should flap vascularity appear to be compromised.

A rhytidectomy lasts for life, in that the skin removed at surgery never returns. Patients should always appear younger than their chronologic age. However, the aging process is ongoing and brings with it *additional* sags and bulges to the skin and tissues that were left behind with the first operation.

Secondary lifting or "tuck-ups" are often beneficial to help maintain a more youthful appearance. Timing of secondary surgery varies from surgeon to surgeon and from patient to patient. Some techniques require earlier secondary intervention than others. Some patients age more rapidly than others, causing the appearance of new sags and bulges sooner than in their peers. Stress and chronic illness seem to play a part in premature aging.

Skin resurfacing (chemical peeling, dermabrasion, and laser surgery) several months after rhytidectomy produces new collagen and elastic fibers, creating a more youthful look that seems to last for years.

9.4.3 Brow and Forehead Lifting

◆ Key Features

- The initial consultation should be used to evaluate the orbital complex, the upper third of the face, and the position of the hairline.
- Brow ptosis not only creates aesthetic concerns but also may be associated with a functional visual field deficit.
- If there is concern for a functional deficit, an ophthalmologic evaluation with visual field testing should be requested.

Over time, the aging face bears the cumulative effects of sun exposure, loss of soft tissue volume and elasticity, and dermal atrophy in a predictable manner. The resultant brow ptosis not only creates aesthetic issues but also may be associated with a functional visual field deficit. The muscular elevators of the forehead become hypertonic in an effort to combat brow ptosis. This results in prominent horizontal forehead wrinkling. These interdependent processes produce a tired facial appearance. The skilled aging-face surgeon has multiple brow-lifting techniques and surgical approaches that can be tailored to the individual patient.

◆ Anatomy

Forehead and Scalp

The forehead is the region from the superior brow to the anterior hairline (trichion). The layers of the scalp, from superficial to deep, include the skin, subcutaneous fat, galea fascia, a loose areolar layer, and the periosteum. Galea fascia envelops the frontalis muscle and connects it to the occipitalis muscle. The galea aponeurotica is contiguous with the superficial musculoaponeurotic system (SMAS) of the face below and the temporoparietal fascia (TPF) laterally. The periosteum of the frontal bone merges with the arcus marginalis of the orbit inferiorly. Laterally, at the temporal line, the periosteum fuses with the galea, TPF, and deep temporal fascia to form the conjoined tendon.

Paired frontalis muscles are the principal elevator of the forehead. They originate from the galea and insert onto the overlying skin. They are responsible for the transverse frontal rhytids. The corrugator supercilii muscles originate from the periosteum along the medial supraorbital rim. They insert laterally onto the skin along with the frontalis and orbicularis oculi. They are primarily responsible for the vertical rhytids of the glabella. The procerus muscles originate from the periosteum over the nasal bones and insert onto the skin between the eyebrows. They are principally responsible for the transverse rhytids of the glabella.

The sensory innervation of the forehead is supplied by the supratrochlear and supraorbital nerves. These represent terminal branches of the first division of the trigeminal nerve. In most skulls, the supraorbital nerve exits from a supraorbital notch along the medial supraorbital rim. However, 10% of nerves will exit from a true foramen located 1 to 2 cm superior to the orbit. In either case, these nerves should be identified and preserved during the browlift dissection (**Fig. 9.22**).

Temporal Area

The layers of the temporal area include the skin, subcutaneous fat, superficial temporal fascia (also known as the TPF), and deep temporal fascia, which splits and envelops the temporalis muscle. The temporal branch of the facial nerve travels with the temporal artery and vein within the TPF.

◆ Evaluation

At initial consultation the orbital complex, the upper third of the face, and the position of the hairline are evaluated. The patient's wishes and expectations are addressed. Any asymmetries, including those of brow position,

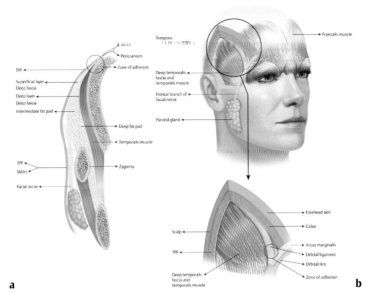

Fig. 9.22 Fascial planes over the temporalis muscle, temporal line, and superior orbital rim. **(a)** Coronal view at the level of midzygomatic arch. **(b)** Note that all layers of the temporalis fascia converge with the galea and pericranium forming the zone of adhesion, which is tightly adherent to the underlying bone. This area, along with the orbital ligament, must be properly released in order to elevate the brow. (Used with permission from Papel ID, ed. *Facial Plastic and Reconstructive Surgery*. 4th ed. New York, NY: Thieme;2016:160.)

should be documented and discussed with the patient. The classic brow is described in its relationship to other structures of the face. The medial limit is positioned through a vertical line originating at the alar–facial groove. The lateral limit is through an oblique line from the alar–facial groove through the lateral canthus of the eye. The medial and lateral brow should lie at the same horizontal position. The ideal female brow possesses an arc over the supraorbital rim. Classically, the maximal peak of the arc is over the lateral limbus of the eye, but many believe that a more natural peak is located above the lateral canthus. The ideal male brow is more horizontal than arced. It should rest along the orbital rim rather than extending above it.

The entire periorbital region should be assessed. The presence of excess upper eyelid skin (dermatochalasis), drooping of the eyelid itself (blepharoptosis), and status of the lower eyelid should be discussed with the patient. These may need to be addressed at the same time as the brow lift. Patients should be asked about dry eye symptoms or use of lubricating drops.

◆ Surgical Approaches and Techniques

Elevation of the brow is performed via with a few main approaches. Although many surgeons currently favor the endoscopic approach, other techniques are available that can be tailored to the individual patient.

Coronal Approach

This technique employs a coronal incision placed 4 to 6 cm posterior to the anterior hairline. The incision is beveled parallel to the hair shafts to minimize trauma and alopecia. Dissection proceeds inferiorly to the level of the supraorbital rims. It occurs within a subgaleal, supraperiosteal plane. The supraorbital neurovascular bundles are identified and preserved. The procerus, frontalis, and corrugator supercilii muscles can be scored or incised. This helps to address prominent forehead and glabellar rhytids.

The lateral dissection occurs in a plane between the TPF and deep temporal fascia. This protects the temporal branch of the facial nerve as well as the temporal artery and vein, which are superficial to the dissection. Once sufficient elevation is achieved, 15 to 25 mm of skin and soft tissue is excised from the length of the incision.

Candidates for this procedure include patients with a low frontal hairline. This approach should not be used on anyone who is losing frontal hair or who is expected to do so. Advantages of the coronal approach are camouflaging of scar, ability to perform myoplasty, and excellent exposure. Limitations include elevation of the hairline, possible alopecia and hypoesthesia along the incision, and requirement of the most extensive dissection.

The *pretrichial lift* is a modification using a coronal incision anterior or just within the frontal border of the hairline. This approach is favored for those with a high hairline or a long forehead. During a *trichophytic lift*, a coronal incision is placed just posterior to the border of the hairline. This has the advantage of superior camouflaging compared with the pretrichial lift.

Midforehead Approach

A transverse incision is placed within a prominent rhytid of the central forehead. The dissection is initially supragaleal and later deepened to a subgaleal plane as the supraorbital margins are approached. This allows for myoplasty of the procerus, corrugator supercilii and the inferior aspect of the frontalis muscles, while minimizing the risk of hypoesthesia to the forehead.

Candidates for this approach are men with thinning hair and prominent forehead rhytids. Advantages of the midforehead approach are that it does not alter the level of the hairline, it allows for myoplasty, and a limited dissection is required. Disadvantages include a potentially unsatisfactory scar, limited lateral elevation, and an inability to address the upper forehead.

Direct Brow Approach

The direct brow approach is a transverse excision of skin and subcutaneous tissue parallel and immediately superior to each brow. The orbicularis oculi is suspended to the periosteum above. This approach is seldom employed. Its application is limited to those with a functional brow ptosis who place little emphasis on aesthetic results or in patients with unilateral brow ptosis secondary to facial paralysis. Advantages are that it is applicable for the very elderly and otherwise poor surgical candidates. It employs a limited dissection and has excellent control of brow position. The limitations of this approach are an unsatisfactory scar, an inability to perform myoplasty, and an inability to address the upper or lateral forehead.

Endoscopic Approach

This is the most recently described and currently favored approach. It employs four to six 1- or 2-cm incisions placed posterior and perpendicular to the hairline. Dissection is carried inferiorly in a subperiosteal plane. Blind dissection may be used until a level 2 cm above the supraorbital rim. A 30° endoscope is then employed to visualize the supraorbital neurovascular bundles. Gentle elevation is used to release the periosteum of the forehead from the arcus marginalis of the orbit. The corrugator supercilii, procerus, and frontalis muscles may be scored if necessary. The lateral dissection occurs in a plane between the TPF and deep temporal fascia. At the temporal line the conjoined tendon is released with sharp and blunt instrumentation joining the central and lateral pockets. The inferior limit is the zygoma, which approximates the level of the lateral canthus. Following sufficient elevation, the flap is suspended to the calvaria using a variety of techniques. Though many advocate suture fixation through cortical bone tunnels, miniplates, microscrews, and other methods are also commonly used.

The endoscopic approach is the preferred approach for most patients. Advantages of the endoscopic approach are that it is the least invasive, provides excellent scar camouflaging, allows myoplasty, and can address the entire upper one-third of the face. It is limited by the need for special training and a lack of long-term results.

◆ Complications

Complications of brow lift include alopecia of scars placed within the hairline, or visible scars in a direct brow, midforehead, or pretrichial lift. Hypoesthesia of the forehead may occur due to injury to the supratrochlear or supraorbital nerves. Weakness of the frontal branch of the facial nerve is uncommon and may be avoided by proper plane of dissection. Overelevation of the brow may lead to lagophthalmos (inability to close the eye), particularly if combined with an upper eyelid blepharoplasty. Proper preoperative diagnosis and meticulous technique are the key to avoiding this complication. If this procedure is performed with a blepharoplasty, the brow lift should be performed first to avoid overresection of eyelid skin. Brow asymmetry may require revision. Inadequate elevation with poor patient satisfaction may occur. Overelevation of the medial brow will produce an unnatural, surprised look and should be carefully avoided.

◆ Outcome and Follow-Up

Suction drains are rarely necessary. Sutures or staples are typically removed ~ 7 days after surgery. Patients may note a "tightness" to their forehead initially that will resolve with time. Bruising and periorbital edema may take 2 weeks to resolve. Patients should be followed until satisfactory healing and results have been achieved.

9.4.4   Chemical Peels and Laser Skin Resurfacing

◆ Key Features

- Resurfacing is useful for improving the quality and texture of the skin.
- Options for facial resurfacing include chemical peeling, dermabrasion, and laser surgery.
- Resurfacing techniques are to be individualized based on skin character as well as patient and surgeon preferences.
- Appropriate measures should be taken to reduce toxic systemic and local side effects with deep chemical peels.

For many years, various methods of resurfacing aged skin have been used, including mechanical resurfacing with dermabrasion, chemical peeling with various agents (e.g., salicylic acid, trichloroacetic acid, phenol), and laser thermal exfoliation. The type of chemical formula used will affect the depth of the peel, and the degree of laser injury may be varied by altering the type of laser technology (wavelength) used and individualizing settings. The type of resurfacing technique selected will depend on patient characteristics and wishes as well as surgeon experience and availability of technology.

◆ Clinical

Patients with wrinkled, sun-damaged, weathered skin are the best candidates for an exfoliative procedure. Resurfacing will also address fine wrinkles that may be present after other rejuvenation procedures (e.g., blepharoplasty). Pigmented lesions (lentigo, freckles, etc.) and diffuse keratotic lesions (seborrheic and actinic keratosis) may also show improvement after chemical exfoliation or laser skin resurfacing. Limited improvement may sometimes be seen when peeling is used for superficial acne scars; however, deeper lesions may require other modalities (dermabrasion, excision, or laser resurfacing).

◆ Evaluation

Patients must be in appropriate physical and mental condition, must be compliant with posttreatment care, and must have realistic expectations. Female patients with a fair complexion are ideal candidates. Pigment change may be more obvious in dark-skinned patients and the risk of postprocedural pigment complications will increase with darker-skinned individuals. Care must be taken in higher Fitzpatrick skin types (**Table 9.7**).

A general facial aesthetic evaluation should be performed evaluating skin character and degree of photoaging, volume loss or redistribution, and presence of sagging skin. As resurfacing techniques will improve the surface appearance of the skin, other signs of aging may need to be addressed concomitantly based on the concerns of the patient. A general health history will determine whether the patient is a candidate for a resurfacing procedure, and a history of recurrent herpes viral outbreaks may require prophylaxis. If a deep peel is selected (e.g., phenol), because of the risk of cardiotoxicity, nephrotoxicity, and hepatotoxicity, a preoperative work-up of electrocardiogram (ECG), liver function panel, and blood urea nitrogen (BUN)/creatinine assay may be considered. Ideal candidates are light-skinned patients with photodamaged skin, facial rhytids, dyschromias, and even irregular scars.

Table 9.7 Fitzpatrick skin type scale

Phototype	Characteristics	Risk of pigmentary dyschromia after resurfacing
I	Pale white skin. Blond or red hair. Blue eyes. Always burns, never tans.	Minimal
II	White skin. Usually burns, tans with minimally. Blue/green/hazel eyes.	Minimal
III	Tans uniformly, burns moderately. Light brown or olive skin.	Intermediate
IV	Burns rarely, tans easily. Moderate brown skin.	High
V	Very rarely burns, tans profusely. Dark brown skin.	High
VI	Never burns or tans. Always deeply pigmented dark brown to black skin.	High

◆ Treatment Options

Chemical Peel

Chemical peeling involves applying an agent or formula to the skin that damages the skin in a predictable manner followed by reepithelialization from the epidermal appendages and wound edges. Many peeling solutions exist (**Table 9.8**) with differing depths of injury. The type of solution to be used will vary based on patient skin characteristics, desired outcome and recovery time, and surgeon experience.

Table 9.8 Depth of chemical peels

Depth of peel	Sample agents	Outcome	Time to healing
Superficial	Trichloroacetic acid (TCA) 10–25% Glycolic acid 40–70% Salicylic acid 5–15% Jessner solution	Exfoliates stratum corneum up to entire epidermis Subtle results Requires repetition	1–4 days

continued

Table 9.8   Depth of chemical peels *(Continued)*

Medium	Trichloroacetic acid 35–50% Combination (glycolic acid or Jessner + 35% TCA)	Moderate reduction of facial rhytids and dyschromias Removal of epidermal lesions	4–10 days
Deep	Trichloroacetic acid > 50% Phenol Combination phenol (e.g., Gordon-Baker)	Improvement in severely photodamaged skin Increased risk of adverse effects	10–14 days

Superficial peels are intended to treat varying degrees of the epidermal layer, from stratum corneum alone to full-thickness epidermal sloughing. For the deeper superficial peels, the end point of treatment is frosting. These peels are well tolerated with minimal downtime and complete resolution of erythema and exfoliation within 1 to 4 days. Results tend to be subtle, and repetitive treatments are required to obtain a satisfactory result.

Medium-depth peeling agents provide a controlled injury down to the papillary dermis, thereby producing more improvement in photoaged skin. The skin is cleansed and degreased prior to applying the peeling agent. Patients will experience more discomfort, which may require pretreatment with an anxiolytic or sedative, and pain medication may be used. After appropriate application, a white frost (indicative of keratocoagulation) with erythema showing through will be apparent for most medium-depth peels.

Deep peels should be reserved for patients with severely photodamaged skin and should be performed by an experienced provider with good preoperative counseling of patients regarding the lengthy recovery period and increased risks associated. The most commonly used deep peel solution is the Baker-Gordon peel (phenol USP 88%, croton oil, Septisol soap [Steris, Mentor, OH], and distilled water), but other solutions exist. More dilute solutions of phenol may penetrate more deeply. As mentioned, phenol has cardiotoxic, nephrotoxic, and hepatotoxic properties, and careful preoperative evaluation and intraoperative monitoring should be performed. This procedure is performed under sedation, and intravenous hydration should be provided to decrease serum phenol concentration. For full face peels, a delay of 15 minutes between applications for each aesthetic unit should be allowed to ensure that the blood level of phenol remains safe, with a total time to full face application of 60 to 90 minutes.

After adequate preparation (for full facial peels), the patient is usually given light sedation while the local anesthesia is administered. The entire face is then cleansed and surface oils are removed. The removal of the surface oils will allow for a deeper, more evenly distributed peel. After a light coating of solution is applied with a cotton-tipped applicator, a light frost should appear immediately and will usually fade within a few minutes. Feathering of the peel at the margins of the peel area helps avoid obvious demarcation lines at the edge of a treated area. If hair is adjacent to the peeled area, then feathering should be performed into hair-bearing areas.

When deep wrinkles extend onto the lips, the application of additional peel may be needed to improve these creases. This is done by dipping the broken end of a wooden cotton-tipped applicator into the peel, then applying a small amount directly onto the crease. When peeling the eyelids, the peel should be applied within 2 to 3 mm of the lid margin. Care should be taken in the canthal regions to dry any tearing that occurs. Tears can draw the peeling fluid into the eye, which could result in ocular damage. Tears may also dilute the peeling formula, which could result in deeper penetration and scarring.

The effect of the peel may be altered by the type of solution used, appropriate cleansing and degreasing of the face, and the postoperative care, including whether occlusive dressings are used.

Laser Skin Resurfacing Procedure

Currently, two lasers are in common use for facial skin resurfacing: the carbon dioxide (CO_2) laser, and the erbium:yttrium-aluminum-garnet (Er:YAG) laser. These two may also be used in combination, and both recognize water as their chromophore. The ultimate depth of injury will vary based on type of laser selected, whether it is fractionated, whether the laser is ablative or nonablative, and the settings selected by the surgeon. These should be customized based on individual patient characteristics. For information on these and other lasers, see **Chapter 1.7**.

Contraindications for laser skin resurfacing include active acne or infection, deep acne pits, and isotretinoin use in the past 6 months.

Prophylactic antibiotics are not uniformly employed, but in patients with a history of herpes viral infection, prophylactic antivirals may be used for 7 to 10 days. Nerve blocks and local anesthetic are used, and an anxiolytic (e.g., lorazepam) or pain medication (e.g., hydrocodone) may be given to patients. No intravenous or intramuscular medications are typically necessary. Skin lesions and actinic regions are removed by sequential ablative passes. The end point is reached when the lesion base has been removed or when a depth to the midreticular dermis has been achieved. Deep wrinkles and scars are treated by direct lasering into the furrows or scar. When treating the whole face or a facial region, each aesthetic unit should be blended within its boundaries for optimal camouflage, and smooth, symmetric passes are made. Following laser skin resurfacing, patients may experience erythema and edema with sloughing for a week while reepithelialization occurs.

Dermabrasion

Dermabrasion is a technique to mechanically resurface by removing the epidermis and into the papillary dermis using a rotating wire brush or diamond fraise. The end point is when pinpoint bleeding is visible followed by faint parallel collagen bands. Reepithelialization occurs from the epidermal appendages as well as wound edges, and there is an increase in type I and III collagen. In patients treated with isotretinoin for acne, pilosebaceous gland atrophy may occur, which increases the risk of adverse scarring. Dermabrasion should be delayed for at least 6 months after stopping therapy to minimize this risk.

◆ Complications

All resurfacing techniques require meticulous postoperative care to prevent complications. Common complications include formation of milia or small inclusion cysts that may require treatment with tretinoin or unroofing, acne outbreaks that may require use of tetracycline, or prolonged erythema treated with topical steroids.

Wound infection may occur in the form of a cutaneous herpes simplex outbreak, bacterial infection, or fungal infection. The incidence of herpes outbreak can be decreased in carriers with perioperative systemic antiviral therapy until reepithelialization has occurred. Bacterial infections (such as with *Staphylococcus* or *Pseudomonas* spp.) are rare when patients follow the postoperative instructions faithfully. Should infection develop, vigorous cleaning and antibiotic therapy are important to prevent any long-term sequelae. Fungal infections typically develop later and should be treated with an antifungal agent.

Other local complications include pigmentary changes. The risk of hyperpigmentation is increased in patients with high postprocedure estrogen states (such as hormone replacements or pregnancy) and in higher Fitzpatrick skin types. Treatment often involves use of hydroquinone, tretinoin, and sunscreen. Hypertrophic scarring has been known to occur and can be treated with intralesional and topical steroids. Scar revision might be needed in some situations. Complications of laser skin resurfacing include hyperpigmentation, erythema, infection, and scarring.

Systemic complications associated with phenol use include hepatotoxicity, nephrotoxicity, and cardiotoxicity. Adequate hydration and judicious time spacing between peeling the aesthetic regions are the keys to keeping blood levels at a tolerable level and avoiding toxicity. Caution should be exercised when using the phenol-containing formulas in patients with abnormal ECGs or with patients with elevated liver or kidney function studies. It may be wise to obtain medical clearance in these patients before proceeding.

◆ Outcome and Follow-Up

Postoperative care regimens vary widely. In general, cool saline sponges are applied to help reduce discomfort. Patients are instructed to cleanse their face 6 to 10 times daily, often with hydrogen peroxide or 0.013% acetic acid (1 teaspoon white vinegar in 1 pint of water). A thick layer of emollient is applied (e.g., Vaseline [Unilever, London, UK], Aquaphor [Beiersdorf AG, Hamburg, Germany]) until reepithelialization occurs. Scabs should not be allowed to form.

Close patient follow-up is of key importance in the first few weeks after resurfacing. Swelling usually begins to subside by the fourth day, whereas the associated erythema may take 8 to 12 weeks or longer for deeper resurfacing procedures. Desquamation usually begins at 24 to 48 hours after surgery, and most is completed by 10 to 14 days postoperatively for even the deepest treatments. Ideally, sun exposure should be avoided for 6 months after peeling, to reduce any undesirable pigmentary changes. Sunscreen should also be used for added protection.

9.4.5 Blepharoplasty

◆ Key Features

- Blepharoplasty is indicated for correction of laxity and redundancy of eyelid skin with removal or repositioning of pseudoherniated fat.
- It may be performed at the same time with correction of abnormal eyelid position or treatment of blepharoptosis.
- The entire brow-lid complex should be assessed and a brow lift performed if necessary.

The aging face often reflects changes in the periorbital region. The goals of blepharoplasty are to provide restoration and rejuvenation of the eyelids, and it may involve addressing the following problems:

- *Blepharochalasia* occurs in young women and is characterized by eyelid edema leading to progressive tissue breakdown. This may be associated with a relatively uncommon variant of angioneurotic edema.
- *Dermatochalasis* consists of excess eyelid skin and is indicative of the aging process, with a genetic predisposition.
- *Blepharoptosis* occurs when the inferior portion of the upper eyelid margin sits over the iris and is due to levator muscle dysfunction. In this case, a ptosis repair will be performed at the time of blepharoplasty.
- Finally, if *brow ptosis* is evident, this may lead to a heavy and fatigued appearance of the periorbital complex and should be addressed at the time of blepharoplasty (see **Chapter 9.4.3**).

◆ Anatomy

Eyelids

The eyelid is a trilamellar structure with thin skin (average thickness 0.13 inches [3.3 mm]) that is adherent to underlying orbicularis oculi muscle, especially in the region of the tarsal plates, with progressive loosening in the area of the orbital rims.

- The anterior lamella consists of skin and orbicularis muscles.
- The middle lamella consists of the orbital septum.
- The posterior lamella consists of the eyelid retractors, tarsus, and conjunctiva. In the upper eyelid this includes the levator aponeurosis, tarsus, Müller muscle (superior tarsal muscle), and the conjunctival lining. In the lower eyelid, it is composed of the inferior retractor muscles, tarsus, conjunctiva, and associated capsulopalpebral fascia (**Fig. 9.23**).

Orbicularis Oculi Muscle

The striated orbicularis oculi muscle encircles the orbit and acts to close the eyes and facilitate tear flow. It is divided into the palpebral portion and

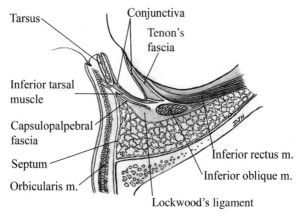

Fig. 9.23 Cross-section of the lower eyelid demonstrating connective tissue expansion of inferior rectus into its terminal insertions. (Used with permission from Papel ID, ed. *Facial Plastic and Reconstructive Surgery*. 3rd ed. New York, NY: Thieme;2009:273.)

the orbital part, which overlies the orbital rim. The palpebral part is further divided into the pretarsal portion over the tarsal plates and the preseptal portion over the orbital septum. The medial canthal tendon is formed via attachment of the superficial heads of the pretarsal muscle and attaches to the lacrimal crest. The lateral canthal tendon is formed by the upper and lower pretarsal muscles joining laterally and inserts on the orbital tubercle (Whitnall's tubercle).

Orbital Septum

The orbital septum attaches to the bony orbital cavity and is anatomically continuous with the periosteum. It acts to support the orbital contents, including orbital fat, and serves as a physical barrier to the spread of infection and tumor. The upper orbital septum fuses with the levator aponeurosis, whereas the lower orbital septum fuses with the capsulopalpebral fascia.

Levator Muscle

The levator palpebrae superioris muscle is the principal elevator of the upper eyelid, originating in the superior orbital apex and inserting in the upper eyelid. As it courses anteriorly, it thins to form the levator aponeurosis.

Capsulopalpebral Fascia

The capsulopalpebral fascia is a fibroelastic structure in the lower eyelid, similar to the levator aponeurosis, which fuses with the orbital septum ~ 5 mm below the inferior boundary of tarsus. This functions, in combination with inferior palpebral muscles, to retract the conjunctiva and tarsus on downward gaze.

Tarsus

The tarsus is dense connective tissue providing support for the eyelid that attaches to trochlear fascia medially and fascia of the orbital lobe of the lacrimal gland laterally. The height of the superior tarsal plate is 8 to 9 mm, and the height of the inferior tarsal plate is 4 to 5 mm.

Orbital Fat Compartments

In the lower eyelid, three fat compartments exist: medial, central, and lateral. The lateral and medial compartments are separated by a fascial barrier, while the medial and central compartments are separated by the inferior oblique muscle. In the upper eyelid there are two fat pads: the central and medial compartments. The lateral compartment of the upper eyelid consists of the lacrimal gland.

◆ Evaluation

A history with focus on aging and ocular history should be performed. In particular, a history of visual field disturbance or dry eye syndrome should be elucidated and further evaluated. An ophthalmologic examination should at least include visual acuity, ocular motility, and general eye health. The presence of Bell phenomenon, in which the eyes rotate upward on attempted closure of the eyelids, should be noted. This normal rotation ensures corneal protection if blepharoplasty results in suboptimal lid closure. The presence of pseudoherniation of orbital fat should be noted. If the upper eyelid extends inferiorly over the iris, indicating blepharoptosis, this should be addressed at the time of surgery.

Lid distraction test should be performed (snap test) to assess for lower lid laxity. This is performed by outwardly displacing the lower lid and observing for a normal snap (lid settling quickly back in place with less than 10 mm displacement). If the test is positive, the patient may need a lid-tightening procedure. A *lid retraction test* also tests the laxity of the lower eyelid via inferior displacement. If the puncta moves > 3 mm, this indicates a lax canthal tendon and the possible need for a tendon plication to avoid ectropion or scleral show.

Any history of dry eye symptoms or use of lubricating drops warrants further evaluation with a *Schirmer test*. This involves placing a strip of filter paper in the fornix of the lower eyelid at the lateral edge of the limbus. More than 10 to 15 mm of moisture on the paper in 5 minutes is normal. Care should be taken in patients with an abnormal test, as blepharoplasty may increase dry eye symptoms.

Finally, the brow position should be assessed and considered as a separate entity. The brow should be at the orbital rim in males or just above the orbital rim in females. If brow ptosis is present, a brow repositioning procedure may be needed as well. In complex cases or if abnormal testing is noted, a formal ophthalmologic evaluation may be warranted.

◆ Contraindications

Contraindications for a cosmetic blepharoplasty include severe heart or lung disease and psychological factors. Blepharoplasty is cautioned in patients with any of the following:

- Bleeding disorder or recent use of anticoagulants
- Previous facial palsy, as it may lead to persistent weakness of the periorbital musculature with inadequate corneal lubrication and recurrent periorbital edema
- Chronic renal disease and diabetes, as they may lead to wound-healing problems
- Thyroid disease including dry eyes syndrome and myxedema; eyelid manifestations may be eliminated by treating hypothyroidism
- Severe dry eyes
- Unrealistic patient expectations

◆ Surgical Goals

Upper Eyelid Blepharoplasty

Goals include addressing fat herniation, skin redundancy, and muscle hypertrophy. Note the asymmetry of the upper eyelids and the position of the superior orbital sulcus: the "tarsal crease" should be < 10 mm from lid margin and below the bony margin of the orbital rim.

The incision is marked with the patient in an upright position. The medial point of incision is 4 mm medial and 4 mm cephalad to the medial canthal tendon, taking care to avoid the concavity of the medial orbital rim, as this leads to webbing. The lower incision is marked along the tarsal crease ~ 9 to 10 mm from the lid margin. Incisions may be carried laterally 3 to 4 mm past the lateral canthal tendon, or farther for severe lateral hooding. An elliptical-shaped skin specimen is incised, followed by blunt dissection with scissors and elevation off the orbicularis muscle. An orbicularis strip may then be removed, followed by conservative fat removal if necessary. The skin is closed with a single layer of running permanent or absorbable suture.

Lower Eyelid Blepharoplasty

Goals include maintaining a sharp, well-defined lateral canthal angle, maintenance of a good lower-eyelid position with an absence of scleral show, resolution of fat bulging and infraorbital hollows, and treatment of excess skin. Surgical incisions are designed to avoid scar contracture in the vertical dimension, lower eyelid retraction, and ectropion.

Two popular surgical approaches include the subciliary and transconjunctival:

Subciliary Approach

The transcutaneous subciliary approach employs an external incision just below the eyelashes (high, immediately subciliary, or relatively lower to preserve the pretarsal orbicularis muscle). A skin-muscle flap technique is the preferred method when resection of the orbicularis muscle and skin is indicated; the incision is through the skin, followed by elevation and possible fat removal. Fat removal requires the discrete separation of muscle fibers over each fat compartment and incising through the orbital septum. Fat may be removed from the lateral compartment first, followed by the central and then medial compartments. Alternatively, the medial and central fat pads may be pedicled and repositioned into a prominent infraorbital hollow. Closure involves lateral and superior elevation with resuspension of the orbicularis muscle.

Advantages of the subciliary approach include a relatively avascular plane with a minimal risk of skin penetration, and additional tightening via skin muscle suspension using sutures from the lateral orbicularis muscle to the lateral orbital region.

Limitations of the subciliary approach include a possible increased risk of ectropion and a visible scar. The surgeon may use surgical tape to counter the gravitational effect of postoperative edema, external scar, hematoma, or bruising as a result of orbicularis muscle dissection. There may be scar contracture with rounding of the eyelid.

Transconjunctival Approach

Lower eyelid blepharoplasty is centered on the removal or repositioning of redundant pseudoherniated fat with incision on the inner aspect of the eyelid. The ideal candidate is young with significant pseudoherniation of fat, minimal skin excess, and minimal orbicularis hypertrophy. This approach is especially helpful to use in patients with tight, inelastic lower eyelids exhibiting scleral show, as this approach transects and releases inferior retractor muscles.

The incision is in the lower eyelid conjunctiva with avoidance of disruption of orbicularis muscle. The preseptal approach involves placing the incision high along the inner eyelid conjunctiva, with dissection anterior to the orbital septum and under the orbicularis muscle. Exposure of the surgical site and globe protection are facilitated with the use of nonconducting retractors. The dissection is continued downward and forward until all the pseudoherniated fat is exposed and either removed or pedicled and repositioned. Skin may be resected as necessary using the "pinch" technique or may be combined with chemical peel or laser resurfacing to address superficial rhytids. The transconjunctival incision does not require closure.

Advantages of the transconjunctival approach include avoidance of external scar, and potentially less risk of ectropion. Limitations include lack of addressing skin excess or hypertrophy of the orbicularis muscle and the potential for entropion.

◆ Surgical Pearls

- Meticulous hemostasis is a must. Lower eyelid blepharoplasty is associated with a higher rate of hematoma formation.
- Avoid braided sutures for closure, as they may lead to inflammation and rejection.

- Avoid a retracted or "hollow" look in patients due to excessive fat removal.
- Fat may be repositioned into the infraorbital hollow in the lower eyelids to improve contour.

◆ Complications

Acute Complications

Milia are inclusion cysts that often require unroofing for treatment. Hematoma is more common in the lower lid, and fat removal may predispose to a retrobulbar hematoma with increased intraocular pressure, requiring urgent surgical intervention to prevent vision loss. It may occur up to a few days postoperatively and is treated with a lateral canthotomy and inferior cantholysis. An ophthalmologic consultation should be sought. Blindness is a rare complication of periorbital surgery.

Chronic Complications

Eyelid malposition with either ectropion or entropion may occur. Immediate treatment consists of eyelid massage for several months. If the abnormality persists it may require surgical revision. Lagophthalmos is the inability to completely close the eye and may be temporary or permanent. This will accentuate dry eye symptoms and may lead to corneal abrasion and vision loss in severe cases. Aggressive lubrication is critical and if it persists intervention is necessary. Injury to the upper lid levator muscle or aponeurosis may lead to blepharoptosis and requires revision surgery for repair. Epiphora, or tearing, may occur if injury to the lacrimal system occurs. Finally, inadequate excision of skin and fat may lead to a dissatisfied patient and require revision.

9.4.6 Otoplasty

◆ Key Features

- An otoplasty entails the changing or reshaping of the auricle, usually applied to congenitally prominent or protruding ears; it should be differentiated from the operations used to repair the congenital condition of microtia.
- Techniques include cartilage scoring, removal, and varied suture techniques.
- Proper diagnosis is critical to successful outcome.

Otoplasty can aesthetically improve the shape, position, or proportion of the auricle (external ear). See **Chapter 3.0** for the embryology and anatomy of the normal ear; **Fig. 3.2** in that chapter illustrates the anatomical landmarks of the auricle. The auricle is composed of fibroelastic cartilage with overlying skin. The lateral skin is tightly adherent to the cartilage, whereas the medial or postauricular skin has loose connective tissue subcutaneously and thus can be easily separated and peeled from the underlying concha and scapha. The lobule has no cartilage and can have several anatomic configurations and positions.

The abnormal development that results in deformities of the auricle usually originates from the second branchial arch. These abnormalities usually manifest themselves before the end of the first trimester of pregnancy; the frequency of variants is from 3 to 5% of the Western population. Auricular deformities are often inherited in an autosomal dominant fashion.

Also, aging makes the auricle appear larger, in part due to elongation of the lobule.

◆ Evaluation of Aesthetic Deformities of the Auricle

The helix, scapha/antihelix, posterior conchal wall, and conchal floor make up the four planes of the auricle. The angles between these planes and the auricle or scalp determine the degree of protrusion of the ear. The degree of protrusion or malformation is described as a variant from the normal concha–scapha angle. Normal ears have a concha–scapha angle of 75° to 105°, with 90° most common. The scalp–concha angle also is typically ~ 90°. This sets the helix approximately parallel to and 2.0 to 2.5 cm from the scalp. The typical angle from the scalp to the helix is 20° to 30°. An ear is classified as "protruding" when the concha–scapha angle > 110°, the angle of the ear to scalp > 40°, or the helical rim protrudes > 3 cm (**Fig. 9.24**).

◆ Surgical Techniques

Treatment of abnormally shaped ears commonly addresses two concerns: the lack of development of the antihelical fold and the deep concha cavum, respectively. Treatment of the underdeveloped antihelical fold is divided into two concepts. The Mustarde-type approach utilizes permanent sutures to re-create the antihelical fold. The second approach utilizes scoring incisions, abrading, or filing the cartilage to alter its shape, thus reestablishing a fold. A combination of the techniques may be utilized, particularly if the scapha is resistant to reshaping via suture placement. The conchal bowl is likewise treated with two different approaches. One is the Furnas-type approach of suturing posterior conchal cartilage to the mastoid periosteum. The other techniques involve excisions of conchal cartilage, usually performed through the postauricular incision. The excisions can be elliptical or crescent-shaped with reapproximation of the cartilage, or they can be disk-shaped when combined with conchal setback techniques. The goal is to reduce the height of the posterior conchal wall, thus reducing the prominence of the ear.

In the majority of patients, the permanent suture technique is utilized with or without scapha weakening. Deep conchal bowls are reduced by elliptical posterior cartilage excisions of 3 to 5 mm and usually followed by a conchal setback procedure. The procedure is done under general anesthesia in children and under local anesthesia with sedation in adults. The procedure is performed with vasoconstricting local anesthesia. The incision is placed above the postauricular sulcus in an intermediate location between the mastoid and postauricular skin and the edge of the auricle.

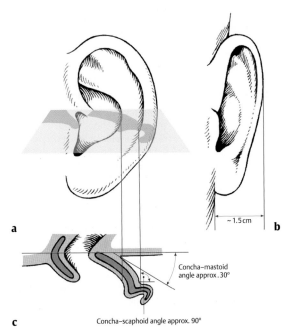

Fig. 9.24 Position of the auricle and angular measurements in cross-section (left auricle). **(a)** Lateral view showing the transverse plane at the level of the ear canal. Corresponding vertical lines indicate the position of the antihelix and scapha. **(b)** Normally the helix projects no more than 1.5 cm from the head when viewed from the front. **(c)** Cross section at the level of the ear canal. The retroauricular angle between the concha and scapha (scaphoconchal angle) is approximately 90°, and the angle between the auricle and mastoid plane (concha–mastoid angle) is approximately 30°. (Used with permission from Theissing J, Rettinger G, Werner JA. *ENT—Head and Neck Surgery: Essential Procedures*. Stuttgart/New York: Thieme; 2011:321.)

When reducing the conchal bowl, perform this first by excision of 3 to 5 mm and reapproximating the edges with 5-0 clear Prolene suture. The edges are undermined to avoid bunching of the skin, but not so extensively as to create conditions for hematoma formation. To create the antihelical fold, the auricle is folded and the location for suture placement necessary to make the fold permanent is noted.

The locations are then marked externally and internally prior to suture placement. The sutures are placed (usually two or three) in horizontal mattress fashion and are tied after all are placed. The knots are triply placed so that the suture can be "cinched" into its ideal position. The protrusion of the ear from the scalp is measured and set to approximately 2.0 cm so that the ear is not bound to the scalp, nor will it be inadequately repositioned. After completing the conchal bowl and antihelical fold portions of the procedure, excess skin may be trimmed and additional maneuvers to reposition the lobule by postauricular skin excision completed if deemed necessary. A cotton ball impregnated with mineral oil or topical ointment is then suture-fixated to the conchal bowl by placing 3–0 nylon on a long Keith needle to secure the bolster. A mastoid dressing is applied. The patient is discharged with a pain medication and a broad spectrum prophylactic antibiotic based on surgeon preference.

◆ Complications

Complications of otoplasty are rare but include the possibility of hematoma formation, incision dehiscence, and a permanent suture dehiscence that would require a secondary procedure to replace the suture. Delayed extrusion of permanent suture can occur. If this should develop after 6 months, the suture can be removed without a significant change to the auricular contour; thus, it is usually not necessary to replace an extruded suture at this point of the recovery. Wound infection is uncommon but should be treated aggressively to avoid the long-term complication associated with chondritis. Although not commonly recognized as a complication, under- or overcorrection of the auricular deformity may occur. This should be managed individually to promote patient and family satisfaction with the surgical outcome, with consideration of the risk-benefit ratio of further intervention.

Revision surgery should not be considered until long-term healing has occurred, with the exception of short-term suture failure, which should be addressed by suture replacement.

◆ Outcome and Follow-Up

After discharge of the patient, a postoperative visit is scheduled 48 hours after the procedure to evaluate the surgical site specifically for a conchal bowl hematoma. The appropriate use of the cotton bolster combined with conservative elevation of the overlying skin of the conchal bowl should make this complication rare. Any hematoma should be promptly evacuated by aspiration or evacuation. It is common at this point to see significant swelling as well as some bruising of the auricle. The dressing is reapplied and left in place for another 48 hours. Upon the patient's revisit, the patient is advised to apply an elastic bandage over the ears at bedtime for one month. Suture removal is done at 7 to 10 days if necessary.

9.4.7 Rhinoplasty

◆ Key Features

- Careful preoperative nasal analysis and clear patient communication are important to success.
- Open or closed approaches can be utilized, depending on the exposure required and preference.
- Meticulous surgical technique is required.

Rhinoplasty is surgery to reshape the nose, the most prominent and central facial feature. Common requests include making a nose smaller, reducing the bridge of the nose, narrowing the nose, making changes to the nasal tip, lifting a droopy nose, improving nasal breathing, revising a previous rhinoplasty, and others. What bothers one person about his or her nose may not bother another person. Still, most rhinoplasty patients know what they do not like about their nose. In addition to cosmetic concerns, deformities may contribute to problems with nasal function, such as an obstruction from valve collapse, requiring repair. The great majority of patients benefit emotionally and psychologically from rhinoplasty.

◆ Anatomy

Although the anatomy of the nose has been fundamentally understood for many years, only relatively recently has there been an increased understanding of the long-term effects of surgical changes upon the function and appearance of the nose. A detailed understanding of nasal anatomy is critical for successful rhinoplasty (**Fig. 9.25**).

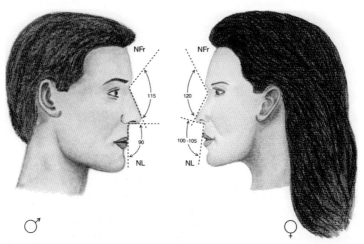

Fig. 9.25   Differences between male and female ideals for the nasofrontal (NFr) and nasolabial (NL) angles. (Used with permission from Papel ID, ed. *Facial Plastic and Reconstructive Surgery.* 3rd ed. New York, NY: Thieme; 2009:122.)

Accurate assessment of the anatomic variations presented by a patient allows the surgeon to develop a rational and realistic surgical plan. Furthermore, recognizing variant or aberrant anatomy is critical to preventing functional compromise or untoward aesthetic results. It is critical to consider the soft tissue and skin of the nose, which is thickest usually at the nasal tip, thinnest at the rhinion, and thick also at the nasion. The main underlying structures are the paired nasal bones, the upper lateral cartilages, the nasal septum, and the lower lateral (alar) cartilages, which include a medial, intermediate, and lateral crus.

✦ Evaluation

It is critically important that the facial plastic surgeon develop skills of facial and nasal analysis. This requires an understanding of the "aesthetic ideal." A nose that is considered "ideal" is one that is harmonious with a patient's other favorable facial features. Our perception of beauty helps define what makes an ideal shape for a female or male nose, so there is also always a bit of an artistic element to this concept. Although the "aesthetic ideal" cannot be completely boiled down to simple lines and numbers, guidelines or proportions do exist that represent primarily the Caucasian aesthetic ideal. Examples include the nasolabial angle (ideally ~ 90–105°) and the nasofrontal angle (ideally ~ 115–120°), though many other angulations and calculations also exist. These are only general guidelines for determining appropriate proportions, and surgeons must have an underlying artistic ability to conceptualize beauty to create a harmonious result. Preoperative photographic documentation is important, in frontal, in right and left oblique, and in right and left lateral and basal views. Again, good communication regarding surgical goals is imperative, bearing in mind these relative contraindications to rhinoplasty:

- Continued intranasal cocaine use
- Psychiatric or mental instability
- Body dysmorphic disorder
- Unrealistic patient expectations
- Significant medical comorbidities
- History of too many previous rhinoplasties

✦ Incisions and Approaches

Incisions are methods of gaining access to the bony and cartilaginous structures of the nose and include transcartilaginous, intercartilaginous, marginal, and transcolumellar incisions. Approaches provide surgical exposure of the nasal structures and include cartilage-splitting (transcartilaginous incision), retrograde (intercartilaginous incision with retrograde dissection), delivery (intercartilaginous and marginal incisions), and external (transcolumellar and marginal incisions) approaches. Based on an analysis of the individual patient's anatomy and surgeon preference, appropriate incisions, approaches, and tip sculpturing techniques may be selected.

An operative algorithm may provide a helpful starting point in selecting the incisions, approaches, and techniques used in nasal surgery. In every case, the patient's anatomy directs the selection of appropriate technique. As the anatomic deformity becomes more abnormal, a graduated, stepwise approach is taken. Other factors, however, such as the need for spreader grafts, complex nasal deviation, and surgeon preference, among other things, may also appropriately affect the ultimate selection of approach.

The endonasal approaches may be generally preferred for patients requiring conservative profile reduction, conservative tip modification, selected revision rhinoplasty, or other situations in which conservative changes are being undertaken. Advantages of less invasive approaches include less dissection, less edema, and less "healing." However, less invasive approaches provide by their very nature less exposure, which in some cases may be a disadvantage.

Indications for external rhinoplasty approach generally include asymmetric nasal tip, crooked nose deformity (lower two-thirds of nose), saddle nose deformity, cleft-lip nasal deformity, secondary rhinoplasty requiring complex structural grafting, and septal perforation repair. Other indications may include complex nasal tip deformity, middle nasal vault deformity, and selected nasal tumors. Some surgeons prefer the open approach for less complex nasal tip deformities because of the precision that they feel it offers them, in their hands, compared with the endonasal approach.

Advantages of the external approach include the maximal surgical exposure available, potentially allowing more accurate anatomic diagnosis. The external approach also provides the opportunity for precise tissue manipulation, suturing, and grafting. Disadvantages include the transcolumellar incision, wide-field dissection resulting in potential loss of support, and nasal tip edema.

Regardless of approach, one must be mindful of the need to maintain appropriate structural support. When the approach is disruptive of tip support, countermeasures, such as the placement of a columellar strut, are warranted. When the support to the upper lateral cartilages has been disrupted, spreader grafts may be appropriate.

◆ Surgical Techniques in Rhinoplasty

Techniques in surgery can be seen as tools to help achieve a specific task. These tools on their own are not necessarily enough, but rather the right combination of techniques must be well applied in a particular situation.

There are a variety of techniques available for various rhinoplasty goals, including hump reduction, profile augmentation, osteotomies, tip modification, and structural graft placement. There are a wide variety of grafts that may be required based on functional and aesthetic goals. Most commonly, spreader grafts may be used to widen the midvault statically and provide internal valve support; batten and rim grafts will help support nasal sidewalls to decrease dynamic valve collapse; a columellar strut will improve tip support, radix and dorsal onlay grafts will augment a low dorsum; and tip grafts may be used to improve tip contour. Graft material may be obtained from the septum, ear, or rib (autologous or homologous). Some surgeons favor alloplastic materials primarily for dorsal augmentation, although many surgeons believe that the nose fulfills few of the criteria needed for the safe use of alloplastic grafts due to the risk of infection and extrusion.

Although a surgeon must master several individual techniques for rhinoplasty, he/she must also have the judgment, skill, and ability to choose the right techniques for each individual situation. A detailed discussion of the different techniques and approaches used in rhinoplasty are beyond the scope of this book.

Septoplasty may be performed at the same time as rhinoplasty (known as septorhinoplasty); see **Chapter 9.4.8**. Surgical considerations include the following:

- Informed consent: Should include the risks of pain, infection, bleeding, septal perforation, nasal airway obstruction, intranasal and columellar scarring, loss or warping of grafts, decreased smell, numbness in the skin of the nose or teeth, irregularities or asymmetries, failure to meet expectations, and need for revision. This consent process should also include a discussion of the healing process as nasal edema and soft tissue contracture may occur for a year or more after rhinoplasty.
- Anesthesia: Most surgeons prefer general anesthesia; however, a local with IV sedation can be used.
- Approach: Closed versus open
- Profile surgery: Hump reduction via rasp, powered rasp, or scalpel and Rubin osteotome; the need for dorsal augmentation
- Tip surgery: May address projection, rotation, and dome refinements
- Osteotomies: May correct the twisted nose, narrow the nose, or close an open roof deformity. Consideration should be given to the type of osteotomies required for each individual, including: medial, lateral, transverse, and intermediate. In addition, osteotomies may be intranasal or via a transcutaneous postage stamp approach.
- Septoplasty: Cartilage harvest for grafting if needed and to straighten a deviated septum. Consider auricular cartilage and rib grafts as alternatives.
- Grafts: Graft choice should be predicted based on the preoperative nasal analysis and may include spreader grafts, alar battens, rim grafts, a columellar strut, tip or shield grafts, dorsal grafts, and camouflage grafts amongst others.
- Closure: The transcolumellar incision is closed precisely with 5–0 or 6–0 permanent or dissolvable suture. The intranasal incisions are generally closed with 4–0 or 5–0 chromic. A quilting suture or intranasal splints may be used if a septoplasty was performed and an external tape dressing and cast may be applied. Nasal packing is rarely required.

◆ Complications

Infection is uncommon and should be treated with antibiotics if it occurs. Infection may delay wound healing, may lead to prolonged edema, and risks viability of grafts. Septal perforation may occur if there has been injury to the mucoperichondrial flaps. This may lead to whistling or crusting and may need to be repaired if symptoms are not improved with nasal hygiene. Decreased smell is common, particularly after more invasive rhinoplasties, and is generally temporary, with resolution as intranasal edema resolves. Grafts may resorb if they do not have an adequate vascular bed with increased risk in smokers, diabetics, and in other immune compromised states. Grafts may warp or be visible/palpable. Visible asymmetries or irregularities that persist often require surgical revision.

◆ Outcome and Follow-Up

Any nasal packing should be removed as soon as possible. Intranasal splints, dorsal nasal cast, and any permanent sutures should be around at 5 to 7 days. Nasal hygiene is paramount (cleansing and hydrating with nasal saline spray and lubricating ointment). Revision may be necessary in up to 8 to 10% of rhinoplasty procedures. Tissue remodeling is gradual; therefore, long-term follow-up is required to monitor final results.

9.4.8   Deviated Septum and Septoplasty

◆ Key Features

- Deviated nasal septum is a common cause of nasal obstruction.
- A detailed nasal analysis should be performed to rule out other causes of obstruction that may need to be addressed.
- An adequate dorsal and caudal strut must be maintained.

The nasal septum is a central support structure for the nose. When significantly deformed, the septum may cause dysfunction and cosmetic deformity, potentially having an impact on the many functions of the nasal cavity. As many as one-third of people have some nasal obstruction, and up to one-quarter of these patients pursue surgical treatment.

◆ Anatomy

The nasal septum is composed of cartilaginous and bony parts. The bones that make up the septum are the perpendicular plate of the ethmoid bone posterosuperiorly and the vomer, together with the crests of the maxillary and palatine bones, posteroinferiorly. The perpendicular plate of the ethmoid unites superiorly with the cribriform plate and anterosuperiorly with the frontal and nasal bones.

◆ Epidemiology

The patient may provide a history of trauma to the nose; however, often there is no clear history of an inciting event. The initial insult to the nasal septum may have been caused by birth trauma or by microfractures occurring early in life that have led to asymmetric growth of the septal cartilage (**Fig. 9.26**).

◆ Clinical

With a complaint of nasal obstruction, a full history and nasal evaluation are necessary to identify other structural or functional contributions aside from septal deviation. A crooked nose, static or dynamic internal or external valve

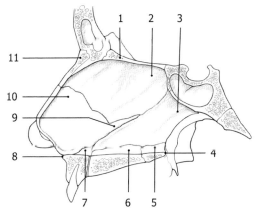

Fig. 9.26 Sagittal section through the facial skeleton with depiction of the nasal septum. 1. cribriform lamina; 2, perpendicular plate of the ethmoid bone; 3, vomer; 4, posterior nasal spine; 5, palatine crest; 6, maxillary crest; 7, premaxilla; 8, anterior nasal spine; 9, (sphenoidal recess of septa) cartilage; 10, septal cartilage; 11, nasal bone. (Used with permission from Sclafani AP, ed. *Rhinoplasty: The Experts' Reference.* New York, NY: Thieme;2015:4.)

dysfunction, ptosis of the tip due to poor support, inferior turbinate hypertrophy, polyps, infection, concha bullosa, and tumors may all contribute to nasal obstruction.

◆ Evaluation

History

The diagnosis of septal deviation begins with taking an adequate history from the patient. This history should include a history of inciting event such as trauma to the nose, presence of nasal airway problems, laterality and fluctuation of obstruction, prior therapies tried, and any history of sinonasal surgeries. Seasonal changes should be elucidating, as allergic rhinitis may also be present. A general health exam is important to determine surgical candidacy and confounding factors (e.g., obstructive sleep apnea), and a review of systems will help guide a potential diagnosis.

Physical Exam

A complete head and neck exam with focus on inspection and palpation of the external and internal nose is critical. The nasal cavity should be inspected before and after nasal decongestion. Anterior rhinoscopy is helpful in diagnosing the location, type, and severity of septal deformity. Both the anterior and posterior septum should be evaluated. A 0° or 30° 4-mm rigid nasal endoscope (e.g., Karl Storz 7200A, Tuttlingen, Germany) may be used by some surgeons to facilitate inspection of the posterior septum. Note the presence of polyps or masses, the severity and extent of septal deviation and bony spurs, presence of a septal perforation, and the presence of mucopus. The size and position of the inferior conchae should be noted during the inspection of the nasal mucosa both before and after the decongestant spray. Bulbous middle conchae may suggest a concha bullosa. Assess the nasal valve areas for cartilage derangement or dynamic collapse.

Imaging

Imaging is not typically required to diagnose a nasal or septal deformity. A sinus computed tomography (CT) scan may be obtained if there are associated symptoms concerning for rhinosinusitis, concha bullosa, polyps, or masses.

◆ Treatment Options

Indications for septoplasty include nasal obstruction, epistaxis, sinus ostium obstruction, trauma, cosmetic deformity, and surgical access (transseptal-transsphenoidal approach). There are various techniques, individualized to the specific problem. If performing open rhinoplasty, the columella and marginal incisions enable one to separate the domes and separate the upper lateral cartilages from the septum, permitting open direct exposure to the entire septal cartilage and bone. Another approach involves a hemitransfixion incision through the lining at the caudal septum, with elevation of mucoperichondrium and mucoperiosteum. The caudal septum can be exposed followed by elevation of the contralateral muco-perichondrial flap. Deviated cartilage or bone is removed and is sometimes replaced. It is critical to leave an adequate dorsal and caudal strut of septum to maintain tip support. Caudal septal deviations should be addressed at the time of septoplasty. Severe deviations may require an external approach. Mucoperichondrial flaps should be carefully elevated, as tears increase the risk of septal perforation. A running quilting suture or intranasal splints may be used to reapproximate the mucoperichondrial flaps.

For more limited deformities, a more posteriorly placed Killian incision may be used to expose cartilaginous or bony deformity. The flap is elevated, cartilage is incised, and a contralateral flap is dissected. The deformity is then removed. If endoscopic sinus surgery is being performed, an endoscopic approach with either incisional approach may be performed using nasal endoscopes. A suction Freer elevator is very useful in this technique.

◆ Complications

Regardless of approach, care must be taken to minimize mucosal tears. Small unopposed tears rarely create problems and heal well without intervention. Large or bilateral tears should be repaired with absorbable suture. In some cases, an interposition graft of acellular human dermis, cartilage replacement, or fascia may be used. Dissection posteriorly and superiorly should be done carefully to avoid transmission of force to the ethmoid roof to prevent cerebrospinal fluid (CSF) leakage. If conchal surgery is done along with septoplasty, the use of Silastic (Dow Corning, Auburn, MI) splints will help prevent intranasal synechiae. Leaving an inadequate dorsal or caudal septal strut predisposes to loss of tip support, nasal obstruction, and nasal deformity (including a saddle deformity). Persistent nasal obstruction after septoplasty is most likely due to incorrect preoperative diagnosis of etiology of nasal obstruction, such as unrecognized valve collapse. This may also arise from failure to treat caudal septal deformities. Septal hematoma may lead to pain, infection, and cartilage loss with deformity. Complaints of pain or swelling must be evaluated promptly, and hematoma or abscess must be drained and antibiotics given. Severe epistaxis is rare but may require cautery, packing or return to the OR for definitive management.

◆ Outcome and Follow-Up

If intranasal splints are used, they should be removed between 5 and 7 days postoperatively. The septum should be evaluated for straightness and presence of septal perforation. Nasal hygiene is important in the recovery period with nasal saline spray and lubricating ointment or saline gel. Patients are followed until a satisfactory result is obtained.

9.4.9   Liposuction of the Head, Face, and Neck

◆ Key Features

- Liposuction of the head, face, and neck involves the use of negative pressure to remove subcutaneous fat.
- The goal of liposuction is improved facial contouring.
- Small incisional punctures in the skin are used to gain access to the subcutaneous plane, and then the cannula is inserted back and forth in different directions (usually radially) and some of the fat extracted.
- This should not be performed as a solitary procedure in older patients with poor skin elasticity.

The use of negative pressure to remove subcutaneous fat has for many years been a popular cosmetic surgical procedure in the United States and elsewhere. This has evolved over the past couple of decades, and various hollow cannulas combined with aspiration machines had been used in many parts of the body to remove unwanted subcutaneous fat. The primary purpose is to help "sculpt" the neck, jowl, and sometimes the face. Liposuction may be performed under local anesthesia, or it may be added to another surgery as an adjunct. The purpose is never to remove all the fat in an area, but rather to thin and partially remove. The fat that is aspirated will be removed permanently, additional fat will be traumatized, and later some of the latter will necrose and dissolve.

◆ Indications

Patients with diet-resistant cervicofacial fat deposits and maintained skin elasticity are candidates for liposuction as a solitary procedure. Of course, realistic expectations must be set.

◆ Contraindications

- Absolute: none
- Relative: Prior trauma or surgery in the area; scar tissue and fibrosis, heavy smokers, and those who have dermatologic, collagen, vascular, or other systemic diseases, psychiatric instability or those who have unrealistic expectations

◆ Procedure

Cervicofacial liposuction may be performed under local anesthesia, intravenous (IV) sedation, or under general anesthesia in conjunction with other surgical procedures. It is often combined with rhytidectomy to improve contour and outcomes. When fat is suctioned as part of a rhytidectomy, the technique might be "open," as it is under direct visualization via the skin flaps. When performed using small puncture incisions, then the technique is "closed."

The procedure is performed traditionally by making several small stab incisions (typically at the base of the earlobes and in the submental crease). The suction cannula is then inserted without suction, and subcutaneous tunnels are created in a radial or fanlike fashion. Suction is then applied to the cannula, and subcutaneous tissue is removed to contour the neck, jowls, and occasionally the face. It is important to leave a layer of normal subcutaneous fat, which acts somewhat as a "carpet pad" between the skin "carpet" and the underlying deeper anatomy. Too superficial liposuctioning may lead to visible irregularities, dimpling, or injury to the dermis.

Over the past few years, the size of cannulas has decreased. Some early cannulas were 10 to 12 mm in diameter or even larger. Although aspiration machines may generate negative pressure close to 1 atmosphere (960 mm Hg), handheld syringes are thought to generate pressures of ~ 600 mm and empirically work well. The negative pressure produced by a handheld syringe combined with a small 2-mm cannula attached to a 3-mL syringe (or 10 mL if preferred) is sufficient for removal of most subcutaneous fat in the submental plane. Additional negative pressure can be utilized for more aggressive or speedier fat removal if necessary. Skin elasticity must be sufficient to redrape in a superior direction (unless it is supported with an additional procedure, such as a facelift). Simply removing fat from a face with poor skin turgor will result in worsening of the appearance (submental "turkey gobbler" deformity, for example). Younger patients (20s–30s) are ideal. Patients in their forties sometimes retain sufficient elasticity. Patients in their fifties will be risky, and patients still older will very rarely be good candidates for liposuction alone.

◆ Complications

Postoperative edema and ecchymosis are common and typically resolve by 1 to 2 weeks postoperatively. Hematoma is rare but should be treated with evacuation. Infection is likewise uncommon and should be treated with appropriate antibiotic therapy. Proper technique is critical to minimize the chance of adverse scarring, dimpling, or other contour irregularities. Proper patient selection is necessary to minimize the chance of poor skin redraping with excess skin and an aged neck appearance. To assist in skin redraping, many surgeons will apply a gentle pressure dressing in the immediate postoperative period. Excess skin or unsatisfactory final contour may require revision surgery. Care must be taken during the operative procedure when liposuction is performed in the face or along the margin of the mandible, as this places branches of the facial nerve (particularly the marginal mandibular branch) at risk. Paresthesias may occur if injury to the great auricular nerve occurs.

◆ Outcome and Follow-Up

Following liposuction, a light compression dressing can be worn by the patient for a week or so and worn at night for perhaps 2 weeks to facilitate redraping of skin. There is some mild discomfort once local anesthesia wears off, which may last a few days, but pain is not usually great. In fair-skinned patients, those who bruise easily, or those taking aspirin or nonsteroidal anti-inflammatory drugs (NSAIDs), there often will be some bruising that may last a week or so.

Healing is gradual, and effects may not be fully appreciated for several months as the remaining fat shrinks, edema resolves, and the skin continues to contract. In properly selected patients, judicious liposuction can be a valuable adjunct to improving the contoured appearance of the face and neck. It is not indicated for facial weight loss and should be used conservatively. It is usually easy to remove additional fat later, if need be, but replacing it is more difficult.

9.4.10 Hair Restoration

◆ Key Features

- Hair loss is a very common cosmetic issue in both men and women.
- Medical therapy includes topical minoxidil and/or oral finasteride and dutasteride.
- Hair transplantation is performed by transferring follicular units from the relatively permanent donor fringe of hair to the area susceptible to alopecia.
- Areas of patterned hair loss may be treated, as well as areas alopecic secondary to trauma, surgery, or radiation.
- The grafts may be produced by microscopic dissection from a single elliptical excision or via follicular unit extraction (FUE).
- The results of hair transplant surgery are natural and long-lasting.

Male pattern baldness (MPB) and female pattern hair loss (FPHL) are extremely prevalent in the population. The genetic basis for alopecia is still not completely defined, but it is polygenetic, with incomplete penetrance, and multifactorial. The approach should ideally include medical treatment in addition to surgical. Hair transplantation can also successfully treat areas that are alopecic following radiation, surgery, or trauma.

◆ Anatomy

The hair follicle is divided into three parts: the infundibulum, the isthmus, and the inferior portion. Hair grows naturally in groupings of one to four hairs known as follicular units (FU), which are bound by adventitial tissue with an associated sebaceous gland and arrector pili muscle. Although hair stem cell cloning is possible in vitro, there remain many obstacles to this technology becoming a reality for use in vivo. The bulge region contains the most active stem cells, and it is believed that a complex communication occurs within the follicular unit to produce ongoing hair growth.

◆ Clinical

The differential diagnosis for alopecia is extensive. Systemic causes of hair loss and possible influences of drugs should be considered as possible causes of telogen effluvium. Alopecia areata, central centrifugal alopecia, folliculitis decalvans, and hair styling products should be considered. There is also an increase in the incidence in inflammatory alopecias, including lichen planopilaris (LPP) and frontal fibrosin alopecia (FFA). The inflammatory alopecias are contraindications to surgery, unless they have been quiescent for a period of at least 1 to 2 years, and ongoing treatment will be necessary. Alopecia secondary to trauma, radiation, or surgery is amenable to hair restoration surgery.

◆ Evaluation

Physical Exam

The Norwood classification is most commonly used to quantify the extensiveness of the hair loss (**Fig. 9.27**). Class I means no alopecia, while class VII is the most severe, with only occipital and parietal rim hair remaining. The Ludwig or Hamilton scales are used to describe FPHL. The pattern of alopecia can sometimes help in the diagnosis. Severe diffuse loss is more commonly secondary to telogen effluvium but may also be diffuse alopecia areata (areata incognita) and diffuse unpatterned alopecia (DUPA). Such patients are not surgical candidates.

The relatively permanent fringe of hair varies in size and density between patients and at various ages. The surgical candidate should ideally have approximately 80 FU per square centimeter and corresponding realistic goals based on his or her likely long-term pattern of hair loss.

Imaging

The development of better imaging has been important in determining candidacy and following treatment. The dermatoscope allows physicians to

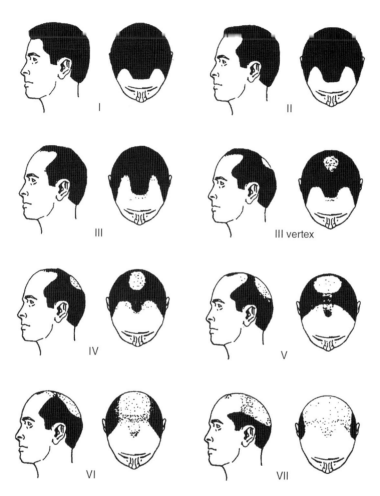

Fig. 9.27 The Norwood classification of male pattern baldness. (Modified with permission from Unger R, Shapiro R, eds. *Hair Transplantation.* 6th ed. New York, NY: Thieme;2018.)

examine the scalp carefully to rule out other potential diseases that should be treated medically. Alopecia areata will clearly show exclamation point hairs and yellow dots. LPP and its frontal variant (FFA) will show perifollicular scale and inflammation, areas devoid of hair and follicular ostia, and sometimes polytrichia.

Perioperative photos should include frontal, three-quarter, lateral, and posterior views. Occasionally it is helpful to part the hair to highlight areas being treated.

◆ Treatment Options

Medical

Medical treatment has actually changed very little in the last 10 years. Topical minoxidil may be utilized for both MPB and FPHL. Minoxidil opens K^+ channels and produces peripheral vasodilation. Both men and women utilize the 5% solution or foam; however, men are instructed to use it twice daily. A recent study showed that nonresponders may benefit from a higher concentration preparation of 15%; no additional side effects were reported. Minoxidil is generally well tolerated, and the response rate is up to 80% when 5% or higher concentrations are used.

Finasteride and dutasteride are the other medications commonly prescribed for MPB (they are not approved for use in women, although some physicians feel comfortable prescribing for FPHL as well). These block the conversion of testosterone to dihydrotestosterone: the former is a 5-α II reductase inhibitor, while the latter inhibits Type I as well. These medications are very effective in treating MPB and are generally well tolerated. However, widely publicized reports of sexual side effects have instilled fear of these in many patients. It is important for the physician to present the facts in an educational and rational manner.

Adjunctive

Patients may not be suitable for surgery and may not respond to medical therapy. These patients may be counseled regarding hair pieces, wigs, and topical color powders. There is also an increase in scalp micropigmentation being performed, with tiny dots that look like hair stubble and color the scalp to match the root color. This may be a good option for some patients; however, the nonpermanent method is superior: the patient does not need to be concerned with change in the tattoo color or hair color, nor the possibility that the tiny dots will spread and coalesce into a solid color.

Platelet-rich plasma (PRP) is also being utilized both as a stand-alone treatment for MPB and FPHL and also to improve the results achieved with surgery. Studies to date are limited, and clinical evidence is not conclusive, but anecdotal reports from some physicians are encouraging.

Surgical

Hair restoration surgery may include alopecia reduction, but the term almost exclusively refers to the transplantation of FUs from the more permanent hair-bearing rim (donor) to the alopecic area (recipient). The FUs may be harvested in a single elliptical excision that is then divided microscopically into the individual units. They may also be harvested utilizing FUE, in which a small punch (0.8 to 1.1 mm) is utilized to extract one follicle at a time. Both harvest methods have advantages and disadvantages, and a good surgeon should be able to offer the patient choices and honestly present the pros and cons. Briefly, the elliptical excision allows for the maximum number of grafts to be harvested from the center of the most permanent region of the donor area; the defect is surgically closed, and usually only a thin linear scar remains, with little impact on the apparent density in the donor. A large number of FUs can be transplanted in one surgery, and the survival of the grafts is well proven.

FUE eliminates the linear scar, which is of benefit to those who wish to wear very short hair styles, and is more comfortable postoperatively. FUs are also harvested from the relatively permanent fringe, but only every third or fourth unit should be removed in order to prevent obvious thinning and future problems. This often leads surgeons to harvest outside the permanent fringe and/or overharvest within the fringe. FUE is ideal for patients with tight scalps, with short hair styles, or in need of smaller surgeries. It can also be used to harvest from other body areas to expand the potential donor hair bank; beard hair grows best, while leg hair has the poorest survival.

The recipient area design is the most important aspect of the surgical plan. Both current and future areas of alopecia should be considered in formulating the design. The goal is to create the look of an early stage of thinning maximizing the illusion of density artistically, not to create true density throughout the alopecic area (which, given donor hair limitations, is impossible). The transplanted hair should follow the angle and direction of the preexisting hair, especially in patients with early MPB and FPHL. This creates a natural appearance and protects the preexisting hair. The hairline zone ideally should be made up of one to two hair FUs approximately 1 cm in depth; posteriorly the density can be increased. A central frontal tuft further back, with even higher hair density, can be especially helpful in creating the illusion of density; this may be created with three to five hair grafts. Hair transplant surgery in women usually focuses on the area of greatest cosmetic significance, and grafts are concentrated in that region.

The first surgery most commonly consists of 1,500 to 2,500 FUs in a man and 1,200 to 1,800 FUs in a female, while subsequent surgeries are generally somewhat smaller. Men will frequently need two to three procedures over their lifetime to cover an average-size alopecic area; however, this varies depending on the pattern of alopecia. Some surgeons believe there is no real upper limit to the size that can be performed in one procedure, although this opinion is not shared by many.

◆ Outcome and Follow-Up

The patient must care for the donor and recipient areas after surgery to ensure proper healing. The closure of the elliptic excision may be done with sutures, absorbable sutures, or staples: surgeons' recommendations for removal vary from 8 days to 3 weeks.

The transplanted hair usually falls out after 2 to 4 weeks, and the new hairs begin to grow 3 to 4 months after surgery. Full growth is achieved 12 to 18 months after surgery. Hair transplantation performed by a well-trained surgeon produces an excellent and lasting result.

Appendix A Basic Procedures and Methods of Investigation

◆ A1 Bronchoscopy

Two methods of bronchoscopy are available: rigid and flexible.

Rigid Bronchoscopy

Historically, rigid bronchoscopy is the older method. Rigid bronchoscopy is performed under general anesthesia. Rigid bronchoscopes are tubes of different calibers with a proximal cold light source. The bronchoscope has direct connection to the anesthetic and respiratory apparatus, so it is called the *respiratory bronchoscope*. A rigid bronchoscope can be combined with other instrumentation, including aspiration, lavage, cytologic diagnosis, and swabs for culture. A rigid bronchoscope may be used in conjunction with a laser.

Indications

Rigid bronchoscopy as a therapeutic measure:

- Emergency bronchoscopy done to bypass sudden obstructive respiratory insufficiency
- Removal of tracheal or bronchial foreign body; arrest of bleeding of the trachea or bronchi

Rigid bronchoscopy as a diagnostic procedure:

- To treat tracheal or bronchial stenosis
- To biopsy a tracheal tumor
- To investigate hemoptysis
- To assess upper airway trauma

Advantages
- It is a versatile procedure.
- It can be used on a bleeding patient.
- It can be used to extract a foreign body.

Disadvantages
- It is technically more difficult with abnormal cervical anatomy.
- It places limitations on neck extension.
- It must be performed under general anesthetic.

Flexible Bronchoscopy

Flexible bronchoscopes are thinner than rigid bronchoscopes, usually having a diameter of 4 to 5 mm. Their distal end is controlled externally, so they can be introduced into the low bronchi or segmental bronchi. The instrument may be introduced via the nose, the mouth, or a tracheotomy. Flexible bronchoscopy may be performed under local or general anesthetic with the patient sitting or lying. When using general anesthetic, at intubation the bronchoscope may be introduced through the endotracheal tube.

Indications
- Bronchial or upper airway tumors
- Hemoptysis
- Undiagnosed disorders such as unresolved pneumonia
- Middle lobe syndrome

Advantages
- The flexible bronchoscope can be introduced far into the periphery as far as the fifth-generation bronchi; therefore, it complements the rigid endoscope.
- Flexible bronchoscopy can be performed under local anesthetic with a conscious patient.

Disadvantages
- It has a relatively narrow working radius; therefore, it cannot be used for large foreign bodies or in the presence of profuse bleeding.

Complications

Complications of rigid and flexible bronchoscopy include:

- Damage to vocal folds
- Perforation of tracheobronchial tree
- Pneumothorax
- Laryngospasm
- Death

◆ A2 Esophagoscopy

Esophagoscopy can be performed with either a rigid or a flexible esophagoscope. The rigid esophagoscope is a rigid tube that is usually used under general anesthesia. It has a high-powered cold light source at the proximal or distal end. Extraction, excision, and coagulation instruments can be used in conjunction with the rigid esophagoscope. Lasers may also be used. Flexible esophagoscopy has a narrow caliber, is suitable for foreign body extraction, and can be used in conjunction with air insufflation and be attached to air insufflation and suction. It also typically provides good photographic documentation for permanent record keeping. Percutaneous endoscopic gastroscopy (PEG) feeding tube placement may also be done via flexible esophagoscopy. Seven PEG kits are available.

Indications

Rigid esophagoscopy as a therapeutic measure:

- Removal of foreign bodies
- Removal of polyps and fibromas
- Division of hypopharyngeal rings and diverticulum
- Dilation stenosis
- Injection of esophageal varices

Rigid esophagoscopy as a diagnostic procedure:

- To diagnose diseases of the esophagus
- To diagnose tumors of the hypopharynx and esophagus
- To evaluate dysphagia

Flexible esophagoscopy as a diagnostic procedure:

- In cases where rigid esophagoscopy is contraindicated or impossible because the patient is unable to flex or extend the neck as a result of cervical spine disease, panendoscopy is indicated.
- General indications are otherwise similar to those for rigid esophagoscopy.

Advantages

Advantages of rigid esophagoscopy include versatility and superior ability to remove large foreign bodies from the esophagus. It is very efficient for both diagnostic and therapeutic usage.
Advantages of flexible esophagoscopy include:

- Simultaneous panendoscopy of the stomach and duodenum may be performed.
- The flexible esophagoscope is a good screening instrument.
- The procedure is less traumatic for the patient than rigid esophagoscopy.

Complications

- Esophageal perforation
- False passage
- Mediastinitis
- Pneumomediastinum
- Oral and dental injury, especially with use of rigid instrumentation
- Death

◆ A3 Rigid Direct Microscopic Laryngoscopy with or without Biopsy

Rigid direct microscopic laryngoscopy is used for larynx and hypopharynx evaluation and biopsy.

Indications

- Suspected or known malignancy
- Treatment of cancer through endoscopic resection
- Together with esophageal endoscopy, bronchoscopy (collectively, panendoscopy)
- Evaluation and treatment of hoarseness
- Endotracheal intubation for difficult airway

Contraindications

- Unstable cervical spine
- Inability to obtain exposure of the larynx

Laryngoscope Types

- Dedo laryngoscope: widely used for laryngeal biopsy procedures including working diameter
- Holinger anterior commissure scope: used for better exposure anteriorly
- Lindholm laryngoscope
- Weerda laryngoscope: bivalve design; useful for endoscopic management of Zenker diverticulum
- Jackson "sliding" laryngoscope

Steps

1. Patient is placed in the supine position with the head extended and with the eyes protected.
2. General anesthesia is used.
3. A tooth or mouth guard is in place.
4. A rigid laryngoscope is placed through the mouth, and with the use of an operating microscope or fiberoptic telescope, the entire throat and affected area are magnified and evaluated.
5. In suspension laryngoscopy, suspending the laryngoscope allows the surgeon to use both hands for procedures within the larynx.
6. Lasers, a microdébrider, a monopolar cautery, and cold microdissection or biopsy instrument tools can be introduced through the laryngoscope.

Complications

- Loss of airway and obstruction
- Damage to teeth, mouth, and gums
- Numb tongue, altered taste, temporomandibular joint disorders
- Hoarseness
- Perforation
- Airway fire; if using laser or cautery

◆ A4 Tonsillectomy

Indications

Absolute indications include:

- Enlarged tonsils with an upper airway obstruction
- Severe dysphagia
- Sleep disorders thought to be related to obstructive tonsil hypertrophy
- Peritonsillar abscess unresponsive to medical management
- Tonsillitis resulting in febrile convulsions

Relative indications include:

- Three or more tonsil infections per year despite adequate medical therapy
- Persistent foul taste or breath
- Chronic tonsillitis in a streptococcal carrier
- Unilateral tonsil hypertrophy presumed to be neoplastic

Contraindications

- Bleeding diathesis, unless managed with appropriated perioperative medical therapy
- Poor anesthetic risk or uncontrolled medical illness
- Acute infection

Steps

1. Place patient on shoulder roll.
2. Induce general anesthesia and intubation in most cases.
3. Insert a mouth prop, open, and suspend.
4. Apply a tonsil clamp to the tonsil to allow medial traction during dissection.
5. Dissect and remove tonsil, taking care to preserve the posterior pillar fully and stay in the capsular plane.

Dissection Instruments

- Cold steel instruments
- Monopolar cautery
- Bipolar cautery with or without a microscope
- Radiofrequency ablation or coblation
- Harmonic scalpel
- Microdébrider

Complications

- Hemorrhage
- Pain

- Dehydration
- Weight loss
- Fever
- Postoperative airway obstruction
- Pulmonary edema
- Local trauma to oral tissues
- Tonsillar remnant regrowth
- Vocal changes
- Temporomandibular joint dysfunction
- Death

◆ A5 Adenoidectomy

Indications

- Adenoid enlargement with nasal airway obstruction
- Obstructive sleep apnea symptoms
- Chronic mouth breathing
- Recurrent or persistent otitis media in children ≥ 3 years old
- Recurrent and/or chronic sinusitis

Contraindications

- Severe bleeding disorder (relative)
- True cleft palate
- Muscle weakness or hypotonia (relative)
- Atlantoaxial joint laxity (relative)

Steps

1. Use a mouth appliance to open the mouth and retract the palate.
2. A mirror can be used to see the adenoids, because they are behind the nasal cavity.
3. The adenoid is removed through the mouth.

Dissection Instruments

- Adenoid curette
- Adenoid punch
- Electrocautery with a suction Bovie
- Microdébrider

Complications

- Hemorrhage
- Velopharyngeal insufficiency
- Torticollis
- Nasopharyngeal stenosis

- Atlantoaxial subluxation from infection (Grisel's syndrome)
- Eustachian tube injury
- Death

◆ A6 Open Surgical Tracheotomy

Indications

- Prolonged intubation with mechanical intubation
- To bypass upper airway obstruction
- To provide pulmonary toilet
- Prophylaxis for anticipated need for ventilator support
- Sleep apnea

Steps

1. Place patient supine, with neck extended on a shoulder roll if possible.
2. Palpate the neck landmarks.
3. Infiltrate lidocaine/epinephrine.
4. Incise the skin between the cricoid and sternal notch (horizontal or vertical).
5. Separate strap muscles and retract laterally.
6. Divide or retract thyroid isthmus.
7. Verify hemostasis.
8. Alert the anesthesiologist of impending airway entry.
9. Tracheal opening (window, trap door flap, slit)
10. Have anesthesiologist withdraw endotracheal tube under direct visualization.
11. Insert the tracheotomy tube into the trachea.
12. Connect circuit and inflate balloon.
13. Verify end tidal CO_2.
14. Secure the tracheotomy tube to the skin with four sutures and a tracheotomy collar.

Complications

- Hemorrhage
- Pneumothorax
- False passage
- Obstruction or decannulation
- Infection
- Tracheoesophageal fistula
- Tracheocutaneous fistula
- Tracheo–innominate artery fistula
- Death

◆ A7 Cricothyroidotomy

Steps

1. Palpate the cricoid in the midline with a neck extension; the thyroid cartilage is stabilized superiorly with a nondominant hand. Move your index finger down until you palpate the cricoid cartilage.

2. The space between the thyroid and cricoid cartilages is the location of the cricothyroid membrane (**Fig. A.1**). Use the scalpel to make a 1.0 to 1.5-cm vertical incision through the skin and subcutaneous tissue (**Fig. A.2**).

3. Use the curved hemostat to make a blunt dissection in the subcutaneous tissue.

4. Next, use the scalpel to make a horizontal incision through the cricothyroid membrane (**Fig. A.3**).

5. You may feel a pop as the trachea is entered.

6. Extend the incision laterally, turn the blade, and extend it in the opposite direction.

7. Once the trachea has been entered, make sure the blade stays within the incision, so that communication with the trachea is never lost.

8. Insert a tracheal hook, and pull superiorly on the upper portion of the incision, elevating the larynx. Once the tracheal hook is in place, you may remove the blade.

9. Insert a Trousseau dilator and open the membrane vertically, then insert the tracheotomy tube; see **Fig. 2.6** in Chapter 2.1.

Because the cricothyroid membrane is situated between two rigid bodies (the thyroid cartilage above and the cricoid cartilage below), there is little flexibility in the size of the opening that can be made in the membrane. A tracheotomy tube or endotracheal tube with an internal diameter of 6 mm should be used. A tube with an internal diameter > 7 mm would be difficult to insert into the cricothyroid membrane. Cricothyroidotomy is a *temporizing technique* only, and in these cases the patient should have a formal tracheotomy performed as soon he or she is stabilized.

Complications

- Esophageal perforation
- Subcutaneous emphysema
- Hemorrhage
- False route
- Injury to larynx

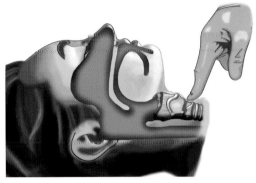

Fig. A.1   The cricothyroid membrane is located and palpated.

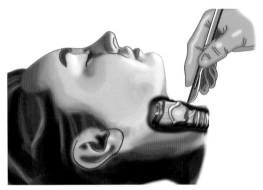

Fig. A.2   Using a scalpel, a midline incision approximately 1.0- to 1.5-cm long is made directly over the cricoid and thyroid cartilages. The incision should cut through the skin and subcutaneous tissues.

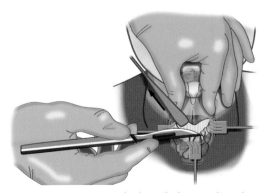

Fig. A.3   A horizontal incision is made through the cricothyroid membrane. A tracheal hook may be used to elevate the thyroid cartilage to provide greater exposure.

Appendix B   The Cranial Nerves

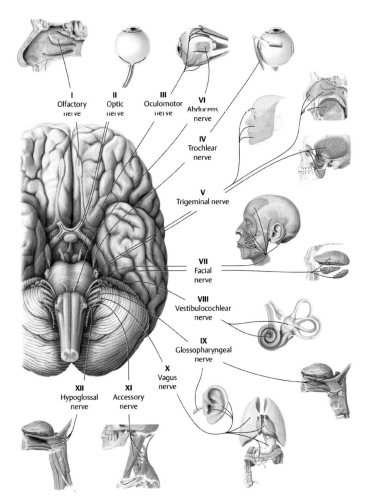

Fig. B.1   The twelve pairs of cranial nerves are designated by Roman numerals according to the order of their emergence from the brain (CN I–II) or brainstem (CN III–XII). (From THIEME Atlas of Anatomy, Head and Neuroanatomy, © Thieme 2010, Illustrations by Markus Voll and Karl Wesker.)

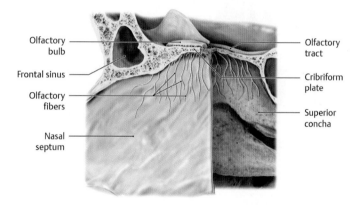

Fig. B.2 The olfactory nerve (cranial nerve I). (From THIEME Atlas of Anatomy, Head and Neuroanatomy, © Thieme 2010, Illustration by Karl Wesker.)

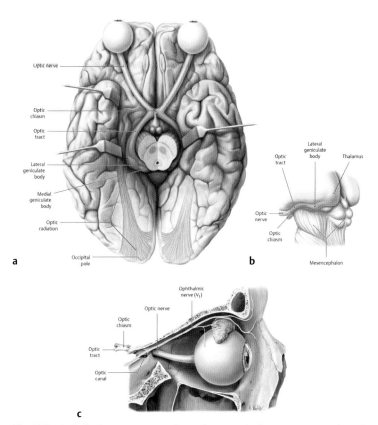

Fig. B.3 (a,b,c) The optic nerve (cranial nerve II). (From THIEME Atlas of Anatomy, Head and Neuroanatomy, © Thieme 2010, Illustrations by Markus Voll and Karl Wesker.)

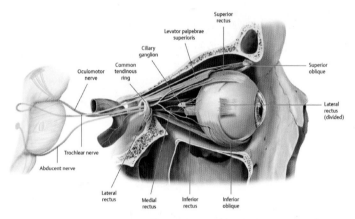

Fig. B.4   The oculomotor nerve (cranial nerve III), trochlear nerve (cranial nerve IV), and abducens nerve (cranial nerve VI). (From THIEME Atlas of Anatomy, Head and Neuroanatomy, © Thieme 2010, Illustration by Karl Wesker.)

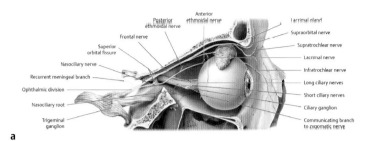

a

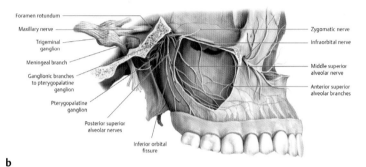

b

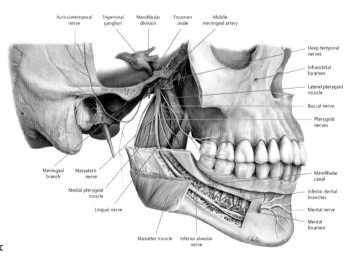

c

Fig. B.5 (a,b,c) The trigeminal nerve (cranial nerve V). (From THIEME Atlas of Anatomy, Head and Neuroanatomy, © Thieme 2010, Illustrations by Karl Wesker.)

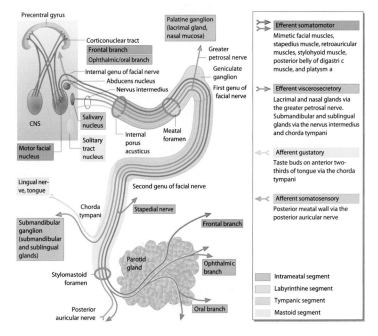

Fig. B.6 The course, segments, and functions of the facial nerve (cranial nerve VII). (Used with permission from Probst R, Grevers G, Iro H. *Basic Otorhinolaryngology: A Step-by-Step Learning Guide*. Stuttgart/New York: Thieme;2006:291.)

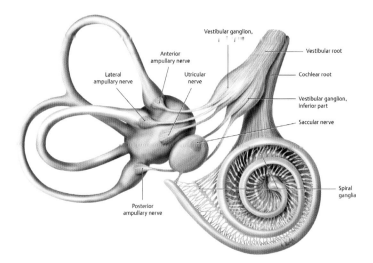

Fig. B.7 The vestibulocochlear nerve (cranial nerve VIII). (From THIEME Atlas of Anatomy, Head and Neuroanatomy, © Thieme 2010, Illustration by Markus Voll.)

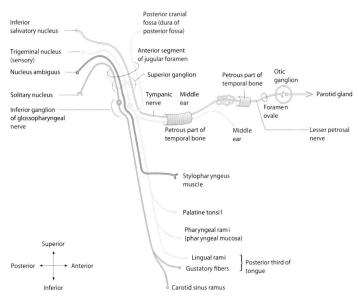

Fig. B.8 The course of the glossopharyngeal nerve (cranial nerve IX). (Used with permission from Probst R, Grevers G, Iro H. *Basic Otorhinolaryngology: A Step-by-Step Learning Guide*. Stuttgart/New York: Thieme;2006:315.)

b N. vagus

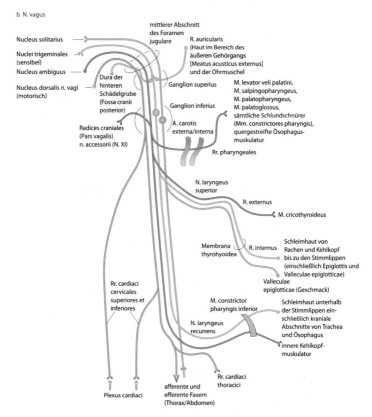

Fig. B.9   The course of the vagus nerve (cranial nerve X). (Used with permission from Probst R, Grevers G, Iro H. *Basic Otorhinolaryngology: A Step-by-Step Learning Guide*. Stuttgart/New York: Thieme;2006:316.)

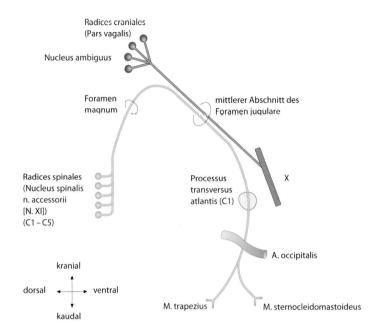

Fig. B.10 The course of the accessory nerve (cranial nerve XI). (Used with permission from Probst R, Grevers G, Iro H. *Basic Otorhinolaryngology: A Step-by-Step Learning Guide*. Stuttgart/ New York: Thieme;2006:317.)

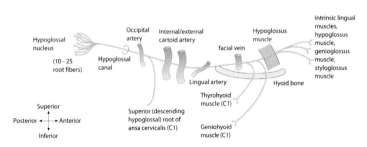

Fig. B.11 The course of the hypoglossal nerve (cranial nerve XII). (Used with permission from Probst R, Grevers G, Iro H. *Basic Otorhinolaryngology: A Step-by-Step Learning Guide*. Stuttgart/New York: Thieme;2006:317.)

Cranial nerve (CN)	Name	Function		Comments
I	Olfactory nerve	Special sensory	Smell	
II	Optic nerve	Special sensory	Sight	
III	Oculomotor nerve	Motor	Skeletal motor to 4 extrinsic eye muscles and levator palpebrae superioris muscle	Visceral motor, parasympathetic; preganglionic fibers synapse in *ciliary ganglion*; innervate ciliary muscle and sphincter pupillae muscle in eye
IV	Trochlear nerve	Motor	Innervates superior oblique muscle (an extrinsic eye muscle)	
V	Trigeminal nerve	Somatic sensory: skin of the face	Visceral sensory: mucous membranes of the nose and mouth	Skeletal motor: mastication (chewing) muscles	Three divisions: ophthalmic (V_1), maxillary (V_2), mandibular (V_3)

continued

Cranial nerve (CN)	Name	Function		Comments
VI	Abducens nerve	Motor	Innervates lateral rectus muscle (an extrinsic eye muscle)	
VII	Facial nerve	Somatic sensory: skin of external ear (small contribution)	Visceral sensory: taste buds on anterior 2/3 of tongue	Nervus intermedius carries general sensory fibers, taste fibers, and visceral motor (parasympathetic) fibers
			Visceral motor (parasympathetic): salivary and lacrimal glands	
			Skeletal motor: muscles of facial expression	
VIII	Vestibulocochlear nerve	Special sensory	Hearing and balance	Vestibular nerve (balance): receptors in semicircular ducts, utricle, saccule
				Cochlear nerve (hearing): receptors in spiral organ (organ of Corti)
IX	Glossopharyngeal nerve	Visceral sensory: mucous membranes of middle ear, posterior tongue, throat	Visceral sensory: taste buds on posterior 1/3 of tongue	
			Visceral motor (parasympathetic): parotid gland	
			Skeletal motor: stylopharyngeus muscle	

continued

Cranial nerve (CN)	Name	Function			Comments
X	Vagus nerve	Somatic sensory: skin of the external ear and eardrum	Visceral sensory: mucous membranes of lower throat and larynx	Visceral motor (parasympathetic): cardiac and smooth muscle in organs of thorax and abdomen	Motor fibers from CN XI to palate, pharynx, and larynx carried by CN X
XI	Spinal accessory nerve	Skeletal motor: trapezius, sternocleidomastoid, pharyngeal and laryngeal muscles except cricothyroid			
XII	Hypoglossal nerve	Skeletal motor: innervates all muscles of the tongue, both intrinsic and extrinsic, except palatoglossus muscle			C1 motor fibers "hitch a ride" on CN XII

Appendix C   ENT Emergencies Requiring Immediate Diagnostic and/or Therapeutic Intervention

Emergency	See Chapter:
Airway obstruction	[Ch. 2.1]
Airway obstruction (pediatric)	[Ch. 8.1]
Anaphylaxis	[Ch. 4.3.2]
Anesthetic emergency	[Ch. 2.2.4]
Aspiration	[Ch. 5.4.3]
Carotid artery blowout	[Ch. 2.4]
Caustic ingestion	[Ch. 5.1.3]
Cerebrospinal fluid rhinorrhea	[Ch. 4.1.4]
Choanal atresia	[Ch. 8.17]
Confusion	[Ch. 2.4]
Deep neck infection	[Ch. 6.1.3]
Delirium tremens	[Ch. 2.4]
Ear foreign body	[Ch. 3.1.4]
Ear trauma	[Ch. 3.1.2]
Epistaxis	[Ch. 4.1.5]
Facial paresis or paralysis (acute)	[Ch. 3.1.3]
Facial reanimation	[Ch. 9.2]
Frontal sinus fracture	[Ch. 9.1.4]
Fungal infection (acute invasive)	[Ch. 4.1.1]
Infectious neck mass	[Ch. 8.12]
Laryngeal fracture	[Ch. 5.1.2]
Laryngeal infection	[Ch. 5.1.4]
Laryngomalacia	[Ch. 8.2]
Ludwig's angina	[Ch. 6.1.2]

continued

Emergency	See Chapter:
Mandible fracture	[Ch. 9.1.6]
Midface fracture	[Ch. 9.1.5]
Nasal fracture	[Ch. 9.1.1]
Naso-orbito-ethmoid fracture	[Ch. 9.1.2]
Neck trauma	[Ch. 6.1.4]
Necrotizing soft tissue infection of the head and neck	[Ch. 6.1.1]
Orbital fracture	[Ch. 9.1.3]
Otitis externa (malignant)	[Ch. 3.3.2]
Otitis media complication	[Ch. 3.2.3]
Postobstructive pulmonary edema	[Ch. 2.4]
Pulmonary embolism	[Ch. 2.4]
Sinusitis complication (intracranial)	[Ch. 4.1.3]
Sinusitis complication (orbital)	[Ch. 4.1.2]
Stridor	[Ch. 5.1.1]
Subglottic stenosis	[Ch. 8.7]
Sudden hearing loss	[Ch. 3.1.1]
Temporal bone trauma	[Ch. 3.1.2]
Thyroid storm	[Ch. 7.6]
Vestibular neuritis	[Ch. 3.6.4]
Vocal fold paralysis	[Ch. 8.3]
Zygomaticomaxillary fracture	[Ch. 9.1.3]

Index

Note: Page numbers followed by *f* and *t* indicate figures and tables, respectively.

A

ABCDE of melanoma, 424
ABCs of neck examination, 615
Abducens nerve, 724*f*, 731*t*
ABI. *See* Auditory brainstem implants
    (ABI)
ABR. *See* Auditory brainstem response
    (ABR)
Abscess
  Bezold, 133
  brain abscess, 137–138
  in children, 585
  drainage, 336*t*
  epidural abscess, 138–139, 231
  intracranial, 233
  periapical, 31
  periodontal, 31
  peritonsillar, 34, 64, 561
  subdural, 231
  subperiosteal, 132, 228
  wound, 95
Abducens nerve, 724*f*, 731*t*
Accessory nerve, 729*f*
Achondroplasia, 553
Acid reflux disorders, 318–320
Acquired hearing loss, pediatric,
    577–579
Acquired immunodeficiency syndrome
    (AIDS), 217
ACT. *See* Activated clotting time (ACT)
Actinomycosis, 287
Activated clotting time (ACT), 18
Acupuncture and CAM, 49
Acute bacterial sialadenitis, 453–454,
    453*f*
Acute facial paresis and paralysis,
    115–120. *See also* Bell's palsy
Acute invasive fungal rhinosinusitis,
    224–227
  treatment algorithm, 226*f*
Acute postobstructive pulmonary
    edema, 93–94
Acute rhinosinusitis, 241–244
  antibiotic therapy, 243*t*

Acute sialadenitis, 452–453
Adenoidectomy, 716–717
Adentonsillar hypertrophy, pediatric,
    563–567
Adenotonsillitis, pediatric, 560–563,
    562*t*
Adjuvant radiotherapy rationale,
    358–359
Adjuvant therapy, 353–354
Advanced oral cavity cancer, 375
Advancement flaps, 653–654, 653*f*, 654*f*
AIDS. *See* HIV/acquired immunodefi-
    ciency syndrome (AIDS)
Airway
  anatomy, 54
    innervation, 55
  assessment and management, 54–70
    cervical spine movements, 57
    Cormack and Lehane grade, 58, 58*f*
    Mallampati classification, 57, 57*f*
    mouth opening, 57
    preoperative endoscopic airway
      evaluation, 58
    temporomandibular joint (TMJ)
      mobility, 58
    thyromental distance, 57
  equipment, 55–56
    facemasks, 55
    laryngoscopes, 55
    oral and nasal airways, 55
  management, 58–65
    complications, 60–65
    endotracheal intubation, 58–60
    pediatric evaluation and management,
      525–528
  size by age, 547*t*
Airway complications, 60–65
  conscious intubation 62
  fiber optic-assisted tracheal
    intubation, 62–63
  GlideScope, 65
  laryngeal mask airway (LMA), 63
  nasotracheal intubation, 61
  orotracheal intubation, 60–61
  rapid-sequence intubation, 61–62

surgical laryngoscopes, 65
transtracheal ventilation, 63
Airway, difficulty, 65–71, 66t
cricothyroidotomy, 67, 67f
stable but compromised airway, 68
extubation criteria, 70
percutaneous dilation tracheotomy, 69
tracheometry, awake, 68
tracheometry, indications for, 68t
Airway, foreign body
difficult airway and intubation, 64t
AJCC Stage Groupings. *See* American Joint Committee on Cancer (AJCC) Stage Groupings
Alcohol
withdrawal, 94
preoperative assessment, 53t
Alkaloids, 354
Allergic rhinitis, acute sinusitis, and asthma and CAM, 48
Allergy, 253–256
anaphylaxis, 255
angioedema, 256
chronic allergy management, 256
Gell and Coombs classification of allergic reactions, 254t
Alexander deafness, 573
American Joint Committee on Cancer (AJCC) Stage Groupings
anaplastic thyroid cancers, 507
Hodgkin and non-Hodgkin, 436t
malignant salivary tumors, 466
medullary thyroid cancers, 511t
melanomas of head, face, and neck, 427
mucosal malignant melanoma, 428–429
non-melanoma cutaneous malignancy, 416
oral cavity cancers, 377
prognostic stage groupings, 423t
sinonasal cancers, 364–365
supraglottis, glottis, and subglottis, 400–401
thyroid cancers, differentiated, 507t
American Society of Anesthesiologists (ASA)
Difficult Airway Algorithm (DAA), 56f
NPO guidelines, 54t
Physical Status Classification System, 54t
American Society of Geriatric Otolaryngology (ASGO), 42
Amnesia/anxiolysis, 71

Amyloidosis laryngeal manifestation, 322
Analgesia, 71
Anaphylactic reaction, 15
Anaphylaxis treatment for allergy, 255
Anaplastic thyroid cancer, 502
Anatomic variations
difficult airway and intubation, 64t
Ancillary techniques for facial paralysis, 647
Anesthesia, 70–89
factors, 71
amnesia/anxiolysis, 71
analgesia, 71
antiemetics, 71
muscle relaxation, 71
modes, 70–71
general anesthesia, 70
regional anesthesia, 71
sedation, 71
phases, 71–72, 72t
regional techniques, 73–76
benefits, 73
complications, 73
contraindications, 73
neck blocks, 74–75
scalp and face blocks, 73–74
upper airway blocks, 75–76
stages, 72–73
Anesthesia drugs, 76–86
benzodiazepine reversal, 80
flumazenil, 80
benzodiazepines, 79–81
diazepam, 80
effect on organ systems, 79t
lorazepam, 80
midazolam, 80
induction medications, 81–83
etomidate, 82, 82t
ketamine, 82t, 83
propofol, 81, 81t
inhaled, 83–84
desflurane, 84
isoflurane, 84
nitrous oxide, 84
sevofluane, 84
muscle relaxation, 84–86
depolarizing muscle relaxants, 85, 85t
isoflurane, 85t
nondepolarizing muscle relaxants, 86, 86t
opioid reversal, 78–79
naxolone, 78–79
opioids, 76–79, 77t
fentanyl, 78

meperidine, 78
morphine, 77
receptors, 78t
remifentanil, 78
Anesthetic emergencies, 86–89
  airway fires, 87
  malignant hyperthermia, 87t
Angioedema treatment for allergy, 256
Angioneurotic edema laryngeal
      manifestation, 323
Anosmia and other olfactory disorders,
      260–262
  conductive anosmia, 261
  sensorineural anosmia, 262
Anterior compartment, 408
Antiemetics, 71
Antimetabolites, 353
Antitumor antibiotics, 353
Apert syndrome, 576
Apocrine phenotype and cartilaginous
      stoma, 459f
Argon laser, 46
Armored endotracheal tubes, 59
Arnold's reflex, 104
Arthrocentesis, 37
Arthroplasty, 37
Arthroscopic surgery, 37
ASA. *See* American Society of
      Anesthesiologists (ASA)
ASGO. *See* American Society of Geriatric
      Otolaryngology (ASGO)
Asymmetric hearing loss, 171–172
Audiology, 153–164
  assessments, 153–159
    pure-tone threshold audiometry, 155f
    Rinne test, 157, 158f
    tuning fork tests, 157
    tympanogram patterns, normal and
        abnormal, 156t
    Weber test, 157, 157f
  electrophysiologic/objective
      assessments, 163–164
  pediatric audiologic assessments,
      159–162
Audiometric hearing loss, pediatric,
      assessment by age, 581t
Auditory brainstem implants (ABI), 181
Auditory brainstem response (ABR), 109,
      581
Auditory neuropathy/dyssynchrony and
      postnatal acquired hearing
      loss, 579
Autonomic nervous system, 450–451
Autosomal recessive hearing loss,
      pediatric, 574

B

Bacterial laryngitis, 286
Balloon, 240
Barium esophagram, 10–11
Basal cell carcinoma (BCC), 413–417
Basaloid squamous cell carcinomas, 384f
Battle sign, 111
BBB syndrome. *See* Opitz G syndrome
      (BBB syndrome)
BCC. *See* Basal cell carcinoma (BCC)
Beahrs triangle, 473
Bell's palsy, 115
Benign paroxysmal positional vertigo
      (BPPV), 186–189
Benign salivary gland tumors, 456–459,
      457t
Bethesda Diagnostic Categories, nodules
      and cysts, 481–482t
Bezold abscess, 133
Bilateral vocal fold paralysis, pediatric,
      531–534
Bing-Siebenmann dysplasia, 574
Blepharoplasty, 687–692
  lower eyelid cross-section, 688f
Blood. *See* Hematology
Blood component therapy, 14
  cryoprecipitate, 14
  fresh frozen plasma (FFP), 14
  PBRCs, 14
  platelets, 14
  whole blood, 14
Blood supply to neck, 328f
BOF syndrome. *See* Branchio-oculo-facial
      (BOF) syndrome
Bone and cartilage grafts for facial
      reconstruction, 661–665
  calvarial bone grafts, 662
  cartilage grafts, 663–664
  iliac crest grafts, 663
  tibial bone grafts, 663
BPPV. *See* Benign paroxysmal positional
      vertigo (BPPV)
Brain abscess, 137–138
Branchial cleft cysts, 589–593, 590t, 591f
Branchio-oculo-facial (BOF) syndrome,
      553
Branchio-Oto-renal syndrome, 575
Broder classification, 371t
Broder classification, tumor differentia-
      tion grading, 346t
Bronchoscopy, 711–712
  flexible bronchoscopy, 711–712
  rigid bronchoscopy, 711
Buccal mucosa cancers, 374

Burning mouth syndrome, 263
Burns, 634–638
    burn depth and skin layer
        involvement, 634f
    classification based on severity, 635t

C

Calcium disorders, 518–521
    hypercalcemia, 520–521, 521t
    hypocalcemia, 519–520
Calcium disturbances, 91
Calvarial bone grafts for facial
        reconstruction, 662
CAM otolaryngological medicine. *See*
        Complementary and alterna-
        tive (CAM) otolaryngological
        medicine
Cancer of unknown primary (CUP), 350,
        385–387
Cancer stage groupings, 352t, 364t
Carbon dioxide laser, 44–45
Cardiac
    preoperative assessment, 53t
Cardiovascular system
    benzodiazepines, effect on, 79t
    etomidate, effect on, 82t
    isoflurane, effect on, 85t
    ketamine, effect on, 82t
    opioids, effect on, 77t
    propofol, effect on, 81t
Carotid artery blowout, 96–97
Cartilage grafts for facial reconstruction,
        663–664
Catel-Manzke syndrome, 553
Caustic ingestion, 282–284, 284t
Central nervous system
    benzodiazepines, effect on, 79t
    etomidate, effect on, 82t
    isoflurane, effect on, 85t
    ketamine, effect on, 82t
    opioids, effect on, 77t
    propofol, effect on, 81t
Cerebellopontine angle tumors, 203–209
    postoperative complications, 208t
    surgical approaches, 206f
    vestibular schwannoma management,
        205t
Cerebrospinal fluid rhinorrhea, 233–236
    diagnostic studies, 235t
Cervical fascial planes, 327f
Cervical spine movements, airway
        assessment, 57
Cervical vestibular evoked myogenic
        potentials (cVEMP), 184
Chandler classification, 228

CHARGE association, 553
Chemical peels and laser skin
        resurfacing, 682–686
    depth of chemical peels, 683–684t
    dermabrasion, 685
    Fitzpatrick skin type scale, 685t
Chemical sensitivity rhinitis, 252
Chemotherapy agents, 355–356t
Chemotherapy, head and neck cancer,
        352–355
    adjuvant therapy, 353–354
    alkaloids, 354
    antimetabolites, 353
    antitumor antibiotics, 353
    chemotherapy agents, 355–356t
    concomitant chemoradiotherapy,
        353
    EGFR inhibitors, 354–355
    neoadjuvant chemotherapy, 353
    PD-1 inhibitors, 355
    platinum-based alkylating agents,
        353
    taxanes, 354
CHL. *See* Conductive hearing loss (CHL)
Choanal atresia, 599–601
Cholesteatoma, 140–145
Chondrosarcoma, 431
Chordoma, 431
Chronic allergy management, 256
Chronic discoid lupus erythematous
        otologic manifestation, 215
Chronic rhinosinusitis, 244–249
    exam findings, 246t
    preoperative review of coronal CT
        scan, 249t
    treatment strategies, 248t
Churg-Strauss's disease with sinonasal
        manifestations, 265
Chylous fistula, 96
Cisatracurium, 86t
Cleft lip and palate, 601–607
    Furlow palate lengthening procedure,
        607f
    Millard rotation advancement lip
        repair, 605f
    palatal flap, 609f
    Tennison-Randa triangular flap lip
        repair, 605f
    Von Langenbeck repair, 604f
Clinical staging of HPV+ head and neck
        cancer, 385t
CMV. *See* Cytomegalovirus (CMV)
Coagulopathies, 17
Cochlear aqueduct, 106
Cochlear implants, 177–180

Complementary and alternative (CAM) otolaryngological medicine, 47–50
  acupuncture, 49
  allergic rhinitis, acute sinusitis, and asthma, 48
  head and neck cancer, 48–49
  herbal and nutritional supplements and surgery, 49, 50t
  tinnitus and vertigo, 49
  upper respiratory infections, 48
Computed tomography (CT) scan, 6–8, 7t
Concomitant chemoradiotherapy, 353
Conductive anosmia, 261
Conductive hearing loss (CHL), 165–168
Congenital conductive hearing loss, pediatric, 573–574, 577
Congenital midline nasal masses, 596–598, 597t
Congenital midline neck masses, 593–595, 595f
Conscious intubation, 62
Cormack and Lehane grade, airway assessment, 58, 58f
Coronal approach to brow and forehead lifting, 680
Cosmetic surgery, 669–709
  blepharoplasty, 687–692
    lower eyelid cross-section, 688f
  brow and forehead lifting, 677–681
    coronal approach, 680
    direct brow approach, 680–681
    endoscopic approach, 681
    fascial planes, 681f
    midforehead approach, 680
  chemical peels and laser skin resurfacing, 682–686
    depth of chemical peels, 683–684t
    dermabrasion, 685
    Fitzpatrick skin type scale, 683t
  deviated septum and septoplasty, 700–703
    sagittal section, 701f
  hair restoration, 705–709
    Norwood classification, male pattern baldness, 707f
  liposuction, 703–705
  neurotoxins, fillers, and implants, 669–674
    injectable fillers, 671–672t
    muscles of facial expression, 671f
    neurotoxins, 670t
  otoplasty, 692–695
    measurement positions, 694f
  rhinoplasty, 695–700

    male and female ideal, differences, 696f
    rhytidectomy, 674–677
Costello syndrome, 554
Cotton-Meyer grading system for subglottic stenosis, 546t
Cranial nerves, 721–732, 721f
  abducens nerve, 724f, 731t
  accessory nerve, 729f, 732t
  facial nerve course, segments, and functions, 726f, 731t
  glossopharyngeal nerve, 727f, 731t
  hypoglossal nerve, 729f, 732t
  oculomotor nerve, 724f, 730t
  olfactory nerve, 722f, 730t
  optic nerve, 727f, 731t
  spinal accessory nerve, 732t
  trigeminal nerve, 725f, 730t
  trochlear nerve, 724f, 730t
  vagus nerve, 728f, 732t
  vestibulocochlear nerve, 727f, 731t
Craniomaxillofacial trauma, 611–638
  burns, 634–638
    burn depth and skin layer involvement, 634f
    classification based on severity, 635t
  frontal sinus fractures, 621–624
    anterior and lateral views, 622f
  mandible fractures, 628–633
    adult occlusion variants, 631f
    favorable and unfavorable, 629f
    mandible anatomy and incidence of fracture sites, 629f
  midface fractures, 624–628
    Le Fort classification of, 625f
    masticatory force transmission, 625f
  nasal fractures, 611–614
    nose cross-section, 612f
  naso-orbito-ethmoid (NOE) fractures, 614–617
    intercanthal distance and telecanthus, 616f
    medial canthal tendon, 616f
  zygomaticomaxillary complex (ZMC) fractures, 618–620
Cricothyroidotomy, 67, 67f, 718
Cri du chat syndrome, 554
Croup, 285–286
Crouzon syndrome, 576
Cryoprecipitate, 14
CT scan. *See* Computed tomography (CT) scan
CUP. *See* Cancer of unknown primary (CUP)

Cutaneous squamous cell carcinoma (SCC), 417–424
 treatment options, 420*t*
cVEMP. *See* Cervical vestibular evoked myogenic potentials (cVEMP)
Cytomegalovirus (CMV), 16
Cytomegalovirus and acquired prenatal hearing loss, 578

D

DAA. *See* Difficult Airway Algorithm (DAA)
da Vinci Surgical System (dVSS), 410
Deep cervical plexus block, 74–75
Dermabrasion, 685
Desflurane, 84
Deviated septum and septoplasty, 700–703
 sagittal section, 701*f*
Diagnostic imaging, 6–13
 barium esophagram, 10–11
 computed tomography (CT) scan, 6–8, 7*t*
 magnetic resonance imaging (MRI), 8–9, 8*t*
 nuclear medicine imaging, 11–13
  four-dimensional parathyroid CT (4D-CT), 13
  parathyroid scintigrahy, 12
  positron emission tomography with computed tomography (PET-CT), 11–12
  single-photon-emission computed tomography (SPECT), 13
  thyroid scintigraphy, 12
 ultrasound, 9–10, 10*f*
Diarrhea, 97–98
Diazepam, 80
Difficult Airway Algorithm (DAA), 56*f*
Dilutional thrombocytopenia, 17
Diode laser, 46
Disseminated intravascular coagulation, 17
Down syndrome, 554
Drainage of abscess, 336*t*
Drug-induced rhinitis, 251
Drug-induced thyroiditis, 495
Drug interactions
 benzodiazepines, effect on, 79*t*
 opioids, effect on, 77*t*
dVSS. *See* da Vinci Surgical System (dVSS)
Dye laser, 46

E

EA. *See* Tracheoesophageal fistula (TEF) and esophageal atresia (EA), pediatric

Ear, 101–107
 anatomy, 103–107
  auricle, 103*f*
  external auditory canal, 104
  inner ear, 106–107
  middle ear, 104–105, 105*f*
  tympanic membrane, 104
 embryology of ear, 101–103, 102*f*
  auricle, 101*t*
EBV. *See* Estimated blood volume (EBV)
ECF. *See* Extracellular fluid (ECF)
Ectopic parathyroid adenoma, 514*f*, 515*f*
Ectrodactyly–ectodermal dysplasia–clefting (EEC) syndrome, 554
EEC syndrome. *See* Ectrodactyly–ectodermal dysplasia–clefting (EEC) syndrome
EGFR. *See* Epidural growth factor receptor (EGFR)
EGFR inhibitors, 354–355
Electrolarynx, 402–403
Electrolyte requirements, daily, 90
Electronystagmography (ENG), 183
Electrophysiologic/objective assessments, 163–164
Elliptical recess, 106
Endocrine system
 and geriatric otolaryngology, 40
 opioids, effect on, 77*t*
Endolymphatic duct, 106
Endolymphatic sac, 106
Endoscopic exam, 4–5
Endotracheal intubation, 58–60
Endotracheal tube types, 59–60
 armored endotracheal tubes, 59
 laser-resistant endotracheal tubes, 60
 nerve-monitoring endotracheal tubes, 60
 Ring-Adair-Elwin (RAE) tubes, 60
ENG. *See* Electronystagmography (ENG)
Enlarged vestibular aqueduct, 573
Eosinophilic granuloma otologic manifestation, 215
Epidermolysis bullosa laryngeal manifestation, 322
Epidural abscess, 138–139, 231
Epidural growth factor receptor (EGFR), 354–355
Epineural nerve repair for facial paralysis, 643*f*
Epitaxis, 237–241
 causes, 238*t*
Epley repositioning maneuver, 188*f*
Epstein-Barr virus, 16
Erosive mucosal lesions, 29–31

Esophageal speech, 403
Esophagoscopy, 712–713
Esophagus anatomy and physiology, 276–277
Estimated blood volume (EBV), 13
Etomidate, 82, 82*t*
Exophytic mucosal lesions, 26–27
External carotid artery, 449–450
Extracellular fluid (ECF), 89

F

Facemasks, 55
Facial nerve course, segments, and functions, 726*f*, 731*t*
Facial nerve neurorrhaphy for facial paralysis, 643
Facial paralysis, facial reanimation, and eye care, 639–648
  dynamic procedures, 643–645
    epineural nerve repair, 643*f*
    facial nerve neurorrhaphy, 643
    greater auricular and transverse cervical nerve grafts, 644
    interpositional graft, 643–644
    nerve crossovers, 644
  facial nerve involvement tests, 640*f*
  muscle transfer techniques, 645
    free-muscle transfer, 645
    regional muscle transfer, 645
    temporalis tendon/muscle transfer, 645
  static procedures, 646–647
    ancillary techniques, 647
    gold or platinum weights, 646
    lower eyelid shortening, 646
    palpebral spring implant, 646
    static sling, 647
    tarsorrhaphy, 646
    temporalis sling, 647
    temporalis tendon transfer, 647
    wedge resection and canthoplasty, 646
  Sunderland classification of nerve injury, 641*t*
Facial reconstruction, 648–668
  bone and cartilage grafts, 661–665
    calvarial bone grafts, 662
    iliac crest grafts, 663
    tibial bone grafts, 663
    cartilage grafts, 663–664
  incision planning and scar revision, 665–668
    etiology of unfavorable scar formation, 667*t*
    relaxed-skin tension lines, 666*f*

Z-plasty, 668*f*
  local cutaneous flaps, 651–657
    advancement flaps, 652*t*, 653–654, 653*f*, 654*f*
    hinged flaps, 652*t*
    pivotal flaps, 652*t*, 654
    transpositional flaps, 654, 655*f*
  microvascular free tissue transfer, 657–661
  skin grafts, 648–651, 650*f*
Factor deficiencies, 19–20
Factor depletion, 17
Febrile reaction, 15
Fentanyl, 78
FFP. *See* Fresh frozen plasma (FFP)
Fiber optic-assisted tracheal intubation, 62–63
Fibrous dysplasia, 217
Fibrous thyroiditis, 495
Fitzpatrick skin type scale, 685*t*
Flexible bronchoscopy, 711–712
Flexible fiberoptic nasopharyngoscopy, 22
Floor of mouth cancer, 374
Fluids and electrolytes, 89–91
  calcium disturbances, 91
  daily electrolyte requirements, 90
  functional compartments
    extracellular fluid (ECF), 89
    intracellular fluid (ICF), 89
    total body water (TBW), 89
  perioperative fluid management, 90–91
Follicular thyroid cancer, 499–500
Foramen of Huischke, 104
Foreign bodies in ear, 120–122
4D-CT. *See* Four-dimensional parathyroid CT (4D-CT)
Four-dimensional parathyroid CT (4D-CT), 13
Fractures, laryngeal, 280–282
Fragile X syndrome, 554–555
Fraser (cryptophthalmos) syndrome, 555
Free-muscle transfer for facial paralysis, 645
Fresh frozen plasma (FFP), 14
Frontal sinus fractures, 621–624
  anterior and lateral views, 622*f*
Fungal laryngitis, 286–287
Furlow palate lengthening procedure, 607*f*

G

Gastrointestinal system, opioids, effect on, 77*t*

Gell and Coombs classification of allergic
　reactions, 254*t*
General anesthesia, 70
GERD. *See* Acid reflux disorders
Geriatric otolaryngology, 38–42, 39*t*
　conditions used to identify patients at
　　risk, 42*t*
　diseases, 39–40
　　endocrine, 40
　　head and neck, 40
　　laryngology and oropharyngeal, 40
　　otology, 39–40
　　rhinology, 40
Glandular tumors, 431–432
GlideScope, 65
Glossopharyngeal nerve, 727*f*, 731*t*
Glossopharyngeal nerve block, 75–76
Glottis cancers, 393
Goldenhar syndrome, 575
Gold or platinum weights for facial
　　paralysis, 646
Gout, 216
Graft-versus-host disease, 16
Greater and lesser occipital nerve blocks,
　　73–74
Greater auricular and transverse cervical
　　nerve grafts for facial paralysis,
　　644
Gustatory rhinitis, 251

H

Hair restoration, 705–709
　Norwood classification, male pattern
　　baldness, 707*f*
Hard palate cancer, 375
Hashimoto thyroiditis, 494–495
Head and neck and geriatric otolaryn-
　　gology, 40
Head and neck cancer, 346–348
　and CAM, 48–49
　cancer of unknown primary, 350
　cervical lymph node metastases
　　incidence, 347*t*
　squamous cell carcinoma, 346–350
　tumor differentiation grading, Broder
　　classification, 346*t*
Hearing aids, 174–176
Hearing loss, 165–182
　asymmetric hearing loss, 171–172
　　Ménière's disease, 171
　conductive hearing loss, 165–168
　cochlear implants, 177–180
　　ossicular disease, 168
　　otosclerosis, 168
　implantable hearing devices, 180–182

　　auditory brainstem implants, 181
　　middle ear implants, 182
　　osseointegrated bone conduction
　　　implants, 181
　　sensorineural hearing loss, 169–173
　　　hearing loss at birth overview, 170*f*
　　　otoxic drugs, 170*t*
Hearing loss, pediatric, 571–582
　acquired, 577–579
　audiometric assessment by age, 581*t*
　congenital, 573–574
　　dysmorphologies, 573–577
　　inherited, 574–577
　congenital conductive, 577
　evaluation, 580*t*
Heerfordt syndrome, 455
Hemangiomas, vascular malformations,
　　lymphatic malformations,
　　neck, 586–589
Hematology, 13–20
　blood loss management, 13–14
　　blood component therapy, 14
　　compatibility testing, 14
　　estimated blood volume (EBV), 13
　　PBRC transfusion guidelines, 13
　coagulation studies, 18
　　activated clotting time (ACT), 18
　　international normalization rate
　　　(INR), 18
　　partial thromboplastin time (PTT), 18
　　platelet function, 18
　　prothrombin time (PT), 18
　disorders, 19–20
　　factor deficiencies, 19–20
　　sickle cell anemia, 19
　　von Willebrand disease, 20
　massive transfusions, 14
　transfusion complications, 15–17
　　anaphylactic reaction, 15
　　coagulopathies, 17
　　dilutional thrombocytopenia, 17
　　disseminated intravascular coagu-
　　　lation, 17
　　factor depletion, 17
　　febrile reaction, 15
　　graft-versus-host disease, 16
　　hemolytic reactions, 15
　　hypothermia, 17
　　immune suppression, 16
　　infectious complications, 16
　　metabolic abnormalities, 16–17
　　microaggregates, 17
　　posttransfusion purpura, 16
　　transfusion-related lung injury
　　　(TRALI), 16

urticarial reaction, 15
treatment of transfusion reactions, 17
universal blood donor, 15
Hematoma and seroma, 95
Hemolytic reactions, 15
Hepatitis, 16
Herbal and nutritional supplements and surgery and CAM, 49, 50*t*
Hinged flaps, 654*t*
Histopathologic types of BCC, 414–415
HIV/acquired immunodeficiency syndrome (AIDS), 16
HL. *See* Hodgkin lymphoma (HL)
Hoarseness. *See* Papillomatosis
Hodgkin lymphoma (HL), 434–440
Holmium: Yttrium-Aluminum-Garnet laser (Ho:YAG) laser, 45
Hormonal rhinitis, 251
House-Brackmann facial nerve grading scale, 117*t*
Ho:YAG laser. *See* Holmium: Yttrium-Aluminum-Garnet laser (Ho:YAG) laser
HPV. *See* Human papillomavirus (HPV)
Human papillomavirus (HPV), 382
Human papillomavirus (HPV) and head and neck cancer, 382–385
  basaloid squamous cell carcinomas, 384*f*
  clinical staging of HPV+ head and neck cancer, 385*t*
  pathologic staging of HPV+ head and neck cancer, 385*t*
Hyperbilirubinemia and acquired prenatal hearing loss, 578
Hyperparathyroidism, 512–517
  ectopic parathyroid adenoma, 514*f*, 515*f*
  multiple endocrine neoplasia, 512*t*
  secondary hyperparathyroidism, 516
  tertiary hyperparathyroidism, 517
Hyperthyroidism, 483–487
  Graves disease, 485–486
Hypoglossal nerve, 729*f*, 732*t*
Hypoparathyoidism, 517–518
Hypopharyngeal cancer, 388–392
Hypothermia, 17
Hypothyroidism, 487–490
  Hashimoto thyroiditis, 490
Hypoxia and acquired prenatal hearing loss, 578

I

ICF. *See* Intracellular fluid (ICF)
Idiopathic midline destructive disease (IMDD), 440–442

Iliac crest grafts for facial reconstruction, 663
IMDD. *See* Idiopathic midline destructive disease (IMDD)
Immune suppression, 16
Implantable hearing devices, 180–182
Inadequate neck extension
  difficult airway and intubation, 64*t*
Incision planning and scar revision 667–670
  etiology of unfavorable scar formation, 667*t*
  relaxed-skin tension lines, 666*f*
  Z-plasty, 668*f*
Incus, 105
Infections
  difficult airway and intubation, 64*t*
  postoperative, 95
Infectious complications, 16
Infectious neck masses, pediatric, 582–586
Infectious thyroiditis, 493–494
Infraorbital nerve block, 74
Innervation, 55
INR. *See* International normalization rate (INR), 18
International normalization rate (INR), 18
Interpositional graft for facial paralysis, 643–644
Intracellular fluid (ICF), 89
Intracranial abscess, 233
Intracranial complications of sinusitis, 230–233
  interpretation of cerebrospinal fluid findings, 232*t*
Intubation, 60–61, 61*f*
Inverted papillomas, 256–259
Isoflurane, 84

J

Jervell and Lange-Nielsen syndrome, 574
Jugular-digastric region, 407

K

Ketamine, 82*t*, 83
KTP laser. *See* Potassium Titanyl Phosphate (KTP) laser

L

Larsen syndrome, 555
Laryngeal and esophageal emergencies, 277–289
  caustic ingestion, 282–284, 284*t*
  fractures, 280–282

infections, 285–289
  actinomycosis, 287
  bacterial laryngitis, 286
  croup, 285–286
  fungal laryngitis, 286–287
  leprosy, 287–288
  syphilis, 287
  tuberculosis, 287
  viral laryngitis, 285
  stridor, 277–280, 278*t*
Laryngeal cancer, 392–401
  glottis cancers, 393
  subglottic cancer, 393
  supraglottic cancers, 393
Laryngeal clefts, pediatric, 534–537, 536*f*
Laryngeal manifestations of systemic
       diseases, 321–323
  amyloidosis, 322
  angioneurotic edema, 323
  epidermolysis bullosa, 322
  neuromuscular disease, 323
  pemphigoid, 322–323
  relapsing polychondritis, 321
  rheumatoid arthritis, 321
  sarcoidosis, 322
  Wegener's granulomatosis, 321–322
Laryngeal mask airway (LMA), 63
Laryngology and oropharyngeal and
       geriatric otolaryngology, 40
Laryngomalacia, pediatric, 529–531
Laryngoscopes, 55
Larynx anatomy and physiology,
       273–276, 274*f*, 275*f*
Laser-resistant endotracheal tubes, 60
Lasers, 43–47
  applications, 44
    facial plastic surgery, 44
    general otolaryngology, 44
    laryngology, 44
    otology, 44
    rhinology, 44
  biophysics, 43–44
  types, 44–46, 45*t*
    carbon dioxide laser, 44–45
    diode laser, 46
    argon laser, 46
    dye laser, 46
    Ebrium: Yttriium-Aluminum-Garnet
      (Er:YAG) laser, 45
    Holmium: Yttrium-Aluminum-
      Garnet (Ho:YAG) laser, 45
    Neodymium: Yttrium-Aluminum-
      Garnet (Nd:YAG) laser, 45
    Potassium Titanyl Phosphate (KTP)
      laser, 45

Leprosy, 287–288
Lethal midline granuloma with sinonasal
      manifestations, 265
Leukemia, 216
Lip cancer, 372
Liposuction, 703–705
LMA. *See* Laryngeal mask airway (LMA)
Longitudinal fracture, 111
Lorazepam, 80
Lower eyelid shortening for facial
      paralysis, 646
Lower jugular region, 407
LPR. *See* Acid reflux disorders
Ludwig's angina, 332–334
Lyme disease otologic manifestation,
    214
Lymphatics, 450
Lymphomas, 434–440, 436–437*t*
  Hodgkin lymphoma, 434–440
  non-Hodgkin lymphoma, 434–440
  World Health Organization
    classification, 438*t*

M

Magnetic resonance imaging (MRI),
    8–9, 8*t*
Malignant hyperthermia (MH), 87*t*,
    88*t*, 88
Malignant neoplasms of ear and tempo-
    ral bone, 430–433
  anatomic illustrations, 433
  chondrosarcoma, 432
  chordoma, 432
  glandular tumors, 442
  melanoma, 432
  metastasis, 432
  sarcoma, 432
Malignant otitis externa (MOE), 149–153
Malignant salivary gland tumors,
    460–466, 461*t*, 464*f*, 464*f*
Mallampati and tonsil staging, 22*t*
Mallampati classification, airway
    assessment, 57, 57*f*
Malleus, 105
Mandible fractures, 628–633
  adult occlusion variants, 631*f*
  favorable and unfavorable, 629*f*
  mandible anatomy and incidence of
    fracture sites, 629*f*
Marshall syndrome, 555
Massive transfusions, 14
Measles otologic manifestation, 214
Medrobotics Flex Robotic System, 410
Medullary thyroid cancer (MTC),
    502–504

Melanomas, head, face, and neck, 423–429, 431
MEN. *See* Multiple endocrine neoplasia (MEN)
Ménière's disease, 171
Meningitis and postnatal acquired hearing loss, 578
Mental confusion, 92–94
 acute postobstructive pulmonary edema, 93–94
 alcohol withdrawal, 94
 psychiatric disorders, 94
 pulmonary embolism, 93
Meperidine, 78
Metabolic abnormalities, 16–17
Metabolic preoperative assessment, 53*t*
Metastasis, 432
Metastatic neoplasms, 216
MH. *See* Malignant hyperthermia (MH)
Michel aplasia, 573
Microaggregates, 17
Microbiome, 247
Microvascular free tissue transfer for facial paralysis, 657–661
Midazolam, 80
Middle ear implants, 182
Middle jugular region, 407
Midface fractures, 624–628
 Le Fort classification of, 625*f*
 masticatory force transmission, 625*f*
Migraine-associated vertigo, 196–199
Millard rotation advancement lip repair, 605*f*
Miller syndrome (postaxial acrofacial dysostosis), 555
Mixed fracture, 111
Möbius syndrome, 555
MOE. *See* Malignant otitis externa (MOE)
Mohs micrographic excision, 416*t*
Mondini deformity, 573
Morphine, 77
Mouth opening, airway assessment, 57
MRI. *See* Magnetic resonance imaging (MRI)
MTC. *See* Medullary thyroid cancer (MTC)
Mucopolysaccharidoses, 216, 556
Multiple endocrine neoplasia (MEN), 512*t*
Multiple myeloma otologic manifestation, 215
Mumps otologic manifestation, 214
Muscle relaxation, 71

N

Nager syndrome (Nager acrofacial dysostoses), 556

NARES. *See* Nonallergic rhinitis with eosinophilia (NARES)
Nasal fractures, 611–614
 nose cross-section, 612*f*
Nasal obstruction, congenital, pediatric, 567–571
Naso-orbito-ethmoid (NOE) fractures, 614–617
 intercanthal distance and telecanthus, 616*f*
 medial canthal tendon, 616*f*
Nasopharyngeal cancer, 365–369, 368*f*
Nasotracheal intubation, 61
Naxolone, 78–79
Nd:YAG laser. *See* Neodymium: Yttrium-Aluminum-Garnet (Nd:YAG) laser
Neck anatomy, 327–329
 blood supply, 328*f*
 cervical fascial planes, 327*f*
 cervical plexus, 329*f*
 nodal levels I–IV, 327*f*
Neck dissection, 406–409
 classification, neck dissections, 407–408
 classifications, neck levels, 406–408
  anterior compartment, 408
  jugular-digastric region, 407
  lower jugular region, 407
  middle jugular region, 407
  posterior triangle, 408
  submandular and submental triangles, 407
Neck emergencies, 330–342
 deep neck infections, 334–337
  surgical approaches for drainage, 336*t*
 Ludwig's angina, 332–334
 neck trauma, 337–342
  management algorithm, 341*f*
  specific injuries sought and treated during neck exploration, 341*t*
  types of injuries, 342*t*
  zones of neck for management of penetrating trauma, 339*f*, 339*t*
 necrotizing soft tissue infections of head and neck, 330–332
Neck masses approaches, 342–346, 343*f*, 344*t*
Neoadjuvant chemotherapy, 353
Neodymium: Yttrium-Aluminum-Garnet (Nd:YAG) laser, 45
Nerve crossovers for facial paralysis, 644
Nerve-monitoring endotracheal tubes, 60

Nervous intermedius, 451*f*
Neurofibromatosis, 576
Neurolaryngology, 289–295
  cerebrovascular accident (stroke), 293
  progressive degeneration, 293
  spasmodic dysphonia, 293
  vocal fold dysfunction, 293–294
  vocal tremor, 293
Neuromuscular disease laryngeal
      manifestation, 323
Neuromuscular system
  isoflurane, effect on, 85*t*
Neurotoxins, fillers, and implants,
      669–674
  injectable fillers, 671–672*t*
  muscles of facial expression, 672*f*
  neurotoxins, 670*t*
NHL. *See* non-Hodgkin lymphoma (NHL)
Nitrous oxide, 84
Nocturnal polysomnography (PSG), 22
Nodal levels I–IV, 327*f*
NOE fractures. *See* Naso-orbito-ethmoid
      (NOE) fractures
Nonallergic rhinitis, 250–253
  chemical sensitivity, 252
  drug-induced, 251
  gustatory, 251
  hormonal, 251
  nonallergic rhinitis with eosinophilia,
      251
  occupational, 251
  vasomotor, 252
Nonallergic rhinitis with eosinophilia
      (NARES), 251
Non-Hodgkin lymphoma (NHL), 434–440
Noonan syndrome, 556
Norrie disease, 577
Norwood classification, male pattern
      baldness, 707*f*
NPO status preoperative assessment, 53*t*

O

Obesity
  difficult airway and intubation, 64*t*
Oblique fracture, 111
Obstructive sleep apnea (OSA), 20–25
  flexible fiberoptic nasopharyngoscopy,
      22
  Mallampati and tonsil staging, 22*t*
  nocturnal polysomnography (PSG), 22
  respiratory disturbance index (RDI), 23
Occupational rhinitis, 251
Ochronosis, 216
Oculomotor nerve, 724*f*, 730*t*
Odontogenic lesions, 31

Odontogenic tumors and cysts, 31–32
Olfactory nerve, 722*f*, 730*t*
Öhngren's plane, 362, 363*f*
Olfactory neuroblastoma tumor, 362*f*
Open surgical tracheotomy, 717
Opitz G syndrome (BBB syndrome), 556
Optic nerve, 727*f*, 731*t*
Oral and nasal airways equipment, 55
Oral and odontogenic disorders, benign,
      25–34
  erosive mucosal lesions, 29–31
  exophytic mucosal lesions, 26–27
  odontogenic lesions, 31
  odontogenic tumors and cysts, 31–32
  surface mucosal lesions, 28–29
  systemic disorders, 32–33
  vitamin deficiencies, 31
Oral cavity anatomy and physiology,
      271–272
Oral cavity cancer, 370–377
  advanced oral cavity cancer, 375
  buccal mucosa cancers, 374
  floor of mouth cancer, 374
  hard palate cancer, 375
  lip cancer, 373
  oral tongue cancer, 373
  retromolar trigone cancer, 375
  squamous cell carcinoma, 376*f*
  tumor differentiation grading, Broder
      classification, 371*t*
Oral tongue cancer, 373
Oral tongue cancer, 373
Orbital complications of sinusitis,
      228–230
  Chandler classification, 228
Oro-facial-digital syndrome, 556–557
Oropharyngeal cancer, 378–381
Orotracheal intubation, 60–61
OSA. *See* Obstructive sleep apnea (OSA)
Osseointegrated bone conduction
      implants, 181
Ossicular disease, 168
Osteogenesis imperfecta, 216, 576
Osteopetosis, 217
Otic-sparing fractures, 111
Otic-violating fractures, 111
Otitis externa, 145–153
  malignant, 149–153
      antibiotic therapy, 153*t*
      diagnostic tests, 151*t*
  uncomplicated, 145–149
      topical preparations, 148*t*
Otitis media, 122–145
  acute, 122–126
  cholesteatoma, 140–145

chronic, 126–131
  topical therapy, 129*t*
complications, 132–140
  acute suppurative labyrinthitis, 135
  Bezold abscess, 133
  brain abscess, 137–138
  coalescent mastoidititis, 134
  epidural abscess, 138–139
  facial paralysis, 135
  labyrinthine fistula, 133–134
  lateral sinus thrombosis, 138
  meningitis, 136, 137*t*
  otitic hydrocephalus, 139–140
  petrous apicitis, 134
  subdural empyema, 139
  subperiosteal abscess, 132
Otologic emergencies, 108–122
  acute facial paresis and paralysis,
      115–120
  algorithm for differential diagnosis,
      116*t*
  ear and temporal bone trauma,
      110–115, 112*f*
  foreign bodies, 120–122
  House-Brackmann facial nerve grading
      scale, 117*t*
  sudden hearing loss, 108–110
Otologic manifestations of systemic
      diseases, 213–217
  autoimmune, 215
    chronic discoid lupus erythematous,
        215
    polyarteritis nodosa, 215
    relapsing polychondritis, 214
    rheumatoid arthritis, 215
  bone diseases, 216–217
    fibrous dysplasia, 217
    osteogenesis imperfecta, 216
    osteopetrosis, 217
    Paget's disease, 216
  immunodeficiencies, 217
    acquired immunodeficiency
        syndrome, 217
    primary/congenital, 217
  infectious/granulomatous processes,
      213–215
    eosinophilic granuloma, 215
    Lyme disease, 214
    measles, 214
    mumps, 214
    sarcoidosis, 214
    syphilis, 214
    tuberculosis, 213
    Wegener's granulomatosis, 214
  metabolic, 216

    gout, 216
    mucopolysaccharidoses, 216
    ochronosis, 216
  neoplastic, 215–216
    leukemia, 216
    metatastic neoplasms, 216
    multiple myeloma, 215
Otology and geriatric otolaryngology,
      39–40
Oto-palatal-digital syndrome, 557
Oto-palato-digital syndrome, 577
Otoplasty, 692–695
  measurement positions, 696*f*
Otosclerosis, 168
Otoxic drugs, 170*t*

P

Paget's disease, 216
Palatal flap, 609*f*
Palliative radiotherapy rationale, 359
Palpebral spring implant for facial
      paralysis, 646
Pancuronium, 86*t*
Papillary thyroid cancer, 497–499
Papillomatosis, 295–298
Paragangliomas, 442–444, 444*f*
Parathyroid glands, 509–511, 512*f*
  vitamin D parathyroid hormone
      integration, 511*f*
Parotid glands, 448–449
Pars tensa, 104
Partial thromboplastin time (PTT), 18
Pathologic staging of HPV+ head and
      neck cancer, 385*t*
PBRCs, 14
PBRC transfusion guidelines, 13
PD. *See* Progressive degeneration (PD)
Pediatric audiologic assessments,
      159–162
Pediatric otolaryngology, 525–607
  adenoids and palatine tonsils diseases,
      560–567, 566*t*
    adentonsillar hypertrophy, 563–567
    adenotonsillitis, 560–563, 562*f*
  airway evaluation and management,
      525–528
    subjective assessment, respiratory
        distress, 526*t*
  bilateral vocal fold paralysis, 531–534
  branchial cleft cysts, 589–593, 590*t*,
      591*f*
  choanal atresia, 599–601
  cleft lip and palate, 601–607
    furlow palate lengthening proce-
        dure, 607*f*

Millard rotation advancement lip repair, 605*f*
   palatal flap, 607*f*
   Tennison-Randall triangular flap lip repair, 605*f*
   Von Langenbeck repair, 606*f*
congenital midline nasal masses, 596–598, 597*t*
congenital midline neck masses, 593–595, 595*f*
genetics and syndromes, 552–559
hearing loss, 571–582
   congenital, 573–577
   types, 572*f*
hemangiomas, vascular malformations, lymphatic malformations, neck, 586–589
infectious neck masses, 582–586
laryngeal clefts, 534–537, 536*f*
laryngomalacia, 529–531
nasal obstruction, congenital, 567–571
Pierre Robin sequence, 549–552
   treatment strategies, 551*t*
subglottic stenosis, 545–548
   Cotton-Meyer grading system, 546*t*
   normal airway size by age, 545*t*
tracheoesophageal fistula and esophageal atresia, 537–540
   classifications, 538*f*
vascular rings, 541–544
Pemphigoid laryngeal manifestation, 322–323
Pendred syndrome, 574
Percutaneous dilation tracheotomy, 69
Periapical abscess, 31
Periodontal abscess, 31
Perioperative fluid management, 90–91
Peripheral nerve sheath tumors, 445–447
Peritonsillar abscess, 34, 64, 561
Pharyngocutaneous fistula, 95–96
Pharynx anatomy and physiology, 272–273, 273*f*
Physical exam, 3–4, 5*t*
Pierre Robin sequence, pediatric, 549–552, 557
Pivotol flaps, 652*t*, 654
Platelet function, 18
Platelets, 14
Platinum-based alkylating agents, 353
Pleomorphic adenomas, 456
Polyarteritis nodosa otologic manifestation, 215

Positron emission tomography with computed tomography (PET-CT), 11–12
Posterior triangle, 408
Postoperative problems, 91–98
   carotid artery blowout, 96–97
   fever, 91–92, 92*t*
   gastrointestinal and genitourinary problems, 97–98
      diarrhea, 97–98
      hypocalcemia, 98
      renal failure, 97
   mental confusion, 92–94
      acute postobstructive pulmonary edema, 93–94
      alcohol withdrawal, 94
      psychiatric disorders, 94
      pulmonary embolism, 93
   wound problems, 95
      chylous fistula, 96
      hematoma and seroma, 95
      infection, 95
      pharyngocutaneous fistula, 95–96
Posttransfusion purpura, 16
Posturography balance test, 184
Potassium Titanyl Phosphate (KTP) laser, 45
Preoperative assessment, 53, 53*t*, 54*t*
Preoperative endoscopic airway evaluation, 58
Procedures and methods of investigation, 711–718
   adenoidectomy, 716–717
   bronchoscopy, 711–712
      flexible bronchoscopy, 711–712
      rigid bronchoscopy, 711
   cricothyroidotomy, 718
   esophagoscopy, 712–713
   open surgical tracheotomy, 717
   rigid direct microscopic laryngoscopy, 713–714
   tonsillectomy, 715–716
Progressive degeneration (PD), 293
Propofol, 81, 81*t*
Prothrombin time (PT), 18
Prussak's space, 104
PSG. *See* Nocturnal polysomnography (PSG)
Psychiatric disorders, 94
PT. *See* Prothrombin time (PT)
PTT. *See* Partial thromboplastin time (PTT)
Pulmonary embolism, 93
Pure-tone threshold audiometry, 155*f*

R

Radiation thyroiditis, 104
Radiotherapy for head and neck cancer,
        355–359
    adjuvant radiotherapy rationale,
        358–359
    definitive (curative) radiotherapy
        rationale, 357
    palliative radiotherapy rationale, 359
RAE tubes. *See* Ring-Adair-Elwin (RAE)
        tubes
Raccoon eyes, 111
Ranula, 456
Rapid-sequence intubation, 61–62
RDI. *See* Respiratory disturbance index
        (RDI)
Referred otalgia in head and neck
        diseases, 404–406
    sources, 404*f*
Regional anesthesia, 71
Regional muscle transfer for facial
        paralysis, 645
Relapsing polychondritis laryngeal
        manifestation, 321
Relapsing polychondritis otologic
        manifestation, 214
Relapsing polychondritis with sinonasal
        manifestations, 265
Relaxed-skin tension lines (RSTLs), 666*f*
Remifentanil, 78
Renal system
    isoflurane, effect on, 85*t*
    postoperative failure, 97
Resection of upper jaw, 361
Respiratory distress, pediatric, 528*t*
Respiratory disturbance index (RDI), 23
Respiratory system
    benzodiazepines, effect on, 79*t*
    etomidate, effect on, 82*t*
    isoflurane, effect on, 85*t*
    ketamine, effect on, 82*t*
    opioids, effect on, 77*t*
    preoperative assessment, 53*t*
    propofol, effect on, 81*t*
Retromolar trigone cancer, 375
Rheumatoid arthritis laryngeal
        manifestation, 321
Rheumatoid arthritis otologic
        manifestation, 215
Rhinitis, 250–256
    allergy, 253–256
        anaphylaxis, 255
        angioedema, 256
        chronic allergy management, 256

        Gell and Coombs classification of
                allergic reactions, 254*t*
    nonallergic rhinitis, 250–252
        chemical sensitivity, 252
        drug-induced, 251
        gustatory, 251
        hormonal, 251
        nonallergic rhinitis with eosino-
                philia, 251
        occupational, 251
        vasomotor, 252
Rhinologic emergencies, 224–241
    acute invasive fungal rhinosinusitis,
            224–227
        treatment algorithm, 226*f*
    cerebrospinal fluid rhinorrhea,
            233–236
        diagnostic studies, 235*t*
    epitaxis, 237–241
        causes, 238*t*
    intracranial complications of sinusitis,
            230–233
        interpretation of cerebrospinal fluid
                findings, 232*t*
    orbital complications, 228–230
        Chandler classification, 228
Rhinologic manifestations of systemic
        diseases, 264–267, 265
Rhinology, 221–224
    blood supply, 222
        vasculature of nasal cavity, 223*f*
    geriatric otolaryngology, 40
    innervation, 222–223
    nose and paranasal anatomy and
            physiology, 221–224
        nasal sinuses, 222*f*
        nasal skeleton, 221*f*
    physiology, 223–224, 224*f*
Rhinoplasty, 695–700
    male and female ideal, differences,
            698*f*
Rhinosinusitis, 241–249
    acute rhinosinusitis, 241–244
        antibiotic therapy, 243*t*
    chronic rhinosinusitis, 244–249
        exam findings, 246*t*
        preoperative review of coronal CT
                scan, 249*t*
        treatment strategies, 248*t*
Rhinosporidiosis with sinonasal
        manifestations, 265
Rhytidectomy, 674–677
Rigid bronchoscopy, 711
Ring-Adair-Elwin (RAE) tubes, 60
Rinne test, 157, 158*f*

RLN. *See* Recurrent laryngeal nerve (RLN)
Robotic-assisted head and neck surgery, 409–412
  da Vinci Surgical System, 410
  Medrobotics Flex Robotic System, 410
  transoral robotic-assisted surgery, 386, 410–411
  transaxillary thyroidectomy, 411–412
  robotic facelift thyroidectomy, 412
Robotic facelift thyroidectomy, 412
Rocuronium, 86*t*
Rotary chair balance test, 184
RSTLs. *See* Relaxed-skin tension lines (RSTLs)
Rubella and acquired prenatal hearing loss, 577

S

Salivary glands, 447–468
  anatomy, 448–452, 449*f*
    autonomic nervous system, 450–451
    external carotid artery, 449–450
    lymphatics, 450
    nervous intermedius, 451*f*
    parotid glands, 448–449
    salivary gland secretory unit, 451, 452*t*
  benign salivary gland tumors, 456–459, 457*t*
    pleomorphic adenomas, 456
    Warthin tumor, 457, 459*f*
    apocrine phenotype and cartilaginous stoma, 459*f*
  embryology, 447–448
  malignant salivary gland tumors, 460–466, 464*f*
    classification, 461*t*
    histologic grading, 463*t*
  salivary gland disease, 450–454, 453*f*
    acute bacterial sialadenitis, 453–454, 453*f*
    acute sialadenitis, 452–453
    Heerfordt syndrome, 455
    ranula, 456
    sialolinthiasis, 455–456
    Sjögren syndrome, 454–455
  sialendoscopy, 467–468
Salivary gland secretory unit, 451, 452*t*
Sarcoidosis laryngeal manifestation, 322
Sarcoidosis otologic manifestation, 214
Sarcoidosis with sinonasal manifestations, 265
Sarcoma, 432
SCC. *See* Squamous cell carcinoma (SCC)

Scheibe aplasia, 573
Secondary hyperparathyroidism, 516
Sedation, 71
Sensorineural anosmia, 262
Sensorineural hearing loss (SNHL), 169–173
Sevofluane, 84
Sialendoscopy, 467–468
Sialolinthiasis, 455–456
Sickle cell anemia, 19
Simon triangle, 473
Single-photon-emission computed tomography (SPECT), 13
Sinonasal cancer, 360–365
  cancer stage groupings, 364*t*
  Öhngren's plane, 363*f*
  olfactory neuroblastoma tumor, 362*f*
  resection of upper jaw, 361
Sino-Nasal Outcome Test (SNOT-20), 245
SIRS. *See* Systemic inflammatory response syndrome (SIRS)
Sjögren syndrome, 454–455
  basal cell carcinoma, 413–417
  histopathologic types of BCC, 414–415
  Mohs micrographic excision, 416*t*
Skin grafts, 648–651, 650*f*
SNHL. *See* Sensorineural hearing loss (SNHL)
SNOT-20. *See* Sino-Nasal Outcome Test (SNOT-20)
Sonographic features warranting thyroid nodule biopsy, 481*t*
SPECT. *See* Single-photon-emission computed tomography (SPECT)
Speech options after laryngectomy, 401–404
  electrolarynx, 402–403
  esophageal speech, 403
  tracheoesophageal puncture voice prosthesis, 403
Spherical recess, 106
Spinal accessory nerve, 732*t*
Squamous cell carcinoma (SCC), 346–350, 376*f*, 417–424
  treatment options, 420*t*
  variants, 419
    adenoid SCC, 419
    Bowen disease, 419
    keratoacanthoma, 419
    spindle cell SCC, 419
    verrucous carcinoma, 419
SSCD. *See* Superior semicircular canal dehiscence syndrome (SSCD)
Stable but compromised airway, 68
  extubation criteria, 70

percutaneous dilation tracheotomy, 69
tracheometry, awake, 68
Stapes, 105
Static sling for facial paralysis, 647
Stickler syndrome, 575
Stridor, 277–280, 278*t*
Subacute thyroiditis, 493
Subdural abscess, 231
Subglottic cancer, 393
Subglottic stenosis, 545–548
Submandular and submental triangles, 407
Subperiosteal abscess, 132, 228
Sudden hearing loss, 108–110
Superficial cervical plexus block, 74
Superior semicircular canal dehiscence syndrome (SSCD), 210–213
Superior laryngeal branch of vagus nerve block, 76
Supraglottic cancers, 393
Supraorbital and supratrochlear nerve blocks, 73
Surface mucosal lesions, 28–29
Surgical laryngoscopes, 65
Swallowing disorders, 307–318
aspiration, 313–318, 316–317*t*
dysphagia, 310–313
Zenker's diverticulum, 307–309, 308*f*
Syphilis, 214, 287
Syphilis and acquired prenatal hearing loss, 578
Syphilis with sinonasal manifestations, 265
Systemic disorders and oral and odonto-genic disorders, benign, 32–33
Systemic inflammatory response syndrome (SIRS), 92

T

Taste disorders, 262–264
Taxanes, 354
TBW. *See* Total body water (TBW)
TEF. *See* Tracheoesophageal fistula (TEF) and esophageal atresia (EA), pediatric
Temporal bone trauma, ear, 110–115, 112*f*
Temporalis tendon/muscle transfer for facial paralysis, 645
Temporalis tendon transfer for facial paralysis, 647
Temporomandibular joint (TMJ) disorders, 34–38
articular temporomandibular disease, 36

myogenous temporomandibular disease, 36
surgery
arthrocentesis, 37
arthroplasty, 37
arthroscopic surgery, 37
Temporomandibular joint (TMJ) mobil-ity, airway assessment, 58
Tennison-Randall triangular flap lip repair, 607*f*
Tertiary hyperparathyroidism, 517
Thyroid cancer, 496–509
anaplastic thyroid cancer, 502, 505*f*
lymphomas, 504–505
medullary thyroid cancer, 502–504
overview, 496–497*t*
staging, 505–509
well-differentiated thyroid carcino-mas, 496–501
follicular thyroid cancer, 499–500
papillary thyroid cancer, 497–499
Thyroid gland, 471–473
anatomy, 472–473
Beahrs triangle, 473
recurrent laryngeal nerve, 472–473
Simon triangle, 473
tubercle of Zuckerkandl, 473
embryology, 471, 473*f*
evaluation, 475–478
conditions affecting protein concen-tration, 476*t*
thyroid function tests, 476
thyroid function workup summary, 477*t*
thyrotoxicosis causes, 477*t*
nodules and cysts, 479–483
Bethesda Diagnostic Categories, 481–482*t*
sonographic features warranting biopsy, 481*t*
ultrasound patterns of thyroid nodule and malignancy, 480*t*
physiology, 472–475, 474*f*
hormone regulation, 474–475
Thyroiditis, 492–495
drug-induced thyroiditis, 495
fibrous thyroiditis, 495
Hashimoto thyroiditis, 494–495
infectious thyroiditis, 493–494
radiation thyroiditis, 494
subacute thyroiditis, 493
types, 494*t*
Thyroid storm, 491–492
Thyromental distance, airway assessment, 57

Tibial bone grafts for facial
reconstruction, 663
Tinnitus, 200–203
Tinnitus and vertigo and CAM, 49
TMJ disorders. *See* Temporomandibular
joint (TMJ) disorders
Tonsillectomy, 715–716
Topical anesthesia of subglottic airway
block, 76
Total body water (TBW), 89
Tracheoesophageal fistula (TEF) and
esophageal atresia (EA),
pediatric, 537–540
Tracheoesophageal puncture voice
prosthesis, 403
Tracheometry, awake, 68
TRALI. *See* Transfusion-related lung
injury (TRALI)
Transaxillary thyroidectomy, 411–412
Transfusion-related lung injury (TRALI), 16
Transoral robotic-assisted surgery
(TORS), 386, 410–411
Transpositional flaps, 654, 656*f*
Transtracheal ventilation, 63
Trauma
difficult airway and intubation, 64*t*
and postnatal acquired hearing loss,
579
Traverse fracture, 111
Treacher Collins syndrome, 575
Trigeminal nerve, 725*f*, 730*t*
Trochlear nerve, 724*f*, 730*t*
Tubercle of Zuckerkandl, 473
Tuberculosis, 287
Tuberculosis otologic manifestation, 213
Tumors
difficult airway and intubation, 64*t*
Tuning fork tests, 157
Tympanogram patterns, normal and
abnormal, 156*t*

U

Ultrasound, 9–10, 10*f*
Ultrasound patterns of thyroid nodule
and malignancy, 480*t*
Uncomplicated otitis externa, 145–149
Universal blood donor, 15
Upper aerodigestive tract anatomy and
physiology, 271–277
esophagus, 276–277
larynx, 273–276, 274*f*, 275*f*
oral cavity, 271–272
pharynx, 272–273, 273*f*
Upper airway blocks, 75–76
glossopharyngeal nerve block, 75–76

superior laryngeal branch of vagus
nerve block, 76
topical anesthesia of subglottic airway
block, 76
Upper respiratory infections and CAM, 48
Urticarial reaction, 15
Usher syndrome, 574, 576*t*

V

Vagus nerve, 728*f*, 732*t*
Van der Woude syndrome, 558
Vascular rings, pediatric, 541–544
Vasomotor rhinitis, 252
Vecuronium, 86*t*
Velocardiofacial syndrome (Shprintzen
syndrome, 22q11 deletion
syndrome), 558
Vertigo, 182–199
balance assessment, 182–186
cervical vestibular evoked myogenic
potentials, 184
electronystagmography, 183
posturography, 184
rotary chair, 184
videonystagmography, 183
benign paroxysmal positional vertigo,
186–189
Epley repositioning maneuver, 188*f*
Ménière's disease, 190–193
diagnostic guidelines, 191*t*
migraine-associated vertigo, 196–199
diagnostic criteria, 197*t*
management strategies, 199*t*
vestibular neuritis, 193–196
management options, 195*t*
Vestibular aqueduct, 106
Vestibular neuritis (VN), 193–196
Vestibulocochlear nerve, 727*f*, 731*t*
VFD. *See* Vocal fold dysfunction (VFD)
Videonystagmography (VNG), 183
Viral laryngitis, 285
Vitamin deficiencies and oral and odon-
togenic disorders, benign, 31
VN. *See* Vestibular neuritis (VN)
VNG. *See* Videonystagmography (VNG)
Vocal fold cysts, nodules, and polyps,
298–300
Vocal fold dysfunction (VFD), 293–294
Vocal fold motion impairment, 300–303
Voice disorders, 295–307
papillomatosis, 295–298
vocal fold cysts, nodules, and polyps,
298–300
vocal fold motion impairment,
300–303

voice rehabilitation, 303–307, 304*t*
Voice rehabilitation, 303–307
Von Langenbeck repair, 606*f*
Von Willebrand disease, 20

W

Waardenburg syndrome, 575
Warthin tumor, 457, 459*f*
Weber test, 157, 157*f*
Wedge resection and canthoplasty for facial paralysis, 640
Wegener's disease with sinonasal manifestations, 265
Wegener's granulomatosis laryngeal manifestation, 321–322
Wegener's granulomatosis otologic manifestation, 214
Whole blood, 14

Wildervanck syndrome, 577
World Health Organization classification for Hodgkin lymphoma, 438*t*
Wound problems, 95
  abscess, 95
  chylous fistula, 96
  hematoma and seroma, 95
  infection, 95
  pharyngocutaneous fistula, 95–96

X

X linked hearing loss, 577

Z

Z-plasty, 668*f*
ZMC fractures. *See* Zygomaticomaxillary complex (ZMC) fractures
Zygomaticomaxillary complex (ZMC) fractures, 618–620